Cleft Lip and Palate Treatment

Nivaldo Alonso
Cassio Eduardo Raposo-Amaral
Editors

Cleft Lip and Palate Treatment

A Comprehensive Guide

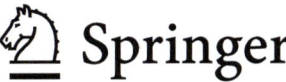

Editors
Nivaldo Alonso, M.D., Ph.D.
University of São Paulo Medical School
São Paulo, SP, Brazil

Cassio Eduardo Raposo-Amaral, M.D., Ph.D.
SOBRAPAR Hospital
Campinas, SP, Brazil

ISBN 978-3-319-63289-6   ISBN 978-3-319-63290-2 (eBook)
https://doi.org/10.1007/978-3-319-63290-2

Library of Congress Control Number: 2017961998

© Springer International Publishing AG 2018
This work is subject to copyright. All rights are reserved by the Publisher, whether the whole or part of the material is concerned, specifically the rights of translation, reprinting, reuse of illustrations, recitation, broadcasting, reproduction on microfilms or in any other physical way, and transmission or information storage and retrieval, electronic adaptation, computer software, or by similar or dissimilar methodology now known or hereafter developed.
The use of general descriptive names, registered names, trademarks, service marks, etc. in this publication does not imply, even in the absence of a specific statement, that such names are exempt from the relevant protective laws and regulations and therefore free for general use.
The publisher, the authors and the editors are safe to assume that the advice and information in this book are believed to be true and accurate at the date of publication. Neither the publisher nor the authors or the editors give a warranty, express or implied, with respect to the material contained herein or for any errors or omissions that may have been made. The publisher remains neutral with regard to jurisdictional claims in published maps and institutional affiliations.

Printed on acid-free paper

This Springer imprint is published by Springer Nature
The registered company is Springer International Publishing AG
The registered company address is: Gewerbestrasse 11, 6330 Cham, Switzerland

In memory of my parents, Nelson and Maria Apparecida, who dedicated their lives to my education.

I have had many mentors in my life, and three of them, Daniel Marchac, William Magee, and John Persing, guided me toward craniofacial surgery and the treatment of patients with cleft lip and palate.

These men showed a passion for plastic surgery and the treatment of congenital deformities. Daniel Marchac gave me a grounding in technical skills and passed on his knowledge, and William Magee and John Persing shared with me their great passion for teaching and for the treatment of cleft lip and palate.

But none of my work in this field would have happened had I not had a beautiful and patient family. So this dedication is made with all my love to Elci, Catherine, Ligia and Alexandre; they are the reason for all that I have accomplished

Nivaldo Alonso

This book is dedicated to my late father, Cassio Raposo do Amaral, a pioneer in the craniofacial field in Brazil, who, together with my mother, Vera Raposo do Amaral, established the SOBRAPAR hospital in 1979. Regrettably, my father did not live long enough to see our family's achievements. When he passed away, I was a senior plastic surgery resident and my brother Cesar was a senior resident in general surgery. Currently, we are both plastic and reconstructive surgeons working together to offer an opportunity to the underprivileged population in Brazil who were born with craniofacial deformities. SOBRAPAR has been a project of two generations, and it recruits excellent professionals for the same cause as that espoused by its founder. Some of these professionals are contributors to this book.

I feel fortunate and grateful to have gained additional experience in craniofacial surgery and surgery for cleft lip and palate at the Institute of Reconstructive Plastic Surgery under the direction of Dr. Joseph McCarthy. In the same year I also gained additional experience as an international fellow at University of California Los Angeles (UCLA) under the leadership of Dr. Henry K. Kawamoto. This was a life-changing experience that helped me to mold some of the principles I had acquired during my residency.

Lastly, I thank my wife Tatiana for providing loving support during the hours of night work, and I thank our 3-year old son, Marc, for being our source of joy and happiness.
      Cassio Eduardo Raposo-Amaral

Foreword I

Almost to the end of the twentieth century, medical/surgical practice was confined to individual clinicians functioning in isolated offices. The concept of multidisciplinary or team care had not yet evolved. However, with the explosion of diagnostic and therapeutic advances resulting from biomedical research, it became apparent that a new model was needed as optimal medical/surgical care was beyond the expertise of a single practitioner or only one discipline. Moreover, the required technological support system was available only in a modern hospital setting.

By the early twenty-first century the concept of true multidisciplinary care under hospital auspices had gained wide acceptance, especially in the treatment of heart disease and cancer. For example, a patient with coronary artery disease is potentially evaluated or treated by a radiologist skilled in cardiac imaging, an adult cardiologist, an electrophysiologist, or interventional cardiologist or cardiothoracic surgeon.

It should be noted that the concept of multidisciplinary or team care was pioneered by clinicians caring for children with cleft lip/palate. I believe the first such integrated center was founded in 1938 in Lancaster, Pennsylvania, by a dentist, Dr. Herbert K. Cooper. He was joined in his early efforts by experts in speech and communication and by Dr. Robert H. Ivy, the first Chief of Plastic Surgery at the University of Pennsylvania. In organizing their team, they recognized that multidisciplinary care provided the optimal outcomes by addressing all aspects of the medical problem on behalf of the patient and family, the latter eventually leading decades later to a new expression in the medical lexicon—holistic medicine. Moreover, it was efficient, as well as caring. Being evaluated in a single setting during one visit by all of the requisite specialists obviated the need for multiple visits at different locations—a scheduling nightmare.

For the team members this model is likewise beneficial. There is direct, face-to-face communication among the members. A discussion with a member from another specialty or discipline is invariably a learning experience. Treatment plans are formulated collectively and presented to the patient in a concise and sympathetic manner. Team meetings also promote clinical research projects, the development of treatment protocols and clinical trials. Moreover, professional meetings are organized more and more along clinical conditions rather than specialty groups.

This text, authored by Drs. Nivaldo Alonso and Cassio Eduardo Raposo-Amaral, reflects the historic heritage and modern evolution of the cleft team.

Organized in a concise and well-written style, the book defines the full spectrum of multidisciplinary cleft care:

- The promotion of cleft care as an important component of every integrated national health care system, as well as the evolving field of international or global health.
- The genetics of cleft lip and palate—an especially important topic in the era of genomics research. The latter has to be correlated with a rigorous classification of cleft phenotypes.
- An overview of clinical protocols and outcome studies—a requisite metric by government agencies and insurance companies in a time when health care costs are skyrocketing.
- The details of treatment, including surgical, protocols for patients with unilateral cleft lip, bilateral cleft lip, and cleft palate.
- Speech therapy and the treatment of velopharyngeal insufficiency.
- Longitudinal orthodontic therapy.
- Closure of alveolar clefts with bone grafts and substitutes.
- The role of orthognathic surgery and cleft rhinoplasty.
- Standardized record keeping with two-dimensional photography and the newer imaging technique of three-dimensional digital stereophotogrammetry.

This book highlights the role and activities of a well-functioning modern-day cleft team as it helps the patient and family navigate a complex clinical trial that often begins before birth with the ultrasonic diagnosis and continues for almost two decades until the face is fully grown. While the treatments may be many and the required resources large, the rewards are enormous—a young person facing life with increased self-confidence and determination to lead a full and productive life.

Joseph G. McCarthy, M.D.
Wyss Department of Plastic Surgery
NYU Langone Medical Center
New York, NY, USA

Foreword II

Cleft lip and palate is the most prevalent congenital anomaly in Brazil that affects 1 per 650 live births, according to our government data.

Cleft Lip and Palate Treatment: A Comprehensive Guide has brought useful knowledge and information to those involved in the rehabilitation of this expressive group of patients in our country.

This twenty-three chapter book aims to cover the diagnosis and treatment of the broad clinical spectrum of cleft, from an incomplete cleft lip to the rarest Tessier facial clefts.

Twenty-seven coauthors were invited to collaborate with this meticulous work planned by Nivaldo Alonso and Cassio Eduardo Raposo-Amaral, who always passionately dedicated themselves to the treatment of these patients, in a feverish search for something that would seem simple—the normalcy. That is definitely not!

The achievements in various areas of health (medicine, dentistry, nursing, speech therapy, psychology, etc.) associated with the new technologies have led the Craniofacial Surgery to become a fascinating specialty. Great refinements in both aesthetic and functional morphology have been amply demonstrated by the authors of this work. In spite of the evolution and consolidation of several surgical techniques in the treatment of cleft lip and palate over the years, many basic precepts regarding the care of this group of patients remain the same. Compassion is undoubtedly one of the most important among these precepts.

Indeed, a coordinated effort in the longitudinal care of this cohort is of paramount importance aiming to avoid excessive scars in the soft tissue envelope that may cause impairment of craniofacial growth. All this must be understood by families who may be afflicted by the burden of multiple surgeries along the years.

The authors have admirably worked in providing a text that demonstrates the results that can be obtained with cooperation between numerous experts, with special emphasis on the most modern and established surgical techniques to correct various problems related to cleft.

I have absolute conviction that this book will represent an excellent source of information to guide experienced professionals and students and even collaborate for understanding basic care issues connected with craniofacial anomalies. In this way, I am pleased to commend the editors and authors for this wonderful effort to present a succinct and practical text to the readers.

Ricardo Cruz, M.D.
National Institute of Traumatology
and Orthopedics
Rio de Janeiro, Brazil

Contents

1 **Introduction**.. 1
Nivaldo Alonso and Cassio Eduardo Raposo-Amaral

2 **Promoting Comprehensive Cleft Care into a Unified Heath System in Brazil: Challenges and Achievements**................. 3
Cassio Eduardo Raposo-Amaral and Nivaldo Alonso

3 **Global Cleft Lip and Palate Care: A Brief Review**............... 15
Benjamin B. Massenburg, Johanna N. Riesel, Christopher D. Hughes, and John G. Meara

4 **Genetics of Cleft Lip and Cleft Palate: Perspectives in Surgery Management and Outcome**........................ 25
Gerson Shigeru Kobayashi, Luciano Abreu Brito, Joanna Goes Castro Meira, Lucas Alvizi, and Maria Rita Passos-Bueno

5 **Classification of Cleft Phenotypes**........................... 37
Cassio Eduardo Raposo-Amaral, Rafael Denadai, and Nivaldo Alonso

6 **An Overview of Protocols and Outcomes in Cleft Care**........... 47
Rafael Denadai and Cassio Eduardo Raposo-Amaral

7 **Unilateral Cleft Lip Repair**................................. 83
Cassio Eduardo Raposo-Amaral and Nivaldo Alonso

8 **Treatment of Bilateral Cleft Lip and Palate: Protocol for Surgical Treatment**..................................... 111
Nivaldo Alonso and Julia Amundson

9 **Current Management of Bilateral Cleft Lip**.................... 123
Cassio Eduardo Raposo-Amaral and Cesar Augusto Raposo-Amaral

10 **Cleft Palate: Anatomy and Surgery**.......................... 139
Nivaldo Alonso, Jonas Eraldo Lima Jr., Hagner Lucio de Andrade Lima, and Hillary E. Jenny

11	**Buccinator Myomucosal Flap in Cleft Palate Repair: The SOBRAPAR Hospital Experience** .... Rafael Denadai, Cassio Eduardo Raposo-Amaral, and Cesar Augusto Raposo-Amaral	155
12	**Velopharyngeal Insufficiency: Etiopathology and Treatment** ...... Nivaldo Alonso, Jonas Eraldo Lima Jr., and Hillary E. Jenny	183
13	**Surgical Management of Velopharyngeal Insufficiency: The SOBRAPAR Hospital Algorithm** .... Rafael Denadai, Cassio Eduardo Raposo-Amaral, Anelise Sabbag, and Cesar Augusto Raposo-Amaral	199
14	**Speech Therapy in Cleft Patients** .... Laura Davison Mangilli and Anelise Sabbag	215
15	**Robin Sequence**.. Nivaldo Alonso, Cristiano Tonello, Ilza Lazarini Marques, Arturo Frick Carpes, Marco Maricevich, and Renata Maricevich	225
16	**Bone Graft in Alveolar Cleft Lip and Palate** .... Nivaldo Alonso, Renato da Silva Freitas, Julia Amundson, and Cassio Eduardo Raposo-Amaral	247
17	**Bone Substitute: Alveolar Bone Grafting (ABG) with rhBMP-2 (Recombinant Bone Morphogenic Protein-2)**....... Nivaldo Alonso and Julia Amundson	263
18	**Orthodontic Treatment of Patients with Orofacial Cleft** .... Paulo Camara, Endrigo Oliveira Bastos, Daniel Curi, and Nivaldo Alonso	269
19	**Orthognathic Surgery in Cleft Patients** .... Nivaldo Alonso, Endrigo Oliveira Bastos, and Geraldo Capuchinho Jr.	279
20	**Secondary Unilateral Cleft Rhinoplasty**........................ Cesar Augusto Raposo-Amaral, Rafael Denadai, Cassio Eduardo Raposo-Amaral, and Celso Luiz Buzzo	297
21	**The Rare Facial Cleft** .... Cassio Eduardo Raposo-Amaral, Reza Jarrahy, Rizal Lim, and Nivaldo Alonso	325
22	**Three-Dimensional Digital Stereophotogrammetry in Cleft Care**... Rafael Denadai and Cassio Eduardo Raposo-Amaral	363
23	**Standardized Two-Dimensional Photographic Documentation of Cleft Patients** .... Rafael Denadai and Cassio Eduardo Raposo-Amaral	379

Contributors and Editors

Contributors

Nivaldo Alonso, M.D., Ph.D. Divisao de Cirurgia Plastica e Queimaduras, Hospital das Clínicas da Faculdade de Medicina da Universidade de São Paulo, São Paulo, Brazil

Lucas Alvizi, Ph.D. Centro de Pesquisas Sobre o Genoma Humano e Células-Tronco, Instituto de Biociências, Universidade de São Paulo, São Paulo, Brazil

Julia Amundson, B.S. Miller School of Medicine, University of Miami, Miami, FL, USA

Hagner Lucio de Andrade Lima, M.D. Plastic Surgeon in a Private Clinic, Bauru, São Paulo, Brazil

Endrigo Oliveira Bastos, M.D., D.D.S., M.Sc. Divisao de Cirurgia Plastica e Queimaduras, Hospital das Clínicas da Faculdade de Medicina da Universidade de São Paulo, São Paulo, SP, Brazil

Luciano Abreu Brito, Ph.D. Centro de Pesquisas sobre o Genoma Humano e Células-Tronco, Instituto de Biociências, Universidade de São Paulo, São Paulo, Brazil

Celso Luiz Buzzo, M.D. Institute of Plastic and Craniofacial Surgery, SOBRAPAR Hospital, Campinas, São Paulo, Brazil

Paulo Camara, D.D.S. Divisao de Cirurgia Plastica e Queimaduras, Hospital das Clínicas da Faculdade de Medicina da Universidade de São Paulo, São Paulo, Brazil

Geraldo Capuchinho Jr., M.D. Department of Plastic and Reconstructive Surgery, Hospital Universitário Risoleta Tolentino Neves, Universidade Federal de Minas Gerais, Belo Horizonte, Brazil

Arturo Frick Carpes, M.D., Ph.D. Department of Plastic Surgery, University of São Paulo Hospital, São Paulo, Brazil

Daniel Curi, M.D., D.D.S. Fellow Craniofacial Surgery, Department of Plastic Surgery at University of São Paulo, São Paulo, Brazil

Rafael Denadai, M.D. Institute of Plastic and Craniofacial Surgery, SOBRAPAR Hospital, Campinas, São Paulo, Brazil

Christopher D. Hughes, M.D., M.P.H. Program in Global Surgery and Social Change, Harvard Medical School, Boston, MA, USA

Harvard Combined Plastic Surgery Residency, Boston, MA, USA

Reza Jarrahy, M.D. Division of Plastic and Reconstructive Surgery, Department of Pediatrics David Geffen School of Medicine at UCLA, Los Angeles, California, USA

Hillary E. Jenny, M.D. Plastic Surgery Resident in the Program at John Hopkins, Baltimore, MD, USA

University of São Paulo, São Paulo, Brazil

Gerson Shigeru Kobayashi, Ph.D. Centro de Pesquisas sobre o Genoma Humano e Células-Tronco, Instituto de Biociências, Universidade de São Paulo, São Paulo, Brazil

Rizal Lim, M.D. Division of Plastic and Reconstructive Surgery, Department of Pediatrics David Geffen School of Medicine at UCLA, Los Angeles, California, USA

Jonas Eraldo Lima Jr., M.D. Board Certified Brazilian Society of Plastic Surgery, Federal University of Tocantins, Palmas, Tocantins, Brazil

Laura Davison Mangilli, Ph.D. Faculdade de Ceilândia, University of Brasilia, Brasilia, Brazil

Marco Maricevich, M.D. Department of Plastic Surgery, Baylor College of Medicine, Houston, TX, USA

Renata Maricevich, M.D. Department of Plastic Surgery, Texas Children's Hospital – Baylor College of Medicine, Houston, TX, USA

Ilza Lazarini Marques, M.D., Ph.D. Department of Craniofacial Surgery, Hospital for Rehabilitation of Craniofacial Anomalies, University of São Paulo, São Paulo, Brazil

Benjamin B. Massenburg, M.D. Division of Plastic Surgery, University of Washington, Seattle, WA, USA

Program in Global Surgery and Social Change, Harvard Medical School, Boston, MA, USA

Department of Plastic and Oral Surgery, Boston Children's Hospital, Boston, MA, USA

John G. Meara, M.D., D.M.D., M.B.A. Program in Global Surgery and Social Change, Harvard Medical School, Boston, MA, USA

Department of Plastic and Oral Surgery, Boston Children's Hospital, Boston, MA, USA

Joanna Goes Castro Meira, Ph.D. Centro de Pesquisas sobre o Genoma Humano e Células-Tronco, Instituto de Biociências, Universidade de São Paulo, São Paulo, Brazil

Maria Rita Passos-Bueno, Ph.D. Centro de Pesquisas sobre o Genoma Humano e Células-Tronco, Instituto de Biociências, Universidade de São Paulo, São Paulo, Brazil

Cassio Eduardo Raposo-Amaral, M.D., Ph.D. Institute of Plastic and Craniofacial Surgery, SOBRAPAR Hospital, Campinas, São Paulo, Brazil

Universidade de São Paulo, São Paulo, Brazil

Cesar Augusto Raposo-Amaral, M.D. Institute of Plastic and Craniofacial Surgery, SOBRAPAR Hospital, Campinas, São Paulo, Brazil

Johanna N. Riesel, M.D. Program in Global Surgery and Social Change, Harvard Medical School, Boston, MA, USA

Harvard Combined Plastic Surgery Residency, Boston, MA, USA

Anelise Sabbag, S.L.P. Institute of Plastic and Craniofacial Surgery, SOBRAPAR Hospital, Campinas, São Paulo, Brazil

Renato da Silva Freitas, M.D., Ph.D. Plastic Surgery Department at Federal University of Parana, Curitiba, Parana, Brazil

Cristiano Tonello, M.D., Ph.D. Department of Craniofacial Surgery, Hospital for Rehabilitation of Craniofacial Anomalies, University of São Paulo, São Paulo, Brazil

About the Editors

Nivaldo Alonso trained in plastic surgery at the University of São Paulo. At the end of his plastic surgery residency he stayed as chief resident for one more year. After this, he went to France for a fellowship in craniofacial surgery with Daniel Marchac, and during this period he was an observer at the Clinique Belvedere Paris France with Paul Tessier. Dr. Alonso returned to Brazil in 1987 and decided to follow an academic career. He completed his Ph.D. in 1992 and later became Associate Professor in the Department of Surgery at the University of São Paulo. Since 1997 he has been an international volunteer for Operation Smile, an organization devoted to the treatment of cleft lip and palate. With many years dedicated to craniofacial surgery, and with his hard work in giving more visibility to the treatment of congenital deformities, he was elected President of the Brazilian Association of Cranio Maxillofacial Surgery and served in that position for 4 years. In 1993 he established the Service of Craniofacial Surgery in the Plastic Surgery Department of the Hospital das Clinics Hospital on Medical School at University of São Paulo, and since then more than 50 fellows have trained there in craniofacial surgery. Dr. Alonso has had more than 250 papers published and has an international reputation. He was invited to be a Visiting Professor at two important American universities, Yale and Harvard. Because of his vast international surgical activities in developing countries he was invited to serve on the Lancet Commission for Global Surgery, which works in close cooperation with Harvard Medical School, Boston, USA, Sweden's Lund University, and King's College of Surgery, London, UK; currently he is still serving on this Commission. He is an active member of the International Society of Craniofacial Surgery and an International Member of the American Society of Plastic Surgeons (ASPS), and he is now a member of the ASPS Volunteers in Plastic Surgery Steering Committee. For more than 20 years Dr. Alonso has been dedicated to the treatment of patients with cleft lip and palate.

Cassio Eduardo Raposo-Amaral completed his plastic surgery training at the University of Campinas, Brazil, under the leadership of Dr. Cassio Raposo do Amaral in 2005. The following year he went to the United States to gain additional experience in craniofacial surgery and surgery for cleft lip and palate at the Institute of Reconstructive Plastic Surgery at New York University (NYU) with Drs. Joseph G. McCarthy and Court B. Cutting. He extended his period in the United States with an International fellowship at UCLA under the leadership of Drs. Henry K. Kawamoto and James P. Bradley. In 2008 he was a recipient of the ASPS International scholar award and returned to the United States to visit world-renowned craniofacial centers. He completed his Ph.D. at the University of São Paulo, working in the field of bone tissue engineering under the leadership of Dr. Nivaldo Alonso. After his return to Brazil, to SOBRAPAR, a hospital established by his late father Cassio Raposo do Amaral in 1979 and totally devoted to craniofacial surgery and surgery for cleft lip and palate, he organized all protocols and data collection, and restructured a very busy practice based on congenital craniofacial anomalies. Dr. Cassio Eduardo Raposo-Amaral is a leading plastic and craniofacial surgeon in Brazil, and with his brother, Cesar Augusto Raposo do Amaral, also a plastic surgeon, has been responsible for the pilgrimage of patients with congenital craniofacial abnormalities from all over the country to Campinas, where SOBRAPAR is located. Dr. Cassio Eduardo Raposo-Amaral has authored more than 100 articles in the English and Portuguese medical literature and has written ten book chapters. He is a member of seven professional societies: the Brazilian Society of Plastic Surgery, Brazilian Association of Cranio-Maxillo-Facial Surgery, Brazilian Cleft Palate Association, Brazilian Burn Society, the American Society of Plastic Surgeons (international member), the International Society of Craniofacial Surgery, and the American Cleft Palate Association. He is a recipient of 13 awards of the Brazilian Society of Plastic Surgery and the Brazilian Association of Cranio-Maxillo-Facial Surgery. Currently, Dr. Raposo is the President of the Brazilian Association of Cranio-Maxillo-Facial Surgery.

Introduction

Nivaldo Alonso and Cassio Eduardo Raposo-Amaral

Cleft lip and palate represent one of the great challenges of craniofacial surgery, with initial descriptions of the condition and surgical repair dating back to ancient times. Despite many diagnostic and technical aspects remaining unclarified, much progress has been achieved in understanding and treating this deformity. From more complex genetic studies clarifying its etiology to less mutilating surgical techniques, these advances have helped improve prevention and appropriate care. There is still an impressive number of patients with cleft lip or palate: it is estimated that 3.5 million children worldwide have this deformity. The burden of disease and barrier to comprehensive care is disproportionate in low- and middle-income countries. Strengthening surgical and dental treatment infrastructure is necessary to care for these patients throughout their initial development (Mars et al. 2008; Kling et al. 2014).

Treatment of cleft lip and palate is complicated by the complex etiologies of the condition. Development of the normal cephalic segment involves a complex genetic system with more than 25,000 protein codes and more than 17,000 genes contributing to the formation of the complex craniofacial skeleton. It is believed that more than 100 genes are responsible for the formation of the normal face. Presentation of cleft lip and palate is further complicated by being associated with other syndromes in more than 30% of cases, with variations seen in the types of cleft of the palate and lip. Increasing understanding of the genetic mechanisms involved in embryologic facial development, however, is encouraging for prevention efforts. Migration and

N. Alonso, M.D., Ph.D.
Divisao de Cirurgia Plastica e Queimaduras, Hospital das Clínicas da Faculdade de Medicina da Universidade de São Paulo, São Paulo, Brazil
e-mail: nivalonso@gmail.com

C.E. Raposo-Amaral, M.D., Ph.D. (✉)
Institute of Plastic and Craniofacial Surgery, SOBRAPAR Hospital, Campinas, São Paulo 13084-880, Brazil

Universidade de São Paulo, São Paulo, Brazil
e-mail: cassioraposo@hotmail.com

© Springer International Publishing AG 2018
N. Alonso, C.E. Raposo-Amaral (eds.), *Cleft Lip and Palate Treatment*,
https://doi.org/10.1007/978-3-319-63290-2_1

formation of facial processes between 4- and 12-week gestation depend on signaling genes such as sonic hedgehog, BMP, and FGFR. This knowledge can be applied to examine syndromes associated with cleft formation in the palate or lip. For example, van der Woude syndrome is often associated with missing teeth, and the main gene on chromosome 1, IRF6, plays an important role in this presentation (Craniofacial and Oral Gene Expression Network (COGENE) 2016). These ongoing findings are very promising for understanding the various mechanisms of cleft formation.

Ultimately, these data will help to guide strategies for prevention, thus avoiding large expenditures on extensive treatment of these patients. In the meantime, it is essential to continue devising protocols for safe and effective surgical treatment and care, in conjunction with speech and development of the dental arch (Losee and Kirschner 2009). In this book, we focus on all aspects of treatment in patients with this deformity throughout the entire phase of their growth and development, with the goal of facilitating full social integration of these individuals into society.

References

Craniofacial and Oral Gene Expression Network (COGENE) Database. St. Louis: Washington University; 2016. http://hg.wustl.edu/cogene/.

Kling RR, Taub PJ, Ye X, Jabs EW. Oral clefting in China over the last decade: 205.679 patients. Plast Reconstr Surg Glob Open. 2014;2(10):e236.

Losee J, Kirschner RE, editors. Comprehensive cleft care. New York: The McGraw Hill Company; 2009.

Mars M, Sell D, Habel A, editors. Management of cleft lip and palate in the developing world. Hoboken: Wiley; 2008.

Promoting Comprehensive Cleft Care into a Unified Heath System in Brazil: Challenges and Achievements

2

Cassio Eduardo Raposo-Amaral and Nivaldo Alonso

The Brazilian unified health care system (named Sistema Único de Saúde [SUS]) was established in 1988 in the Federal Constitution and determined that "health is a right of every citizen and a duty of the State" (Malik 1997). This complex social program was created based on the tripod of universal access to health care services, equality of access to health care, and comprehensiveness, meaning an integral continuity of health assistance (Tanaka et al. 2012; de Sousa and Mendonca 2014; Pontes et al. 2014).

The primary goal of SUS was to decentralize health policy from a federal cell to state and municipality, which have the responsibility to locally offer the healthy assistance to the population by contracting public and private hospitals or any other needed services to accomplish this task (Cohn 2009; Cortes 2009). Since 1988, the SUS and the decentralization policies have significantly expanded, even though the current health spending is still fewer than 4% of gross domestic product (GDP) (Araujo 2010; Artmann et al. 2013; Ramos et al. 2014; Vincens and Stafstrom 2015). Although philosophically interesting, the SUS fails to achieve its primary goal of offering high-quality pro-bono care to citizen in all Brazilian territory and disparities between services along the country have occurred, impacting quality of life and longevity of Brazilians. Lack of infrastructure and qualified professionals is seen in some regions as the North and Northwest regions of Brazil that coincides with low human development index (HDI) marked by social contrast and poverty. Some Brazilian municipalities have HDI classified as low (<0.500) that correspond to countries such as Laos, Yemen, Haiti, and Madagascar (Carneiro et al. 2012).

C.E. Raposo-Amaral, M.D., Ph.D. (✉)
Institute of Plastic and Craniofacial Surgery, SOBRAPAR Hospital, Campinas, São Paulo 13084-880, Brazil

Universidade de São Paulo, São Paulo, Brazil
e-mail: cassioraposo@hotmail.com

N. Alonso, M.D., Ph.D.
Divisao de Cirurgia Plastica e Queimaduras, Hospital das Clínicas da Faculdade de Medicina da Universidade de São Paulo, São Paulo, Brazil

© Springer International Publishing AG 2018
N. Alonso, C.E. Raposo-Amaral (eds.), *Cleft Lip and Palate Treatment*,
https://doi.org/10.1007/978-3-319-63290-2_2

Public and private hospitals contracted by the Ministry of Health are reimbursed a flat month fee (based on the average production of the immediate past year). The Ministry of Health created values for each procedure that is significantly lower than the market and calculates an average sum of all procedures in the analyzed timeframe to be monthly sent to their contracted hospitals. Thus, the lack of reimbursement generates a monthly deficit for public and private hospitals that exclusively works for SUS. Therefore, many of these hospitals have already presented difficulties of self-sustainability.

The Ministry of Health established their main concerns and policies to tackle the immense diversity of national health problems and cleft care does not sit into their budget priority. Controlling of the Aedes aegypti seems a great priority as it is the vector of the dengue fever, a currently epidemic disease in Brazil (Monteiro et al. 2014).

Twenty-six centers around the country were accredited by the Ministry of Health to offer assistance to cleft population; three of them (although surprisingly accredited) does not have sufficient infrastructure and human resource to offer surgery to patients and end up referring patients to a center in the inner State of São Paulo. Four centers located in São Paulo State are responsible for 67% of Brazilian cleft care, forcing families to continuously travel (from restricted areas of the country to São Paulo State) to obtain a chance to have their children treated.

These populations are supposed to be seen by a cleft team in their own region, avoiding patient migration to other regions. The phenomenon of patient's migration still occurs, owing to the lack of trained plastic surgeons and multidisciplinary teams in the north, northwest, central, and even some Southwest areas of Brazil. The population migration causes a negative and destructive impact on the family household, therefore maintaining the vicious circle of poverty, because only the mother and the affected child travel, leaving behind the rest of the family. Moreover, when patients migrate to have a surgery done in a cleft lip and palate center far away from their homes, they never receive the full benefits of ancillary treatment and full rehabilitation. Thus, it would be extremely important to stimulate a better distribution of cleft teams around the country, and create surgical infrastructure in the three habilitated centers and other places around the country, as well as a better network among centers to avoid treatment delay and poor adherence.

Older patients with late presentation, coming from restricted, underprivileged regions are not uncommon in our centers, and we usually adjust our protocol to maximize rehabilitation that is already delayed (Fig. 2.1).

Cleft should have a compulsory notification like other diseases in Brazil. This would indicate the exact number of newborn babies with cleft, per region, per year. The number of new cases has an expected rate of approximately 5000 new patients each year, and the SUS has identified less than 2000 new cases and only one-fifth has access to comprehensive care, thus creating a backlog of untreated patients in the restrict areas of Brazil, especially those with low human development index as regions of the Northeast of Brazil (e.g., Maranhão and Alagoas States whose HIDs are inferior of 0.65, the lowest in the country) (Figs. 2.2 and 2.3).

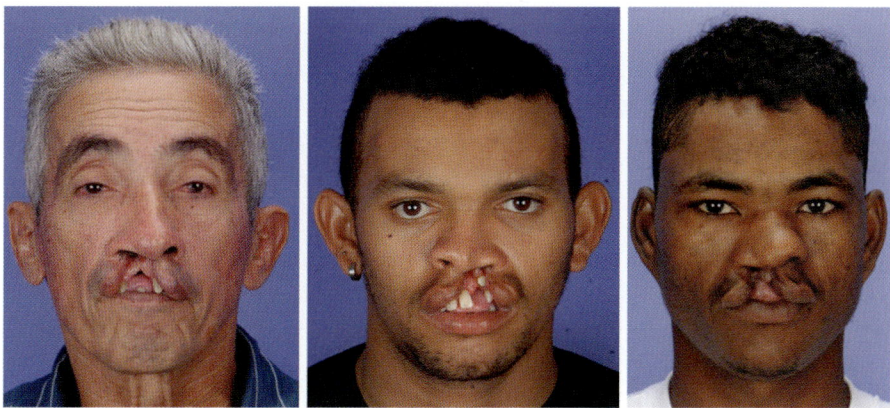

Fig. 2.1 Frontal photography of unrepaired cleft patients without any type of ancillary treatment. Patients in these conditions are commonly seen in Brazil. Note the different type of ethnicity

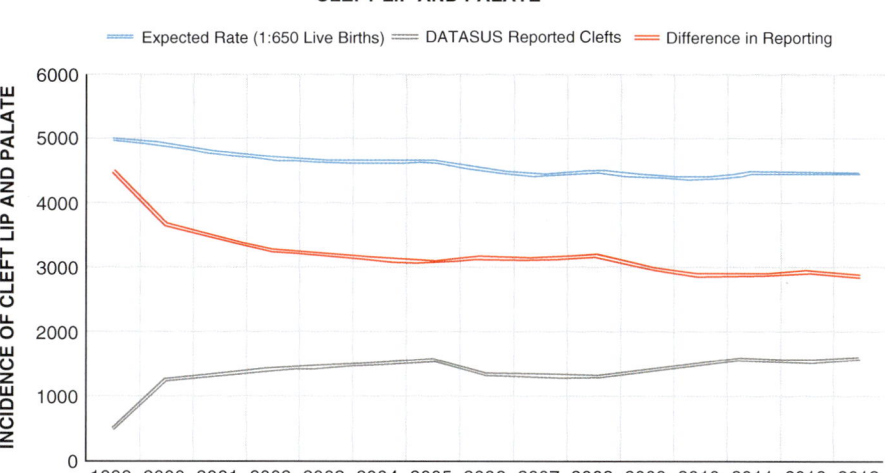

Fig. 2.2 Graph showing the incidence of patients born with cleft lip and palate in Brazil. The expected rate based on the ratio of 1:650 (1 affected child in 650 births) is approximately 5000 new cases (*blue line*). The SUS reported significantly less patients (*grey line*). The red line points out the difference in reporting. This phenomenon might have occurred due to either an overestimation of patients born with cleft (the number could be lower) or the lack of report

Data has shown that 13% of prenatal deaths are patients with congenital craniofacial anomalies, showing an urgent necessity to expand care to the entire country (DATASUS 2003 data). Our team always considers speech as a priority when examining a primary patient with late presentation; therefore, the first operation in an older patient with complete cleft lip and palate is always the palate repair. These nuances are examples of common issues that a cleft team of a developing country

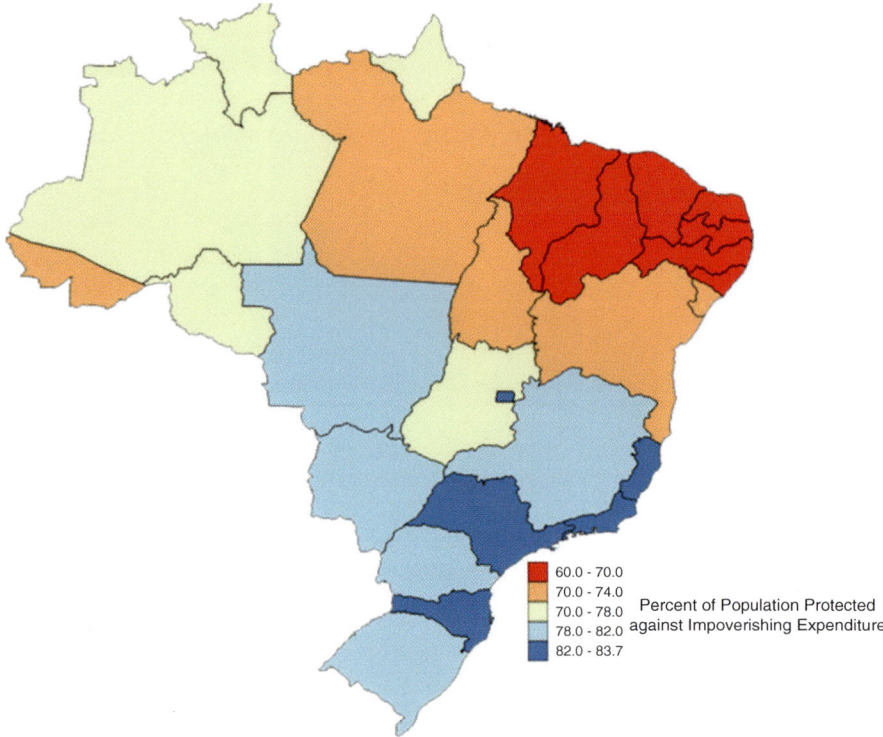

Fig. 2.3 Map of Brazil showing the areas with low human development index (HDI). These areas are located in the Northeast and North regions of Brazil

may have to face. Our both protocols have always been adapted to fit the patients' needs and priorities. Here, the authors lead two different types of facilities: one is SOBRAPAR, a private philanthropic hospital created by a plastic surgeon, late Cassio Raposo do Amaral in 1979 and accredited by the Ministry of Health, and the other is the Service of Craniofacial Surgery from the Department of Plastic Surgery from University of São Paulo (USP), the largest university of South America, a public hospital whose craniofacial surgery has been led by Nivaldo Alonso. Both Brazilian leading institutions have been offering cutting-edge comprehensive care to patients with congenital and acquired craniofacial anomalies and have been served as models for established and new centers around the country. There is another common type of cleft center, those that are exclusively public municipal hospitals, which offer space for a cleft team and have no link with universities. This last type of cleft center is the most common organization distributed across Brazil. The centers that receive accreditation by the government to perform cleft lip and palate surgery are named high complexity (alta complexidade in Portuguese). These are the centers that are paid a higher financial amount by the government each month in comparison to the others named median complexity (media complexidade in Portuguese) (Fig. 2.4).

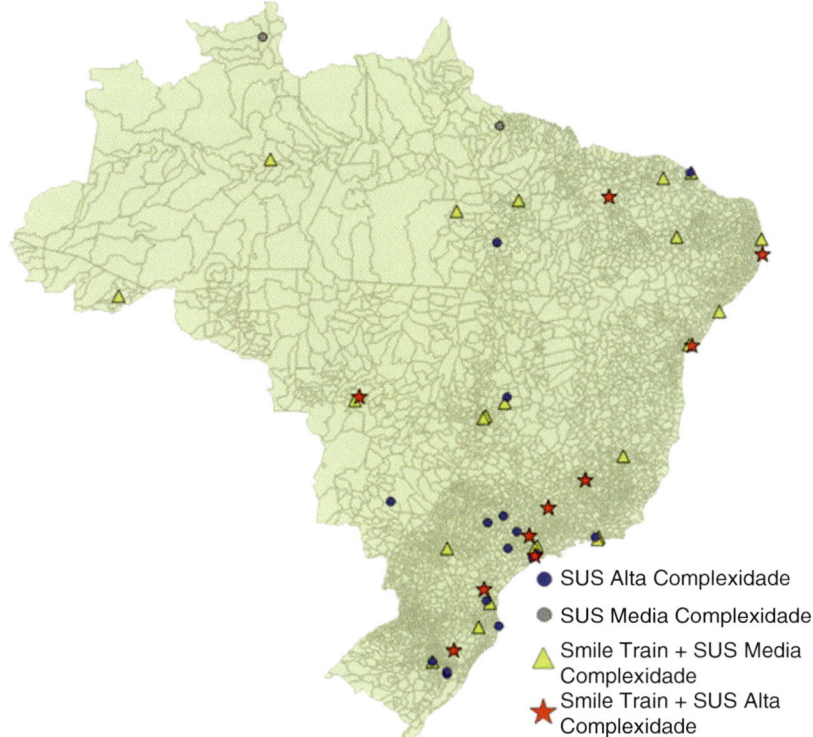

Fig. 2.4 Map of Brazil showing the distribution of the cleft center around the country. High complexity (alta complexidade in Portuguese) and median complexity (media complexidade in Portuguese). Smile Train supports centers of high and median complexity

The Smile Train has its own policy and usually funds centers with high and median complexity regardless of their financial status. The majority of centers of high complexity are located in the South and Southeast region of Brazil as shown in Fig. 2.3.

More recently, the Brazilian Society of Plastic Surgery (Sociedade Brasileira de Cirurgia Plástica [SBCP], in Portuguese) and its associated new foundation IDEAH and the Smile Train foundation created a partnership to expand care in remote areas of the country where some centers are trying to emerge and whose access to care to the cleft population has been continuously overlooked by the government. The project named Cleft Week (Semana da fissura in Portuguese) has been financing cleft and craniofacial surgeons to go to some remote areas of Brazil, where cleft care remains incipient aiming to offer assistance, education, and training to local surgeons. Instead of promoting foreign surgeons to operate on the native patients by International Missions, the Smile Train and SBCP have been strengthening the local surgeons and starting to improve their infrastructure. As described by Pfeifer, cleft charity missions are useful in developing countries that have little or no infrastructure (e.g., Haiti); however, in countries like Brazil, Chile, India, and others, it has been more efficient and sustainable to finance and educationally support the local centers (Pfeifer et al. 2002). Additionally, the charity missions do not create local infrastructure and maintain dependence.

The concept of supporting operative camps in charity missions is opposite to the concept of supporting local centers, specifically for countries with expanding infrastructure. It was described, based on a retrospective study, that cleft palate patients receive less attention in operative camps than patients with cleft lip, meaning that surgeons who work on operative camps prefer to operate a cleft lip than a cleft palate (Patil et al. 2011). Additionally, the same study highlighted that 86.4% of patients operated on in camp settings did not receive information regarding the fundamental importance of the team approach and the necessity of longitudinal follow-up, in opposition of 100% of patients operated on in cleft centers, who received full explanation and were aware of the deleterious consequences of the poor adherence and delayed treatment (Patil et al. 2011).

Ideally, a cleft lip and palate center in a developing country should be based accordingly, with the main philosophy of a multidisciplinary treatment, by means of different specialties acting together in the same physical space, with each specialty guaranteeing their own peculiarities to aim the best result for their patients and family. Additionally, it is our belief that each center, included in a national referral list of local health systems, should receive at least 80–100 new cleft cases per year. This would be the level of activity to maintain the criterion standard of care. Not all the 23 centers of high complexity around the country have attended the minimum criteria regarding the number of specialties and required infrastructure, suggested by the American Cleft Palate Association and Eurocleft that include plastic surgery, general dentistry, psychology, speech–language pathology, and otolaryngology (Shaw et al. 2001; Strauss 1998). A parameter of care for our reality and heterogeneous scenario is warranted (Fig. 2.5).

We have previously established some guidelines for offering care to our patients based on six principles for sustaining a cleft health care system in developing country that can be summarized into longitudinal protocols involving a multidisciplinary approach, with strong infrastructure and competent, educated professionals with research involvement.

Our guidelines are based on the geographic distribution of cleft lip and palate centers around Brazilian territory, in order to achieve the four objectives: first, avoid patient's migration; second, facilitate patient's adherence; third, focus on a global and continuous multidisciplinary treatment; fourth, avoid indiscriminate opening of non-prepared cleft lip and palate centers in our country; fifth, creating a national board of experienced and distinguished professionals to guide and implement comprehensive care across the territory; and sixth, facilitate communication with national board members and government members that can implement and guide directions to new policies.

The description of the two different center types follows: the SOBRAPAR model and the University of São Paulo model.

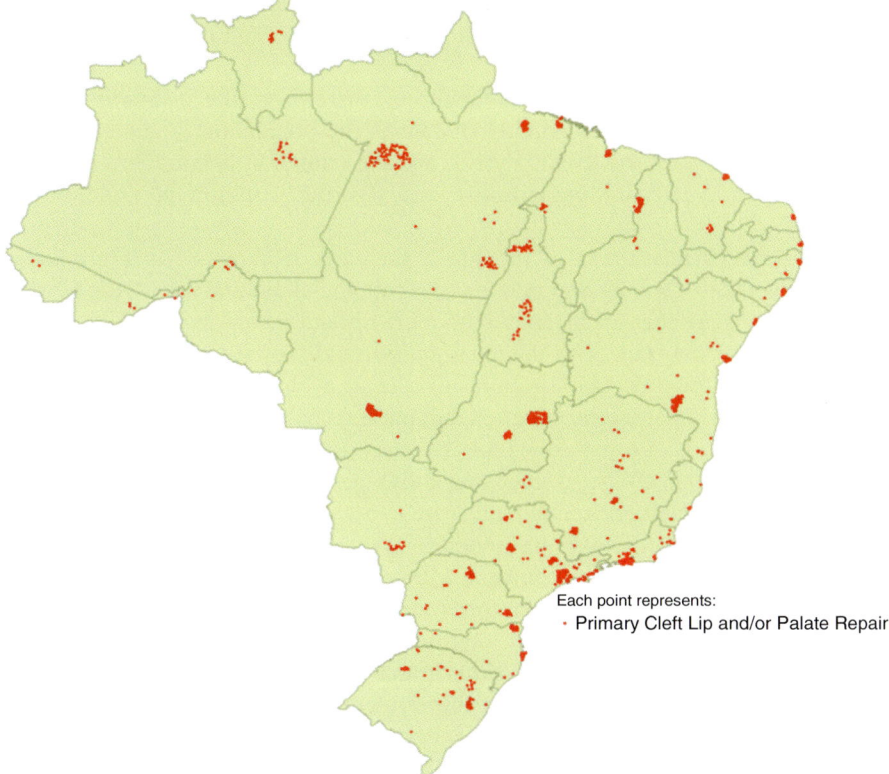

Fig. 2.5 Map of Brazil showing the location of primary cleft lip and/or palate surgeries performed in Brazil. The concentration of surgeries around few centers is evident showing a paucity of a public policy to control patient migration

2.1 SOBRAPAR Model

SOBRAPAR has been serving as a model in Brazil for cleft and craniofacial treatments for over 37 years. The concept of creating a multidisciplinary center to treat congenital and acquired anomalies was brought from the Institute of Reconstructive Plastic Surgery at the New York University Medical Center and its associated fundraising foundation, the former National Foundation for Facial Reconstruction (NFFR). SOBRAPAR hospital, named in Portuguese Hospital de Crânio e Face SOBRAPAR, is a private philanthropic hospital, created in 1979, with 19 beds exclusively devoted to craniofacial care. SOBRAPAR was constructed with the effort of a group of people led by the founder and who received financial support by the former entrepreneur, owner of COFAP automobile industry, Abrahão Kasisnski, and German foundation named Latin America Zentrum at that time headed by Mr. Herman Gorhagan. They both found the project inspiring and put their strength in its materialization.

We received the certificate of philanthropy that spares the institution to pay income taxes and guarantees gratuity of care to the population. The certificate is audited by the government every 3 years, and the criteria to obtain it are based on transparency and account organization and rigorous audition by independent auditors.

SOBRAPAR's mission is to provide a standard of care for underprivileged patients born with cleft lip and palate and craniofacial anomalies. SOBRAPAR's ethical values state that all patients with cleft lip and palate in Brazil should be treated in their local centers by the local multidisciplinary team; thus we strongly support the treatment decentralization in order to avoid patient's migration. Our goals are to provide assistance and rehabilitation to patients and their families, to educate plastic surgeons that are willing to return to their region to help their own people and to strengthen their local team, and to perform clinical and experimental research related to cleft and craniofacial care.

In Brazil, the social worker has a determinant role of providing adherence of the patient in his treatment. A center in a developing country should be responsible for maintaining their patient's return for routine speech, orthodontia, and psychological sessions, as well as their long-term follow-up. We define rehabilitation as a gathering of efforts by the multidisciplinary team, patient, family, and community to correct, minimize, and prevent problems related to cleft lip and palate, therefore offering better conditions for a physical, psychological, and effective social development. As also emphasized by Reddy et al., who developed a cleft center in India, a rehabilitation occurs with patient's integration into society and self-sustainability (Reddy et al. 2009). The mission of an established cleft center should go beyond the surgical repair. Neither a non-prepared center nor a surgeon working alone should operate on a cleft patient. Surgery done by non-trained surgeons may result in a severe deformity. The burdens of cleft sequels for the centers in developing countries are significantly increasing. In most of these patients, multiple surgeries are needed to recreate a minimum aesthetic and functional condition. Additional costs are added to centers in developing countries to treat these gross sequels.

As noted by Mulliken, the cleft lip and palate cause is often of low priority for health care and budgets (Mulliken 2004). In addition, offering little or no reimbursement, the cleft lip and palate cause yearly loses most of the well-trained plastic surgeons for the aesthetic plastic surgery. It is our continuous concern to raise awareness of the cleft lip and palate cause among the plastic surgeons of the Brazilian Society of Plastic Surgery. Over the last 10 years, SOBRAPAR organized more than seven cleft and craniofacial meetings, including the official meeting of the International Society of Craniofacial Surgery and the International Confederation of Cleft Palate and Craniofacial Anomalies, held every 4 years in different parts of the globe. More than 1200 delegates from all over the world attended the meeting (Raposo-Amaral and Warren 2011).

2.2 Striving for Sustainability

In additional to SUS, SOBRAPAR receives support from the Smile Train foundation. Considering that the cost of health care in Brazil is increasing, we could not survive without a further plan. In this direction, we have two full-time professionals to screen and create awareness campaigns in our community that consequently raises interest from local donors and companies.

In 1999, the late Dr. Cassio Raposo do Amaral invited a director of Goodwill Industries International, Inc., who visited SOBRAPAR. Since then, a similar model of selling donated products was established. Throughout these 16 years, our Bazaar has significantly grown. We have developed a picking-up service branch of our Bazaar, which is responsible to pick up and carry all of the used items, at no effort or cost for donors. We fix and sell absolutely everything from books to clothes, to electronics, to furniture. Moreover, this program trains and employs people, and some of them are our own habilitated patients.

A sewing industry was also created to support the center by fixing used clothes and shoes to be sold in the Bazaar, in addition to external contracts with other institutions.

2.3 Ongoing Education and Resident Training

SOBRAPAR offers a 3-year residency program in plastic and reconstructive surgery and 1-year fellowship in craniofacial surgery. Although the residents have an opportunity to rotate in all areas of the field including aesthetic plastic surgery, the training focuses on cleft lip and palate and craniofacial surgery. Our primary goal is to spread plastic surgeons with a craniofacial training, who are willing to devote at least part of their time, to treat underprivileged children with cleft lip and palate and craniofacial anomalies.

2.4 Research

Collecting data at a longitudinal basis allows us to promote clinical research (Raposo-Amaral et al. 2011). Assessment of the surgical outcomes and of our current protocol is done at least on a yearly basis. Supporting continuing education allows local professionals with the opportunity to be exposed to new ideas and technology, as well as to compare our results with our peers.

2.5 University of São Paulo

The multidisciplinary treatment of patients with cleft lip and palate in Brazil started at 1960s when Professor Victor Spina, Associate Professor of the Medical School at University of São Paulo (USP), founded in 1958 the CEFILPA, Center for Cleft Lip and Palate Rehabilitation inserted inside of the University of São Paulo-affiliated Hospital das Clínicas. This was the first attempt to create in Brazil a multidisciplinary care for this population. For the first time in Brazil one surgeon and one orthodontist started to treat a cleft patient together. A team was formed and many publications were pioneering the study for cleft lip and palate repair in Brazil. One of them is still in use in all country for many other services, Spina's Classification for Cleft Lip and Palate (Spina 1973; Spina and Lodovici 1960; Spina et al. 1972). Dr. Orlando Lodovici, former chief of the Plastic Surgery Department just after Dr. Victor Spina, has shown his concern about multidisciplinary care very early, and presented a thesis in (Lodovici 1964) at the University of Sao Paulo about Facial Growth in Children operated on Cleft Lip, very ahead of time at that moment (Spina and Lodovici 1960).

This concept extended throughout the country and generated other centers as "Hospital of Rehabilitation of Craniofacial Anomalies known as Centrinho de Bauru" which is affiliated to the USP. This hospital HRAC—Bauru was responsible for training professionals to work into the multidisciplinary setting around the country.

The basic research and basic education are the main goals of the service. Association with the many different specialties and genetics is the fundamental, created long time ago. The high number of patients and their complexity are the main features of the service.

More recently, the partnership between the Division of Speech Pathology and Division of Plastic and Reconstructive Surgery of USP presents a very interesting association for the future, not just in education but also for the comprehensive care of these patients.

The Division of Plastic and Reconstructive Surgery of USP has a 3-year training on general plastic surgery and one additional year (fellowship) for cleft and craniofacial surgery. USP receives patients from all over the country and most of them have already received a partial or an incomplete treatment in their states. It is not uncommon to see primary adult patients and gross sequels from inappropriate treatment coming from elsewhere.

The description of the Hospital das Clínicas of USP as the largest public hospital of South America and a reference center for diseases and complex syndromes has required creation of a center inside the university hospital devoted to assist this population, considering that association of cleft and craniofacial anomalies is quite frequent. The center of craniofacial anomalies of USP works very close to the Division of Neurosurgery and Genetics of USP; this association not just permits assistance for a great number of patients with high complex facial deformities but also improves the education and research on the field ended by relevant number of publications.

Despite these two excellent centers, Brazil had more than 200 million inhabitants in 2016 with an estimated rate for cleft-born children of 1:750 that gives us around 5000 new babies with cleft lip and palate a year, transforming cleft treatment into a great challenge for all specialties involved.

References

Araujo MA. Results-oriented management and accountability in the Brazilian Unified Health System. Rev Panam Salud Publica. 2010;27(3):230–6.

Artmann E, Andrade MA, Rivera FJ. Challenges for the discussion of a complex institutional mission: the case of a health research institute. Cien Saude Colet. 2013;18(1):191–202.

Carneiro FF, Franco Netto G, Corvalan C, de Freitas CM, Sales LB. Environmental health and inequalities: building indicators for sustainable development. Cien Saude Colet. 2012;17(6):1419–25.

Cohn A. Reflections on Brazilian National Health Reform after 20 years of experience with the Unified National Health System. Cad Saude Publica. 2009;25(7):1614–9.

Cortes SV. The Unified National Health System: decision-making forums and the political arena in health. Cad Saude Publica. 2009;25(7):1626–33.

de Sousa MF, Mendonca AV. Primary Health Care in the Brazilian Unified Health System (SUS): a bequest and a legacy. Cien Saude Colet. 2014;19(2):330–1.

Lodovici O. O crescimento da maxila em criancas com fissura lábio palatina operada – Estudo pela cefalometria radiologica. Tese de Doutorado apresentada à Universidade de São Paulo; 1964.

Malik AM. Quality improvement issues in Brazil. Jt Comm J Qual Improv. 1997;23(1):55–9.

Monteiro FA, Schama R, Martins AJ, Gloria-Soria A, Brown JE, Powell JR. Genetic diversity of Brazilian Aedes aegypti: patterns following an eradication program. PLoS Negl Trop Dis. 2014;8(9):e3167.

Mulliken JB. The changing faces of children with cleft lip and palate. N Engl J Med. 2004;351(8):745–7.

Patil SB, Kale SM, Khare N, Math M, Jaiswal S, Jain A. Changing patterns in demography of cleft lip-cleft palate deformities in a developing country: the Smile Train effect--what lies ahead? Plast Reconstr Surg. 2011;127(1):327–32.

Pfeifer TM, Grayson BH, Cutting CB. Nasoalveolar molding and gingivoperiosteoplasty versus alveolar bone graft: an outcome analysis of costs in the treatment of unilateral cleft alveolus. Cleft Palate Craniofac J. 2002;39(1):26–9.

Pontes AP, Oliveira DC, Gomes AM. The principles of the Brazilian Unified Health System, studied based on similitude analysis. Rev Lat Am Enfermagem. 2014;22(1):59–67.

Ramos LR, Malta DC, Gomes GA, Bracco MM, Florindo AA, Mielke GI, et al. Prevalence of health promotion programs in primary health care units in Brazil. Rev Saude Publica. 2014;48(5):837–44.

Raposo-Amaral CE, Raposo-Amaral CM, Raposo-Amaral CA, Chahal H, Bradley JP, Jarrahy R. Age at surgery significantly impacts the amount of orbital relapse following hypertelorbitism correction: a 30-year longitudinal study. Plast Reconstr Surg. 2011;127(4):1620–30.

Raposo-Amaral CE, Warren SM. Highlights from the 11th international congress on cleft palate and related craniofacial anomalies. J Craniofac Surg. 2011;22(3):781.

Reddy SG, Reddy LV, Reddy RR. Developing and standardizing a center to treat cleft and craniofacial anomalies in a developing country like India. J Craniofac Surg. 2009;20(Suppl 2): 1664–7.

Shaw WC, Semb G, Nelson P, Brattstrom V, Molsted K, Prahl-Andersen B, et al. The Eurocleft project 1996-2000: overview. J Craniomaxillofac Surg. 2001;29(3):131–40. discussion 41-2

Spina V. A proposed modification for the classification of cleft lip and palate. Cleft Palate J. 1973;110:251.

Spina V, Lodovici O. Conservative technique for treatment of unilateral cleft lip : reconstruction of the midline tubercle of the vermelion. Br J Plast Surg. 1960;13:110–7.

Spina V, Psillakis JM, Lapa FS, Ferreira MC. Classificação de Fissuras lábio-palatinas. Sugestão de modificação. Rev Hosp Clin Fac Med SPaulo. 1972;27:5–6.

Strauss RP. Cleft palate and craniofacial teams in the United States and Canada: a national survey of team organization and standards of care. The American Cleft Palate-Craniofacial Association (ACPA) Team Standards Committee. Cleft Palate Craniofac J. 1998;35(6):473–80.

Tanaka OY, Tamaki E, Felisberto E. The challenges of evaluation in the Brazilian Unified Health System (SUS). Cien Saude Colet. 2012;17(4):818–9.

Vincens N, Stafstrom M. Income inequality, economic growth and stroke mortality in Brazil: longitudinal and regional analysis 2002-2009. PLoS One. 2015;10(9):e0137332.

Global Cleft Lip and Palate Care: A Brief Review

3

Benjamin B. Massenburg, Johanna N. Riesel, Christopher D. Hughes, and John G. Meara

In the last decade, surgical care has gained new attention as an "indivisible, indispensable part of health care" (Meara et al. 2015; Kim 2014). No longer limited to short-term interventions, improving access to equitable surgical care is both a movement that is gaining traction and a career path that is earning acceptance (Chao et al. 2015; Dare et al. 2014; Leow et al. 2010). In the last decade, several key initiatives have launched access to equitable surgical care onto social and political agendas: The Bellagio Essential Surgery Group (Luboga et al. 2009), Disease Control Priorities II and III (Jamison et al. 2006, 2015), the Lancet Commission on Global Surgery (Meara et al. 2015), WHO's Global Initiative for Emergency and Essential Surgical Care (Bickler and Spiegel 2010), and World Health Assembly resolution 68.15 on surgical system strengthening (Price et al. 2015). Throughout this evolution, reconstructive surgical care for patients in resource-limited settings around the world, including cleft lip and palate care, has remained a priority to many private and governmental organizations, and now stands to benefit from this

B.B. Massenburg, M.D. (✉)
Division of Plastic Surgery, University of Washington, Seattle, WA, USA

Program in Global Surgery and Social Change, Harvard Medical School, Boston, MA, USA

Department of Plastic and Oral Surgery, Boston Children's Hospital, Boston, MA, USA
e-mail: ben.massenburg@gmail.com

J.N. Riesel, M.D. • C.D. Hughes, M.D., M.P.H.
Program in Global Surgery and Social Change, Harvard Medical School, Boston, MA, USA

Harvard Combined Plastic Surgery Residency, Boston, MA, USA

J.G. Meara, M.D., D.M.D., M.B.A.
Program in Global Surgery and Social Change, Harvard Medical School, Boston, MA, USA

Department of Plastic and Oral Surgery, Boston Children's Hospital, Boston, MA, USA

© Springer International Publishing AG 2018
N. Alonso, C.E. Raposo-Amaral (eds.), *Cleft Lip and Palate Treatment*,
https://doi.org/10.1007/978-3-319-63290-2_3

new focus. As the political landscape changes for access to safe and affordable surgical and anesthesia care worldwide, those that provide reconstructive care for children must understand the context in which this arena is changing as well as what is both possible and expected for the future.

Historically, periods of large-scale conflict and war have been unfortunate innovators in plastic surgery. Worldwide, the art of reconstructive care grew substantially in the periods around and after World Wars I and II. A collaborative effort between the American Society of Plastic and Reconstructive Surgeons Educational Foundation (PSEF) and the Medical International Cooperation Organization (MEDICO) in the 1960s helped to formalize interest and attention in addressing reconstructive surgical needs among the world's poorest populations (Maliniac 1958; Stark 1981; TIME Magazine 1961; Hyland 1981). Children were typically a substantial focus of these collaborations, including an emphasis on the care of cleft lip and palate. Throughout the late 1960s and 1970s, plastic surgeons steadily developed and strengthened their efforts in building comprehensive and sustainable cleft care for populations in resource-poor regions of low- and middle-income countries (LMICs). From Samuel Noordhoff's experiences in Taiwan to Arthur Barsky's iconoclastic development of the Barsky Unit in Saigon, to Tom Rees's development of the Flying Doctors of Africa, the latter half of the twentieth century saw substantial growth in formalized cleft care efforts around the world (Bingham 1991; Rees et al. 1994; Barsky 1978, 1970; Hughes et al. 2013; USA A 2010). Interplast was born in 1969 from Don Laub's work, and, under different names, has grown to develop sustainable care programs for children with cleft lip and palate for the past 45 years. Perhaps the most visible global cleft organizations today, Operation Smile and Smile Train, have been in existence since the 1980s and 1990s, respectively.

The efforts of these and other organizations and individuals have been driven by the ongoing, relatively unchanged need for comprehensive cleft care. Cleft lip and/or palate is estimated to occur in 1 out of every 500–1000 births and represents a large public health burden around the world (Derijcke et al. 1996; World Health Organization 2000; McQueen et al. 2010; Mock et al. 2010). Furthermore, the burden of congenital anomalies is unevenly carried by patients in LMICs, where 94% of all congenital anomalies occur (WHO 2012). With a smaller surgical workforce in low-resource settings, the global unmet need of patients with unrepaired cleft lip and palate is estimated to be between 400,000 and two million (Diana Farmer et al. 2015). The map accompanying this chapter displays the estimated ratio of newborns with cleft lip and/or palate to each member of the surgical workforce—including all surgeons, anesthesiologists, and obstetricians (Fig. 3.1) worldwide. Though most of the physicians in the surgical workforce may not treat patients with cleft lip and palate, this may serve as a proxy to demonstrate the scale of unmet need in resource-limited settings. The inequitable distribution of the surgical workforce in LMICs where disease incidence is highest results in surgical repairs that are performed later in life, if at all—long after pertinent developments in speech and language acquisition have already taken place. For example, in sub-Saharan Africa, the average age of a child receiving primary cleft lip or palate repair has been reported to be 10 years as compared to the recommended standard of 9–12 months found in high-resource

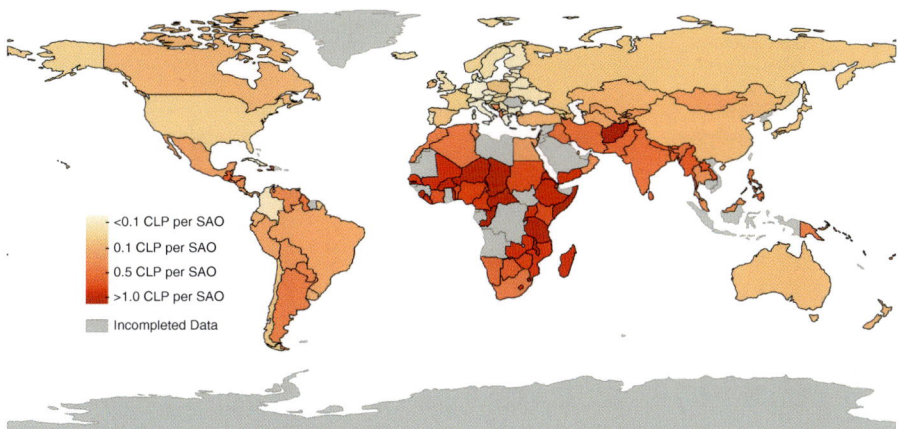

Fig. 3.1 The estimated incidence of cleft lip and/or palate (CLP) per surgeon, anesthesiologist, and obstetrician (SAO) in each country. Darker red represents an increased ratio of newborns with cleft lip and/or palate to members of the surgical workforce. *This map captures only the incidence of CLP and the surgical workforce density at one moment in time. Additionally, SAO density does not truly represent the CLP workforce but is used as a proxy for CLP workforce density. This is a static representation of a dynamic relationship. As surgical systems and our ability to treat and prevent CLP develop, this figure is likely to continue to evolve*

settings (Poenaru 2013). Repair of a cleft lip has substantial benefits at any age, as it removes the social stigma associated with having a visible facial deformity (Petrackova et al. 2015). However, it has been suggested that late cleft palate repair may not improve speech outcomes and may, in fact, worsen speech predictability and nasal regurgitation (Schonmeyr et al. 2015).

Delays in surgical care are not limited to cleft patients alone. In 2015, Alkire et al. found that less than 1% of individuals in low-income countries and less than 5% of those in lower middle-income countries have access to surgical care. In total, five billion people, the majority of the world's population, lack access to safe and affordable surgical care (Alkire et al. 2015a). This inequity is further compounded by the disparate allocation of resources, resulting in a concentration of surgical efforts in urban areas despite significant rural populations worldwide (Meara et al. 2015). Subsequently, the burden of untreated surgical disease continues to grow and, without increasing surgical capacity, is met only with a growing inability to address elective, nonurgent cases, such as cleft lip and palate repair. Providers from nongovernmental organizations (NGOs) and surgically focused mission trips attempt to alleviate this burden by providing scheduled repairs of elective cases, but the number of patients with untreated clefts remains alarmingly high. Thus, efforts to identify and surgically repair cleft lip and palate at an early, appropriate age are warranted, but will require significant investments in surgical system strengthening to take effect.

A growing body of literature proves this to be a wise investment. Quality surgical care, while complex, can yield significant gains for populations and their economies. Estimated economic losses of not investing in surgical care will total to

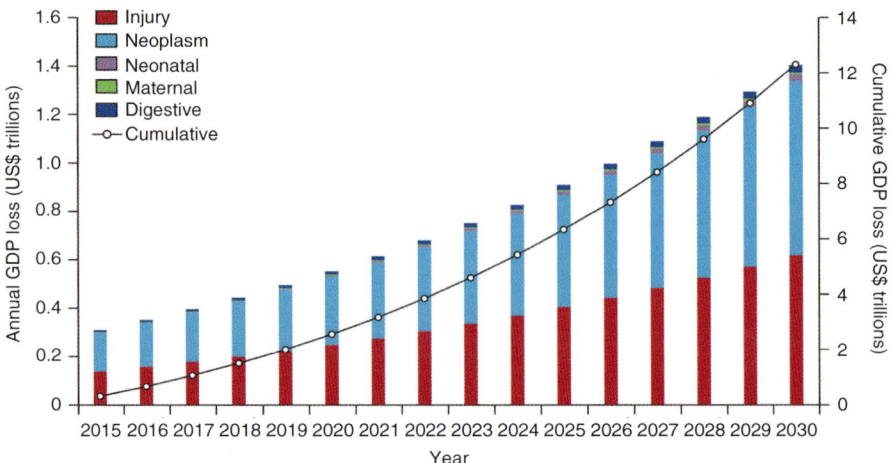

Fig. 3.2 Annual and cumulative GDP lost in low-income and middle-income countries from surgical conditions (image used under the creative commons agreement from The Lancet Commission on Global Surgery (Meara et al. 2015))

US$12.3 trillion in LMICs between 2015 and 2030 (Fig. 3.2) (Alkire et al. 2015b). In 2010, an estimated 16.9 million deaths were due to causes requiring surgical intervention, a number far exceeding the number of deaths from HIV, tuberculosis, and malaria combined (Shrime et al. 2015). Providing surgical care saves lives, often amongst the most economically productive members of society (Meara et al. 2015). For example, using the value of statistical life approach, the lifetime economic benefit for cleft lip repair has been reported to be between $52,000 and $141,000 per patient, with the benefit for cleft palate repair between $145,000 and $390,000 per patient (Hughes et al. 2012). Additionally, cleft repairs have been reported to be more cost effective than the treatment for certain chronic diseases like heart disease and HIV as well as some vaccinations like BCG (Chao et al. 2014). Scaling up surgical services equips healthcare systems with the resources to manage more complex and high-acuity disease processes that otherwise would not be available at health centers without surgical care (Editors 2008; Farmer and Kim 2008). Therein, global investment in surgical care, including the repair of cleft lip and palate, is both prudent and essential.

Addressing the gaps in global cleft care will require a multifaceted approach. Establishing platforms that can sustain surgical care requires, at a minimum, a trained, multidisciplinary team with ongoing platforms for continuing medical education and the training of new providers, a strong supply chain to provide essential equipment and medicines, a safe space within which to provide care, and financial risk protection for patients and families seeking care (Meara et al. 2015; Storeng et al. 2008). To coordinate such large-scale infrastructure improvements, groups such as the Lancet Commission on Global Surgery have recommended that both frontline providers and national stakeholders develop country-specific National

Surgical Plans (Table 3.1). Such a framework yields an infrastructure not only for development of surgical systems but also for measurement of such growth over time. In this way, stakeholders can continue to be informed on where gaps in progress remain and where potential weaknesses in comprehensive surgical systems might exist.

Table 3.1 National surgical plan components and framework

	Recommendations	Assessment methods
Infrastructure		
Surgical facilities; facility readiness; blood supply; access and referral systems	• Track number and distribution of surgical facilities • Negotiate centralized framework purchase agreements with decentralized ordering • Equip first-level surgical facilities to be able to do laparotomy, caesarean delivery, and treatment of open fracture (the Bellwether procedures) • Develop national blood plan • Reduce barriers to access through enhanced connectivity across entire care delivery chain from community to tertiary care • Establish referral systems with community integration, transfer criteria, referral logistics, and protection for first responders and helpful members of the public	• Proportion of population with 2-h access to first-level facility • WHO Hospital Assessment Tool (e.g., assessment of structure, electricity, water, oxygen, surgical equipment and supplies, computers, and Internet) • Proportion of hospitals fulfilling safe surgery criteria • Blood bank distribution, donation rate
Workforce		
Surgical, anesthetic, and obstetric providers; allied health providers (nursing, operational managers, biomedical engineers, and radiology, pathology, and laboratory technician officers)	• Establish training and education strategy based on population and needs of country • Require rural component of surgical and anesthetic training programs • Develop a context-appropriate licensing and credentialing requirement for all surgical workforce • Training and education strategy of ancillary staff based on population and needs of country • Invest in professional healthcare manager training • Establish biomedical equipment training program	• Density and distribution of specialist surgical, anesthetic, and obstetric providers • Number of surgical, anesthetic, and obstetric graduates and retirees • Proportion of surgical workforce training programs accredited • Presence of task-sharing or nursing-accredited programs and number of providers • Presence of attraction and retention strategies • Density and distribution of nurses, and ancillary staff including operational managers, biomedical engineers, and radiology, pathology, and laboratory technicians

(continued)

Table 3.1 (continued)

	Recommendations	Assessment methods
Service delivery		
Surgical volume; system coordination; quality and safety	• All first-level hospitals should provide laparotomy, caesarean delivery, and open fracture treatment (Bellwether procedures) • Integrate public and private NGO providers into common national delivery framework; promote demand-driven partnerships with NGOs to build surgical capacity • Prioritize healthcare management training • Prioritize quality improvement processes and outcomes monitoring • Promote telemedicine to build system-wide connectivity • Promote system-wide connectivity for telemedicine applications, clinical support, and education	• Proportion of surgical facilities offering the Bellwether procedures • Number of surgical procedures done per year • Surgical and anesthetic related morbidity and mortality (perioperative) • Availability of system-wide communication
Financing		
Health financing and accounting; budget allocation	• Cover basic surgical packages within universal health coverage • Risk pool with a single pool; minimize user fees at the point of care • Track financial flows for surgery through national health accounts • Use value-based purchasing with risk-pooled funds	• Surgical expenditure as a proportion of gross domestic product • Surgical expenditure as a proportion of total national healthcare budget • Out-of-pocket expenditures on surgery • Catastrophic and impoverishing expenditures on surgery
Information management		
Information systems; research agenda	• Develop robust information systems to monitor clinical processes, cost, outcomes, and identify deficits • Identify, regulate, and fund surgical research priorities of local relevance	• Presence of data systems that promote monitoring and accountability related to surgical and anesthesia care • Proportion of hospital facilities with high-speed Internet connections

Table adapted with permission from the Lancet Commission on Global Surgery (Meara et al. 2015)

Looking forward, scaling up access to and improving cleft lip and palate care will require an honest appraisal of motivations. What are the long-term goals for addressing the disease burden, and who is responsible for driving this change? Increasing local capacity to identify and treat patients with cleft lip and palate will require an increase in educators and sincere investments in both human and physical capital. Many believe that change should come from the local level, but knowing the constraints that face many LMIC providers, many also believe that appropriate collaborations may be beneficial. Collaborations may be at the local-regional level as well as at the international level between high-resource partners and other academic institutions (Ng-Kamstra et al. 2015). To yield the most impactful results, collaborations should embrace the complexity of care for the child with cleft lip and palate. This should include dentistry, orthodontics, oral surgery, otolaryngology, speech pathology, audiology, nursing, and social work providers. In developing partnerships, participants in global cleft care should define and measure endpoints to encourage local partners to reach independence in these areas. The sustainability of these efforts will be negated if the local "brain drain" that results from inadequate resources, lack of continuing education, and abundant professional isolation that often afflicts the limited resource provider is not addressed (Meara et al. 2015; Hagander et al. 2013). Therefore, equal attention must be paid to the development of safe and sustainable work environments such that returns on investments continue to grow.

Operation Smile's Comprehensive Cleft Care Center in Guwahati, India, represents a collaborative example for addressing the complexities and spectrum of cleft care in the developing world. In 2009, with a backlog of over 30,000 cleft lip and palate surgical patients and a substantial lack of trained healthcare personnel to care for them, Operation Smile, the Government of Assam, the National Rural Health Mission, and the TATA Corporation formed a collaborative effort to address cleft care in the region. Their goals were to increase capacity, decrease costs, and create a cleft-free Assam state (Campbell et al. 2014a). Uniting under their shared objectives, the group created a unique public-private partnership that was able to leverage the strengths of each individual stakeholder to optimize care delivery and training, organizational management, financial efficiency, and ultimately quality of care (Campbell et al. 2014a). Operation Smile provided the initial leadership, healthcare personnel, and supplies to support the evolution of locally based medical staff. The National Rural Health Mission provided budgetary funding to reimburse the center on a fee-for-service basis so that patients were not financially responsible and productivity was incentivized. The local Assam Government provided the physical infrastructure, and the TATA Corporation provided additional charitable contributions with mechanisms for evaluation and auditing. Five years into the partnership, the center has stabilized its clinical output at 250–300 cases per month, it has demonstrated financial self-sufficiency with local governmental and business support, it has a medical staff that is greater than 90% locally based, and it fosters a multidisciplinary system that addresses the spectrum of cleft care both within the center and within the greater community (Campbell et al. 2014b). Although unique to its particular region of the world, the Comprehensive Cleft Care Center model provides a useful example of the potentials in addressing large-scale cleft care worldwide.

Irrespective of the source of financial or structural support, local providers and patients need to be the voices of change based on priorities identified at the local level. Change may come from myriad sources, and measuring the results of any intervention or collaboration will be essential to continued progress. Proposals for progress must incorporate a pathway to provide low-cost, high-quality care—as providing high-quality surgical care that few can afford will serve only to broaden the access gap. This is an achievable goal. The initial investment is significant but the costs of inaction are far more grave. As the global surgery community stands at the forefront of change, it will be imperative to include comprehensive, affordable, quality surgical and anesthesia care with measurable outcomes in our efforts to address both emergent and elective surgical cases. The misconceptions that once left surgical care a neglected area of development have been razed, and future progress waits only for thoughtful and measurable change that is well within our reach.

References

Alkire BC, Raykar NP, Shrime MG, Weiser TG, Bickler SW, Rose JA, et al. Global access to surgical care: a modelling study. Lancet Glob Health. 2015a;3(6):e316–23.

Alkire BC, Shrime MG, Dare AJ, Vincent JR, Meara JG. Global economic consequences of selected surgical diseases: a modelling study. Lancet Glob Health. 2015b;3(Suppl 2):S21–7.

Barsky AJ. Establishing a plastic surgical unit in South Vietnam. Plast Reconstr Surg. 1970;45(5):431–4.

Barsky AJ. A personal memoir: plastic surgery in the twentieth century. Surg Clin N Am. 1978;58(5):1019–29.

Bickler SW, Spiegel D. Improving surgical care in low- and middle-income countries: a pivotal role for the World Health Organization. World J Surg. 2010;34(3):386–90.

Bingham HG. An African experience with the flying doctor of AMREF. African Medical Research and Educational Foundation. Plast Reconstr Surg. 1991;88(2):357–62.

Campbell A, Restrepo C, Mackay D, Sherman R, Varma A, Ayala R, et al. Scalable, sustainable cost-effective surgical care: a model for safety and quality in the developing world, part I: challenge and commitment. J Craniofac Surg. 2014a;25(5):1674–9.

Campbell A, Restrepo C, Mackay D, Sherman R, Varma A, Ayala R, et al. Scalable, sustainable cost-effective surgical care: a model for safety and quality in the developing world, part III: impact and sustainability. J Craniofac Surg. 2014b;25(5):1685–9.

Chao TE, Riesel JN, Anderson GA, Mullen JT, Doyle J, Briggs SM, et al. Building a global surgery initiative through evaluation, collaboration, and training: the Massachusetts General Hospital experience. J Surg Educ. 2015;72(4):e21–8.

Chao TE, Sharma K, Mandigo M, Hagander L, Resch SC, Weiser TG, et al. Cost-effectiveness of surgery and its policy implications for global health: a systematic review and analysis. Lancet Glob Health. 2014;2(6):e334–45.

Dare AJ, Grimes CE, Gillies R, Greenberg SL, Hagander L, Meara JG, et al. Global surgery: defining an emerging global health field. Lancet. 2014;384(9961):2245–7.

Derijcke A, Eerens A, Carels C. The incidence of oral clefts: a review. Br J Oral Maxillofac Surg. 1996;34(6):488–94.

Diana Farmer NS, Katrine Lofberg, Peter Donkor, Doruk Ozgediz. Surgical interventions for congenital anomalies: The World Bank. Essential Surgery. 2015. http://dcp-3.org/chapter/1769/surgical-interventions-congenital-anomalies.

Editors PLM. A crucial role for surgery in reaching the UN millennium development goals. PLoS Med. 2008;5(8):e182.

Farmer PE, Kim JY. Surgery and global health: a view from beyond the OR. World J Surg. 2008;32(4):533–6.

Hagander LE, Hughes CD, Nash K, Ganjawalla K, Linden A, Martins Y, et al. Surgeon migration between developing countries and the United States: train, retain, and gain from brain drain. World J Surg. 2013;37(1):14–23.

Hughes CD, Babigian A, McCormack S, Alkire BC, Wong A, Pap SA, et al. The clinical and economic impact of a sustained program in global plastic surgery: valuing cleft care in resource-poor settings. Plast Reconstr Surg. 2012;130(1):87e–94e.

Hughes CD, Barsky E, Hagander L, Barsky AJ 3rd, Meara JG. Better to light a candle: Arthur Barsky and global plastic surgery. Ann Plast Surg. 2013;71(2):131–4.

Hyland WT. Plastic surgery in Tunisia--an experience with CARE/MEDICO. Ann Plast Surg. 1981;6(2):163–7.

Jamison DT, Breman JG, Measham AR, Alleyne G, Claeson M, Evans DB, et al. Disease control priorities in developing countries. 2nd ed. New York: Oxford University Press; 2006.

Jamison DT, Nugent R, Gelband H, Horton S, Jha P, Laxminarayan R. Disease control priorities: essential surgery. 3rd ed, Vol 1. 2015.

Kim J. Importance of global surgery. 2014. https://www.youtube.com/watch?v=A9v49JpmIK8. Accessed 5 Jan 2016.

Leow JJ, Kingham TP, Casey KM, Kushner AL. Global surgery: thoughts on an emerging surgical subspecialty for students and residents. J Surg Educ. 2010;67(3):143–8.

Luboga S, Macfarlane SB, von Schreeb J, Kruk ME, Cherian MN, Bergstrom S, et al. Increasing access to surgical services in sub-saharan Africa: priorities for national and international agencies recommended by the Bellagio Essential Surgery Group. PLoS Med. 2009;6(12):e1000200.

Maliniac JW. Unsolved problems of the Foundation of the American Society of Plastic and Reconstructive Surgery viewed from the Latin American scene. Plast Reconstr Surg Transplant Bull. 1958;22(1):56–61.

McQueen KA, Ozgediz D, Riviello R, Hsia RY, Jayaraman S, Sullivan SR, et al. Essential surgery: integral to the right to health. Health Hum Rights. 2010;12(1):137–52.

Meara JG, Leather AJ, Hagander L, Alkire BC, Alonso N, Ameh EA, et al. Global Surgery 2030: evidence and solutions for achieving health, welfare, and economic development. Lancet. 2015;386(9993):569–624.

Mock C, Cherian M, Juillard C, Donkor P, Bickler S, Jamison D, et al. Developing priorities for addressing surgical conditions globally: furthering the link between surgery and public health policy. World J Surg. 2010;34(3):381–5.

Ng-Kamstra J, SLM G, Abdullah F, Amado V, Anderson GA, Cossa M, et al. Global Surgery 2030: a roadmap for high income country actors. BMJ Global Health. 2015;1(1):e000011.

Petrackova I, Zach J, Borsky J, Cerny M, Hacklova R, Tvrdek M, et al. Early and late operation of cleft lip and intelligence quotient and psychosocial development in 3-7 years. Early Hum Dev. 2015;91(2):149–52.

Poenaru D. Getting the job done: analysis of the impact and effectiveness of the SmileTrain program in alleviating the global burden of cleft disease. World J Surg. 2013;37(7):1562–70.

Price R, Makasa E, Hollands M. World health assembly resolution WHA68.15: "Strengthening emergency and essential surgical care and anesthesia as a component of universal health coverage"-addressing the public health gaps arising from lack of safe, affordable and accessible surgical and anesthetic services. World J Surg. 2015;39(9):2115–25.

Rees TD, Raassen T, Wachira J, Mustafa O, Adams-Ray B. The flying doctors of east Africa. Bull Am Coll Surg. 1994;79(10):12–20.

Schonmeyr B, Wendby L, Sharma M, Jacobson L, Restrepo C, Campbell A. Speech and speech-related quality of life after late palate repair: a patient's perspective. J Craniofac Surg. 2015;26(5):1513–6.

Shrime MG, Bickler SW, Alkire BC, Mock C. Global burden of surgical disease: an estimation from the provider perspective. Lancet Glob Health. 2015;3(Suppl 2):S8–9.

Stark RB. Early overseas programs of the Educational Foundation. Ann Plast Surg. 1981;6(1):76–82.

Storeng KT, Baggaley RF, Ganaba R, Ouattara F, Akoum MS, Filippi V. Paying the price: the cost and consequences of emergency obstetric care in Burkina Faso. Soc Sci Med. 2008;66(3):545–57.

TIME Magazine. Medicine: what few have done; 1961.

USA A. Our history. 2010. www.amrefusa.org

WHO. Congenital anomalies geneva. 2012. http://www.who.int/mediacentre/factsheets/fs370/en/.

World Health Organization. Global strategies to reduce the health-care burden of craniofacial anomalies. Geneva; 2000.

Genetics of Cleft Lip and Cleft Palate: Perspectives in Surgery Management and Outcome

4

Gerson Shigeru Kobayashi, Luciano Abreu Brito, Joanna Goes Castro Meira, Lucas Alvizi, and Maria Rita Passos-Bueno

Clefts of the lip (with or without palate) and of the palate (CLP) comprise a complex, clinically, and etiologically heterogeneous group of craniofacial malformations that affect around 1:700 live births (Dixon et al. 2011). Expressivity varies from mild defects, such as discreet *orbicularis oris* muscle discontinuity and submucous cleft palate, to more severe phenotypes in which several orofacial tissues are affected. Patients afflicted by CLP often require extensive treatment for their functional rehabilitation and social integration, as they are subject to several surgical interventions and management by a multidisciplinary team for many years (Hamm and Robin 2015). Given the high incidence of CLP and the important psychosocial and health care burden it entails, understanding the etiology of this disorder is of utmost importance, as it may lead to the development or improvement of preventive and therapeutic strategies.

Development of the human face is reliant upon a series of spatiotemporally coordinated morphogenetic events. The critical period for lip and palate development falls within the first trimester of embryonic development, when the facial prominences that will constitute the upper lip and palate must undergo correct orientation, growth, and fusion (Chang et al. 2015). Upper lip and primary palate formation is completed by the end of the sixth gestational week, while secondary palate formation occurs between the 6th and 12th weeks. Completion of these processes is particularly sensitive to perturbations; therefore, the action of genetic or environmental insults during these periods is thought to result in CLP (Dixon et al. 2011; Jiang et al. 2006; Kerrigan et al. 2000).

Historically, CLP has been divided into two major groups: cleft lip with or without cleft palate (CL/P) and cleft palate only (CP) (Dixon et al. 2011). In CL/P, clefts involving the upper lip/primary palate may be associated or not with clefts of the

G.S. Kobayashi, Ph.D. • L.A. Brito, Ph.D. • J.G.C. Meira, Ph.D.
L. Alvizi, Ph.D. • M.R. Passos-Bueno, Ph.D. (✉)
Centro de Pesquisas sobre o Genoma Humano e Células-Tronco, Instituto de Biociências, Universidade de São Paulo, São Paulo, Brazil
e-mail: passos@ib.usp.br

© Springer International Publishing AG 2018
N. Alonso, C.E. Raposo-Amaral (eds.), *Cleft Lip and Palate Treatment*, https://doi.org/10.1007/978-3-319-63290-2_4

secondary palate, while CP is restricted to clefts that only affect the secondary palate. This classification is rooted in epidemiological and embryological data, as CL/P and CP seldom co-segregate within families, and during orofacial morphogenesis CL/P and CP can be caused by insults to different developmental stages (Gorlin et al. 2001). Still, this distinction between CL/P and CP is not absolute, and notable exceptions include families with affected subjects harboring loss-of-function mutations in *MSX1* (CLP and tooth agenesis) and in *IRF6* (van der Woude syndrome; VWS) (Brito et al. 2012a; van den Boogaard et al. 2000).

Appropriate classification of CLP is important to direct surgical procedures, genetic counselling, and inclusion of subjects in research protocols. These different areas require specific information regarding patients, which has led to the creation of distinct classification criteria. While anatomy-based criteria are mostly used by surgeons and dentists, professionals responsible for genetic counselling and evaluation of prognosis and genetic recurrence risks (RR) employ classifications based on the primary cause of the clefts. In this context, CL/P and CP are primarily divided into **syndromic** and **nonsyndromic** forms, and the identification of the etiological factors responsible for these forms of CLP is expected to bring about a more universal classification.

4.1 Syndromic CLP

Syndromic forms of CLP are those occurring in association with other clinical manifestations. These include additional congenital defects such as cardiac malformations or dysmorphic features, which may be accompanied or not by intellectual disability. About 30% of CL/P and about 50% of CP cases are syndromic, with a joint incidence of 1.4:1000 livebirths.

Syndromic CLP can be caused by teratogenic agents, chromosomal alterations, or genetic mutations (Mossey et al. 2009). Many teratogenic agents have been associated with CLP, and they include maternal alcohol intake and use of anticonvulsants during pregnancy (Smith et al. 2014; Tomson and Battino 2012). Chromosomal causes of CLP include trisomies 13, 18, and 21, in addition to deletions or duplications in several genomic *loci* (Berge et al. 2001; Schutte and Murray 1999; Snijders et al. 1995). Further, CLP has been described in over 500 genetic syndromes with Mendelian inheritance (Dixon et al. 2011). Precise diagnosis and identification of the primary cause for the CLP are important for establishing prognosis and estimating RR of the malformation within families; as such, detailed clinical evaluation, including the search of abnormalities in internal organs, is necessary.

The most prevalent syndromic forms of CLP are van der Woude syndrome (VWS), with an incidence of 1:35,000 livebirths (Schutte et al. 1996), and DiGeorge or velocardiofacial syndrome (VCFS), with an incidence of 1:4000 livebirths (Devriendt et al. 1998). As summarized in Table 4.1, both syndromes segregate in an autosomal dominant fashion, implying a RR of about 50% for carriers of the pathogenic variant. Their molecular etiologies are well characterized, and a proportion of cases, particularly of VCFS, are a result of de novo mutations. VWS and VCFS display high clinical

Table 4.1 Clinical features of van der Woude and DiGeorge/velocardiofacial syndromes, the two most common syndromic forms of typical CLP

Syndrome	Cause	Major clinical features	Mode of inheritance and recurrence risk	Genetic test
van der Woude	Mutation in the *IRF6* gene at 1q32 (70% of the cases)	CL/P or CP		
		Lower lip pits	Autosomal dominant, ~50%	Gene sequencing
	Mutation in the *GRHL3* gene on chromosome 1p36 (5% of the cases)	Hypodontia		
DiGeorge/velocardiofacial		CP or submucous cleft		
		Velopharyngeal insufficiency		
		Typical facies		MLPA
	1.5- to 3.0-Mb hemizygous deletion of chromosome 22q11.2	Mental retardation	Autosomal dominant, ~50%	FISH
		Thymic hypoplasia		Array-CGH
		Neonatal hypocalcemia		

variability and high penetrance, besides genetic heterogeneity. Further, phenotype severity is not always correlated with the location of the variant in VWS or with the size of the deletion in VCFS. So, anticipating clinical severity in young patients is not possible solely based on information regarding the pathogenic variant.

It is very important to stress that subjects affected by VWS and VCFS may be prone to surgical complications and worsened postsurgical outcomes. VCFS patients, for example, may show anomalous position of the internal carotid arteries, a decisive factor for selection of surgical procedures to be employed on these patients (Saman and Tatum 2012). Additionally, VWS patients have an increased likelihood of healing complications after cleft repair, in comparison to children with nonsyndromic CLP (Jones et al. 2010).

Differential clinical diagnosis between VWS and nonsyndromic CLP is based on the presence of lower lip pits in at least one relative. If a lip pit is not identified, the only way to distinguish between VWS and nonsyndromic CLP is through genetic tests. The recommendation of genetic tests in these situations should be discussed (Table 4.1), particularly for familial cases co-segregating CL/P and CP, which is more common among VWS cases (Jehee et al. 2009; van den Boogaard et al. 2000). Among isolated VWS cases, genetic test is usually recommended in young non-affected parents, as the syndrome shows incomplete penetrance and most of the cases (about 80%) are inherited (Shprintzen et al. 1980).

Establishing diagnosis of VCFS only based on clinical evaluation is often difficult, particularly in neonates, and a genetic confirmation test is usually recommended. Genetic testing of unaffected parents should be discussed for family planning purposes, as 8–28% of the affected individuals inherit the pathogenic mutation (Driscoll 2001). Several genetic tests are available for VCFS (Table 4.1) and the choice is mostly based on financial grounds.

In addition to VWS and VCFS, Robin sequence (RS) represents a frequent form of CP in craniofacial rehabilitation clinics. RS is characterized by micro- or retrognathia, and glossoptosis, with or without CP. RS is also associated with high morbidity due to upper respiratory tract problems, which cause, in addition to severe respiratory distress, feeding and speech difficulties. RS is usually sporadic, with a very low RR for a second affected child in non-affected parents. However, RS can occur in association with many very-well-characterized genetic syndromes, such as Stickler and Treacher Collins syndromes, and in these cases the recurrence risk varies respectively to their inheritance patterns (Evans et al. 2011; Shprintzen 1992). The mutated genes and inheritance patterns of these and other less frequent clefting syndromes are summarized in Table 4.2.

4.2 Nonsyndromic CLP

In nonsyndromic CLP, the orofacial cleft is the only malformation in the individual, with no other congenital defect and with normal cognitive development. Most of the nonsyndromic CLP cases are believed to follow a multifactorial pattern of inheritance in which the phenotype results from a combination of genetic and environmental factors. Given the different etiological aspects of CL/P and CP, these will be discussed separately.

4.3 Nonsyndromic CL/P (NS CL/P)

About 70% of the CL/P cases are nonsyndromic, corresponding to an average incidence of 0.7:1000 births. Ethnic background, geographic location, and socioeconomic status are factors that contribute to variations in incidence (Mossey et al. 2009).

Maternal smoking, alcohol, retinol, and anticonvulsant usage during early pregnancy are some of the environmental factors associated with NS CL/P. However, replication studies often produce conflicting results.

Indirect evidence suggests an important contribution of genetic factors to NS CL/P, such as phenotype concordance in twins (40–60% in monozygotic vs. 3–5% among dizygotic twins) and familial aggregation (observed in 20–30% of the cases) (Grosen et al. 2010; Jugessur et al. 2009; Murray 2002). In addition, heritability estimates have indicated that, depending on the population, up to 85% of the phenotypic variability observed in NS CL/P is due to genetic variation among individuals (Brito et al. 2011).

4 Genetics of Cleft Lip and Cleft Palate

Table 4.2 Main syndromes associated with typical CLP and causative genes

Syndrome	OMIM[a] number	Gene	Mode of Inheritance
AEC (ankyloblepharon-ectodermal defects-cleft lip/palate)	106260	TP73L	Autosomal dominant
Apert	101200	FGFR2	Autosomal dominant
Branchiooculofacial	113620	TFAP2A	Autosomal dominant
Charge	214800	CHD7	Autosomal dominant
Cornelia de Lange	122470	NIPBL	Autosomal dominant
Crouzon	123500	FGFR2	Autosomal dominant
Desmosterolosis	602398	DHCR24	Autosomal recessive
Campomelic dysplasia	114290	SOX9	Autosomal dominant
Craniofrontonasal dysplasia	304110	EFNB1	X-linked dominant
Diastrophic dysplasia	222600	SLC26A2	Autosomal recessive
EEC (ectrodactyly, ectodermal dysplasia, and cleft lip/palate syndrome)	129900	TP73L	Autosomal dominant
Gorlin	109400	PTCH1	Autosomal dominant
Hydrolethalus	236680	HYLS1	Autosomal recessive
Holoprosencephaly[b]	609637	ZIC2	Autosomal dominant
Cleft lip/palate-ectodermal dysplasia	225060	PVRL1	Autosomal recessive
Cleft palate with or without ankyloglossia, X-linked	303400	TBX22	X-linked recessive
Kabuki	147920	MLL2	Autosomal dominant
Kallmann 2	147950	FGFR1	Autosomal dominant
Larsen; atelosteogenesis	150250	FLNB	Autosomal dominant
Lymphedema-distichiasis	153400	FOXC2	Autosomal dominant
Loeys-Dietz 1	609192	TGFBR1	Autosomal dominant
Loeys-Dietz 4	614816	TGFB2	Autosomal dominant
Miller (postaxial acrofacial dysostosis)	263750	DHODH	Autosomal recessive
Oculofaciocardiodental	300166	BCOR	X-linked dominant

(continued)

Table 4.2 (continued)

Syndrome	OMIM[a] number	Gene	Mode of Inheritance
Otopalatodigital, type I and II	311300 and 304120	*FLNA*	X-linked dominant
Roberts	268300	*ESCO2*	Autosomal recessive
Saethre-Chotzen	101400	*TWIST1*	Autosomal dominant
Stickler 1	108300	*COL2A1*	Autosomal dominant
Stickler 2	604841	*COL11A1*	Autosomal dominant
Stickler 3	184840	*COL11A2*	Autosomal dominant
Smith-Lemli-Opitz	270400	*DHCR7*	Autosomal recessive
Tetraamelia	273395	*WNT3*	Autosomal recessive
Treacher Collins	154500	*TCOF1*	Autosomal dominant

Genetic heterogeneity is a common feature in these syndromes, and genes accounting for the majority of the cases are depicted
[a]OMIM: "Online Mendelian Inheritance in Man"
[b]In this item, only nonsyndromic and Mendelian forms of holoprosencephaly were considered. Mutations in *ZIC2* are more prevalent in nonfamilial forms (70% of cases), which occur de novo. However, in cases with familial history, mutations are more prevalent in *SHH*, *SIX3*, and *TGIF* genes (Mercier et al. 2011)

A variety of approaches have been used to investigate the genetic etiology of NS CL/P. Gene mapping strategies such as linkage and association analyses have historically been the most popular approaches. Linkage analysis relies on the co-segregation between genetic markers and disease in families. Association analysis, on the other hand, relies on the differential distribution of a genetic marker between groups of affected and unaffected individuals. Association analysis was initially restricted to candidate genes, requiring previous knowledge about the genes before including them in the studies (Altshuler et al. 2008). Although many susceptibility loci have been suggested by linkage and candidate gene association analyses, the vast majority were nonreplicable across studies (Dixon et al. 2011; Leslie and Marazita 2013). A single remarkable exception was *IRF6* (1q32), in which heterozygous loss-of-function mutations lead to VWS (OMIM#119300). Common variants in *IRF6* were firstly associated with NS CL/P (Zucchero et al. 2004) and consistently replicated thenceforth (Jugessur et al. 2008; Rahimov et al. 2008). Recently, methodological improvements allowed association analysis to be performed in a genome-wide scale (genome-wide association studies, GWAS), independent of a priori knowledge on gene function. With GWAS, new susceptibility loci have been identified, with consistent replication across populations (e.g., 1p22.1, 1p36, 2p21, 3p11.1, 8q21.3, 8q24, 10q25, 13q31.1, 15q22.2, 16p13, 17p13, 17q22, and 20q12). Among these new loci, the 8q24 region represents the strongest association in a variety of populations of European ancestry (Brito et al. 2012c; Ludwig et al. 2012).

With the advent of next-generation sequencing techniques, exome or whole-genome sequencing has become accessible tools to detect gene variants in individuals affected by NS CL/P. Using this strategy, rare, high-effect mutations in new genes have broadened the spectrum of genes etiologically relevant to NS CL/P. Among these genes, *CDH1*, at 16q22.1 (Brito et al. 2015; Bureau et al. 2014), and *DLX4*, at 17q21.33 (Wu et al. 2015), are prime examples.

Despite these advances, the risk factors currently implicated with NS CL/P do not explain most of genetic contribution attributed to the disease, and the biological mechanisms by which these genetic factors confer susceptibility to NS CL/P are still unclear. To address these questions, functional approaches have shed some light into the etiological mechanisms determining susceptibility to NS CL/P. As an example, transcriptome profiling of cell cultures from NS CL/P individuals has shown that NS CL/P possesses expression signatures characterized by dysregulation of genes involved in extracellular matrix metabolism and DNA damage repair pathways (Baroni et al. 2010; Bueno et al. 2011; Kobayashi et al. 2013).

The RR for NS CL/P is estimated empirically, based on epidemiological data. Reports have shown that RR increases according to the number of affected individuals in the family. In this regard, in families with only one individual with NS CL/P, the RR for a second case in this family can reach 4%. This value rises to 10% if two affected individuals exist in the family. Therefore, in familial cases, it is important to clinically evaluate as many patients as possible in order to establish precise RR estimates and exclude possible monogenic forms of CL/P, such as VWS. In addition, it is also important to discuss the need and relevance of genetic tests with families (Brito et al. 2012b).

4.4 Nonsyndromic Cleft Palate (NS CP)

Worldwide incidence of NS CP has been estimated as 1:4700 livebirths, with no remarkable variation among ethnicities (Tolarova and Cervenka 1998). Maternal smoking and alcohol intake during pregnancy have also been reported as risk factors for NS CP (Cobourne 2004). In contrast to NS CL/P, the genetic risk factors for NS CP remain mostly unexplored, possibly because of its lower prevalence and difficulties in neonatal diagnostics. Several at-risk *loci* have been suggested for NS CP, such as *MSX1*, *TGFA*, *TGFB3*, and *FAF1*, among others (Dixon et al. 2011); however, most of the results are controversial and lack replication.

RR estimates, as for NS CL/P, are also based on empirical data. For families with only one affected child, the RR is lower than in NS CL/P, being estimated as 2%. If one of the progenitors also has CP, the risk increases to 6%, and if the progenitor and another child are both affected by CP, RR increases to 15% (Curtis et al. 1961). In familial cases, detailed clinical examination is recommended to exclude the possibility of syndromic forms, such as VCFS and VWS.

4.5 Genetic Counselling and Final Considerations

Families with CLP children should attend a genetic counselling service preferentially in the children's first semester of life for diagnosis confirmation, discussing the applicability of genetic tests, and for CLP RR estimates. During genetic counselling, CLP cases are initially classified as syndromic or nonsyndromic, and as familial or nonfamilial, based on the presence of other relatives with CLP. It is also important to investigate if the pregnancy was potentially exposed to teratogenic factors, which could indicate an environmental cause for the CLP. Geneticists should always evaluate the need for genetic testing, such as chromosomal analysis (array-CGH, MLPA), disease-specific genetic tests (for typical syndromes, such as VWS), and, in very rare situations, exome analysis (e.g., suspicion of a monogenic form, but with uncertain diagnosis) (Table 4.1).

Identification of the primary cause of syndromic CLP cases allows for more precise RR estimates for the future offspring of the parents with a CLP child as well as for other family members. If enough evidence supports a teratogenic cause for CLP, the RR is low, as exposure to teratogens is unlikely in future pregnancies. Among clefts caused by chromosomal abnormalities, it is important to verify if it has occurred de novo or if it is the product of a balanced chromosomal rearrangement in one of the parents. In these cases, karyotype with FISH analysis is usually the most recommended. If one of the parents has a balanced chromosomal rearrangement, the RR for future children may increase (5–10% or higher) as compared to the population risk.

For Mendelian, syndromic CLP cases, the RR is directly related to the inheritance pattern, which is frequently autosomal dominant (Table 4.2). In these cases, the RR is about 50% for the next child of the affected individual, depending on the penetrance. On the other hand, in recessive forms (autosomal or X-linked), the RR is 25%, and among the recessive X-linked forms only males will present the malformation. These situations illustrate the importance of careful diagnosis for precise RR estimates.

Among the nonsyndromic forms of CLP, the RR is estimated by empirical data which considers the number of affected individuals within the family as well. It is also known that the phenotype severity may influence the RR. Genetic tests for nonsyndromic forms are not recommended, particularly for nonfamilial cases, as the known at-risk alleles are still not good predictive factors for recurrence of the malformation.

Advances in genomic analysis are expected to greatly improve the knowledge on the genetic etiology of CLP. Techniques such as whole-exome and whole-genome sequencing can be employed to clarify the genetic etiology of NS CLP and to identify the remaining causative loci responsible for syndromic CLP forms. Furthermore, these technologies are expected to shed more light on the impact exerted by genetic variants on the rehabilitation of CLP patients. Hopefully, in the next years, we will be able to dissect the main pathways and mechanisms responsible for CLP, which in turn will open new venues for prevention and rehabilitation of this group of malformations.

Acknowledgements Authors were financed by FAPESP/CEPID.
Online resources: OMIM (Online Mendelian Inheritance in Man): http://www.omim.org/.

References

Altshuler D, Daly MJ, Lander ES. Genetic mapping in human disease. Science. 2008;322(5903):881–8.
Baroni T, Bellucci C, Lilli C, Pezzetti F, Carinci F, Lumare E, Palmieri A, Stabellini G, Bodo M. Human cleft lip and palate fibroblasts and normal nicotine-treated fibroblasts show altered in vitro expressions of genes related to molecular signaling pathways and extracellular matrix metabolism. J Cell Physiol. 2010;222(3):748–56.
Berge SJ, Plath H, Van de Vondel PT, Appel T, Niederhagen B, Von Lindern JJ, Reich RH, Hansmann M. Fetal cleft lip and palate: sonographic diagnosis, chromosomal abnormalities, associated anomalies and postnatal outcome in 70 fetuses. Ultrasound Obstet Gynecol. 2001;18(5):422–31.
Brito LA, Bassi CF, Masotti C, Malcher C, Rocha KM, Schlesinger D, Bueno DF, Cruz LA, Barbara LK, Bertola DR, et al. IRF6 is a risk factor for nonsyndromic cleft lip in the Brazilian population. Am J Med Genet A. 2012a;158A(9):2170–5.
Brito LA, Cruz LA, Rocha KM, Barbara LK, Silva CB, Bueno DF, Aguena M, Bertola DR, Franco D, Costa AM, et al. Genetic contribution for non-syndromic cleft lip with or without cleft palate (NS CL/P) in different regions of Brazil and implications for association studies. Am J Med Genet A. 2011;155A(7):1581–7.
Brito LA, Meira JG, Kobayashi GS, Passos-Bueno MR. Genetics and management of the patient with orofacial cleft. Plast Surg Int. 2012b;2012:782821.
Brito LA, Paranaiba LM, Bassi CF, Masotti C, Malcher C, Schlesinger D, Rocha KM, Cruz LA, Barbara LK, Alonso N, et al. Region 8q24 is a susceptibility locus for nonsyndromic oral clefting in Brazil. Birth Defects Res A Clin Mol Teratol. 2012c;94(6):464–8.
Brito LA, Yamamoto GL, Melo S, Malcher C, Ferreira SG, Figueiredo J, Alvizi L, Kobayashi GS, Naslavsky MS, Alonso N, et al. Rare variants in the epithelial cadherin gene underlying the genetic etiology of nonsyndromic cleft lip with or without cleft palate. Hum Mutat. 2015;36(11):1029–33.
Bueno DF, Sunaga DY, Kobayashi GS, Aguena M, Raposo-Amaral CE, Masotti C, Cruz LA, Pearson PL, Passos-Bueno MR. Human stem cell cultures from cleft lip/palate patients show enrichment of transcripts involved in extracellular matrix modeling by comparison to controls. Stem Cell Rev. 2011;7(2):446–57.
Bureau A, Parker MM, Ruczinski I, Taub MA, Marazita ML, Murray JC, Mangold E, Noethen MM, Ludwig KU, Hetmanski JB, et al. Whole exome sequencing of distant relatives in multiplex families implicates rare variants in candidate genes for oral clefts. Genetics. 2014;197(3):1039–44.
Chang C, Schock EN, Billmire DA, Brugmann SA. Craniofacial syndromes: etiology, impact and treatment. In: Moody S, editor. Principles of developmental genetics. Cambridge: Academic Press; 2015. p. 654–71.
Cobourne MT. The complex genetics of cleft lip and palate. Eur J Orthod. 2004;26(1):7–16.
Curtis EJ, Fraser FC, Warburton D. Congenital cleft lip and palate. Am J Dis Child. 1961;102:853–7.
Devriendt K, Fryns JP, Mortier G, van Thienen MN, Keymolen K. The annual incidence of DiGeorge/velocardiofacial syndrome. J Med Genet. 1998;35(9):789–90.
Dixon MJ, Marazita ML, Beaty TH, Murray JC. Cleft lip and palate: understanding genetic and environmental influences. Nat Rev Genet. 2011;12(3):167–78.
Driscoll DA. Prenatal diagnosis of the 22q11.2 deletion syndrome. Genet Med. 2001;3(1):14–8.
Evans KN, Sie KC, Hopper RA, Glass RP, Hing AV, Cunningham ML. Robin sequence: from diagnosis to development of an effective management plan. Pediatrics. 2011;127(5):936–48.
Gorlin RJ, Cohen MMH Jr, Hennekam RCM. Syndromes of the head and neck. New York: Oxford University Press; 2001.
Grosen D, Bille C, Pedersen JK, Skytthe A, Murray JC, Christensen K. Recurrence risk for offspring of twins discordant for oral cleft: a population-based cohort study of the Danish 1936-2004 cleft twin cohort. Am J Med Genet A. 2010;152A(10):2468–74.
Hamm JA, Robin NH. Newborn craniofacial malformations: orofacial clefting and craniosynostosis. Clin Perinatol. 2015;42(2):321–36. viii

Jehee FS, Burin BA, Rocha KM, Zechi-Ceide R, Bueno DF, Brito L, Souza J, Leal GF, Richieri-Costa A, Alonso N, et al. Novel mutations in IRF6 in nonsyndromic cleft lip with or without cleft palate: when should IRF6 mutational screening be done? Am J Med Genet A. 2009;149A(6):1319–22.

Jiang R, Bush JO, Lidral AC. Development of the upper lip: morphogenetic and molecular mechanisms. Dev Dyn. 2006;235(5):1152–66.

Jones JL, Canady JW, Brookes JT, Wehby GL, L'Heureux J, Schutte BC, Murray JC, Dunnwald M. Wound complications after cleft repair in children with Van der Woude syndrome. J Craniofac Surg. 2010;21(5):1350–3.

Jugessur A, Rahimov F, Lie RT, Wilcox AJ, Gjessing HK, Nilsen RM, Nguyen TT, Murray JC. Genetic variants in IRF6 and the risk of facial clefts: single-marker and haplotype-based analyses in a population-based case-control study of facial clefts in Norway. Genet Epidemiol. 2008;32(5):413–24.

Jugessur A, Shi M, Gjessing HK, Lie RT, Wilcox AJ, Weinberg CR, Christensen K, Boyles AL, Daack-Hirsch S, Trung TN, et al. Genetic determinants of facial clefting: analysis of 357 candidate genes using two national cleft studies from Scandinavia. PLoS One. 2009;4(4):e5385.

Kerrigan JJ, Mansell JP, Sengupta A, Brown N, Sandy JR. Palatogenesis and potential mechanisms for clefting. J R Coll Surg Edinb. 2000;45(6):351–8.

Kobayashi GS, Alvizi L, Sunaga DY, Francis-West P, Kuta A, Almada BV, Ferreira SG, de Andrade-Lima LC, Bueno DF, Raposo-Amaral CE, et al. Susceptibility to DNA damage as a molecular mechanism for non-syndromic cleft lip and palate. PLoS One. 2013;8(6):e65677.

Leslie EJ, Marazita ML. Genetics of cleft lip and cleft palate. Am J Med Genet C Semin Med Genet. 2013;163C(4):246–58.

Ludwig KU, Mangold E, Herms S, Nowak S, Reutter H, Paul A, Becker J, Herberz R, AlChawa T, Nasser E, et al. Genome-wide meta-analyses of nonsyndromic cleft lip with or without cleft palate identify six new risk loci. Nat Genet. 2012;44(9):968–71.

Mercier S, Dubourg C, Garcelon N, Campillo-Gimenez B, Gicquel I, Belleguic M, Ratie L, Pasquier L, Loget P, Bendavid C, et al. New findings for phenotype-genotype correlations in a large European series of holoprosencephaly cases. J Med Genet. 2011;48(11):752–60.

Mossey PA, Little J, Munger RG, Dixon MJ, Shaw WC. Cleft lip and palate. Lancet. 2009;374(9703):1773–85.

Murray JC. Gene/environment causes of cleft lip and/or palate. Clin Genet. 2002;61(4):248–56.

Rahimov F, Marazita ML, Visel A, Cooper ME, Hitchler MJ, Rubini M, Domann FE, Govil M, Christensen K, Bille C, et al. Disruption of an AP-2alpha binding site in an IRF6 enhancer is associated with cleft lip. Nat Genet. 2008;40(11):1341–7.

Saman M, Tatum SA 3rd. Recent advances in surgical pharyngeal modification procedures for the treatment of velopharyngeal insufficiency in patients with cleft palate. Arch Facial Plast Surg. 2012;14(2):85–8.

Schutte BC, Murray JC. The many faces and factors of orofacial clefts. Hum Mol Genet. 1999;8(10):1853–9.

Schutte BC, Sander A, Malik M, Murray JC. Refinement of the Van der Woude gene location and construction of a 3.5-Mb YAC contig and STS map spanning the critical region in 1q32-q41. Genomics. 1996;36(3):507–14.

Shprintzen RJ. The implications of the diagnosis of Robin sequence. Cleft Palate Craniofac J. 1992;29(3):205–9.

Shprintzen RJ, Goldberg RB, Sidoti EJ. The penetrance and variable expression of the Van der Woude syndrome: implications for genetic counseling. Cleft Palate J. 1980;17(1):52–7.

Smith SM, Garic A, Flentke GR, Berres ME. Neural crest development in fetal alcohol syndrome. Birth Defects Res C Embryo Today. 2014;102(3):210–20.

Snijders RJ, Sebire NJ, Psara N, Souka A, Nicolaides KH. Prevalence of fetal facial cleft at different stages of pregnancy. Ultrasound Obstet Gynecol. 1995;6(5):327–9.

Tolarova MM, Cervenka J. Classification and birth prevalence of orofacial clefts. Am J Med Genet. 1998;75(2):126–37.

Tomson T, Battino D. Teratogenic effects of antiepileptic drugs. Lancet Neurol. 2012;11(9):803–13.

van den Boogaard MJ, Dorland M, Beemer FA, van Amstel HK. MSX1 mutation is associated with orofacial clefting and tooth agenesis in humans. Nat Genet. 2000;24(4):342–3.

Wu D, Mandal S, Choi A, Anderson A, Prochazkova M, Perry H, Gil-Da-Silva-Lopes VL, Lao R, Wan E, Tang PL, et al. DLX4 is associated with orofacial clefting and abnormal jaw development. Hum Mol Genet. 2015;24(15):4340–52.

Zucchero TM, Cooper ME, Maher BS, Daack-Hirsch S, Nepomuceno B, Ribeiro L, Caprau D, Christensen K, Suzuki Y, Machida J, et al. Interferon regulatory factor 6 (IRF6) gene variants and the risk of isolated cleft lip or palate. N Engl J Med. 2004;351(8):769–80.

Classification of Cleft Phenotypes

5

Cassio Eduardo Raposo-Amaral, Rafael Denadai, and Nivaldo Alonso

The beginning of wisdom is to call things by their right name.
Chinese proverb reference unknown.

5.1 Classification of Cleft Phenotypes

Cleft is about to become a compulsory notification like other diseases in Brazil by a new law. Every child born with cleft must be reported and the exact number of newborn babies with cleft, per region, per year will be known soon. The number of new cases has been estimated by the government by around 5000 new cases each year and only 150 has access to comprehensive care. The cleft epidemiology through the notification report will be performed by pediatricians and social workers at primary care around public and philanthropic maternities around the country contracted by the unified health care system (*Sistema Único de Saúde* [SUS]; Ministry of Health, Brazil). Thus, having a unified cleft classification will be of paramount importance as cleft epidemiology can be known in order to create strategies of care, direct public investments by allocating human resources and building infra-structure, and generating public awareness for this health problem (Raposo-Amaral and Raposo-Amaral 2012).

To date there is no consensus regarding the ideal classification, and several ones have been proposed and adopted around the continent (Table 5.1). The criteria to determine the ideal elements that a classification should present has been described

---

C.E. Raposo-Amaral, M.D., Ph.D. (✉) • R. Denadai, M.D.
Institute of Plastic and Craniofacial Surgery, SOBRAPAR Hospital, Campinas, São Paulo, Brazil
e-mail: cassioraposo@hotmail.com

N. Alonso, M.D., Ph.D.
Divisao de Cirurgia Plastica e Queimaduras, Hospital das Clínicas da Faculdade de Medicina da Universidade de São Paulo, São Paulo, Brazil

© Springer International Publishing AG 2018
N. Alonso, C.E. Raposo-Amaral (eds.), *Cleft Lip and Palate Treatment*,
https://doi.org/10.1007/978-3-319-63290-2_5

Table 5.1 Some classification systems of cleft patients

Classification systems	Description
Davis and Ritchie	
Group 1	Clefts of the lip (without the inclusion of the maxillary alveolus), unilateral, bilateral, or median
Group 2	Clefts inclusive from the maxillary alveolus to the palate, hard and soft
Group 3	Cleft including the alveolus, unilateral, bilateral, or median being complete or incomplete
Veau	
Class I	Cleft of the soft palate
Class II	Clefts of the soft and hard palates, posterior to the incisive foramen
Class III	Complete unilateral cleft lip and cleft palate
Class IV	Complete bilateral cleft lip and cleft palate
Fogh-Andersen	
Group 1	Clefts of the primary palate, including lip, alveolus, and incisive foramen
Group 2	Unilateral and bilateral clefts of the lip (complete or incomplete) that extend into the hard palate
Group 3	Midline clefts of the secondary palate, posterior to the incisive foramen
Group 4	Median cleft lip
Kernahan and Stark	
Group 1	Cleft affecting the primary palate
Group 2	Cleft affecting the secondary palate
Group 3	Cleft affecting primary and secondary palates
ACPA	
Group 1	a. Cleft lip; b. cleft alveolus; c. cleft lip, alveolus, and primary palate
Group 2	a. Cleft of the hard palate; b. cleft of the soft palate; c. cleft of the hard and soft palates
Group 3	Clefts of the prepalate and palate
Group 4	a. Cleft of the mandibular process; b. naso-ocular clefts; c. oro-ocular clefts; d. oroaural clefts

ACPA American Cleft Palate–Craniofacial Association

based on three pillars by the Nomenclature Committee of American Association for Cleft Palate Rehabilitation (Harkins et al. 1962): concise clear definitions of terms, convenience of use, and stimulation of scholarly and clinical research. Although described in 1962, this description is still valid as it guides authors to elaborate new classifications that can persist the span of time and new features, characteristics and findings that may occur in new patients over the years. This aforementioned guide postulated that every new classification should be based on embryology concept as a landmark reference for the division among groups.

In the craniofacial care, one example of a classification that persists the span of time (maintaining updated for almost four decades) as it kept the original characteristic described by the author is the Tessier Rare Facial Cleft Classification (Tessier 1976). Interestingly, even though a cleft lip and palate may show less clinical features and are also less complex compared to the entire scope of rare facial clefts, attempts to describe a cleft lip and palate classification that fill previous weakness, aiming enhanced intelligibility and embracing different anatomic features and severity grades, are still being described.

Looking back to former classifications one can easily understand why the initial classifications did not resist the test of time. In 1922, Davis and Ritchie (1922) described a classification divided on three groups of cleft types morphologically based on the alveolus (Table 5.1). However, patients born either with cleft of the lip and posterior palate with intact cleft alveolus or bilateral with similar characteristics may fail to fit into a single group. Thus, after receiving the criticism of cleft surgeons, this classification was discontinued.

In 1931, Victor Veau (1931) published his book in French named "*Division Palatine*" and described a simple classification anatomically dividing the clefts into four types (Table 5.1). Although widely used and universally accepted at that time, this classification did overlook the cleft patients born with cleft lip alveolus as it also did not embrace in a single classification some rare forms such as cleft of the lip and soft palate. However, it was a redirection and progress of a line of thinking as he used the incisive foramen as an anatomic landmark for division of types II, III, and IV. Poul Fogh-Andersen, plastic surgeon from Copenhagen, went one step further in 1942, by using the incisive foramen as anatomic reference of a cleft type division, showing a more complete comprehensive (or an intuition) toward the marriage between anatomy and embryology, as the concept of primary and secondary palate had been completely overlooked by his predecessors. He additionally included the submucous cleft, a cleft of soft palate, and a cleft of hard palate with intact oral and nasal mucous membrane. Additional modification was done by him (Fogh-Andersen 1971) in 1971 and he added a new group to feature the median clefts (Table 5.1).

Kernahan and Stark (1958) from New York consolidated the concept of embryology and anatomy as they described and defined the primary and secondary palate. They emphasized the embryology knowledge as a requirement for a useful cleft classification. They both were credited for being the first who consolidated the embryological concepts into the description of a cleft classification, by creating the term primary and secondary palate even though it was previously intuitively used by Poul Fogh-Andersen. Cleft of primary palate was defined as a cleft of all anatomic structures anterior to the incisive foramen, whereas cleft of secondary palate was defined as cleft of hard and soft palates posterior to the incisive foramen, occurring at 7–12 weeks of gestation. This classification divided the cleft into three groups (Table 5.1).

In 1962, Vilar-Sancho (1962) classified and coded congenital cleft lip and cleft palate based on Greek nomenclature. Lip was represented by "K" (*keilos*), alveolus by "G" (*gnato*), hard palate by "U" (*urano*), and soft palate by "S" (*stafilos*). Complete cleft was represented in capitals and partial in small letters. "2" was used to represent bilateral, "d" indicated right, "l" indicated left, "I" indicated incomplete, and "o" indicated operated. Being in Greek, it could not be adapted worldwide. It also could not classify many of the cleft subtypes.

In 1962, Harkins et al. (1962) were appointed by American Cleft Palate Association (ACPA) to design a classification of cleft lip and palate. Anatomic segmentation into the prepalate and the palate permitted separation into four major categories of orofacial clefts in the ACPA classification: clefts of the prepalate (cleft of lip and embryologic primary palate); clefts of the palate (cleft of the embryologic secondary palate);

clefts of the prepalate and palate; and facial clefts other than prepalatal and palatal (Table 5.1). Each cleft could be further characterized by laterality (left, right, bilateral, or median) and severity. With regard to severity, the committee chose to use quantitative measurement of the width of the cleft and semiquantitative description of the extent of the cleft. Extent was denoted as 1/3, 2/3, or 3/3 the length or area of the involved structure. Specific criteria were attached to these descriptors for each condition on a case-by-case basis, but they may be thought of as corresponding roughly with minor form, incomplete, and complete, respectively.

In 1969, Santiago (1969) proposed a classification using four digits (0 = no cleft; 1 = midline cleft; 2 = cleft on right side; 3 = cleft on left side; 4 = bilateral cleft) to indicate the presence of cleft and its location. Each digit is followed by a letter to indicate the condition of cleft (complete, incomplete, or submucous). The first digit refers to the lip, the second to the alveolus, the third to the hard palate, and the fourth to the soft palate. The letters indicate more specifically the type of cleft: A = An incomplete midline cleft; B = An incomplete cleft of right side; C = An incomplete cleft of left side; D = Bilateral incomplete cleft; and E = Submucous cleft. When a cleft is not described as being complete or incomplete, it is always assumed as complete cleft. When clefts of lip, hard, and soft palate are described without giving any information about alveolus, it is assumed that it is completely affected by cleft. All cases will be considered midline cleft unless otherwise specified. An example was "4411" which should be interpreted as follows: the first digit indicates bilateral cleft lip, second digit represents bilateral cleft alveolus, third digit shows a midline cleft in hard palate, and last digit shows midline cleft of soft palate. Further example was "001A1" which should be interpreted as follows: The first digit indicates no cleft in lip, second digit indicates no cleft in alveolus, and third digit represents midline cleft of hard palate. The letter A shows that midline cleft is incomplete and last digit indicates a complete midline cleft of soft palate. This classification encompasses a whole range of defects and by the use of machine coding data can be retrieved and used for research purposes.

In 1972, Victor Spina (1973), a Brazilian plastic surgeon, described a terminology modification of a previous classification (namely, International Classification, 1967) by using the Latin term "foraminal" Silva Filho et al. (1992) (Table 5.2). Although it was considered a minor modification of a previous classification that has used the embryologic concept (by using the incisive foramen as an anatomic landmark), it added the rare facial cleft into the cleft lip and palate scheme. It is the most used classification in the Brazilian cleft centers, as it unifies the terms in a simply and clear manner, facilitating verbal communication and referral among centers of SUS. For example, by classifying the cleft patient as post-foraminal, two different pieces of information are communicated; this is a cleft of soft and hard palates extended up to the anterior limit of the incisive foramen and this cleft results from failure of the union of the secondary palate during embryonic period. In addition, although Spina has stated "a partial cleft of lip and of the palate not transversing the incisive foramen would be termed a pre-incisive and pos-incisive foramen cleft," this particular cleft population cannot be included in the numerical order (groups I–IV) established in this particular classification system. Since 2007, we

5 Classification of Cleft Phenotypes

Table 5.2 Spina and modified Spina's classification systems of cleft patients

Classification systems	Description
Spina	
Group I	Pre-foraminal cleft
a	Unilateral (right or left)
1	Total
2	Partial
b	Bilateral
1	Total
2	Partial
c	Median
1	Total
2	Partial
Group II	Transforaminal cleft
a	Unilateral (right or left)
b	Bilateral
Group III	Post-foraminal cleft
1	Total
2	Partial
Group IV	Rare facial cleft
Modified Spina (SOBRAPAR classification)	
Spina group I	Pre-foraminal cleft[a]
Spina group II	Transforaminal cleft[b]
Spina group III	Post-foraminal cleft[c]
Modified group I/III	Pre-foraminal[a] and post-foraminal[c] cleft without alveolar ridge involvement
Spina group IV	Rare facial cleft

[a]Unilateral (right or left), total or partial; bilateral, total or partial; or median, total, or partial
[b]Unilateral (right or left) or bilateral
[c]Total or partial

have adopted a modified Spina classification with the inclusion of group I/III as it allows the stratification of cleft patients presenting both the pre-foraminal and post-foraminal clefts, but without alveolar ridge involvement. This modified Spina classification has been termed as SOBRAPAR classification (Table). Although this is only a minor modification, we could fit a broad spectrum of cleft patients, therefore facilitating communication between the cleft centers and professionals, only with the description of the group that the patient is included.

In this context, the main criticism related to this system is the absence of assessment of cleft severity (cleft size) and the capacity for prognosis estimation. The Spina classification does not inform if the cleft is 1 mm or 1 cm wide and this specific information might be of major prognostic importance or determine the best approach to be followed. This deficiency is solved by complementing the classification with a parameter of extend, so by listening or receiving the description of a patient, the appearance of the cleft might be visualized as most accurately as possible as well as the best therapeutic options and challenges to be encountered during patient's rehabilitation. The terminology used in this system favors a quick and intuitive interpretation for healthcare professionals less familiarized with the cleft care. We believe that it will be indispensable for creating accurate epidemiology in

Brazil as a reliable tool for compulsory notification done by pediatricians around Brazilian maternities in the future.

A schematic diagram described as Y-shaped diagram was introduced by Kernahan (1971) in 1971 due to the need for optimizing registration and research of cleft types in patient's record. This diagram derived from the perception that most severe, extensive form of cleft lip and palate has the shape resembling this letter, representing the lip, palate, and maxillary alveolus. This Y-shaped system can be divided into nine areas: areas one and four—lip; areas two and five—alveolus; areas three and six—hard palate between the alveolus and the incisive foramen; areas seven and eight—hard palate; and area nine—soft palate. Therefore, this system is merely visual with no applications other than to medical records. In 1998, Smith et al. (1998) proposed a modified classification to compensate the shortcomings of Kernahan striped "Y" classification. It provided more detailed description of the cleft deformities. Cleft lip was divided into additional types denoted "a" to "d" depending on the extent of involved lip. Similarly, cleft of the secondary palate was subdivided into three segments and the submucous cleft of the palate was denoted by the letter "a." In the Smith-modified Kernahan "Y" classification, the submucous cleft palate was denoted by "a" but it did not describe the different varieties of the submucous cleft palate because it can involve the hard palate to different levels. Therefore, in 2013, Khan et al. (2013) proposed a revised Smith-modified Kernahan "Y" classification of the cleft lip and palate, incorporating different varieties of the submucous cleft, which can provide an anatomical basis for the severity of velopharyngeal insufficiency. The submucous cleft palate was denoted by number "7," which was subdivided into four segments: A—submucous cleft palate with involvement of the primary hard palate lying anterior to the incisive foramen and posterior to the alveolus; B—submucous cleft palate with involvement of the palatine process of the maxillary bone of the secondary hard palate; C—submucous cleft palate with involvement of the palatine process of the palatine bone of the secondary hard palate; and D—submucous cleft of the soft palate including occult submucous cleft palate.

Another principle was used by LAHSHAL classification proposed by Kriens in 1985 (Kriens 1989). This term is a palindrome, a projection of the first letters of the names of involved anatomic structures written in English (Lip, Alveolus, Hard palate, Soft palate). The first three letters represent the right side and the last three, the left side. Complete malformations are written in capitals and incomplete in lower case letters. Although it has been suggested that LAHSHAL classification is reliable and reproducible as it has been used by many associations and society of specialties for coding and epidemiology, it eventually became limited because of the ongoing necessity of verbally communicating the classification in different languages. The LAHSN (lip, alveolus, hard and soft palate, and nose) system proposed by Koch et al. (1995) further elaborates on the severity of all single or combined cleft malformations based on the extent of the defect in transverse, vertical, and sagittal directions.

In 1993, Schwartz et al. (1993) introduced an RPL system for numerical coding with 0–3 numbers to simplify the representation of the clefts. In 2001, Ortiz-Posadas et al. (2001) developed a mathematical expression to characterize clefts of the primary palate, including the magnitude of palatal segment separation and the added complexity of bilateral clefts, yielding a numerical score that reflects overall complexity of the cleft; clefts of the secondary palate were also considered in a separate score. In 2004, Castilla and Orioli (2004) presented ECLAMC (Latin-American Collaborative Study of Congenital Malformations) system for numeral coding. This recording system for oral clefts is based on a simple annotation scheme, or formula, including four fields, representing four clinical topographic areas: lip, alveolar, hard palate, and soft palate; two numbers are to be written into each field, representing the right and left sides; and the numbers express cleft extent in thirds: 0 no cleft, 1 and 2 incomplete cleft, and 3 complete cleft. If only one figure is written within a given field, it means a midline location. Further working definitions for cleft extent are given in a procedure manual. LIP—1: cleft does not go beyond the vermillion; 2: cleft goes beyond the vermillion; and 3: cleft penetrated the nostril. GUM—1: cleft affects less than half of the alveolar height; 2: cleft affects more than half of the alveolar height; and 3: cleft breaks the maxillary arch, which is dislocated. HARD PALATE, as well as SOFT PALATE—1, 2, 3, meaning one, two, or three thirds extension. Numbers other than 0, 1, 2, and 3 are used to specify rare situations such as discontinuous cleft lip and palate, gum notch, submucous cleft palate, healed cleft lip (frustre, or Simonart's band), and other specified anomalies (Castilla and Orioli 2004).

In 2005, Rossell-Perry (2009) from Peru presented a new cleft classification and subsequently published the classification of severity and diagram for cleft description (the clock diagram), which includes the palatal index, a method of evaluation of the cleft palate. This palatal index is adopted to classify cleft palate deformity and select a proper surgical technique based on the severity of the cleft palate and tissue deficiency. This index is the proportion between the width of the cleft (cleft severity) and the sum of the width of the two palatal segments (tissue deficiency) measured at the level of the hard and soft palate junction. The index indicates the amount of soft tissue available for palatal flaps and its relation to the width of the cleft to be repaired. Based on these measurements, the index classifies three degrees of severity for the cleft palate: mild (palatal index of 0–0.2), moderate (0.2–0.4), and severe (>0.4).

In 2007, Liu et al. (2007) from China developed a five-digit numerical recording system for the identification of cleft lip and palate according to the existing classifications, especially the Kernahan "Y" classification, the Smith-modified Kernahan "Y" classification, and the RPL system. The descriptions of the cleft components were anatomically denoted with five Arabic numerals in order of right lip (L), right alveolus and primary palate (A), secondary palate (P), left alveolus and primary palate (A), and left lip (L), otherwise known as the LAPAL system. The extent of cleft deformity is represented by the Arabic numerals 0–4 (i.e., intact through complete cleft). Associated descriptions for cleft lip, cleft alveolus and primary palate, and cleft palate were also provided. In addition, rare atypical craniofacial clefts can also be represented by the LAPAL system by using additional numerals: 5 denotes a median cleft of the upper lip; 6 and 7 denote an oblique facial cleft and transversal facial cleft, respectively; and 8 denotes a median cleft of the lower lip.

Also in 2007, Koul (2007) proposed the expression system that comprises two components, namely anatomical nomenclature (text) and symbols. It is based on the phrase "lip and palate." Uppercase letters signify normal structures and lowercase letters signify cleft. Laterality of clefts is expressed by + for right side, − for left side, = for median, and ± for bilateral. Absence of an anatomical unit is denoted by #, with the segment denoted by small letters, and submucosal cleft by (), defining the extent of cleft and surface structures represented by uppercase letters. The described examples were "LIP AND PALATE," "liP," "±lip and palate," and "=liP" which should be interpreted as "intact structures without cleft," "incomplete lip cleft," bilateral complete cleft, and median incomplete cleft of upper lip, respectively.

In 2008, Yuzuriha and Mulliken (2008) described lesser form labial clefts (those at the far end of the unilateral incomplete spectrum) as minor form (notched vermillion-cutaneous junction extending 3 mm or more above the normal Cupid's bow peak), microform (notch less than 3 mm above the normal Cupid's bow peak), or mini-microform (disrupted vermilion-cutaneous junction without elevation of Cupid's bow peak). For each, nasal severity reflects that of the lip. Yuzuriha and Mulliken's classification Yuzuriha and Mulliken (2008) is practical because it guides optimal operative technique by cleft severity.

In 2014, Agrawal (2014) proposed a modified Indian classification based on the Indian Classification initially described by Balakrishan (1975). Combinations of clefts were marked with "+" sign, and the abbreviation part of this classification was divided into four parts. Part 1: group ("Gp"). Part 2 (cleft organ): lip ("L"); lip and alveolus ("LA"); cleft lip (1); cleft palate (2); cleft lip, alveolus, and palate (3); and protruding premaxilla ("Pmax"). Part 3 (details): complete (there is no specific notation/abbreviation); partial ("P"); submucosal ("S"); Simonart's band ("sb"); and microform ("m"). Part 4 (side): right ("R"); left ("L"); bilateral ("R + L"); and median ("M"). The described example was "Gp 1R + Gp 3 L" which should be interpreted as "complete cleft lip on right side with cleft lip, alveolus and palate on left side." Further example was "Gp 1R + Gp 3L sb" which should be interpreted as "complete cleft lip on right side with cleft lip, alveolus and palate on left side with Simonart's band on left side."

Luijsterburg et al. (2014) presented, also in 2014, a classification based on patho-embryological events of the primary and secondary palates resulting in various subphenotypes of common oral clefts. Patients within the three categories cleft lip/alveolus (CL/A), cleft lip/alveolus and palate (CL/AP), and cleft palate (CP) were divided into three subgroups: fusion defects, differentiation defects, and fusion and differentiation defects. This classification provides new cleft subgroups that may be used for clinical and experimental research.

In 2015, Allori et al. (2015) from the Cleft Kit Collaboration proposed a universal structured form (a longhand structured form and a complementary shorthand notation) for description of cleft lip and/or palate phenotypes. Based on previously described classification systems, this universal structured form included anatomical involvement (pre-foraminal [lip/alveolus] and post-foraminal [palate] descriptions), side (right/left), laterality (unilateral/bilateral/median), severity (complete/incomplete; minor-form/microform/mini-microform; asymmetric), and morphology of the post-foraminal component. It proposed the CLAP notation as acronymic shorthand for the longhand structured form. Uppercase letters summarize the part of the anatomy involved (L, lip; A, alveolus; P, palate).

A lowercase prefix describes the laterality and severity of the pre-foraminal component (lip) (laterality = u, unilateral; b, bilateral; med, median; severity = c, complete; i, incomplete; m, minor-form, microform, or mini-microform; a, asymmetric). A lowercase suffix designates morphology of the post-foraminal component (secondary palate; bu, bifid uvula; sm, submucous; v1, v2, v3, and v4, Veau I–IV, respectively). CLAP notation should be read from left to right and translates directly to the structured form. The described example was "right ucCLAPv3" which should be interpreted as "right unilateral complete cleft of the lip and alveolus with a palate that is Veau III."

5.2 Summary

Cleft lip and palate are marked by a wide diversity in terms of clinical types, making classification difficult. In this chapter we included an overview of the classification of cleft phenotypes to facilitate diagnosis, management, surgical treatment, and research.

Classifications are very important not only for clinical diagnostic of syndromic and nonsyndromic cleft patients but also to define the long-term prognostic of these patients. The size and localization of the cleft would preview the facial growth and also the final result for speech. The new classification with the localization in the primary palate or only in the secondary palate with the severity could predict the final rehabilitation of these patients with or without final good speech.

References

Agrawal K. Classification of cleft lip and palate: an Indian perspective. J Cleft Lip Palate Craniofac Anomal. 2014;1:78–84.
Allori AC, Mulliken JB, Meara JG, Shusterman S, Marcus JR, CleftKit Collaboration. Classification of cleft lip/palate: then and now. Cleft Palate Craniofac J. 2015;54(2):175–88.
Balakrishnan C. Indian classification of cleft lip and palate. Indian J Plast Surg. 1975;8:23–4.
Castilla EE, Orioli IM. ECLAMC: the Latin-American collaborative study of congenital malformations. Community Genet. 2004;7:76–94.
Davis JS, Ritchie HP. Classification of congenital clefts of the lip and palate. JAMA. 1922;79:1323–7.
Fogh-Andersen P. Epidemiology and etiology of clefts. Birth Defects Orig Artic Ser. 1971;7:50–3.
Harkins CS, Berlin A, Harding RL, Longacre JJ, Snodgrasse RM. A classification of cleft lip and cleft palate. Plast Reconstr Surg Transplant Bull. 1962;29:31–9.
Kernahan DA. The striped Y — a symbolic classification for cleft lip and palate. Plast Reconstr Surg. 1971;47:469–70.
Kernahan DA, Stark RB. A new classification for cleft lip and cleft palate. Plast Reconstr Surg Transplant Bull. 1958;22:435–41.
Khan M, Ullah H, Naz S, Iqbal T, Ullah T, Tahir M, Ullah O. A revised classification of the cleft lip and palate. Can J Plast Surg. 2013;21:48–50.
Koch H, Grzonka M, Koch J. Cleft malformation of lip, alveolus, hard and soft palate, and nose (LAHSN)--a critical view of the terminology, the diagnosis and gradation as a basis for documentation and therapy. Br J Oral Maxillofac Surg. 1995;33:51–8.
Koul R. Describing cleft lip and palate using a new expression system. Cleft Palate Craniofac J. 2007;44:585–9.

Kriens O. Lahshal: a concise documentation system for cleft lip, alvolus and palate diagnoses. In: Kriens O, editor. What is cleft lip and palate? A multidisciplinary update workshop, Bremen 1987. Stuttgart: Thieme; 1989.

Liu Q, Yang ML, Li ZJ, Bai XF, Wang XK, Lu L, Wang YX. A simple and precise classification for cleft lip and palate: a five-digit numerical recording system. Cleft Palate Craniofac J. 2007;44:465–8.

Luijsterburg AJ, Rozendaal AM, Vermeij-Keers C. Classifying common oral clefts: a new approach after descriptive registration. Cleft Palate Craniofac J. 2014;51:381–91.

Ortiz-Posadas MR, Vega-Alvarado L, Maya-Behar J. A new approach to classify cleft lip and palate. Cleft Palate Craniofac J. 2001;38:545–50.

Raposo-Amaral CE, Raposo-Amaral CA. Changing face of cleft care: specialized centers in developing countries. J Craniofac Surg. 2012;23:206–9.

Rossell-Perry P. New diagram for cleft lip and palate description: the clock diagram. Cleft Palate Craniofac J. 2009;46:305–13.

Santiago A. Classification of cleft lip and palate for machine record coding. Cleft Palate J. 1969;6:434–9.

Schwartz S, Kapala JT, Rajchgot H, Roberts GL. Accurate and systematic numerical recording system for the identification of various types of lip and maxillary clefts (RPL system). Cleft Palate Craniofac J. 1993;30:330–2.

Silva Filho OG, Ferrari FM Jr, Rocha DL, Souza Freitas JA. Classificação das fissuras lábio-palatais. Breve histórico, considerações clínicas e sugestão de modificação. Rev Bras Cir. 1992;82(2):59–65.

Smith AW, Khoo AK, Jackson IT. A modification of the Kernahan "Y" classification in cleft lip and palate deformities. Plast Reconstr Surg. 1998;102:1842–7.

Spina V. A proposed modification for the classification of cleft lip and cleft palate. Cleft Palate J. 1973;10:251–2.

Tessier P. Anatomical classification of facial, cranio-facial and laterofacial clefts. J Maxillofac Surg. 1976;4:69–92.

Veau V. Division palantine. Paris: Masson et Cie; 1931.

Vilar-Sancho B. A proposed new international classification of congenital cleft lip and cleft palate. Plast Reconstr Surg Transplant Bull. 1962;30:263–6.

Yuzuriha S, Mulliken JB. Minor-form, microform, and mini-microform cleft lip: anatomical features, operative techniques, and revisions. Plast Reconstr Surg. 2008;122:1485–93.

An Overview of Protocols and Outcomes in Cleft Care

6

Rafael Denadai and Cassio Eduardo Raposo-Amaral

6.1 Protocols in Cleft Care

Highly specialized primary cleft surgery must ensure that normalized nasolabial esthetic appearance; intact primary and secondary palate; normalized speech, language, and hearing; nasal airway patency; class I occlusion with normal masticatory function; good dental and periodontal health; and normal psychosocial development are obtained (Ranganathan et al. 2015; Sitzman et al. 2014; Shaye 2014; Jones et al. 2014; Campbell et al. 2010). Interestingly, approaches to cleft care vary considerably between cleft centers (Table 6.1) and achieving optimal standards of cleft care across different countries and cleft centers remains an outstanding challenge (Persson et al. 2015; Dissaux et al. 2015, 2016; Long et al. 2011; Alonso et al. 2010; Semb et al. 2005a; Shaw et al. 2001; Sandy et al. 2001). Relevant examples of this diversity in cleft practices can be seen from the Eurocleft and Americleft intercenter outcome studies (Long et al. 2011; Shaw et al. 2001).

The Eurocleft study (Shaw et al. 2001) identified that 201 competent centers adopt 194 different surgical protocols for one cleft subtype. Seventeen possible sequences of operation to close the cleft were practiced. Though 86 (42.8%) of cleft teams repaired the lip at the first operation and the hard and soft palate together at the second, almost every other conceivable sequence appears to be practiced somewhere. The total number of operations taken to complete the closure of the cleft varied from one (5%), two (71.1%), three (21.9%), and four (2%). Around half the

---

R. Denadai, M.D. (✉)
Institute of Plastic and Craniofacial Surgery, SOBRAPAR Hospital,
Campinas, São Paulo, Brazil
e-mail: denadai.rafael@hotmail.com

C.E. Raposo-Amaral, M.D., Ph.D.
Institute of Plastic and Craniofacial Surgery, SOBRAPAR Hospital,
Campinas, São Paulo, Brazil

Universidade de São Paulo, São Paulo, Brazil

Table 6.1 Some examples of the wide diversity of surgical protocols (sequence, technique, and timing) adopted for unilateral cleft forms at different cleft centers worldwide

Cleft centers	Treatment Presurgical orthopedics	Lip repair	Primary bone graft	Hard palate repair	Soft palate repair	Secondary bone grafting	Nose/lip revisions
Eurocleft study (Shaw et al. 2001)							
Center A	Yes	3–4 m Millard, Skoog	No	6–9 y	9–15 m Von Langenbeck, Perko, Wardill, Kriens	9 y	–
Center B	No	2 m Tennison	No	2 m Vomer plasty; 22 m Wardill pushback		9 y	–
Center C	No	≤ 6 m Variable	No	12 m Variable		9 y	–
Center D	Yes	≤ 6 m Variable	No	≤ 24 m Variable		9 y	–
Center E	No	3 m Millard	No	3 m Vomer plasty; 18–20 m modified von Langenbeck		9 y	–
Center F	Yes	4–6 m Modified Skoog, Tennison-Randall	Yes	12 m Veau-Wardill-Kilner		9 y	–
Americleft study (Long et al. 2011)							
Center A	No	6–12 wk. Millard or 5–6 wk. Delaire	No	9–12 m Bardach or Delaire		6–7 y	4–5 y
Center B	Yes	2–3 m Millard	Yes	11–15 m Wardill-Kilner	11–15 m IVP or some Furlow	8–9 y	4 y
Center C	No	3 m Tennison	No	12 m Vomer flap	18 m Median suture with IVP	9 y	14–20 y
Center D	Yes	3 m Millard	No	12 m Wardill and Vomer flap		7–10 y	4–5 y
Center E	Yes	3–4 m Millard	No	12–14 m Vomer flap/ von Langenbeck	12–14 m Veau pushback	9–11 y	4–7 y
French centers (Dissaux et al. 2015)							
Center A	–	3 m Skoog	–	6–8 m Veau-Wardill and straight veloplasty		–	–

Cleft centers	Treatment						
	Presurgical orthopedics	Lip repair	Primary bone graft	Hard palate repair	Soft palate repair	Secondary bone grafting	Nose/lip revisions
Center B	–	2 m Lip adhesion; 5 m Skoog	–	5 m Free tibial periosteum graft (Stricker)	9–11 m Straight veloplasty	–	–
Center C	–	5 m Malek	–	5 m Malek	3 m IVP	–	–
Center D	–	6–8 m Millard modified Talmant	–	9–14 m Talmant (without raising flaps)	6–8 m Sommerland IVP	–	–
Brazil centers							
HCFMUSP (Alonso et al. 2010)	No	3 m Modified Millard	No	12 m von Langenbeck with extended IVP		8–12 y	–
SOBRAPAR hospital	No	3–4 m Cutting extended Mohler	No	12 m Vomer flap/von Langenbeck, Veau or Wardill-Kilner with IVP		7–10 y	4–5 y

wk weeks, *m* months, *y* years, *IVP* intravelar veloplasty, – data not provided

registered teams employ presurgical orthopedics, of whom 67 (65%), use it routinely. Mostly passive plates were used by 74 (70%) and some teams also used the plate as a feeding plate. The Americleft study (Long et al. 2011) also showed a wide range of protocols within five well-established North American cleft centers. One (20%) center used primary bone grafting, three (60%) centers used variations of presurgical orthopedic treatment, and one (20%) center used two-stage palate repair. There was also a wide and representative range of lip and palate repair techniques.

Difficulties and obstacles for implementation of standardized protocols in different cleft centers were approached in previous seminal articles (Persson et al. 2015; Dissaux et al. 2015, 2016; Scott et al. 2014; Long et al. 2011; Alonso et al. 2010; Semb et al. 2005a; Shaw et al. 2001; Sandy et al. 2001) and are beyond the scope of this chapter.

6.2 Measuring Outcomes in Cleft Care

The use of outcome measures is essential in the auditing and drive for continued improvements in the standards of care for cleft patients (Ranganathan et al. 2015; Sitzman et al. 2014; Shaye 2014; Jones et al. 2014; Campbell et al. 2010). In cleft care, a large number of outcome measures (namely, surgical, orthodontic, dental, speech, and patient satisfaction measures) (Table 6.2) have been available as a reflection of the complex, multidisciplinary, and longitudinal nature of the cleft care provided (Ranganathan et al. 2015; Sitzman et al. 2014; Shaye 2014; Jones et al. 2014; Campbell et al. 2010). In addition, new outcome measures are constantly being developed and tested in an attempt to more accurately demonstrate the success, or otherwise, of different therapeutic interventions.

Outcomes of interest in the Eurocleft, Americleft, CSAG (Clinical Standards Advisory Group), and Cleft Care UK studies (Persson et al. 2015; Dissaux et al.

Table 6.2 Some outcome measures for evaluating cleft treatment outcomes

Endpoints	Outcome measures
Aesthetic	Asher-McDade system, VLS classification, craniofacial proportion indices, aesthetic index, and cleft lip evaluation profile (CLEP) index
Craniofacial form	Two-dimensional and three-dimensional cephalometrics
Dental arch relations	Goslon yardstick, 5-year-olds' index, modified Huddart/Bodenham system, and EUROCRAN index
Speech	Cleft Audit Protocol for Speech-Augmented (CAPS-A), Universal Parameters, Great Ormond Street Speech Assessment (GOS. SP. ASS), aerodynamic vocal tract measurements (e.g., nasometry and pressure-flow testing), videofluoroscopy, and nasopharyngoscopy
Dental	DMFS(T)/Dmfs(t) index and Care Index
Bone grafting	Two-dimensional radiographs and three-dimensional technologies
Oral health, psychosocial, and comprehensive	Child Oral Health Impact Profile, CLEFT-Q, and CLP-360°

2015, 2016; Long et al. 2011; Semb et al. 2005a, b; Shaw et al. 2001, 2005; Sandy et al. 2001; Al-Ghatam et al. 2015; Smallridge et al. 2015; Sell et al. 2015, 2001; Waylen et al. 2015; Hathaway et al. 2011; Daskalogiannakis et al. 2011; Mercado et al. 2011; Russell et al. 2011; Brattström et al. 2005; Mølsted et al. 2005; Williams et al. 2001; Bearn et al. 2001) were dental arch relationships, craniofacial form, nasolabial appearance, speech, oral health and audiology, orthognathic outcomes at skeletal maturity, burden of care, and patient satisfaction. Although some of these outcome measures could successfully discriminate between the results of different cleft interventions in the major intercenter outcome studies (Persson et al. 2015; Dissaux et al. 2015, 2016; Long et al. 2011; Semb et al. 2005a, b; Shaw et al. 2001, 2005; Sandy et al. 2001; Al-Ghatam et al. 2015; Smallridge et al. 2015; Sell et al. 2015, 2001; Waylen et al. 2015; Hathaway et al. 2011; Daskalogiannakis et al. 2011; Mercado et al. 2011; Russell et al. 2011; Brattström et al. 2005; Mølsted et al. 2005; Williams et al. 2001; Bearn et al. 2001), there are no unanimous results in favor of a protocol rather than other. In fact, the heterogeneity among patient populations, surgical techniques, and outcome assessment strategies makes comparisons an arduous work in cleft care (Ranganathan et al. 2015; Sitzman et al. 2014; Shaye 2014; Jones et al. 2014; Campbell et al. 2010).

In this context, as each outcome of interest can be viewed from a different vantage point and may be measured in a different way (Ranganathan et al. 2015; Sitzman et al. 2014; Shaye 2014; Jones et al. 2014; Campbell et al. 2010), we will provide a description and brief appraisal of the three outcomes of interest (midfacial growth, speech development, and nasolabial appearance) widely used within modern cleft care, primarily adopted for measuring primary cleft surgery outcomes. It is important to highlight that as some of the cleft patients have been evaluated between ages 9 and 17 years, part of the results of different primary surgery techniques were biased by the interaction of different orthodontic treatments or secondary surgeries, occurring at different times.

6.3 Midfacial Growth

The maxillofacial growth on cleft patients is influenced by a myriad of variables, basically influenced by pathogenesis from intrinsic growth deficiency and iatrogenesis from surgical and nonsurgical maneuvers (Shi and Losee 2015; Berkowitz 2015). Essentially every cleft surgical intervention has been reported to be associated with maxillary hypoplasia due to disruption of growth centers and scar tissue formation; early cleft palate repair led to maxilla growth inhibition in all dimensions; cleft lip repair inhibited maxilla sagittal length in cleft lip and palate patients; Veau's pushback and Langenbeck's cleft palate repairs with relaxing incisions were most detrimental to growth; Furlow's cleft repair showed little detrimental effect on maxilla growth; and timing of hard palate closure, instead of the sequence of hard or soft palate repair, determined the postoperative growth (Shi and Losee 2015). In addition, lateral incisor agenesis and canine substitution (a nonsurgical, orthodontic maneuver to close dental spaces) have demonstrated as significant independent predictors of maxillary hypoplasia in the anteroposterior dimension and need for Le Fort I advancement surgery (Lai et al. 2015; Lee et al. 2014). However, surgeons performing the same repairs can have significantly different midfacial growth outcomes, and if unoperated clefts have normal growth potential or not and if presurgical intervention and pharyngoplasty inhibited maxillofacial growth or not remain as controversial viewpoints (Shi and Losee 2015; Berkowitz 2015). In addition, systematic reviews (Liao and Mars 2006; Lee and Liao 2013) have demonstrated that further well-designed, well-controlled, and long-term studies are needed. Contradictory results with lack of high-quality and long-term outcomes of reviewed studies provided no conclusive scientific evidence about the effects of timing of hard palate repair (or techniques) on facial growth in cleft patients.

Independent of the main cause of midfacial hypoplasia in cleft patients that continues to be a controversy (Shi and Losee 2015; Berkowitz 2015), midfacial growth and Le Fort I maxillary advancement surgery rate have been adopted as major outcomes of interest in cleft care. Outcome measures to assess the effects of primary surgery on midfacial growth largely focus on dental arch relationships. Some scoring study models (e.g., GOSLON [Great Ormond Street, London and Oslo, Norway] Yardstick, an occlusal index) (Mars et al. 1987) exist to assess the relationship of the maxilla and the mandible and the resulting occlusion (Table 6.2).

The applicability of these study methods in cleft literature is undeniable. However, as the categorization of the dental arch relationships ultimately represents the severity of the malocclusion, it can create the false impression that excellent or good scores (which theoretically require no additional treatments or only minor orthodontic adjustments) should always be obtained without Le Fort I advancement surgery as this surgical intervention has been interpreted as a negative aspect of the cleft care (i.e., using the Goslon yardstick assumptions, the cleft center with the best scores would be expected to require end-stage maxillary advancement orthognathic surgery in 20% of its patients (Hathaway et al. 2011)). In addition, this can create a further misimpression that a better quality treatment pattern is to find cleft patients with occlusion Class I based only on the evaluation of the study models.

As a consequence, we have evaluated several skeletal mature cleft patients with Class I occlusion obtained only with orthodontic compensation in different cleft and non-cleft centers. Interestingly, a most accurate characterization of deformity these cleft patients has revealed concaved midfaces and non-harmonious and non-balanced upper lip and nasal region relationships. In fact, these are cleft patients with a skeletal Class III malocclusion managed with exclusive orthodontic compensation (e.g., downward and backward mandibular rotation, advancement of the maxillary incisors, and retraction of the mandibular incisors) until obtaining Class I occlusion. This makes these cleft patients to be well ranked in dental arch relationship on study models and creates a wrong low orthognathic surgery rates.

However, these particular cleft patients with excellent or good dental arch relationships on study models (i.e., occlusion Class I orthodontically compensated) do not represent the true status of the skeletal framework of the midface or the full facial profile (Figs. 6.1–6.8). In addition, some of these skeletally mature cleft patients had their nose surgically treated and it is culminated in suboptimal results as the interplay of anatomic variables between maxillary structure and rhinoplasty is inseparable, and secondary cleft nasal reconstruction should not be performed without first correcting any significant problems with the skeletal base under the nose (additional details on the importance of skeletal base in rhinoplasty can be ascertained in the chapter "Secondary unilateral cleft rhinoplasty" of this book).

Interestingly, the literature has revealed skeletally mature patients with repaired unilateral cleft lip and palate, a flattened midface, and an edge-to-edge anterior occlusion that could have been corrected orthodontically, but which were

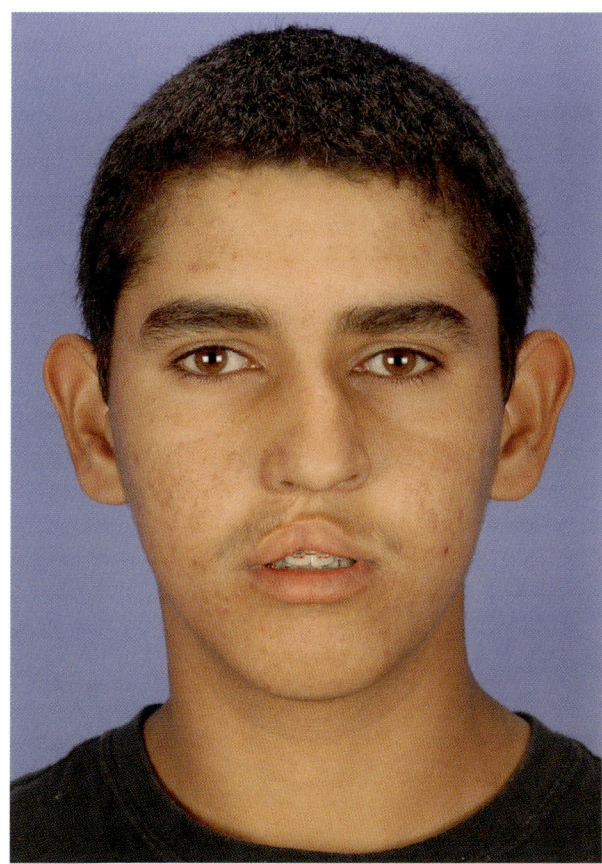

Fig. 6.1 Photograph of the skeletal mature patient with unilateral complete cleft lip and palate and Class I occlusion obtained only with orthodontic compensation. Note that this patient with occlusion Class I orthodontically compensated does not represent the true status of their skeletal framework of the midface or the full facial profile as demonstrated in Fig. 6.2

Fig. 6.2 Left profile view of the patient in Fig. 6.1 illustrating a concaved midface and non-harmonious and non-balanced upper lip and nasal region relationship

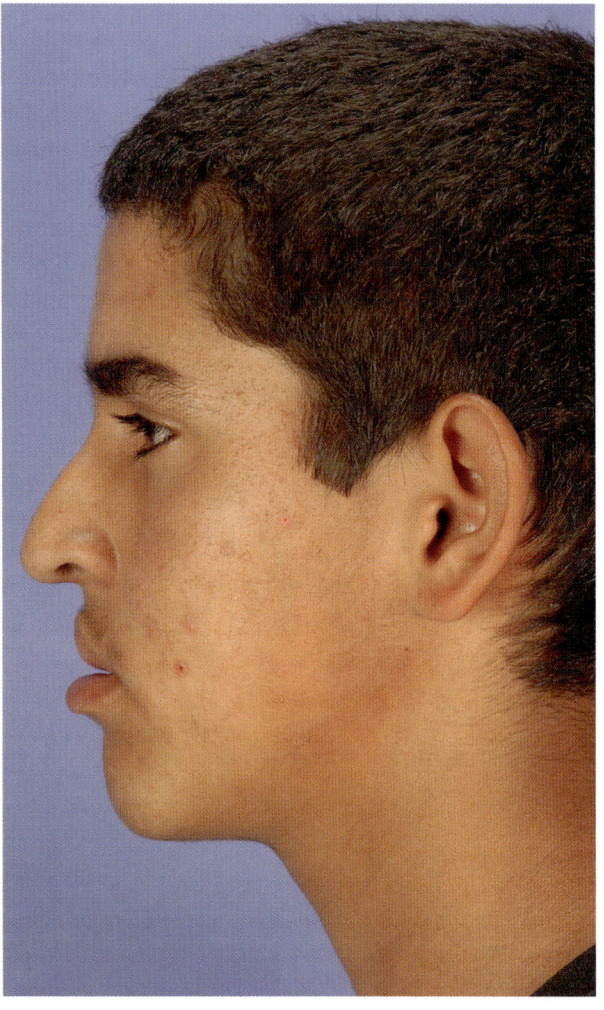

successfully managed (i.e., improvement in midfacial profile) with orthodontic decompensation followed by Le Fort I osteotomy and maxillary advancement (Good et al. 2007). In fact, up to 25% of cleft lip and palate patients present hypoplastic maxilla, concaved midface, and deformed dental arch which cannot be treated orthodontically alone but requires maxillary advancement by distraction or by conventional orthognathic surgery to achieve a global improvement in facial aesthetic (i.e., more convex facial angle and a more harmonious and balanced upper lip, upper incisor, and nasal region relationship) (Yamaguchi et al. 2016; Austin et al. 2015; Susarla et al. 2015; Chua and Cheung 2012; Phillips et al. 2012; Vasudavan et al. 2012; Kumar et al. 2006). These results have been found to be stable, with only minor changes on the long term, and surgical related complications that do not contraindicate the procedure, as it may be due to a variety of reasons, including

Fig. 6.3 Right profile view of the patient in Figs. 6.1 and 6.3 illustrating a concaved midface and non-harmonious and non-balanced upper lip and nasal region relationship. In fact, this patient had a skeletal Class III malocclusion managed with exclusive orthodontic compensation until obtaining Class I occlusion

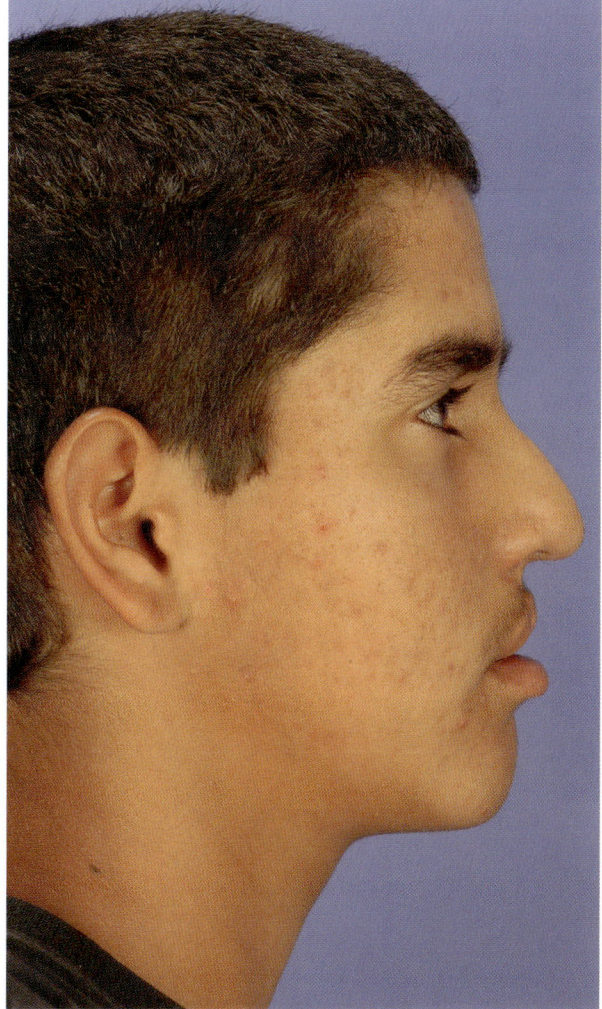

Fig. 6.4 Frontal occlusal view of the patient in Figs. 6.1–6.3 illustrating a Class I occlusion obtained only with orthodontic compensation

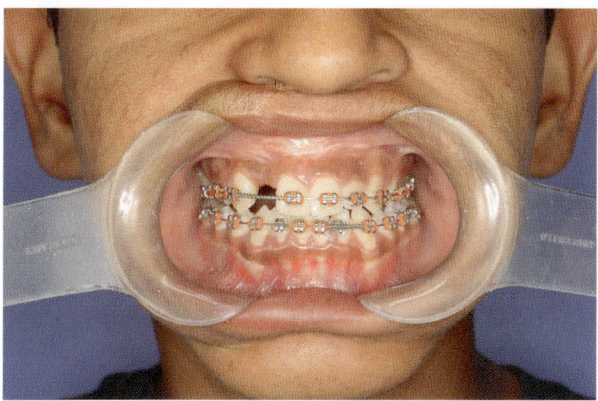

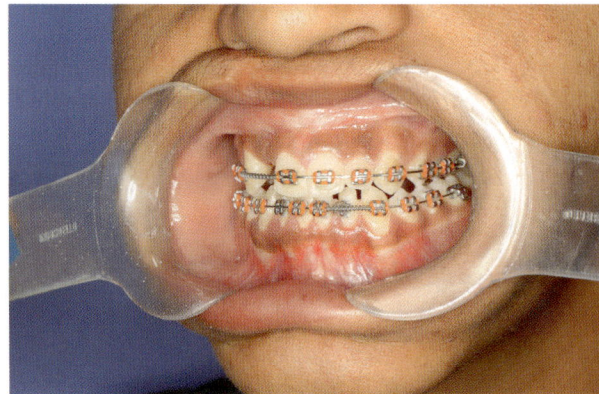

Fig. 6.5 Left profile occlusal view of the patient in Figs. 6.1–6.4 illustrating a Class I occlusion obtained only with orthodontic compensation

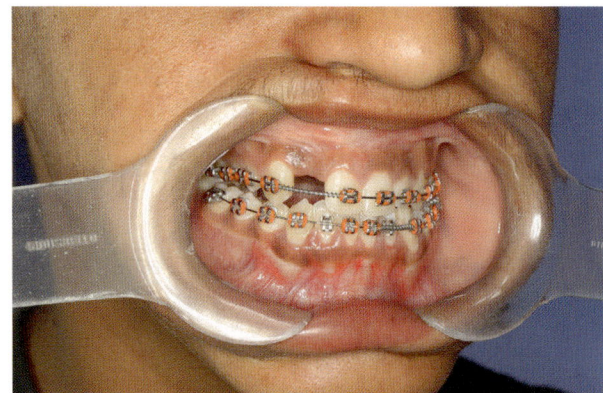

Fig. 6.6 Right profile occlusal view of the patient in Figs. 6.1–6.5. illustrating a Class I occlusion obtained only with orthodontic compensation

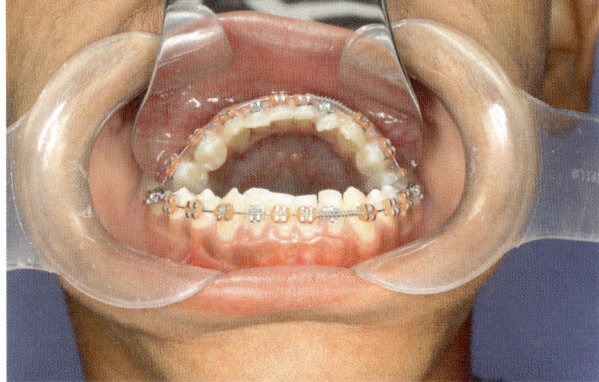

Fig. 6.7 Lower occlusal surface view of the patient in Figs. 6.1–6.6 illustrating the mandibular teeth with lingual inclination

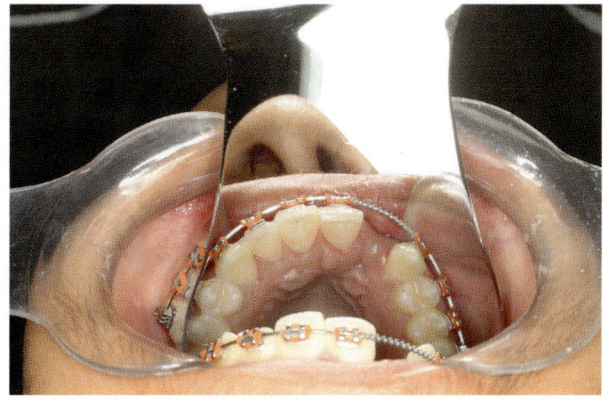

Fig. 6.8 Upper occlusal surface view of the patient in Figs. 6.1–6.7 illustrating the maxillary teeth with lip inclination

institution, surgeon, operative technique, treatment protocol, differences in reporting cleft populations, and hypoplasia (Yamaguchi et al. 2016; Austin et al. 2015; Susarla et al. 2015; Chua and Cheung 2012; Phillips et al. 2012; Vasudavan et al. 2012; Kumar et al. 2006).

In this context, the relevance of orthodontic treatments within the multidisciplinary cleft care is unquestionable, although there were many discrepancies from country to country and region to region. We also recognize the significance of facial growth in craniofacial and cleft care (Raposo-Amaral et al. 2011, 2013; Denadai et al. 2016). However, we interpret Le Fort I maxillary advancement surgery at skeletal maturity following preoperative orthodontic preparation removing dental compensations as a key therapeutic procedure in the longitudinal cleft care (Raposo-do-Amaral et al. 2008), instead of interpreting it as a poor outcome; the midfacial growth, the Class III malocclusion, and the Le Fort I maxillary advancement surgery rate have only been adopted as secondary endpoints in our cleft practice. Since 2007, we have discouraged the therapeutic option for compensatory treatment of the skeletal Class III malocclusion (even minor discrepancies) without orthognathic surgery in different craniofacial, cleft, and plastic surgery round tables and meetings. Although a statistically significant negative correlation exists between GOSLON scores and ANB angle (a cephalometric index of maxillomandibular sagittal discrepancy) (Daskalogiannakis et al. 2011), we believe that an individualized evaluation and treatment planning should be the basis for the cleft treatment, instead of adopting one outcome measurement alone (namely, study models). So, the additional information on craniofacial form/midfacial status (e.g., lateral cephalograms) should be incorporated into dental arch relationship assessments (Figs. 6.9–6.11). As a ripple effect, this rational can potentially reduce the number of skeletal Class III cleft patients that have been misdiagnosed and undertreated in Brazil.

American cleft centers ratify our therapeutic rationale (Lai et al. 2015; Lee et al. 2014; Good et al. 2007). The UCLA group (Lai et al. 2015; Lee et al. 2014) stated

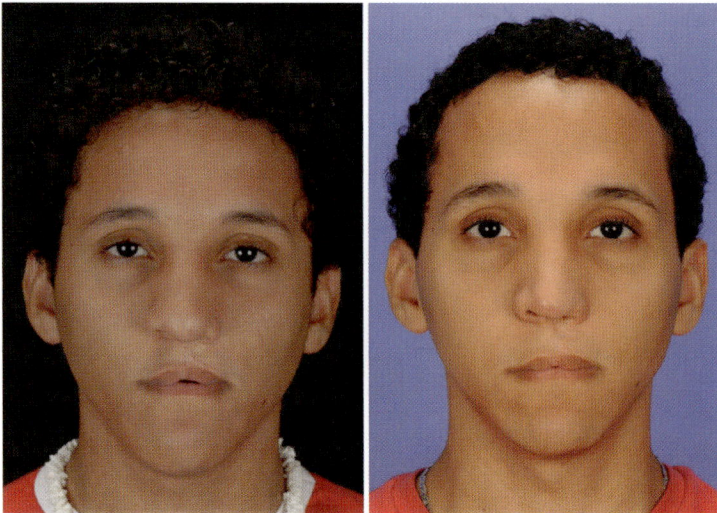

Fig. 6.9 (*Left*) Preoperative full-face view of a skeletal mature patient with unilateral complete cleft lip and palate. (*Right*) Late postoperative full-face view after the Le Fort I maxillary advancement

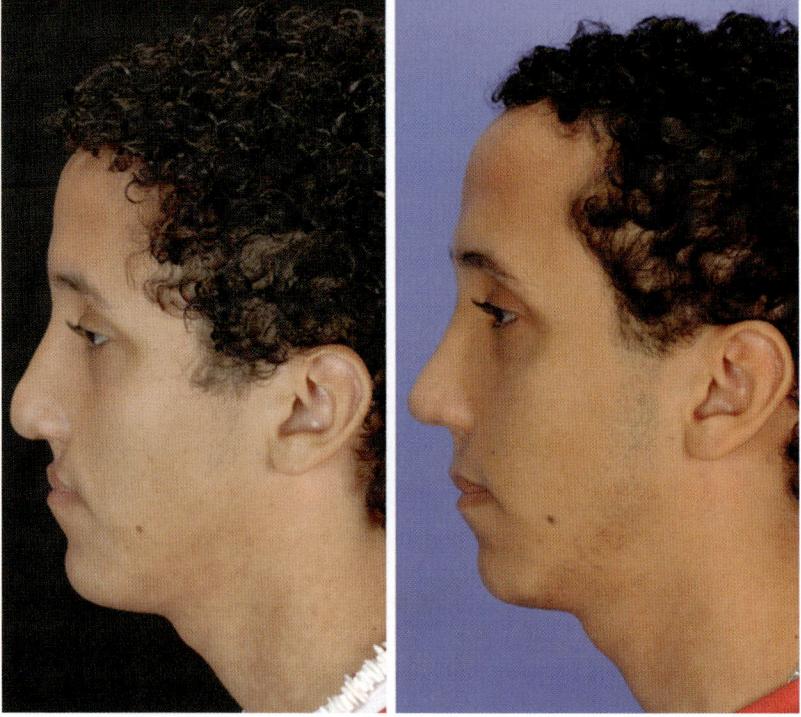

Fig. 6.10 (*Left*) Preoperative and (*right*) late postoperative profile views of the patient in Fig. 6.9

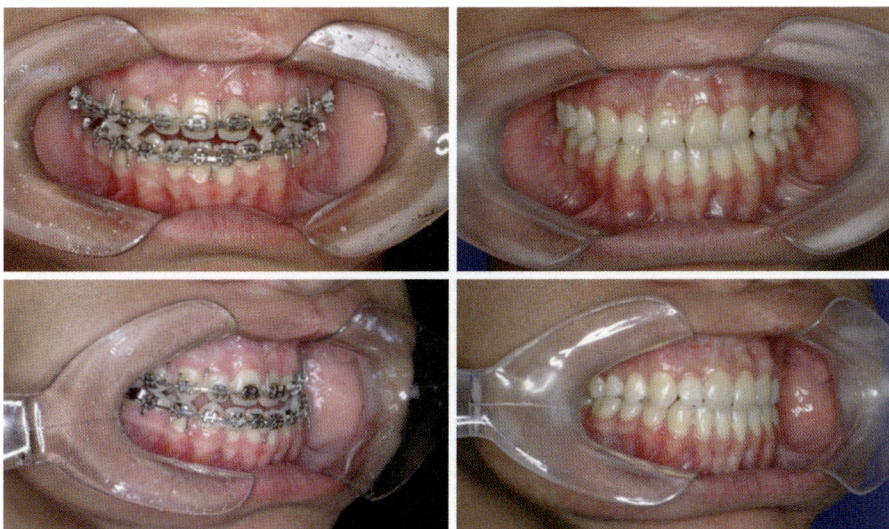

Fig. 6.11 (*Left*) Preoperative occlusal view of the patient in Figs. 6.9 and 6.10 illustrating a Class III malocclusion. The preoperative overall analysis of this patient (Figs. 6.9–6.11, left) reveals a concaved midface, a non-harmonious and non-balanced upper lip and nasal region relationship, and a severe skeletal Class III malocclusion which was surgically managed with the Le Fort I maxillary advancement. (*Right*) Late postoperative occlusal view showing a satisfactory occlusion. The postoperative analysis (Figs. 6.9–6.11, right) illustrates a harmonious and balanced upper lip, lower lip, and nasal region relationship, and a stable Class I occlusion

that the need for Le Fort I maxillary advancement surgery should not be subjected to bias as a failure but as a common consequence of treatment that requires consideration in planning surgical and orthodontic maneuvers, and the Boston Children's Hospital group (Good et al. 2007) justify that the their higher frequency of Le Fort I osteotomy may reflect the preference for operative correction for all cleft patients who have poor midfacial aesthetics despite their occlusal relationship.

Finally, although there are these precedents in the literature (Lai et al. 2015; Lee et al. 2014; Good et al. 2007), we emphasize that our rationale refers primarily to a regional problem with inconsistent multidisciplinary cleft care across the different cleft centers (Raposo-Amaral and Raposo-Amaral 2012; Denadai et al. 2015a, b) and should be interpreted with caution by American and European cleft centers with well-established rehabilitative process.

6.4　Speech Development

Enabling cleft patients to have normal speech (e.g., resonance, nasality, and intelligibility) should be a major functional outcome of interest in cleft care; unintelligible speech of cleft patients affects social and personal attribute judgments made by typically developing peers (Lee et al. 2017), and cleft children with less severe speech problems had higher total Pediatric Quality of Life Inventory scores as well as higher physical and psychosocial health domain scores (Damiano et al. 2007). Therefore, cleft surgeons are obligated to intermittently and critically assess their cleft repair outcomes including speech quality (e.g., velopharyngeal insufficiency rate and secondary speech surgery rate) and palatal integrity (fistula rate) (Smith and Losee 2014) and then redirect treatment protocols accordingly (Sullivan et al. 2009). In fact, speech outcomes represent a cleft team's multidisciplinary outcome, encompassing timely and effective primary surgery, well-coordinated follow-up, proactive hearing management, effective speech and language therapy, prompt and appropriate revision surgery where necessary, as well as recognition of a family's commitment to care (Britton et al. 2014).

6.4.1 Timing Protocols

The palate is divided functionally into the hard palate (serving as structural support and a growth center for the maxilla) and the soft palate (providing velopharyngeal competence) (Smith and Losee 2014; Sadove et al. 2004). The most debated issues in cleft palate repair have been how to achieve optimal speech development and how to avoid abnormal midfacial growth after repair as maxillary growth and speech development do not occur in perfect harmony. A wide variety of therapeutic protocols exist at different cleft centers worldwide (Table 6.1) as there are differences of opinion on the optimal timing and technique of cleft palate repair to obtain the best speech and midfacial growth outcomes.

Some cleft centers address this discrepancy by temporally separating (named as two-stage cleft palate repair) soft palate repair (i.e., veloplasty) from hard palate repair to uncouple the perceived deleterious effects of a late soft palate repair (impaired speech development during initial speech acquisition) from those of an early hard palate repair (stunted maxillary growth consequently to the amount of scar in the bony palate). A major stated advantage of this two-stage repairs is the narrowing of the hard palate cleft after primary veloplasty; the reduced defect size allows for closure later in the growth curve, with a tension-free repair and smaller flaps (minimized mucoperiosteal elevation) and, presumably, less of a negative effect on future growth.

Historically, Schweckendiek first proposed this two-staged cleft palate repair (Schweckendiek and Doz 1978). In Schweckendiek's 25-year follow-up study, over 60% of cleft patients demonstrated normal maxillary growth (Schweckendiek and Doz 1978). In 1984, the Marburg project (Schweckendiek's data collected and evaluated by three American specialists) showed similar normal maxillary growth success (Bardach et al. 1984). However, mixed midfacial growth outcomes have been reported in experiences from cleft centers adopting different techniques and timing of the early soft (between 3 and 18 months of age) and delayed hard (between 3 and 12 years of age) palate repairs (Al-Ghatam et al. 2015; Hathaway et al. 2011; Daskalogiannakis et al. 2011; Brattström et al. 2005; Mølsted et al. 2005; Williams et al. 2001; Xu et al. 2015; Bakri et al. 2014; Gundlach et al. 2013; Friede et al. 2012; Zemann et al. 2011; Yamanishi et al. 2011, 2009; Yang and Liao 2010; Liao et al. 2010; Del Guercio et al. 2010; Pradel et al. 2009; Holland et al. 2007; Lilja et al. 2006; Mommaerts et al. 2006; Richard et al. 2006; Semb 1991).

From a speech perspective, further Marburg project examination revealed a high incidence of short palate, poor mobility of the soft palate, velopharyngeal incompetence, and compensatory misarticulations (Bardach et al. 1984). Subsequent mixed speech outcomes have also been demonstrated within cleft centers adopting modified two-stage palate repair protocols (Dissaux et al. 2016; Sell et al. 2015, 2001; Pradel et al. 2009; Holland et al. 2007; Dingman and Argenta 1985; Lohmander-Agerskov et al. 1998; Lohmander-Agerskov 1998; Lohmander et al. 2012; Randag et al. 2014; Klintö et al. 2014; Funayama et al. 2014; Willadsen 2012; Brunnegård and Lohmander 2007; Rohrich and Gosman 2004; Van Lierde et al. 2004; Rohrich et al. 2000; Noordhoff et al. 1987; Witzel et al. 1984; Jackson et al. 1983; Cosman and Falk 1980). In fact, although there were improved speech outcomes at some cleft centers using two-stage protocol, several other cleft centers reported worse speech outcomes (Dissaux et al. 2016; Sell et al. 2015, 2001; Pradel et al. 2009; Holland et al. 2007; Dingman and Argenta 1985; Lohmander-Agerskov et al. 1998; Lohmander-Agerskov 1998; Lohmander et al. 2012; Randag et al. 2014; Klintö et al. 2014; Funayama et al. 2014; Willadsen 2012; Brunnegård and Lohmander 2007; Rohrich and Gosman 2004; Van Lierde et al. 2004; Rohrich et al. 2000; Noordhoff et al. 1987; Witzel et al. 1984; Jackson et al. 1983; Cosman and Falk 1980). In addition, many cleft centers (Pradel et al. 2009; Randag et al. 2014; Klintö et al. 2014; Funayama et al. 2014; Van Lierde et al. 2004; Cosman and Falk 1980) have also demonstrated that one-stage repair cleft palate repair (both the hard and soft palates are closed in a single surgical intervention) results in significantly better speech outcome than the two-stage repair.

Although there are cleft centers in favor of two-stage cleft palate repair, the presently available evidence of impaired midface growth secondary to early cleft repair is not sufficiently convincing to justify sacrificing the opportunity to correct soft palate anatomy and facilitate normal speech development with early cleft palate repair. Interestingly, a survey of 288 American cleft surgeons showed that 88% perform one-stage cleft palate repairs (Katzel et al. 2009).

6.4.2 Velopharyngeal Insufficiency

Velopharyngeal insufficiency, a structural defect (i.e., the inability to completely close the velopharyngeal sphincter), results in the characteristic speech problems of hypernasality (excessive nasal resonance [i.e., too much acoustic energy resonating in the nose during oral—vowel—production]), audible/visible nasal emission (turbulent airflow through the nasal cavities during oral speech—consonant—production), and weak pressure consonants (decreased intraoral pressure for pressure-dependent consonants during speech [i.e., reduced ability to impound oral airflow, which keeps pressures low and results in insufficient aspiration when pressure consonants are released]) and it also results in speech articulation errors (i.e., distortions, substitutions, and omissions) (Kummer 2014; Smith and Guyette 2004).

In this context, it is important to emphasize that speech outcomes have been linked to age at surgical repair, type and timing of surgical repair, surgeon experience, Veau hierarchy, cleft width, and presence of craniofacial syndrome (Sullivan et al. 2009; Yuan et al. 2016; Timbang et al. 2014; Chen et al. 2011; Phua and de Chalain 2008; Salyer et al. 2006; Inman et al. 2005; Sommerlad 2003; Marrinan et al. 1998; Witt et al. 1998; Dorf and Curtin 1982). Velopharyngeal competence, a sine qua non for success in cleft palate repair (Smith and Losee 2014), is directly connected with the age at cleft palate repair as was demonstrated by a significantly increased odds of velopharyngeal insufficiency with each month in advanced age at the time of cleft palate repair (Sullivan et al. 2009, 2014). Cleft centers (Smith and Losee 2014; Sullivan et al. 2009; Pradel et al. 2009; Jackson et al. 2013) adopting one-stage repair highlight the importance of performing palate repair before the acquisition of language (speech sound production and articulation). Based on the available data (Smith and Losee 2014; Sullivan et al. 2009; Pradel et al. 2009; Marrinan et al. 1998; Dorf and Curtin 1982; Jackson et al. 2013; Chapman et al. 2008; Kirschner et al. 2000; Chapman and Hardin 1992), the cleft palate repair should most often be performed between 7 and 15 months of age (Campbell et al. 2010). In addition, nearly 80% of the American cleft surgeons perform cleft palate surgery when the patient is between 6 and 12 months of age (Katzel et al. 2009).

A properly functioning velopharyngeal mechanism is critical to proper speech development. A universal requirement essential to achieve velopharyngeal competence is a two-layer, tension-free, watertight repair of the palate to minimize subsequent scarring and fistula formation (Smith and Losee 2014; Losee et al. 2008). Most surgeons today perform either some modification of a straight-line intravelar veloplasty or a double-opposing z-plasty (Kriens' and Furlow's techniques and subsequent modifications, respectively) of soft palate repair, focusing on either lengthening of the palate, alignment of the muscle, or both. These soft palate repair techniques may be used in isolation or combined with hard palate procedures, as necessary (Timbang et al. 2014; Inman et al. 2005; Marrinan et al. 1998; Jackson et al. 2013; Sommerlad et al. 2002; Furlow 1986; Andrades et al. 2008; Cutting et al. 1995; Kriens 1969; Brothers et al. 1995; Polzer et al. 2006; Williams et al. 2011; Dreyer and Trier 1984; Ito et al. 2006; Koh et al. 2009; Yu et al. 2001).

A recent systematic review (Timbang et al. 2014) revealed that in patients affected by unilateral cleft lip–cleft palate, straight-line repair combined with intravelar veloplasty was significantly associated with an increased risk of a secondary operation compared with the double-opposing Z-plasty. However, there are excellent and poor speech outcomes in both intravelar veloplasty and double-opposing Z-plasty (Timbang et al. 2014; Inman et al. 2005; Marrinan et al. 1998; Jackson et al. 2013; Sommerlad et al. 2002; Furlow 1986; Andrades et al. 2008; Cutting et al. 1995; Kriens 1969; Brothers et al. 1995; Polzer et al. 2006; Williams et al. 2011; Dreyer and Trier 1984; Ito et al. 2006; Koh et al. 2009; Yu et al. 2001). In addition, the variations in the intravelar veloplasty outcomes could be secondary to improper identification, mishandling, or incomplete posterior repositioning of the levator veli palatini muscles as there is much variability among surgeons in how the musculature is dissected and repositioned, and tension of suture in the midline.

There also were reports showing that the extent of retropositioning of the levator muscles achieved with intravelar veloplasty affects velopharyngeal function (Salyer et al. 2006; Sommerlad 2003; Cutting et al. 1995), whereas incomplete muscle mobilization was associated with less favorable speech outcomes (Andrades et al. 2008). Thus, intravelar veloplasty is more operator dependent than the double-opposing Z-plasty (Timbang et al. 2014; Salyer et al. 2006; Sommerlad 2003; Andrades et al. 2008; Cutting et al. 1995). Furthermore, care must be taken when interpreting this systematic review (Timbang et al. 2014) as the selection bias may have impacted with the results (Nardini and Flores 2015). In fact, an reanalysis of data with modifications in the comparative groups (modern intravelar veloplasty versus double-opposing Z-plasty) may reveal equivalent outcomes between the two cleft palate repairs, with the radical intravelar veloplasty demonstrating slightly superior speech outcomes (Nardini and Flores 2015).

6.4.3 Oronasal Fistula

The presence of an oronasal fistula is one of the important factors indicating the early outcomes of the primary cleft palate repair as it can result in significant long-term sequelae that may directly interfere with speech development (nasal air escape and difficulty with articulation) (Witt and D'Antonio 1993), allow regurgitation of food and liquid into the nasal cavity (resulting in halitosis, infection, and chronic inflammation), and be associated with dental decay (Richards et al. 2015). Additionally, patients with oronasal fistula had significantly lower COHIP (Child Oral Health Impact Profile) scores and worse self-reported speech scores (Long et al. 2015).

The reported oronasal fistula rate after primary cleft palate repair varies enormously (Salimi et al. 2017; Bykowski et al. 2015; Hardwicke et al. 2014). Two worldwide systematic reviews with meta-analyses (Bykowski et al. 2015; Hardwicke et al. 2014) reported that oronasal fistulas develop in 8.6 and 4.9% of 9294 and 2505 patients after cleft palate repair, respectively. However, as there were problems of classification of the oronasal fistula and lack of standardization in the reporting of fistulas, possible ambiguity and underreporting may interfere with the establishment of a more realistic oronasal fistulae rate (Salimi et al. 2017; Bykowski et al. 2015; Hardwicke et al. 2014). In this context, although postoperative fistula is an extremely relevant issue within the cleft care, no classification scheme for palatal fistulas had been described until the Pittsburgh group (Smith et al. 2007) proposed, in 2007, the Pittsburgh Fistula Classification System, an anatomically based numerical fistula classification system: fistulas at the uvula, or bifid uvulae (type I); within the soft palate (type II); at the junction of the soft and hard palates (type III); within the hard palate (type IV); at the incisive foramen, or junction of the primary and secondary palates (type V; this designation is reserved for use with Veau type IV clefts); lingual-alveolar (type VI); and labial-alveolar (type VII). In addition, besides anatomic location, oronasal fistulas may be best characterized by whether they are clinically important leading to nasal air emission, hypernasal resonance, decreased intraoral pressure, or regurgitation of fluid and food (Sullivan et al. 2009). So, adopting a standardized scheme for the anatomical and functional description of oronasal fistulas will serve as a prerequisite for meaningful discussion among cleft centers and ongoing cleft palate research (Sullivan et al. 2009; Smith et al. 2007).

Multiple factors have been identified as contributing to the development of postoperative oronasal fistula, including patient (gender, age at operation, type and extent of cleft, associated craniofacial syndromes, inadequate oral hygiene) and surgical (surgeon experience [number of cases], surgical technique, tension at the site of repair, inadequate mobilization, poor handling of tissues, failure to achieve a layered closure, injury at reintubation, inadequate blood supply, bleeding, infection, and postsurgical transverse maxillary orthodontic forces) factors (Yuan et al. 2016; Salimi et al. 2017; Ahmed et al. 2015; Aznar et al. 2015; Rossell-Perry et al. 2014; Lu et al. 2010; Landheer et al. 2010; Parwaz et al. 2009; Emory et al. 1997; Rohrich et al. 1996; Cohen et al. 1991); however, the relevance of these factors is debated as there are mixed results (Yuan et al. 2016; Salimi et al. 2017; Ahmed et al. 2015; Aznar et al. 2015; Rossell-Perry et al. 2014; Lu et al. 2010; Landheer et al. 2010; Parwaz et al. 2009; Emory et al. 1997; Rohrich et al. 1996; Cohen et al. 1991). In addition, pediatric patients undergoing cleft palate repair on surgical missions have higher postoperative odds of oronasal fistula than children treated by local physicians, and pediatric patients in low-resource settings have higher complication rates than do children in high-resource settings (Daniels et al. 2015).

Within the possible risk factors, some deserve further discussion. Surgeon experience and surgical technique can also influence oronasal fistula rates. Both inexperience and choice of inappropriate technique clearly contribute in an intertwined manner to postoperative oronasal fistula development (Losken et al. 2011). Overall, the more occasional cleft palate surgeon will have a higher fistula rate (Cohen et al. 1991). High-volume surgeons have significantly lower oronasal fistula rate when compared with low-volume surgeons (Bearn et al. 2001). Interestingly, on the other hand lower velopharyngeal insufficiency rates have been reported by some cleft groups (Salyer et al. 2006; Sommerlad 2003; LaRossa et al. 2004), with a correspondingly higher fistula rate. It is possible that attempts to improve velar functioning by more extensive dissection increase the likelihood of developing a fistula (Sullivan et al. 2009). In addition, criticisms of the double-opposing Z-plasty have included higher fistula rates when this repair is adopted in wider clefts and without relaxing incisions (Losken et al. 2011; Williams et al. 1998). However, a recent systematic review showed no significant difference in fistula rate between the double-opposing Z-plasty repair and the straight-line repair (Timbang et al. 2014). Based on a particular prior data, it was described that the occurrence of fistula correlated more with the width of the cleft (Veau classification) than with the repair technique (Timbang et al. 2014).

A significant relation between Veau classification and the occurrence of a fistula has been established (Bykowski et al. 2015; Hardwicke et al. 2014; Ahmed et al. 2015; Rossell-Perry et al. 2014; Cohen et al. 1991; Moar et al. 2016), patients with Veau classes III or IV being significantly more likely to develop an oronasal fistula than those with Veau classes I or II. Besides the Veau classification, cleft width has also been associated to oronasal fistula as clefts of the same Veau grade class can vary dramatically in width (Yuan et al. 2016; Rossell-Perry et al. 2014; Parwaz et al. 2009). This association is likely due to the increased tension that comes from repairing a bilateral cleft lip and palate or a wide cleft as compared to other clefts. The explanation of increased tension as the main reason for oronasal fistula formation is supported by the finding that patients had fistulae at the junction of the hard and soft palates, the most common site of fistula formation; this particular location is problematic because it is generally the widest portion of a cleft, and it is associated with the greatest tension for both the nasal and oral mucosal layer closures (Yuan et al. 2016; Losee et al. 2008; Losken et al. 2011).

In this context, as experience alone or the choice of a particular cleft repair technique alone does not guarantee lower fistula rate and as the prevention of postoperative oronasal fistula is a critical goal in cleft palate care, adherence to relevant particular surgical principles is the key to avoiding fistulas as have been adopted by some cleft centers (Losee et al. 2008; Losken et al. 2011; Dec et al. 2013). The NYU group (Dec et al. 2013) highlights that four factors (namely, preoperative nasoalveolar molding, surgeon experience and technique, type of primary lip and palate repair, and well-practiced multidisciplinary team) contributed to a low postsurgical oronasal fistula rate. The UNC Craniofacial Center (Losken et al. 2011) described technical keys to achieving low fistula rate: skeletonization of the vascular pedicle for medialization of the mucoperiosteal flaps, aggressive posterior repositioning of the levator muscle, meticulous two-layer mattress-suture closure, and tension-free midline closure of the palate; it was also recommend that less experienced surgeons should consider doing the Bardach two-flap cleft palate repair for wider clefts (≥ 8 mm), and reserving the Furlow double-opposing Z-plasty repair for narrower clefts (<8 mm wide at the posterior border of the hard palate). The Pittsburgh group (Losee et al. 2008) delineate the following algorithm to limit postoperative oronasal fistulas: use of relaxing incisions, complete intravelar veloplasty, total release of the tensor tendon at the level of the hamulus, complete dissection of the neurovascular bundle with optional osteotomy of the bony foramen, and incorporation of acellular dermal matrix to achieve complete nasal lining reconstruction and adequate two-layer closure in difficult cleft repairs. Postoperative antibiotic prophylaxis can also reduce the incidence of fistulas after primary cleft palate repair primarily in a developing cleft center (Aznar et al. 2015).

6.4.4 The Multidisciplinary SOBRAPAR Team for Cleft Palate Speech Management

Overall, we have prioritized the speech production with the standardization of multidisciplinary SOBRAPAR team for evaluation and management of cleft palate speech development, while the midfacial growth has been a secondary level of importance. Further arguments on our rational and concepts can be found in the midfacial growth, velopharyngeal insufficiency, and oronasal fistula subheads of this chapter.

In our comprehensive approach of the many cleft palate-related issues (i.e., feeding, hearing, and speech), all cleft patients have been managed by a team of healthcare providers including speech-language pathologists, otolaryngologists, and plastic surgeons. All patients have regular feeding, hearing, and speech evaluations, starting in the first consultation at our center (regardless of age at presentation) and often continuing into adulthood according to the individual needs. Particularly these speech evaluations have been established based on specific recommendations (Kummer 2014; Smith and Guyette 2004; Fitzsimons 2014; Henningsson et al. 2008; Alfwaress et al. 2015). Repeated perceptual speech assessment with speech-language pathologists at the preoperative and postoperative periods of cleft palate repair determines if hypernasal speech or concern for velopharyngeal insufficiency persists, and subsequent evaluation with nasoendoscopy measurements has been critical in determining appropriate treatment (e.g., surgery, speech therapy, or both) (Raposo do Amaral et al. 2009; Raposo-do-Amaral 2013).

From the surgical point of view, we (Table 6.1) have adopted the one-stage cleft palate repair at 12 months of age as the speech process in children begins approximately at 1 year of age. In particular in unrepaired cleft lip and palate patients with an advanced age (often adopted patients or from rural and incipient regions in Brazil with low human development index [HDI], further delineated in another chapter (public policies) of this book), we have altered the usual order of surgical interventions to first schedule cleft palate repair followed by cleft lip repair, although there is limited speech improvement after cleft palate repair as the age of patients increases (Sullivan et al. 2009, 2014; Schönmeyr et al. 2015).

In addition, we are proponents of early, single-stage repair as it improves speech outcomes through promotion of proper phonologic development and reduces the development of learned, compensatory misarticulations associated with velopharyngeal insufficiency, and the benefits of improved speech outcome that outweigh potential midfacial growth restriction that may ensue. In fact, midfacial hypoplasia can be repaired surgically (Yamaguchi et al. 2016; Austin et al. 2015; Susarla et al. 2015; Chua and Cheung 2012; Phillips et al. 2012; Vasudavan et al. 2012; Kumar et al. 2006), whereas overcoming velopharyngeal insufficiency at a later age remains a much more challenging endeavor.

The severity of the cleft has determined our decision on the cleft repair technique as also reported by 50% of American cleft surgeons (Katzel et al. 2009). As wide (the distance between the medial edges of the hard palate is >1.5 cm) palatal cleft repair may place the palatal tissue under great tension and product in a higher fistula rate, additional precautions should be taken in the accurate classification of each patient, selection of the appropriate surgical technique, and meticulous tissue manipulation. We have systematically adopted the following surgical rational. Regarding soft palate repair, straight-line closure combined with intravelar veloplasty has been used for both the narrow and wide clefts (Veau I to IV clefts). V-Y pushback technique from the hard palate mucoperiosteum or lateral relaxing incisions in the soft palate to bring the cleft edges may be necessary in clefts of the soft palate (Veau I clefts). V-Y pushback cleft palate repair (Veau–Wardill–Kilner's technique) has been adopted in wider clefts of the soft and hard palates, posterior to the incisive foramen (Veau II clefts), whereas bipedicled flaps (von Langenbeck's technique) may be alternatively adopted in narrow Veau II clefts. The unipedicled hard palate mucoperiosteal flaps (two-flap cleft palate repair such as Veau's technique or Bardach's technique) have been used in complete unilateral cleft lip and palate (Veau III clefts) and complete bilateral cleft lip and palate (Veau IV clefts). The vomer flap has been applied to the anterior (hard palate) closure of nasal layer achieving complete, tension-free, two-layer closure of wide palatal clefts. The mucosal velar relaxing incisions (from the retromolar trigone posteriorly to the maxillary tuberosity anteriorly), further dissection of the hamulus and pedicle region, osteotomy of the bony foramen, and/or breaking of hamulus may also be adopted to allow adequate posterior/medial mobilization and relieve tension on the suture line, primarily in wide clefts and/or if a high tension on the suture is intraoperatively diagnosed. Both lack of government liberation and underfunding from the Brazilian unified healthcare system (*Sistema Único de Saúde* [SUS]; Ministry of Health, Brazil) (Raposo-Amaral and Raposo-Amaral 2012) have limited the incorporation of alternatives such as acellular dermal matrix in our cleft care.

6.5 Nasolabial Aesthetics

Cleft lip and palate patients undergo numerous surgeries throughout their childhood and early adulthood to correct the aesthetic and functional stigmata of their diagnoses (McIntyre et al. 2016). In most cleft centers (Table 6.1), the cleft lip surgical repair (associated or not with primary rhinoplasty) is the first operation with the primary aim of achieving a functionally and aesthetically (balance, symmetry, and proportion) acceptable upper lip and nose appearance which enhance social acceptability. Regardless of the cleft lip repair technique used, three-dimensional and functional anatomic understanding of the cleft (and non-cleft) lip, nose, and alveolus; precise preoperative marking; accurate plan of the surgical maneuvers; restoration of normal surface, muscle, and mucosal anatomy; anticipation of the need for overcorrection of the vertical dimension of the lips and symmetry of nostril; and meticulous tissue manipulations are some of most relevant surgical principles that may interfere with the postoperative outcomes (Raposo-Amaral et al. 2014, 2012). However, the longitudinal follow-up usually revels a residual (from minor to major) nasolabial deformity culminating in an adverse effect on facial attractiveness, which, in turn, may predispose the development of problems in the psychosocial functioning of patients with cleft lip and may also explain, at least partially, some of the social hardships experienced by patients with operated cleft lip (Hunt et al. 2005; Meyer-Marcotty et al. 2010; Millar et al. 2013). Therefore, it is essential to have a reliable outcome measure as it becomes an increasing healthcare priority both politically and professionally (individual surgeons and/or cleft teams). However, while midfacial growth and speech development outcomes have become more objectively assessable, there is no accepted facial aesthetic outcome measure in cleft care (Mosmuller et al. 2013; Sharma et al. 2012; Al-Omari et al. 2005).

There are two principal methods by which nasolabial appearance can be assessed: directly and indirectly. Direct assessment is performed in the clinic setting, whereas indirect is performed using a wide range of tools (e.g., photographs, videotapes, and computer-generated pictures). In addition, the exiting methods can be broadly divided into quantitative and qualitative. Quantitative methods analyze the extent of abnormal morphology and the degree of disproportion through direct or indirect facial measurements (linear or angular dimensions). Dr. Leslie Farkas (Farkas et al. 2000), father of medical anthropometry (measurement of the human individual), provided normative measurements of the lip and nose and Farkas' direct anthropometric measurement methods have been used as a more detailed guideline to objectively measure aesthetic outcomes over time. This method is most accurate and well accepted by anthropologists, but it is problematical to reproduce, especially in large numbers of patients (Nagy and Mommaerts 2007). For children, this is most accurately obtained in the operating room under general anesthesia and then additional measures have been delayed until the next operation (if any). Furthermore, quantitative methods abstract the appearance based on numerical data without evaluating the overall facial and/or nasolabial aesthetic. Therefore, the qualitative method better reflects both the patient's and the public's perception, although it is a subjective method (Johnson and Sandy 2003).

The most adopted methods can also be divided into four groups: direct clinical assessment (e.g., plaster casts of midface with angular, linear, and surface measurements; measures of the nasolabial area using calipers; and live evaluation of vermillion, lip, and scar [VLS classification]), clinical two-dimensional photographic evaluation (e.g., Asher-McDade aesthetic index; rating nasal form, deviation, vermillion border, and profile; measures of 25 craniofacial proportion indices; and computerized measurement), clinical videographic evaluation (e.g., 3-s video recording of cleft patients during four facial movements), and three-dimensional evaluation (e.g., facial anthropometric linear and angular distances; and modified Asher-McDade system) (Mosmuller et al. 2013; Sharma et al. 2012; Al-Omari et al. 2005). Different reviews (Mosmuller et al. 2013; Sharma et al. 2012; Al-Omari et al. 2005) have indicated that reliability tests have been conducted for only a few of the currently available methods used to assess the aesthetic results of cleft surgeries.

The majority of studies use two-dimensional photographs combined with a numerical or ordinal scale for the assessment of the cleft lip and nose surgical repair (Mosmuller et al. 2013; Sharma et al. 2012; Al-Omari et al. 2005). In 1991, Asher-McDade et al. (Asher-McDade et al. 1991) proposed a system using cropped two-dimensional photographs. In this scoring system, the observers are asked to rate each feature (i.e., frontal view photographs [nasal form, nasal symmetry, and vermilion border] and profile view photographs [nasal profile including the upper lip]) on a five-point ordinal scale (1 = very good appearance, 2 = good appearance, 3 = fair appearance, 4 = poor appearance, and 5 = very poor appearance). This particular scoring system has been validated in large multicenter cleft studies, namely the nasolabial aesthetics comparative analyses of the Eurocleft and Americleft studies (Mercado et al. 2011; Brattström et al. 2005).

Various other protocols (e.g., visual analog scale, numerical scale, and visual rating chart) for clinical assessment of aesthetic outcome of cleft surgery have also been proposed (Adeola and Oladimeji 2015; Kim et al. 2011; Ohannessian et al. 2011; He et al. 2009; Prahl et al. 2006; Bongaarts et al. 2008; Tobiasen and Hiebert 1994; Tobiasen et al. 1991). It was found that the numerical scale was more discriminative than the visual analog scale and a visual analog scale can cause problems for interpretation of the results (Prahl et al. 2006). The Prahl scoring system (visual analog scale and a numerical scale [0–200] using a reference photograph) and the modified Prahl scoring system (i.e., a simplified version with a 5-point scale without the use of a reference photograph) were equivalent in their reliability and outcome (Mosmuller et al. 2014); it was advocated to use the least complicated simplified scoring system (i.e., the modified Prahl scoring system), and to assess the lip and nose separately because, when assessed together, the lip was dominating the overall scorings (Mosmuller et al. 2014). In addition, although the Asher-McDade aesthetic index has been superior to the Prahl scoring system and the modified Prahl scoring system, all three scoring systems are reliable, when three or more observers are used. However, there still is a need for a more reliable scoring system using two-dimensional photographs because the most frequently used scoring system (i.e., Asher-McDade aesthetic index) can be considered as not reliable enough when only one observer is used (Mosmuller et al. 2015).

Additionally, different kinds of cropped photographs (triangle (Asher-McDade et al. 1991), circle (Prahl et al. 2006), or oval (Bongaarts et al. 2008) revealing the nose and mouth) have been adopted in cleft outcome measures to reduce the influence of the surrounding facial nasolabial area, because it has been shown that judges are influenced by the overall attractiveness of the face. In fact, previous reports (Asher-McDade et al. 1991; Prahl et al. 2006; Bongaarts et al. 2008) revealed that full-face photographs are scored much more attractive than cropped photographs. However, a most recent report (Kocher et al. 2016) demonstrated that cropping facial images for assessment of nasolabial appearance in complete unilateral cleft lip and palate patients seems unnecessary; instead, aesthetic evaluation can be performed on images of full faces. Further studies with large database and a large number of evaluators should investigate these mixed findings.

Standardized, reference libraries of images of nasolabial appearance in unilateral cleft lip and palate patients were also recently created (Kuijpers-Jagtman et al. 2009; Rubin et al. 2015). In 2009, Kuijpers-Jagtman et al. (Kuijpers-Jagtman et al. 2009) included frontal and profile photographs of 42 postoperative children, matched for age, race, and non-syndromic. It was assessed by four evaluators (senior orthodontists) using the Asher-McDade system, demonstrating good interrater reliability between observers (Kuijpers-Jagtman et al. 2009). For each of the 4 components (i.e., nasal form, nasal deviation, nasal profile, and shape of the vermilion border), 5 photographs were selected to illustrate the whole range of the scale (scores 1–5), resulting in the selection of 20 pictures. In 2015, Rubin et al. (Rubin et al. 2015) proposed further reference photographs for nasal form and nasal symmetry from the basal view to illustrate the Asher-McDade system and facilitate its use. Four raters (2 craniofacial plastic surgeons and 2 craniofacial orthodontists) assessed nasolabial appearance (form and symmetry) on basal view photographs of 50 complete unilateral cleft lip and palate children (average age 8 years) with a repaired cleft lip. Intraclass correlation coefficients show fair to moderate interrater reliability. Cronbach α indicated strong agreement between raters, along with low duplicate measurement error and strong internal consistency between the measures. The photographs with the highest agreement among raters were selected to illustrate each point on the five-point scale for nasal form and for nasal symmetry, resulting in the selection of ten reference photographs. These reference photographs could act as a good benchmark for aesthetic assessment, but this needs significantly more cleft patients and comparison with normative data from controls (Kuijpers-Jagtman et al. 2009; Rubin et al. 2015).

Next to the investigations that use two-dimensional photographs in combination with different grading systems, there are also reports in which indirect linear and angular measurements have been made on digital photographs, most often done by specially designed software programs (e.g., Photoshop (Raposo-Amaral et al. 2014; Raposo-Amaral et al. 2012; Nagy and Mommaerts 2007) and SymNose (Pigott and Pigott 2010; McKearney et al. 2013)). Computerized photogrammetry (i.e., indirect anthropometry) has a combination of advantages, including safety (inexposure to ionizing radiation), accessibility, relatively cheap, and user-friendliness (fast image capture and archival capabilities), compared to new technological equipment (e.g., three-dimensional imaging techniques are more expensive, less available, and painstaking methodology). Another advantage of this method is the reduced time of exposure and embarrassment patients (principally children) may feel during measurements; some measurements, such as those around the eyes, are difficult to obtain directly without risk for discomfort (snap shut of the caliper or contact of its tips on the skin can make the subject uncomfortable) or injury to the patient. It also allows the surgeon to take the measurements under proper conditions at a time other than during a child's visit. The most mentioned disadvantage of two-dimensional photographs is the distortion errors due to projecting a three-dimensional object on a two-dimensional image. Further disadvantage is that measurements on two-dimensional photographs are affected by differences in lighting and head orientation, and the distance between the camera and the subject can vary, which makes the measurements unreliable. The use of standardized photographs has been proposed to overcome this problem; however, it is important to recognize that additional precautions are required to take children photos. Our standardized two-dimensional photographic documentation of cleft patients was delineated in other chapter of this book.

Another way of assessing cleft surgery outcome is the use of clinical video recordings. In 1996, Morrant and Shaw (Morrant and Shaw 1996) described a standardized method of video recording the nasolabial area of 30 children with complete unilateral clefts of the lip and nose. Recordings were taken from six different angles, when each subject was asked to repeat three phrases and make a series of lip movements. The pooled panel scores for different aspects of the nose and the lip had a poor to excellent reliability. This technique could be useful for quality assurance, intercenter comparisons, or outcome studies of surgical techniques.

However, patients must be told enough to cooperate fully and appropriate trained operators are needed to ensure reproducible recording. In 2000, Trotman et al. (Trotman et al. 2000) improved assessment with better video quality, a simplified rating system, and significantly shorter time needed for scoring. In this study, the suitability of a novel modified Procrustes fit method to adjust data for head motion during instructed facial movements was explored and this method allows cleft subjects to move the head naturally without the inconvenience of a splint, while facial movement data are being collected. Results obtained using this method support the view that facial movements in cleft patients may be severely hampered and that assessment of facial animation should be strongly considered when contemplating surgical lip revisions. Years later, Trotman et al. (2007) used the video-based tracking system (it tracks retroreflective markers secured to specific facial landmarks) to measure the circumoral movements of three groups of participants (repaired cleft lip slated to have revision surgery but who had not yet undergone the surgery; repaired cleft lip who did not have surgery; and non-cleft participants) and concluded that to distinguish reliably between a participant with a repaired cleft of the upper lip and a control participant many repeated movements are required. Further Trotman et al. (2013) report demonstrated that the use of videos of cleft patients' faces combined with objective three-dimensional measures altered the surgeon's treatment plan for a significant number of patients; surgeons can more accurately determine areas of the face that are impaired by visually comparing the mean movement of a patient's facial landmarks for an animation superimposed on that of the mean movement of the control-group landmark movement.

A newly introduced three-dimensional imaging technology has also been adopted to assess cleft lip-nose repair outcomes (Mosmuller et al. 2013; Sharma et al. 2012; Al-Omari et al. 2005; Kuijpers et al. 2014). An increasing number of studies adopting a wide variety of different three-dimensional imaging techniques and methods for the evaluation of facial morphology and treatment outcomes in patients with clefts have been published (Mosmuller et al. 2013; Sharma et al. 2012; Al-Omari et al. 2005; Kuijpers et al. 2014). There are some advantages and disadvantages of this particular technology and it was discussed in another chapter ("Three-Dimensional Digital Stereophotogrammetry in Cleft Care") of this book.

In different systematic reviews (Mosmuller et al. 2013; Sharma et al. 2012; Al-Omari et al. 2005; Kuijpers et al. 2014), stereophotogrammetry and laser scanners were the three-dimensional technologies most adopted for asymmetry assessment of the face, nose, and lips as well as for soft tissue changes of the nose, lips, and facial soft tissue before and after surgery. Desmedt et al. (2015) evaluated the relationship between symmetry and aesthetics on cropped three-dimensional stereophotogrammetric facial images and demonstrated that nasolabial appearance was affected by nasolabial asymmetry (i.e., subjects with more nasolabial asymmetry were judged as having a less aesthetically pleasing nasolabial area) and then nasolabial symmetry assessed with three-dimensional facial imaging can be used as an objective measure of treatment outcome in subjects with less severe cleft deformity. The three-dimensional technology has also gained favor as an alternative to direct anthropometry in children because images are captured in as little as 3.5 ms.

Wong et al. (2008) evaluated the validity and reliability of nasolabial anthropometry using three-dimensional stereophotogrammetry compared with direct anthropometry and found that linear measurements were highly correlated and overall precision of three-dimensional measurements was within 1 mm of direct measurements.

In the most recent systematic review (Kuijpers et al. 2014), the maximum reported error for soft tissue measurements with stereophotogrammetry and laser surface scanning was 0.55 mm as described by Hoefert et al. (2010), whereas only van Loon et al. (2010) reported a measurement error for volume measurements of the nose, with a maximum of 147.40 mm^3. Based on the measurement errors in the good-quality studies of this recent systematic review (Kuijpers et al. 2014), laser surface scanning and stereophotogrammetry seem to be reliable methods for quantitatively measuring asymmetry and three-dimensional changes in soft tissues after treatment.

Rating nasolabial appearance and scoring asymmetry on three-dimensional images using a panel of raters has also been performed. Al-Omari et al. (2003) evaluated the reliability of clinical assessment, two-dimensional color transparencies, and three-dimensional imaging for evaluating the residual facial deformity (modified five-point Asher-McDade system) in patients with repaired complete unilateral cleft lip and palate and compared the ratings of facial deformity made by healthcare professionals with those made by lay assessors. It was demonstrated that the equivalence of two-dimensional and three-dimensional imaging versus clinical assessment depended on the area of face being evaluated, and it was concluded that in comparison with lay assessors, clinical assessment among professionals (plastic, maxillofacial, and orthodontic surgeons) was more reproducible. Stebel et al. (2016) compared reliability of rating nasolabial appearance on three-dimensional stereophotogrammetric images and standard two-dimensional photographs in cleft children. Lay observers (junior postgraduate students) were asked to rate nasolabial aesthetics with a visual analogue scale. It was demonstrated that three-dimensional stereophotogrammetric images seem better than two-dimensional images for rating nasolabial aesthetics but raters should familiarize themselves with them prior to rating.

As demonstrated in the findings of these studies (Al-Omari et al. 2003; Stebel et al. 2016), there is a controversy regarding ideal panel composition—lay panel versus professional panel—for assessment of aesthetic outcome in cleft care. A recent systematic review (Zhu et al. 2016) assessed the full facial appearance of cleft patients based on two-dimensional photographs, three-dimensional images, or clinical examination by laypeople and professionals using a visual analog scale or a categorical rating scale. It was concluded that it remains unknown whether laypeople are more or less critical than professionals when rating facial appearance of repaired cleft patients. Professionals are more familiar with the aesthetic outcomes and difficulties of treating patients. The opposite may be true for laypeople; this disparity between what is achievable by professionals and what is expected by laypeople may be a source of dissatisfaction in facial appearance outcome. Further well-designed studies should be carried out to address this question and the clinical significance of the difference in rating scores for cleft patients.

Furthermore, following the same line of reasoning, further efforts should go towards the continuing search for a standardized and universal method for aesthetic outcome measurement in cleft care. Besides permitting easy, objective, and practical assessment of aesthetic outcome of the cleft surgical repair, this outcome measure can enhance communication between the laypersons (e.g., cleft patients, relations, and the general public) and the healthcare professionals (Mosmuller et al. 2013; Sharma et al. 2012; Al-Omari et al. 2005).

6.6 Summary

Cleft lip and palate are marked by the absence of a gold standard protocol to date, making the achievement of optimal standards of cleft care across different cleft centers an outstanding challenge. In this chapter we included an overview of the cleft protocols, emphasizing our rationale to adopt nasolabial aesthetics and speech development as principal outcome of interest in cleft care, instead of midfacial growth.

References

Adeola AO, Oladimeji AA. Developing a visual rating chart for the esthetic outcome of unilateral cleft lip and palate repair. Ann Maxillofac Surg. 2015;5:55–61.

Ahmed MK, Maganzini AL, Marantz PR, Rousso JJ. Risk of persistent palatal fistula in patients with cleft palate. JAMA Facial Plast Surg. 2015;17:126–30.

Alfwaress FS, Khwaileh FA, Khamaiseh ZA. The speech language pathologist's role in the cleft lip and palate team. J Craniofac Surg. 2015;26:1439–42.

Al-Ghatam R, Jones TE, Ireland AJ, Atack NE, Chawla O, Deacon S, Albery L, Cobb AR, Cadogan J, Leary S, Waylen A, Wills AK, Richard B, Bella H, Ness AR, Sandy JR. Structural outcomes in the Cleft Care UK study. Part 2: dento-facial outcomes. Orthod Craniofac Res. 2015;18(Suppl 2):14–24.

Al-Omari I, Millett DT, Ayoub A, Bock M, Ray A, Dunaway D, Crampin L. An appraisal of three methods of rating facial deformity in patients with repaired complete unilateral cleft lip and palate. Cleft Palate Craniofac J. 2003;40:530–7.

Al-Omari I, Millet DT, Ayoub AF. Methods of assessment of cleft-related facial deformity: a review. Cleft Palate Craniofac J. 2005;42:145–56.

Alonso N, Tanikawa DY, Lima-Junior JE, Ferreira MC. Comparative and evolutive of attendance protocols of patients with clef lip and palate. Rev Bras Cir Plást. 2010;25:434–8.

Andrades P, Espinosa-de-los-Monteros A, Shell DH 4th, Thurston TE, Fowler JS, Xavier ST, Ray PD, Grant JH 3rd. The importance of radical intravelar veloplasty during two-flap palatoplasty. Plast Reconstr Surg. 2008;122:1121–30.

Asher-McDade C, Roberts C, Shaw WC, Gallager C. Development of a method for rating nasolabial appearance in patients with clefts of the lip and palate. Cleft Palate Craniofac J. 1991;28:385–90.

Austin SL, Mattick CR, Waterhouse PJ. Distraction osteogenesis versus orthognathic surgery for the treatment of maxillary hypoplasia in cleft lip and palate patients: a systematic review. Orthod Craniofac Res. 2015;18:96–108.

Aznar ML, Schönmeyr B, Echaniz G, Nebeker L, Wendby L, Campbell A. Role of postoperative antimicrobials in cleft palate surgery: prospective, double-blind, randomized, placebo-controlled clinical study in India. Plast Reconstr Surg. 2015;136:59e–66e.

Bakri S, Rizell S, Lilja J, Mark H. Vertical maxillary growth after two different surgical protocols in unilateral cleft lip and palate patients. Cleft Palate Craniofac J. 2014;51:645–50.

Bardach J, Morris HL, Olin WH. Late results of primary veloplasty: the Marburg Project. Plast Reconstr Surg. 1984;73:207–18.

Bearn D, Mildinhall S, Murphy T, Murray JJ, Sell D, Shaw WC, Williams AC, Sandy JR. Cleft lip and palate care in the United Kingdom--the Clinical Standards Advisory Group (CSAG) Study. Part 4: outcome comparisons, training, and conclusions. Cleft Palate Craniofac J. 2001;38:38–43.

Berkowitz S. A review of the cleft lip/palate literature reveals that differential diagnosis of the facial skeleton and musculature is essential to achieve all treatment goals. J Craniofac Surg. 2015;26:1143–50.

Bongaarts CA, Prahl-Andersen B, Bronkhorst EM, Spauwen PH, Mulder JW, Vaandrager JM, Kuijpers-Jagtman AM. Effect of infant orthopedics on facial appearance of toddlers with complete unilateral cleft lip and palate (Dutchcleft). Cleft Palate Craniofac J. 2008;45:407–13.

Brattström V, Mølsted K, Prahl-Andersen B, Semb G, Shaw WC. The Eurocleft study: intercenter study of treatment outcome in patients with complete cleft lip and palate. Part 2: craniofacial form and nasolabial appearance. Cleft Palate Craniofac J. 2005;42:69–77.

Britton L, Albery L, Bowden M, Harding-Bell A, Phippen G, Sell D. A cross-sectional cohort study of speech in five-year-olds with cleft palate ± lip to support development of national audit standards: benchmarking speech standards in the United Kingdom. Cleft Palate Craniofac J. 2014;51:431–51.

Brothers DB, Dalston RW, Peterson HD, Lawrence WT. Comparison of the Furlow double-opposing Z-palatoplasty with the Wardill-Kilner procedure for isolated clefts of the soft palate. Plast Reconstr Surg. 1995;95:969–77.

Brunnegård K, Lohmander A. A cross-sectional study of speech in 10-year-old children with cleft palate: results and issues of rater reliability. Cleft Palate Craniofac J. 2007;44:33–44.

Bykowski MR, Naran S, Winger DG, Losee JE. The rate of oronasal fistula following primary cleft palate surgery: a meta-analysis. Cleft Palate Craniofac J. 2015;52:e81–7.

Campbell A, Costello BJ, Ruiz RL. Cleft lip and palate surgery: an update of clinical outcomes for primary repair. Oral Maxillofac Surg Clin North Am. 2010;22:43–58.

Chapman KL, Hardin MA. Phonetic and phonologic skills of two-year-olds with cleft palate. Cleft Palate Craniofac J. 1992;29:435–43.

Chapman KL, Hardin-Jones MA, Goldstein JA, Halter KA, Havlik RJ, Schulte J. Timing of palatal surgery and speech outcome. Cleft Palate Craniofac J. 2008;45:297–308.

Chen Q, Zheng Q, Shi B, Yin H, Meng T, Zheng GN. Study of relationship between clinical factors and velopharyngeal closure in cleft palate patients. J Res Med Sci. 2011;16:945–95.

Chua HD, Cheung LK. Soft tissue changes from maxillary distraction osteogenesis versus orthognathic surgery in patients with cleft lip and palate--a randomized controlled clinical trial. J Oral Maxillofac Surg. 2012;70:1648–58.

Cohen SR, Kalinowski J, LaRossa D, Randall P. Cleft palate fistulas: a multivariate statistical analysis of prevalence, etiology, and surgical management. Plast Reconstr Surg. 1991;87:1041–7.

Cosman B, Falk AS. Delayed hard palate repair and speech deficiencies: a cautionary report. Cleft Palate J. 1980;17:27–33.

Cutting C, Rosenbaum J, Rovati L. The technique of muscle repair in the cleft soft palate. Oper Tech Plast Reconstr Surg. 1995;2:215–22.

Damiano PC, Tyler MC, Romitti PA, Momany ET, Jones MP, Canady JW, Karnell MP, Murray JC. Health-related quality of life among preadolescent children with oral clefts: the mother's perspective. Pediatrics. 2007;120:e283–90.

Daniels KM, Yu EY, Maine RG, Corlew S, Bing S, Hoffman WY, Gregory GA. Palatal fistula risk after primary palatoplasty: a retrospective comparison of humanitarian operations and tertiary hospitals. Lancet. 2015;385(Suppl 2):S37.

Daskalogiannakis J, Mercado A, Russell K, Hathaway R, Dugas G, Long RE Jr, Cohen M, Semb G, Shaw W. The Americleft study: an inter-center study of treatment outcomes for patients with unilateral cleft lip and palate part 3. Analysis of craniofacial form. Cleft Palate Craniofac J. 2011;48:252–8.

Dec W, Shetye PR, Grayson BH, Brecht LE, Cutting CB, Warren SM. Incidence of oronasal fistula formation after nasoalveolar molding and primary cleft repair. J Craniofac Surg. 2013;24:57–61.

Del Guercio F, Meazzini MC, Garattini G, Morabito A, Semb G, Brusati R. A cephalometric inter-centre comparison of patients with unilateral cleft lip and palate at 5 and 10 years of age. Eur J Orthod. 2010;32:24–7.

Denadai R, Samartine Junior H, Denadai R, Raposo-Amaral CE. The public recognizes plastic surgeons as leading experts in the treatment of congenital cleft and craniofacial anomalies. J Craniofac Surg. 2015a;26:e684–9.

Denadai R, Muraro CA, Raposo-Amaral CE. Residents' perceptions of plastic surgeons as craniofacial surgery specialists. J Craniofac Surg. 2015b;26:2334–8.

Denadai R, Raposo-Amaral CA, Buzzo CL, Raposo-Amaral CE. Isolated autologous free fat grafting for management of facial contour asymmetry in a subset of growing patients with craniofacial microsomia. Ann Plast Surg. 2016;76:288–94.

Desmedt DJ, Maal TJ, Kuijpers MA, Bronkhorst EM, Kuijpers-Jagtman AM, Fudalej PS. Nasolabial symmetry and esthetics in cleft lip and palate: analysis of 3D facial images. Clin Oral Investig. 2015;19:1833–42.

Dingman RO, Argenta LC. The correction of cleft palate with primary veloplasty anddelayed repair of the hard palate. Clin Plast Surg. 1985;12:677–84.

Dissaux C, Bodin F, Grollemund B, Picard A, Vazquez MP, Morand B, James I, Kauffmann I, Bruant-Rodier C. Evaluation of 5-year-old children with complete cleft lip and palate: multicenter study. Part 1: lip and nose aesthetic results. J Craniomaxillofac Surg. 2015;43:2085–92.

Dissaux C, Grollemund B, Bodin F, Picard A, Vazquez MP, Morand B, James I, Kauffmann I, Bruant-Rodier C. Evaluation of 5-year-old children with complete cleft lip and palate: multicenter study. Part 2: functional results. J Craniomaxillofac Surg. 2016;44:94–103.

Dorf DS, Curtin JW. Early cleft palate repair and speech outcome. Plast Reconstr Surg. 1982;70:74–81.

Dreyer TM, Trier WC. A comparison of palatoplasty techniques. Cleft Palate J. 1984;21:251–3.

Emory RE Jr, Clay RP, Bite U, Jackson IT. Fistula formation and repair after palatal closure: an institutional perspective. Plast Reconstr Surg. 1997;99:1535–8.

Farkas LG, Forrest CR, Phillips JH. Comparison of the morphology of the "cleft face" and the normal face: defining the anthropometric differences. J Craniofac Surg. 2000;11:76–82.

Fitzsimons DA. International confederation for cleft lip and palate and related craniofacial anomalies task force report: speech assessment. Cleft Palate Craniofac J. 2014;51:e138–45.

Friede H, Lilja J, Lohmander A. Long-term, longitudinal follow-up of individuals with UCLP after the Gothenburg primary early veloplasty and delayed hard palate closure protocol: maxillofacial growth outcome. Cleft Palate Craniofac J. 2012;49:649–56.

Funayama E, Yamamoto Y, Nishizawa N, Mikoya T, Okamoto T, Imai S, Murao N, Furukawa H, Hayashi T, Oyama A. Important points for primary cleft palate repair for speech derived from speech outcome after three different types of palatoplasty. Int J Pediatr Otorhinolaryngol. 2014;78:2127–31.

Furlow LT Jr. Cleft palate repair by double opposing Z-plasty. Plast Reconstr Surg. 1986;78:724–38.

Good PM, Mulliken JB, Padwa BL. Frequency of Le Fort I osteotomy after repaired cleft lip and palate orcleft palate. Cleft Palate Craniofac J. 2007;44:396–401.

Gundlach KK, Bardach J, Filippow D, Stahl-de Castrillon F, Lenz JH. Two-stage palatoplasty, is it still a valuable treatment protocol for patients with a cleft of lip, alveolus, and palate? J Craniomaxillofac Surg. 2013;41:62–70.

Hardwicke JT, Landini G, Richard BM. Fistula incidence after primary cleft palate repair: a systematic review of the literature. Plast Reconstr Surg. 2014;134:618e–27e.

Hathaway R, Daskalogiannakis J, Mercado A, Russell K, Long RE Jr, Cohen M, Semb G, Shaw W. The Americleft study: an inter-center study of treatment outcomes for patients with unilateral cleft lip and palate part 2. Dental arch relationships. Cleft Palate Craniofac J. 2011;48:244–51.

He X, Shi B, Kamdar M, Zheng Q, Li S, Wang Y. Development of a method for rating nasal appearance after cleft lip repair. J Plast Reconstr Aesthet Surg. 2009;62:1437–41.

Henningsson G, Kuehn DP, Sell D, Sweeney T, Trost-Cardamone JE, Whitehill TL, Speech Parameters Group. Universal parameters for reporting speech outcomes in individuals with cleft palate. Cleft Palate Craniofac J. 2008;45:1–17.

Hoefert CS, Bacher M, Herberts T, Krimmel M, Reinert S, Hoefert S, Göz G. Implementing a superimposition and measurement model for 3D sagittal analysis of therapy-induced changes in facial soft tissue: a pilot study. J Orofac Orthop. 2010;71:221–34.

Holland S, Gabbay JS, Heller JB, O'Hara C, Hurwitz D, Ford MD, Sauder AS, Bradley JP. Delayed closure of the hard palate leads to speech problems and deleterious maxillary growth. Plast Reconstr Surg. 2007;119:1302–10.

Hunt O, Burden D, Hepper P, Johnston C. The psychosocial effects of cleft lip and palate: asystematic review. Eur J Orthod. 2005;27:274–85.

Inman DS, Thomas P, Hodgkinson PD, Reid CA. Oro-nasal fistula development and velopharyngeal insufficiency following primary cleft palate surgery: an audit of 148 children born between 1985 and 1997. Br J Plast Surg. 2005;58:1051–4.

Ito S, Noguchi M, Suda Y, Yamaguchi A, Kohama G, Yamamoto E. Speech evaluation and dental arch shape following pushback palatoplasty in cleft palate patients: supraperiosteal flap technique versus mucoperiosteal flap technique. J Craniomaxillofac Surg. 2006;34:135–43.

Jackson IT, McLennan G, Scheker LR. Primary veloplasty or primary palatoplasty: some preliminary findings. Plast Reconstr Surg. 1983;72:153–7.

Jackson O, Stransky CA, Jawad AF, Basta M, Solot C, Cohen M, Kirschner R, Low DW, Randall P, LaRossa D. The Children's Hospital of Philadelphia modification of the Furlow double-opposing Z-palatoplasty: 30-year experience and long-term speech outcomes. Plast Reconstr Surg. 2013;132:613–22.

Johnson N, Sandy J. An aesthetic index for evaluation of cleft repair. Eur J Orthod. 2003;25:243–9.

Jones T, Al-Ghatam R, Atack N, Deacon S, Power R, Albery L, Ireland T, Sandy J. A review of outcome measures used in cleft care. J Orthod. 2014;41:128–40.

Katzel EB, Basile P, Koltz PF, Marcus JR, Girotto JA. Current surgical practices in cleft care: cleft palate repair techniques and postoperative care. Plast Reconstr Surg. 2009;124:899–906.

Kim JB, Strike P, Cadier MC. A simple assessment method for auditing multi-centre unilateral cleft lip repairs. J Plast Reconstr Aesthet Surg. 2011;64:195–200.

Kirschner RE, Randall P, Wang P, Jawad AF, Duran M, Huang K, Solot C, Cohen M, LaRossa D. Cleft palate repair at 3 to 7 months of age. Plast Reconstr Surg. 2000;105:2127–32.

Klintö K, Svensson H, Elander A, Lohmander A. Speech and phonology in Swedish-speaking 3-year-olds with unilateral complete cleft lip and palate following different methods for primary palatal surgery. Cleft Palate Craniofac J. 2014;51:274–82.

Kocher K, Kowalski P, Kolokitha OE, Katsaros C, Fudalej PS. Judgment of nasolabial esthetics in cleft lip and palate is not influenced by overall facial attractiveness. Cleft Palate Craniofac J. 2016;53:e45–52.

Koh KS, Kang BS, Seo DW. Speech evaluation after repair of unilateral complete cleft palate using modified 2-flap palatoplasty. J Craniofac Surg. 2009;20:111–4.

Kriens OB. An anatomical approach to veloplasty. Plast Reconstr Surg. 1969;43:29–41.

Kuijpers MA, Chiu YT, Nada RM, Carels CE, Fudalej PS. Three-dimensional imaging methods for quantitative analysis of facial soft tissues and skeletal morphology in patients with orofacial clefts: a systematic review. PLoS One. 2014;9:e93442.

Kuijpers-Jagtman AM, Nollet PJ, Semb G, Bronkhorst EM, Shaw WC, Katsaros C. Reference photographs for nasolabial appearance rating in unilateral cleft lip and palate. J Craniofac Surg. 2009;20:1683–6.

Kumar A, Gabbay JS, Nikjoo R, Heller JB, O'Hara CM, Sisodia M, Garri JI, Wilson LS, Kawamoto HK Jr, Bradley JP. Improved outcomes in cleft patients with severe maxillary deficiency after Le Fort I internal distraction. Plast Reconstr Surg. 2006;117:1499–509.

Kummer AW. Speech evaluation for patients with cleft palate. Clin Plast Surg. 2014;41:241–51.

Lai LH, Hui BK, Nguyen PD, Yee KS, Martz MG, Bradley JP, Lee JC. Lateral incisor agenesis predicts maxillary hypoplasia and Le Fort I advancement surgery in cleft patients. Plast Reconstr Surg. 2015;135:142e–8e.

Landheer JA, Breugem CC, van der Molen AB. Fistula incidence and predictors of fistula occurrence after cleft palate repair: two-stage closure versus one-stage closure. Cleft Palate Craniofac J. 2010;47:623–30.

LaRossa D, Jackson OH, Kirschner RE, Low DW, Solot CB, Cohen MA, Mayro R, Wang P, Minugh-Purvis N, Randall P. The Children's Hospital of Philadelphia modification of the Furlow double-opposing z-palatoplasty: long-term speech and growth results. Clin Plast Surg. 2004;31:243–9.

Lee YH, Liao YF. Hard palate-repair technique and facial growth in patients with cleft lip and palate: a systematic review. Br J Oral Maxillofac Surg. 2013;51:851–7.

Lee JC, Slack GC, Walker R, Graves L, Yen S, Woo J, Ambaram R, Martz MG, Kawamoto HK Jr, Bradley JP. Maxillary hypoplasia in the cleft patient: contribution of orthodontic dental space closure to orthognathic surgery. Plast Reconstr Surg. 2014;133:355–61.

Lee A, Gibbon FE, Spivey K. Children's attitudes toward peers with unintelligible speech associated with cleft lip and/or palate. Cleft Palate Craniofac J. 2017;54(3):262–8.

Liao YF, Mars M. Hard palate repair timing and facial growth in cleft lip and palate: a systematic review. Cleft Palate Craniofac J. 2006;43:563–70.

Liao YF, Yang IY, Wang R, Yun C, Huang CS. Two-stage palate repair with delayed hard palate closure is related to favorable maxillary growth in unilateral cleft lip and palate. Plast Reconstr Surg. 2010;125:1503–10.

Lilja J, Mars M, Elander A, Enocson L, Hagberg C, Worrell E, Batra P, Friede H. Analysis of dental arch relationships in Swedish unilateral cleft lip and palate subjects: 20-year longitudinal consecutive series treated with delayed hard palate closure. Cleft Palate Craniofac J. 2006;43:606–11.

Lohmander A, Friede H, Lilja J. Long-term, longitudinal follow-up of individuals with unilateral cleft lip and palate after the Gothenburg primary early veloplasty and delayed hard palate closure protocol: speech outcome. Cleft Palate Craniofac J. 2012;49:657–71.

Lohmander-Agerskov A. Speech outcome after cleft palate surgery with the Göteborg regimen including delayed hard palate closure. Scand J Plast Reconstr Surg Hand Surg. 1998;32:63–80.

Lohmander-Agerskov A, Söderpalm E, Friede H, Lilja J. A comparison of babbling and speech at pre-speech level, 3, and 5 years of age in children with cleft lip and palate treated with delayed hard palate closure. Folia Phoniatr Logop. 1998;50:320–34.

Long RE Jr, Hathaway R, Daskalogiannakis J, Mercado A, Russell K, Cohen M, Semb G, Shaw W. The Americleft study: an inter-center study of treatment outcomes for patients with unilateral cleft lip and palate part 1. Principles and study design. Cleft Palate Craniofac J. 2011;48:239–43.

Long RE, Wilson-Genderson M, Grayson BH, Flores R, Broder HL (2015) Oral health-related quality of life and self-rated speech in children with existing fistulas in mid-childhood and adolescence. Cleft Palate Craniofac J. [Epub ahead of print].

van Loon B, Maal TJ, Plooij JM, Ingels KJ, Borstlap WA, Kuijpers-Jagtman AM, Spauwen PH, Bergé SJ. 3D Stereophotogrammetric assessment of pre- and postoperative volumetric changes in the cleft lip and palate nose. Int J Oral Maxillofac Surg. 2010;39:534–40.

Losee JE, Smith DM, Afifi AM, Jiang S, Ford M, Vecchione L, Cooper GM, Naran S, Mooney MP, Serletti JM. A successful algorithm for limiting postoperative fistulae following palatal procedures in the patient with orofacial clefting. Plast Reconstr Surg. 2008;122:544–54.

Losken HW, van Aalst JA, Teotia SS, Dean SB, Hultman S, Uhrich KS. Achieving low cleft palate fistula rates: surgical results and techniques. Cleft Palate Craniofac J. 2011;48:312–20.

Lu Y, Shi B, Zheng Q, Hu Q, Wang Z. Incidence of palatal fistula after palatoplasty with levator veli palatini retropositioning according to Sommerlad. Br J Oral Maxillofac Surg. 2010;48:637–40.

Marrinan EM, LaBrie RA, Mulliken JB. Velopharyngeal function in nonsyndromic cleft palate: relevance of surgical technique, age at repair, and cleft type. Cleft Palate Craniofac J. 1998;35:95–100.

Mars M, Plint DA, Houston WJ, Bergland O, Semb G. The Goslon Yardstick: a new system of assessing dental arch relationships in children with unilateral clefts of the lip and palate. Cleft Palate J. 1987;24:314–22.

McIntyre JK, Sethi H, Schönbrunner A, Proudfoot J, Jones M, Gosman A. Number of surgical procedures for patients with cleft lip and palate from birth to 21 years old at a single children's hospital. Ann Plast Surg. 2016;76:S205–8.

McKearney RM, Williams JV, Mercer NS. Quantitative computer-based assessment of lip symmetry following cleft lip repair. Cleft Palate Craniofac J. 2013;50:138–43.

Mercado A, Russell K, Hathaway R, Daskalogiannakis J, Sadek H, Long RE Jr, Cohen M, Semb G, Shaw W. The Americleft study: an inter-center study of treatment outcomes for patients with unilateral cleft lip and palate part 4. Nasolabial aesthetics. Cleft Palate Craniofac J. 2011;48:259–64.

Meyer-Marcotty P, Gerdes AB, Reuther T, Stellzig-Eisenhauer A, Alpers GW. Persons with cleft lip and palate are looked at differently. J Dent Res. 2010;89:400–4.

Millar K, Bell A, Bowman A, Brown D, Lo TW, Siebert P, Simmons D, Ayoub A. Psychological status as a function of residual scarring and facial asymmetry after surgical repair of cleft lip and palate. Cleft Palate Craniofac J. 2013;50:150–7.

Moar KK, Sweet C, Beale V. Fistula rate after primary palatal repair with intravelarveloplasty: a retrospective three-year audit of six units (NorCleft) in the UK. Br J Oral Maxillofac Surg. 2016;54(6):634–7.

Mølsted K, Brattström V, Prahl-Andersen B, Shaw WC, Semb G. The Eurocleft study: intercenter study of treatment outcome in patients with complete cleft lip and palate. Part 3: dental arch relationships. Cleft Palate Craniofac J. 2005;42:78–82.

Mommaerts MY, Combes FA, Drake D. The Furlow Z-plasty in two-staged palatal repair modifications and complications. Br J Oral Maxillofac Surg. 2006;44:94–9.

Morrant DG, Shaw WC. Use of standardized video recordings to assess cleft surgery outcome. Cleft Palate Craniofac J. 1996;33:134–42.

Mosmuller DG, Griot JP, Bijnen CL, Niessen FB. Scoring systems of cleft-related facial deformities: a review of literature. Cleft Palate Craniofac J. 2013;50:286–96.

Mosmuller DG, Bijnen CL, Don Griot JP, Kramer GJ, Disse MA, Prahl C, Kuik DJ, Niessen FB. Comparison of two scoring systems in the assessment of nasolabial appearance in cleft lip and palate patients. J Craniofac Surg. 2014;25:1222–5.

Mosmuller DG, Bijnen CL, Kramer GJ, Disse MA, Prahl C, Kuik DJ, Niessen FB, Don Griot JP. The Asher-McDade aesthetic index in comparison with two scoring systems in nonsyndromic complete unilateral cleft lip and palate patients. J Craniofac Surg. 2015;26:1242–5.

Nagy K, Mommaerts MY. Analysis of the cleft-lip nose in submental-vertical view, part I--reliability of a new measurement instrument. J Craniomaxillofac Surg. 2007;35:265–77.

Nardini G, Flores RL. A systematic review comparing furlow double-opposing z-plasty and straight-line intravelar veloplasty methods of cleftpalate repair. Plast Reconstr Surg. 2015;135:927e–8e.

Noordhoff MS, Kuo J, Wang F, Huang H, Witzel MA. Development of articulation before delayed hard-palate closurein children with cleft palate: a cross-sectional study. Plast Reconstr Surg. 1987;80:518–24.

Ohannessian P, Berggren A, Abdiu A. The cleft lip evaluation profile (CLEP): a new approach for postoperative nasolabial assessment in patients with unilateral cleft lip and palate. J Plast Surg Hand Surg. 2011;45:8–13.

Parwaz MA, Sharma RK, Parashar A, Nanda V, Biswas G, Makkar S. Width of cleft palate and postoperative palatal fistula--do they correlate? J Plast Reconstr Aesthet Surg. 2009;62:1559–63.

Persson M, Sandy JR, Waylen A, Wills AK, Al-Ghatam R, Ireland AJ, Hall AJ, Hollingworth W, Jones T, Peters TJ, Preston R, Sell D, Smallridge J, Worthington H, Ness AR. A cross-sectional survey of 5-year-old children with non-syndromic unilateral cleft lip and palate: the Cleft Care UK study. Part 1: background and methodology. Orthod Craniofac Res. 2015;18(Suppl 2):1–13.

Phillips JH, Nish I, Daskalogiannakis J. Orthognathic surgery in cleft patients. Plast Reconstr Surg. 2012;129:535e–48e.

Phua YS, de Chalain T. Incidence of oronasal fistulae and velopharyngeal insufficiency after cleft palate repair: an audit of 211 children born between 1990 and 2004. Cleft Palate Craniofac J. 2008;45:172–8.

Pigott R, Pigott B. Quantitative measurement of symmetry from photographs following surgery for unilateral cleft lip and palate. Cleft Palate Craniofac J. 2010;47:363–7.

Polzer I, Breitsprecher L, Winter K, Biffar R. Videoendoscopic, speech and hearing in cleft palate children after levator-palatopharyngeus surgery according to Kriens. J Craniomaxillofac Surg. 2006;34:52–6.

Pradel W, Senf D, Mai R, Ludicke G, Eckelt U, Lauer G. One-stage palate repair improves speech outcome and early maxillary growth in patients with cleft lip and palate. J Physiol Pharmacol. 2009;60(Suppl 8):37–41.

Prahl C, Prahl-Andersen B, van't Hof MA, Kuijpers-Jagtman AM. Infant orthopedics and facial appearance: a randomized clinical trial (Dutchcleft). Cleft Palate Craniofac J. 2006;43:659–64.

Randag AC, Dreise MM, Ruettermann M. Surgical impact and speech outcome at 2.5 years after one- or two-stage cleft palate closure. Int J Pediatr Otorhinolaryngol. 2014;78:1903–7.

Ranganathan K, Vercler CJ, Warschausky SA, MacEachern MP, Buchman SR, Waljee JF. Comparative effectiveness studies examining patient-reported outcomes among children with cleft lip and/or palate: a systematic review. Plast Reconstr Surg. 2015;135:198–211.

Raposo do Amaral CA, Sabbag A, Ferreira LA, Almeida AB, Buzzo CL, Raposo do Amaral CE. Dissecção radical da musculatura do véu palatino em casos secundários de pacientes fissurados. Rev Bras Cir Plást. 2009;24:432–6.

Raposo-Amaral CE, Raposo-Amaral CA. Changing face of cleft care: specialized centers in developing countries. J Craniofac Surg. 2012;23:206–9.

Raposo-Amaral CE, Raposo-Amaral CM, Raposo-Amaral CA, Chahal H, Bradley JP, Jarrahy R. Age at surgery significantly impacts the amount of orbital relapse following hypertelorbitism correction: a 30-year longitudinal study. Plast Reconstr Surg. 2011;127:1620–30.

Raposo-Amaral CE, Giancolli AP, Denadai R, Marques FF, Somensi RS, Raposo-Amaral CA, Alonso N. Lip height improvement during the first year of unilateral complete cleft lip repair using cutting extended Mohler Technique. Plast Surg Int. 2012;2012:206481.

Raposo-Amaral CE, Denadai R, Camargo DN, Artioli TO, Gelmini Y, Buzzo CL, Raposo-Amaral CA. Parry-Romberg syndrome: severity of the deformity does not correlate with quality of life. Aesthet Plast Surg. 2013;37:792–801.

Raposo-Amaral CE, Giancolli AP, Denadai R, Somensi RS, Raposo-Amaral CA. Late cutaneous lip height in unilateral incomplete cleft lip patients does not differ from the normative data. J Craniofac Surg. 2014;25:308–13.

Raposo-do-Amaral CA. Uso do retalho miomucoso do músculo bucinador bilateral para o tratamento de insuficiência velofaríngea: avaliação preliminar. Rev Bras Cir Plást. 2013;28:455–661.

Raposo-do-Amaral CA, Raposo-do-Amaral CE, Carone DR, Pinheiro AF, Braga EV, Guidi MC, Buzzo CL. Study of the maxillary advancement and complications in cleft and non-cleft patients underwent to orthognathic surgery. Rev Bras Cir Plást. 2008;23:263–7.

Richard B, Russell J, McMahon S, Pigott R. Results of randomized controlled trial of soft palate first versus hard palate first repair in unilateral complete cleft lip and palate. Cleft Palate Craniofac J. 2006;43:329–38.

Richards H, van Bommel A, Clark V, Richard B. Are cleft palate fistulae a cause of dental decay? Cleft Palate Craniofac J. 2015;52:341–5.

Rohrich RJ, Gosman AA. An update on the timing of hard palate closure: a critical long-term analysis. Plast Reconstr Surg. 2004;113:350–2.

Rohrich RJ, Rowsell AR, Johns DF. Timing of hard palatal closure: a critical long-term analysis. Plast Reconstr Surg. 1996;98:236–46.

Rohrich RJ, Love EJ, Byrd HS, Johns DF. Optimal timing of cleft palate closure. Plast Reconstr Surg. 2000;106:413–21.

Rossell-Perry P, Caceres Nano E, Gavino-Gutierrez AM. Association between palatal index and cleft palate repair outcomes in patients with complete unilateral cleft lip and palate. JAMA Facial Plast Surg. 2014;16:206–10.

Rubin MS, Lowe KM, Clouston S, Shetye PR, Warren SM, Grayson BH. Basal view reference photographs for nasolabial appearance rating in unilateral cleft lip and palate. J Craniofac Surg. 2015;26:1548–50.

Russell K, Long RE Jr, Hathaway R, Daskalogiannakis J, Mercado A, Cohen M, Semb G, Shaw W. The Americleft study: an inter-center study of treatment outcomes for patients with unilateral cleft lip and palate part 5. General discussion and conclusions. Cleft Palate Craniofac J. 2011;48:265–70.

Sadove AM, van Aalst JA, Culp JA. Cleft palate repair: art and issues. Clin Plast Surg. 2004;31:231–41.

Salimi N, Aleksejūnienė J, Yen EH, Loo AY. Fistula in cleft lip and palate patients-a systematic scoping review. Ann Plast Surg. 2017;78(1):91–102.

Salyer KE, Sng KW, Sperry EE. Two-flap palatoplasty: 20-year experience and evolution of surgical technique. Plast Reconstr Surg. 2006;118:193–204.

Sandy JR, Williams AC, Bearn D, Mildinhall S, Murphy T, Sell D, Murray JJ, Shaw WC, Cleft lip and palate care in the United Kingdom--the Clinical Standards Advisory Group (CSAG) Study. Part 1: background and methodology. Cleft Palate Craniofac J. 2001;38:20–3.

Schönmeyr B, Wendby L, Sharma M, Raud-Westberg L, Restrepo C, Campbell A. Limited chances of speech improvement after late cleft palate repair. J Craniofac Surg. 2015;26:1182–5.

Schweckendiek W, Doz P. Primary veloplasty: long-term results without maxillary deformity. A twenty-five year report. Cleft Palate J. 1978;15:268–74.

Scott JK, Leary SD, Ness AR, Sandy JR, Persson M, Kilpatrick N, Waylen AE. Centralization of services for children born with orofacial clefts in the United kingdom: a cross-sectional survey. Cleft Palate Craniofac J. 2014;51:e102–9.

Sell D, Grunwell P, Mildinhall S, Murphy T, Cornish TA, Bearn D, Shaw WC, Murray JJ, Williams AC, Sandy JR. Cleft lip and palate care in the United Kingdom--the Clinical Standards Advisory Group (CSAG) Study. Part 3: speech outcomes. Cleft Palate Craniofac J. 2001;38:30–7.

Sell D, Mildinhall S, Albery L, Wills AK, Sandy JR, Ness AR. The Cleft Care UK study. Part 4: perceptual speech outcomes. Orthod Craniofac Res. 2015;18(Suppl 2):36–46.

Semb G. A study of facial growth in patients with unilateral cleft lip and palate treated by the Oslo CLP Team. Cleft Palate Craniofac J. 1991;28:1–21.

Semb G, Brattström V, Mølsted K, Prahl-Andersen B, Shaw WC. The Eurocleft study: intercenter study of treatment outcome in patients with complete cleft lip and palate. Part 1: introduction and treatment experience. Cleft Palate Craniofac J. 2005a;42:64–8.

Semb G, Brattström V, Mølsted K, Prahl-Andersen B, Zuurbier P, Rumsey N, Shaw WC. The Eurocleft study: intercenter study of treatment outcome in patients with complete cleft lip and palate. Part 4: relationship among treatment outcome, patient/parent satisfaction, and the burden of care. Cleft Palate Craniofac J. 2005b;42:83–92.

Sharma VP, Bella H, Cadier MM, Pigott RW, Goodacre TE, Richard BM. Outcomes in facial aesthetics in cleft lip and palate surgery: a systematic review. J Plast Reconstr Aesthet Surg. 2012;65:1233–45.

Shaw WC, Semb G, Nelson P, Brattström V, Mølsted K, Prahl-Andersen B, Gundlach KK. The Eurocleft project 1996-2000: overview. J Craniomaxillofac Surg. 2001;29:131–40.

Shaw WC, Brattström V, Mølsted K, Prahl-Andersen B, Roberts CT, Semb G. The Eurocleft study: intercenter study of treatment outcome in patients with complete cleft lip and palate. Part 5: discussion and conclusions. Cleft Palate Craniofac J. 2005;42:93–8.

Shaye D. Update on outcomes research for cleft lip and palate. Curr Opin Otolaryngol Head Neck Surg. 2014;22:255–9.

Shi B, Losee JE. The impact of cleft lip and palate repair on maxillofacial growth. Int J Oral Sci. 2015;7:14–7.

Sitzman TJ, Allori AC, Thorburn G. Measuring outcomes in cleft lip and palate treatment. Clin Plast Surg. 2014;41:311–9.

Smallridge J, Hall AJ, Chorbachi R, Parfect V, Persson M, Ireland AJ, Wills AK, Ness AR, Sandy JR. Functional outcomes in the Cleft Care UK study--part 3: oral health and audiology. Orthod Craniofac Res. 2015;18(Suppl 2):25–35.

Smith B, Guyette TW. Evaluation of cleft palate speech. Clin Plast Surg. 2004;31:251–60.

Smith DM, Losee JE. Cleft palate repair. Clin Plast Surg. 2014;41:189–210.

Smith DM, Vecchione L, Jiang S, Ford M, Deleyiannis FW, Haralam MA, Naran S, Worrall CI, Dudas JR, Afifi AM, Marazita ML, Losee JE. The Pittsburgh Fistula Classification System: a standardized scheme for the description of palatal fistulas. Cleft Palate Craniofac J. 2007;44:590–4.

Sommerlad BC. A technique for cleft palate repair. Plast Reconstr Surg. 2003;112:1542–8.

Sommerlad BC, Mehendale FV, Birch MJ, Sell D, Hattee C, Harland K. Palate re-repair revisited. Cleft Palate Craniofac J. 2002;39:295–307.

Stebel A, Desmedt D, Bronkhorst E, Kuijpers MA, Fudalej PS. Rating nasolabial appearance on three-dimensional images in cleft lip and palate: a comparison with standard photographs. Eur J Orthod. 2016;38:197–201.

Sullivan SR, Marrinan EM, LaBrie RA, Rogers GF, Mulliken JB. Palatoplasty outcomes in nonsyndromic patients with cleft palate: a 29-year assessment of one surgeon's experience. J Craniofac Surg. 2009;20(Suppl 1):612–6.

Sullivan SR, Jung YS, Mulliken JB. Outcomes of cleft palatal repair for internationally adopted children. Plast Reconstr Surg. 2014;133:1445–52.

Susarla SM, Berli JU, Kumar A. Midfacial volumetric and upper lip soft tissue changes after Le Fort I advancement of the cleft maxilla. J Oral Maxillofac Surg. 2015;73:708–18.

Timbang MR, Gharb BB, Rampazzo A, Papay F, Zins J, Doumit G. A systematic review comparing Furlow double-opposing Z-plasty and straight-line intravelar veloplasty methods of cleft palate repair. Plast Reconstr Surg. 2014;134:1014–22.

Tobiasen JM, Hiebert JM. Facial impairment scales for clefts. Plast Reconstr Surg. 1994;93:31–41.

Tobiasen JM, Hiebert JM, Boraz RA. Development of scales of severity of facial cleft impairment. Cleft Palate Craniofac J. 1991;28:419–24.

Trotman CA, Faraway JJ, Essick GK. Three-dimensional nasolabial displacement during movement in repaired cleft lip and palate patients. Plast Reconstr Surg. 2000;105:1273–83.

Trotman CA, Faraway JJ, Losken HW, van Aalst JA. Functional outcomes of cleft lip surgery. Part II: quantification of nasolabial movement. Cleft Palate Craniofac J. 2007;44:607–16.

Trotman CA, Phillips C, Faraway JJ, Hartman T, van Aalst JA. Influence of objective three-dimensional measures and movement images on surgeon treatment planning for lip revision surgery. Cleft Palate Craniofac J. 2013;50:684–95.

Van Lierde KM, Monstrey S, Bonte K, Van Cauwenberge P, Vinck B. The long-term speech outcome in Flemish young adults after twodifferent types of palatoplasty. Int J Pediatr Otorhinolaryngol. 2004;68:865–75.

Vasudavan S, Jayaratne YS, Padwa BL. Nasolabial soft tissue changes after Le Fort I advancement. J Oral Maxillofac Surg. 2012;70:e270–7.

Waylen A, Ness AR, Wills AK, Persson M, Rumsey N, Sandy JR. Cleft Care UK study. Part 5: child psychosocial outcomes and satisfaction with cleft services. Orthod Craniofac Res. 2015;18(Suppl 2):47–55.

Willadsen E. Influence of timing of hard palate repair in a two-stage procedure on early language development in Danish children with cleft palate. Cleft Palate Craniofac J. 2012;49:574–95.

Williams WN, Seagle MB, Nackashi AJ, Marks R, Boggs SR, Kemker J, Wharton W, Bzoch KR, Dixon-Wood V, Pegoraro-Krook MI, de Souza Freitas JA, Garla LA, de Souza TV, Silva ML, Neto JS, Montagnoli LC, Martinelli AP, Marques IL, Zimmerman MC, Feniman MB, de Azevedo Bento Gonçalves CG, Piazentin SH, Graciano MI, Chinellato MC, Jorge JC, et al. A methodology report of a randomized prospective clinical trial to assess velopharyngeal function for speech following palatal surgery. Control Clin Trials. 1998;19:297–312.

Williams AC, Bearn D, Mildinhall S, Murphy T, Sell D, Shaw WC, Murray JJ, Sandy JR. Cleft lip and palate care in the United Kingdom--the Clinical Standards Advisory Group (CSAG) Study. Part 2: dentofacial outcomes and patient satisfaction. Cleft Palate Craniofac J. 2001;38:24–9.

Williams WN, Seagle MB, Pegoraro-Krook MI, Souza TV, Garla L, Silva ML, Machado Neto JS, Dutka JC, Nackashi J, Boggs S, Shuster J, Moorhead J, Wharton W, Graciano MI, Pimentel MC, Feniman M, Piazentin-Penna SH, Kemker J, Zimmermann MC, Bento-Gonçalvez C, Borgo H, Marques IL, Martinelli AP, Jorge JC, Antonelli P, Neves JF, Whitaker ME. Prospective clinical trial comparing outcome measures between Furlow and von Langenbeck Palatoplasties for UCLP. Ann Plast Surg. 2011;66(2):154–63.

Witt PD, D'Antonio LL. Velopharyngeal insufficiency and secondary palatal management: a new look at an old problem. Clin Plast Surg. 1993;20:707–21.

Witt PD, Wahlen JC, Marsh JL, Grames LM, Pilgram TK. The effect of surgeon experience on velopharyngeal functional outcome following palatoplasty: is there a learning curve? Plast Reconstr Surg. 1998;102:1375–84.

Witzel MA, Salyer KE, Ross RB. Delayed hard palate closure: the philosophy revisited. Cleft Palate J. 1984;21:263–9.

Wong JY, Oh AK, Ohta E, Hunt AT, Rogers GF, Mulliken JB, Deutsch CK. Validity and reliability of craniofacial anthropometric measurement of 3D digital photogrammetric images. Cleft Palate Craniofac J. 2008;45:232–9.

Xu X, Kwon HJ, Shi B, Zheng Q, Yin H, Li C. Influence of different palate repair protocols onfacial growth in unilateral complete cleft lip and palate. J Craniomaxillofac Surg. 2015;43:43–7.

Yamaguchi K, Lonic D, Lo LJ. Complications following orthognathic surgery for patients with cleft lip/palate: a systematic review. J Formos Med Assoc. 2016;115:269–77.

Yamanishi T, Nishio J, Kohara H, Hirano Y, Sako M, Yamanishi Y, Adachi T, Miya S, Mukai T. Effect on maxillary arch development of early 2-stage palatoplasty by modified furlow technique and conventional 1-stage palatoplasty in children with complete unilateral cleft lip and palate. J Oral Maxillofac Surg. 2009;67:2210–6.

Yamanishi T, Nishio J, Sako M, Kohara H, Hirano Y, Yamanishi Y, Adachi T, Miya S, Mukai T. Early two-stage double opposing Z-plasty or one-stage push-back palatoplasty?: comparisons in maxillary development and speech outcome at 4 years of age. Ann Plast Surg. 2011;66:148–53.

Yang IY, Liao YF. The effect of 1-stage versus 2-stage palate repair on facial growth in patients with cleft lip and palate: a review. Int J Oral Maxillofac Surg. 2010;39:945–50.

Yu CC, Chen PK, Chen YR. Comparison of speech results after Furlow palatoplasty and von Langenbeck palatoplasty in incomplete cleft of the secondary palate. Chang Gung Med J. 2001;24:628–32.

Yuan N, Dorafshar AH, Follmar KE, Pendleton C, Ferguson K, Redett RJ 3rd. Effects of cleft width and veau type on incidence of palatal fistula and velopharyngeal insufficiency after cleft palate repair. Ann Plast Surg. 2016;76:406–10.

Zemann W, Kärcher H, Drevenšek M, Koželj V. Sagittal maxillary growth in children with unilateral cleft of the lip, alveolus and palate at the age of 10 years: an inter centre comparison. J Craniomaxillofac Surg. 2011;39:469–74.

Zhu S, Jayaraman J, Khambay B. Evaluation of facial appearance in patients with cleft lip and palate by laypeople and professionals: a systematic literature review. Cleft Palate Craniofac J. 2016;53:187–96.

Unilateral Cleft Lip Repair

7

Cassio Eduardo Raposo-Amaral and Nivaldo Alonso

7.1 Introduction: Overview of the History of Unilateral Cheiloplasty

The history of cleft surgery overrides the history of plastic surgery. The principles outlined for the manipulation of the soft tissues in patients with cleft lip and palate gradually evolved and integrated to the arsenal of principles of modern plastic surgery. The first surgical attempts to correct a cleft lip and palate date from 390 BC year in China, and were carried out with the approximation of the cleft margins (Boo 1966). In the early fourteenth century, Jehan Yperman was the first to describe in detail the primary unilateral and bilateral cheiloplasty (Millard 1976). In 1564, Ambroise Paré illustrated the procedure used to obtain a straight-line closure of cleft lip (Millard 1976) and subsequently wrote the principles of plastic surgery, stating that "surgery is an art" (Paré 1964). In 1597, Gaspar Tagliacozzi described with illustrations surgical steps of primary cheiloplasty (Gnudi and Wester 1976). In the eighteenth century, Lorenz Heister, in his treatise named "*Chirurgie*," emphasized the need for delicate surgical instruments in the proper handling of cleft lip (Millard 1976). In 1843, Malgaigne described the primary cheiloplasty principles with local flaps, and in the following year, Mirault modified Malgaigne technique utilizing lateral segment flaps to establish length of the medial cleft segment (Malgaigne 1861; Mirault 1884).

C.E. Raposo-Amaral, M.D., Ph.D. (✉)
Institute of Plastic and Craniofacial Surgery, SOBRAPAR Hospital,
Campinas, São Paulo 13084-880, Brazil

Universidade de São Paulo, São Paulo, Brazil
e-mail: cassioraposo@hotmail.com

N. Alonso, M.D., Ph.D.
Divisao de Cirurgia Plastica e Queimaduras, Hospital das Clínicas da Faculdade de Medicina da Universidade de São Paulo, São Paulo, Brazil

© Springer International Publishing AG 2018
N. Alonso, C.E. Raposo-Amaral (eds.), *Cleft Lip and Palate Treatment*,
https://doi.org/10.1007/978-3-319-63290-2_7

William Rose, in 1879, described the use of curvilinear incision along the lateral segment from alar base to lip vermilion in order to preserve tissue during cheiloplasty (Rose 1891) and was credited to be the first to observe the necessity to bow the incision in the prolabium to decrease scar contraction and vermilion notch (Rose 1891). James Thompson pointed out the need to build the cleft philtrum column that mirrors the contralateral side and emphasized the importance of repositioning of the alar base (Thompson 1912).

The primary cheiloplasty was constantly evolving and there were still many unanswered questions. At the time, the results showed a short lip and nose with the remaining deformity with cleft stigmata. There was a great avenue for innovation and refinement on cheiloplasty techniques.

Blair and Robinson also made their contributions describing the straight-line cheiloplasty (Blair and Robinson 1948; Blair and Letterman 1950). Nasal region remained as an anatomical paradigm in the lip surgery. It was believed that nasal approach would impair its growth. The first attempt to create a Cupid bow arch was described by Hagedorn (1892). Le-Mesurier in 1949 described a quadrangular flap to fill the medial element and recreate the Cupid bow (LeMesurier 1949).

A Brazilian plastic surgeon described in 1952 a cheiloplasty technique using triangular flaps with preservation of Cupid bow (Cardoso 1952). The Cardoso's concept of a triangular lip repair led Tennison to publish in 1954 the important principles of primary cheiloplasty with *orbicularis oris muscle* repositioning and execution of triangular flaps at the cleft lip margins to avoid scar contraction and lip deformity (Tennison 1952). Interestingly, the principles described by Tennison resisted the span of time and are still being used by some plastic surgeons who adopt the triangular cleft lip repair technique.

Randall modified the Tennison technique changing the direction of the triangular flaps and decreased the number of scars crossing the philtrum dimple (Randall 1959, 1986).

Spina realized important contributions to the field of cleft lip repair as he described the most important classification of cleft lip and palate used in Brazil as well as a cheiloplasty technique using triangular flaps (Spina and Lodovici 1960; Spina et al. 1972). His technique of correcting the bilateral cleft is still being used in most cleft centers in Brazil.

Ralph Millard and Sir Harold Gillies delineated the modern principles of plastic surgery in their famous tretise.[19] Millard developed during the Korean War the principles of primary cheiloplasty based on the rotation and advancement, which is the most popular technique to date worldwide, and his results were presented in 1955 during the International Plastic Surgery Congress held in Stockholm (Millard 1986). After his presentation, Millard was strongly criticized being said that the technique was obsolete (Millard 2003). In the same year, some surgeons in the world have recognized the significant impact of the rotation advancement technique. Millard technique has a significant advantage in comparison to the others, since it allows individual adaptations and modification considering the severity of cleft deformity and surgeon creativity. The principles of the rotation and advancement described by Millard are now widely used throughout the world.

In 1987, Mohler described a modification of Millard technique using a smaller C flap and extended the incision 2 mm vertically in the nasal region, allowing elongation of the columella (Mohler 1987; Cutting and Dayan 2003; Xu et al. 2009). In the Mohler description, the Millard back-cut incision does not extend beyond the contralateral philtral column and generates a straight-line scar that mirrors the contralateral philtrum column direction (Mohler 1987; Cutting and Dayan 2003).

7.2 Primary Rhinoplasty

The primary surgery of the nose started almost four decades ago with the principles of cartilage repositioning. In the early 1970s, Salyer developed the principles of undermining and repositioning the alar cartilages and since that period many authors gradually broke the paradigm that early surgery of the nose would prevent the facial and nasal growth (Xu et al. 2009).

In 1975, McComb emphasized the need for primary rhinoplasty during lip repair by suturing the alar cartilages at a higher anatomical point of the triangular cartilages, providing an overcorrection of anatomical structures (McComb 1975). Currently in Brazil, the vast majority of surgeons working with cleft patients admit the importance of primary rhinoplasty during primary lip repair.

Millard initially placed little emphasis on the nose. The columella "C" flap was built to lengthen the columella and recreate the nasal floor (Millard 1960). After a few years of experience with the rotation advancement technique, the author recognized the importance of increasing efforts in surgical nasal region by proposing maneuvers to improve the alar cartilage positioning, suturing the superior region of quadrangular cartilage and the alar cartilages together, and repositioning the incision on the nasal floor (Millard and Morovic 1998).

Surgical modifications of Cutting and Mulliken for primary rhinoplasty provided a significant improvement in nasal symmetry of cleft patients (Cutting 1994; Wong et al. 2002; Mulliken and Martinez-Pérez 1999). Cutting changed the McComb stitches by using a horizontal mattress suture to elevate the dome and the medial crus of the alar cartilage (Cutting 1994). Mulliken completely undermines the entire region of the alar cartilage and places it in a more anatomically appropriate region. Additionally, he includes an absorbable plate that prevents the recurrence of nasal deformities (Mulliken and Martinez-Pérez 1999).

Despite the great effort to obtain the nasal symmetry there is always a great tendency to recurrence of nasal deformity at the dome and at the nasal floor by the lateral displacement of the nasal base.

7.3 Anatomical Aspects

The anatomical features of a patient with cleft lip and palate delineate their morphological characteristics, both in complete and in incomplete forms. Therefore, the degree of hypoplasia of the craniofacial skeleton associated with the distance

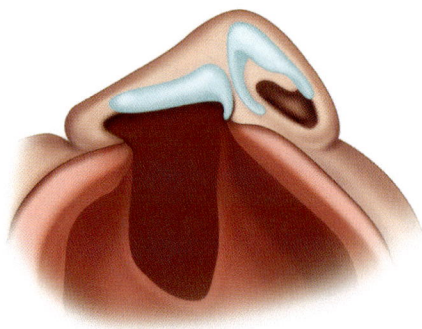
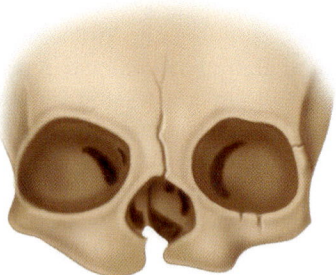

Unilateral complete cleft anatomical aspects

Facial skeleton unilateral

Fig. 7.1 Abnormal anatomic characteristics of soft tissue and skeletal unilateral deformity presented in patients with unilateral complete cleft lip and palate

between the palatine bone plates inherent to the bony cleft leads to a significant distortion in soft-tissue structures, skin, muscle, and cartilage. The main anatomical abnormalities of the nasal region are didactically itemized below:

- The columella is short on the cleft side, and the lateral crus of the alar cartilage and nasal base are posteriorly displaced.
- The base of the columella is deflected to the noncleft side.
- The medial crus of the alar cartilage is shorter in the cleft side and the reflection angle is more obtuse compared to the contralateral side.
- The lateral crus of the alar cartilage is long in the cleft side and deformed in the form of "S" following the asymmetry of the maxillary cleft segment.
- Nasal dome on the cleft side presents a more obtuse angle of reflection compared to the contralateral side.
- The nasal lining is missing or inferiorly located in the cleft side.
- The anterior septum and the anterior nasal spine are deviated to the noncleft side.
- The pyriform aperture can be clefted, without bone continuity, asymmetrically compared to the contralateral side and retro-positioned (Fig. 7.1).

7.4 Surgical Goals

Both authors utilize a variation of Millard repair in their practice. Senior author described his own modification and first author has been using a Cutting-Mohler modification of Millard repair (Stal et al. 2009). Mohler described a more rectilinear incision than the incision generated by Millard and therefore the possibility of using the columellar C flap to fill the space generated by the back-cut incision and rotation of the medial cleft segment (Noordhoff 1984). The final scar tends to mirror the contralateral philtrum column.

7.5 Alonso's Personal Modification of Millard Repair: Markings

The key anatomical points were marked with brilliant green dye. First, the midline and alar contour of the nose and the dome position of both nasal lower lateral cartilages and the transition between dry and wet vermilion were marked. Next, on the medial lip, points of the median tubercle and of the Cupid's bow on the noncleft side and on the cleft side were marked on the white roll. Reference points for the nasal floor were established on the noncleft side, and, by transferring this dimension on the cleft side, other two landmarks were established in this segment. The base of philtrum column on the noncleft side was delimited, observing the philtral column conformation. A rotation incision was marked from the Cupid's bow on the cleft side to the base of the philtral column on the noncleft side and of the medial vertical height, and the marked incision was somewhat arched. Whenever the lip was very short, lengthening at 90° on the philtrum column on the noncleft side was possible, delimiting the rotation flap. An incision on the medial margin of the cleft from the cleft-side Cupid's bow was established delimiting the C flap. On the lateral lip, The Cupid's bow on the cleft side on the white roll coincides with the location in which the narrowing of the vermilion lip begins. Lip height on the noncleft side allows the establishment of the height on the lateral lip. Through a small incision located 1 mm from the naris, the advancement flap was delimited (Figs. 7.2, 7.3, and 7.4; Alonso et al. 2010).

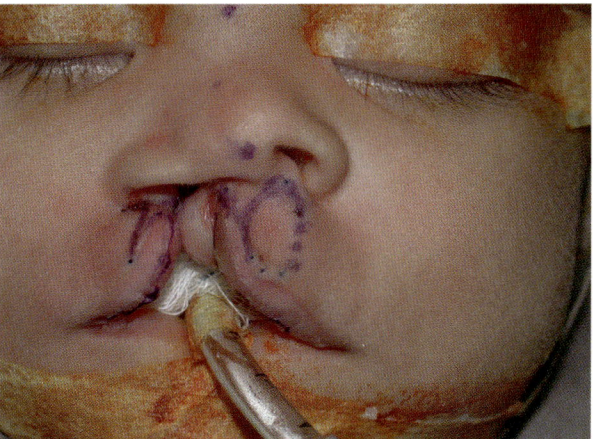

Fig. 7.2 Intraoperative photograph of a patient with right unilateral complete cleft lip and palate showing markings on the medial margin of the cleft from the cleft-side Cupid's bow. On the lateral lip, the Cupid's bow on the cleft side on the white roll coinciding with the location in which the narrowing of the vermilion lip begins. Lip height on the noncleft side allows the establishment of the height on the lateral lip. A rotation incision was marked from the Cupid's bow on the cleft side to the base of the philtral column on the noncleft side and of the medial vertical height, and the marked incision was somewhat arched

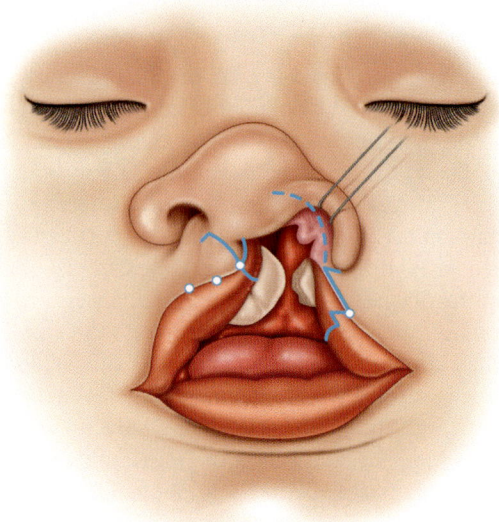

Fig. 7.3 Illustrative drawing showing the markings on medial and lateral lip. A triangular flap is performed in the lip vermilion and markings extent in the nasal vestibular region in the transition of nasal skin and nasal mucosa

7.6 Operative Technique

Initially, on the medial lip, an incision in the cleft margin above the cutaneous roll was made through the skin and subcutaneous tissue and not through the muscle. Cleft marginal tissue was discarded. Dissection of the orbicularis oris muscle from the overlying skin, vermilion, and underlying mucosa was performed. In the skin, to preserve the philtral dimple, the muscle was dissected and limited to 1 mm from the cut edge. Through a small releasing incision in the gingivolabial sulcus, the labial frenulum was sectioned. The orbicularis oris muscle was released from its insertion in the columellar base and from the upper alveolar cleft portion, allowing the exposure of the anterior nasal spine. By positioning the lip and nose, the symmetry between the philtral column and the planned rotation incision was verified. An incision on the previously marked markings was made through the skin creating the rotation and C flap. For those cases in which the downward rotation was insufficient, lengthening on the philtral column could be performed inferiorly.

On the lateral lip, an incision on the cleft margin above the cutaneous roll was made, similarly that it was performed on the medial lip, preserving the

Fig. 7.4 (**a, b**) Pre- and postoperative pictures of Alonso's technique 10 years later showing the stability of the result and good quality of lip scar

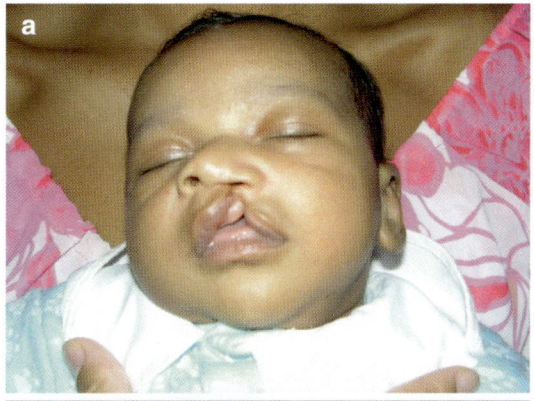

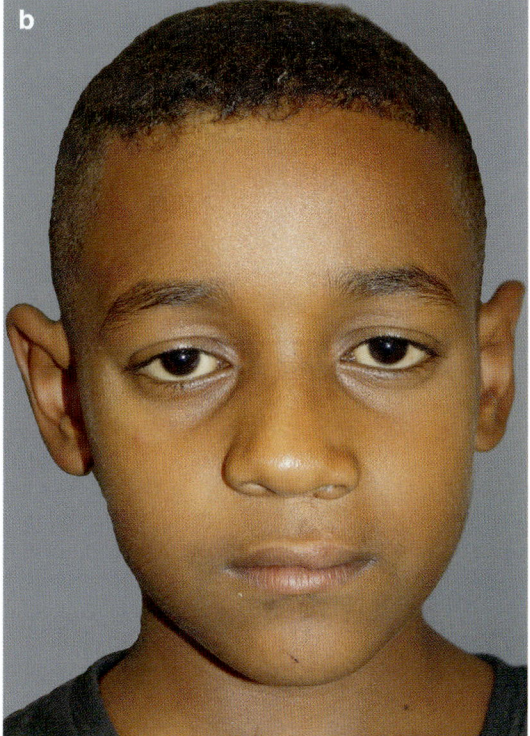

muscle. Below the cutaneous roll, a vermilion flap was created. Cleft marginal tissue was discarded. Dissection of the orbicularis oris muscle from the overlying skin, vermilion, and underlying mucosa was performed. Dissection between the skin and muscle was more extensive in the lateral lip than in the medial lip. Below the alar base, wide dissection of the orbicularis oris muscle was performed. Through an incision in the gingivolabial sulcus, the lip was released relative to the alveolar ridge and to the pyriform aperture. Supraperiosteal dissection on the maxilla released the alar base. Through an intercartilaginous incision, the lateral crus of the lower lateral cartilage and its vestibular portion were released from the posterolateral insertion in the pyriform aperture, allowing anteromedial advancement of the alar base. Cutaneous detachment of the nasal lower lateral cartilages and upper lateral cartilages on the cleft side was performed. After positioning of the cleft-side dome anteromedially, two or three stitches with 5-0 Vicryl (Ethicon, Inc.®, Somerville, NJ) were placed, closing the intercartilaginous incision to maintain the lateral crus advancement of the lower lateral cartilage. To achieve tip symmetry, a U-shaped transdomal suture was made using 5-0 Monocryl (Ethicon, Inc.®). Transfixation sutures around the ala fixed the lower lateral cartilage back, preventing dead space formation. By sectioning the labial frenulum, medial advancement of the mucosa corrected lip height on the medial lip. Closure of medial and lateral mucosa was performed with separate stitches using 5-0 Vicryl. The releasing incision was sutured with two to three stitches of this same thread laterally. The orbicularis oris muscle was sutured with simple stitches using 5-0 Nylon (Ethicon, Inc.®). The nasal band was sutured on the anterior nasal spine, and deep fibers of the vermilion were united. C-flap positioning was adjusted, and the length of the incision delimiting the advancement flap was calculated with a double-hook retraction of the nose and landmark on the cutaneous roll. Regardless of the cleft size, this incision, of short length on all occasions, was positioned 1 mm from the alar base, never exceeding the lateral half of the naris. Three subdermal stitches using 5-0 Monocryl were placed, and, at the end, the cutaneous suture was obtained with simple stitches using 6-0 Vicryl Rapid (Ethicon, Inc.®). Considering the difference of the vermilion height medially and laterally, the laterally based vermilion flap was positioned to correct this difference. By respecting the anatomic reference of the median tubercle, dimension of this flap was modeled, and the flap was medially inserted through a small incision on the transition between the dry and wet vermilion. Suture was obtained with separate stitches using 6-0 Vicryl Rapid, ending the procedure. A silicone nasal stent was placed. An antibiotic ointment was applied to the suture line. The patient was extubated and sent to postanesthetic recovery. Discharge occurred on the first postoperative day. During the first week, the use of bottles and pacifiers was restricted. Outpatient returned at 7, 15, and 30 days and thereafter patients were periodically evaluated with a multidisciplinary approach according to the routine established in the unit (Figs. 7.5, 7.6, 7.7, 7.8, 7.9, 7.10, 7.11, 7.12, and 7.13).

7 Unilateral Cleft Lip Repair

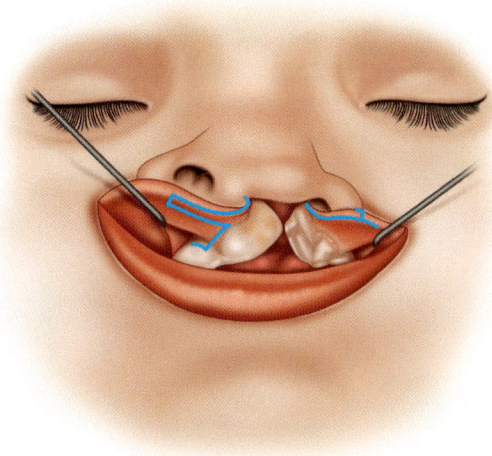

Fig. 7.5 Intraoral view of the markings of Alonso's personal modification of Millard repair

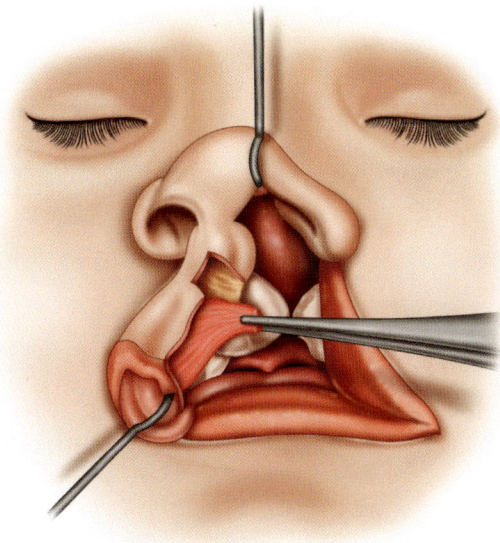

Fig. 7.6 Illustrative drawing showing the dissection of the *orbicularis oris* muscle and the skin back-cut to allow length gain at the medial philtrum column

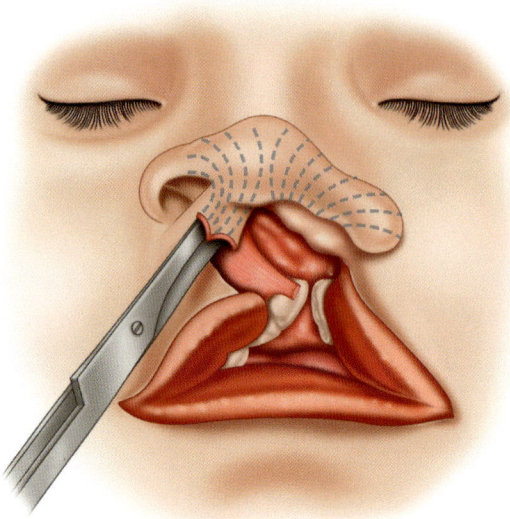

Fig. 7.7 The collumelar incision is used to offer access to the nasal tip and delicate scissor to harvest the medial and lateral crus of the alar cartilage

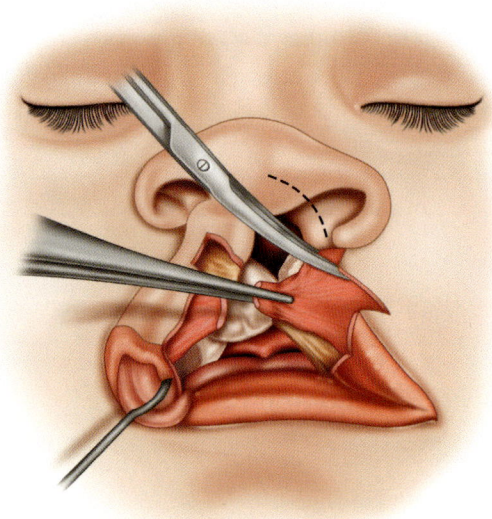

Fig. 7.8 Illustrative drawing showing the rotation of medial and lateral segments and isolation of the *orbicularis oris* muscle

7 Unilateral Cleft Lip Repair

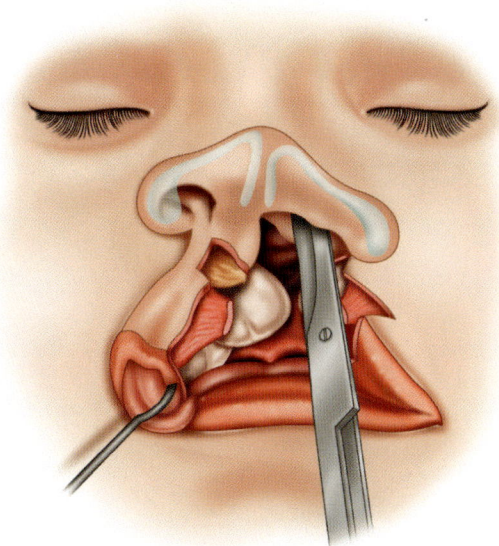

Fig. 7.9 Illustrative drawing showing the upper incision of the lateral segment used to gain acess to lateral crus of lateral cartilage. The wide dissection allow the alar cartilage to be freed of the nasal skin and mucosa and to subsequently be positioned with percutaneous suture

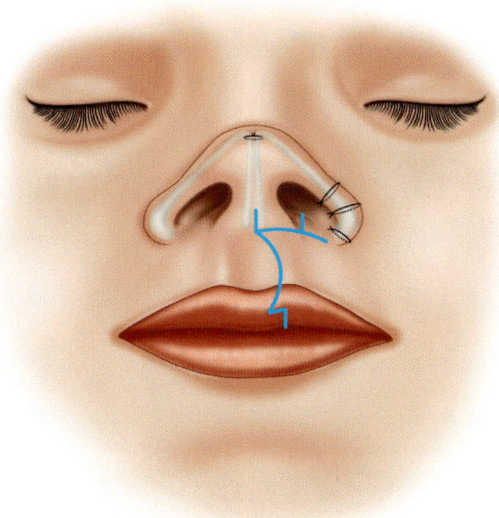

Fig. 7.10 Illustrative drawing showing the final appearance of the lip repair

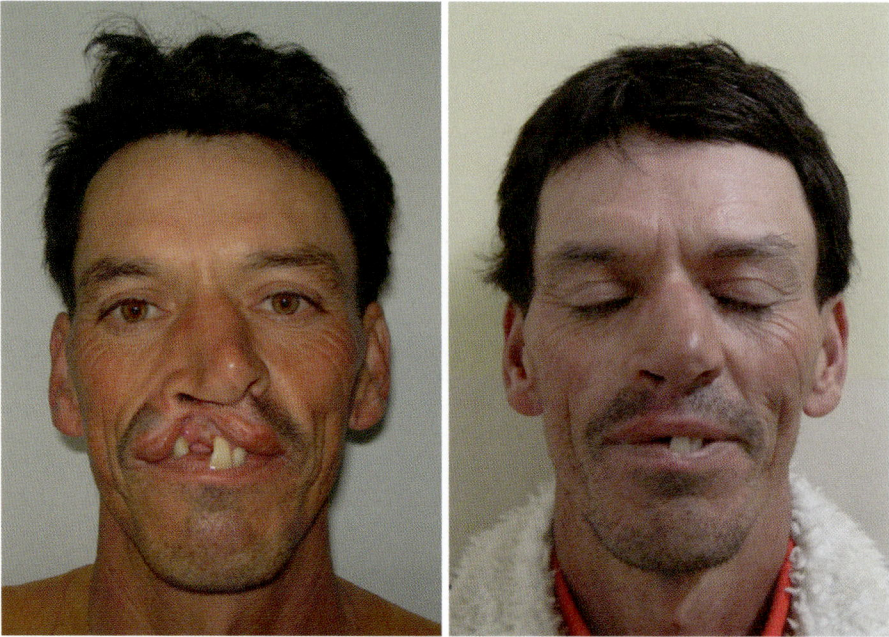

Fig. 7.11 Preoperative frontal photograph of an adult primary right unilateral incomplete cleft lip (*left*). Postoperative photograph of the same patient after Alonso's personal modification of Millard repair (*right*)

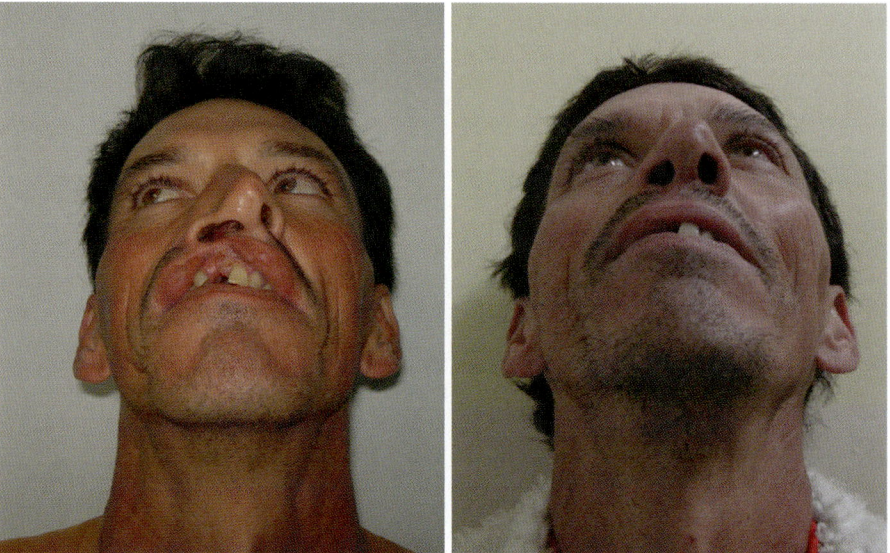

Fig. 7.12 Preoperative basal view photograph of an adult primary right unilateral incomplete cleft lip (*left*). Postoperative basal view photograph of the same patient after Alonso's personal modification of Millard repair (*right*)

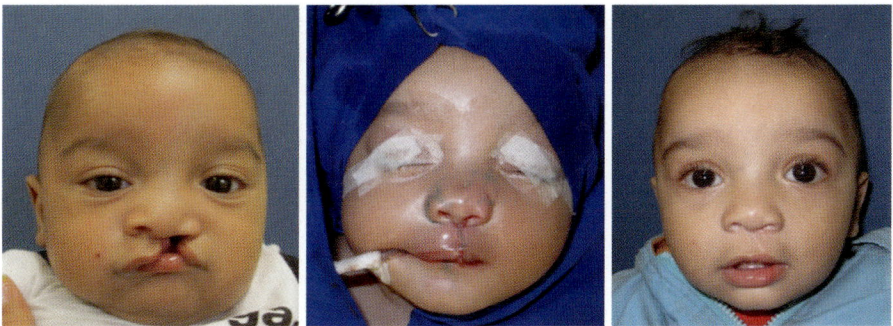

Fig. 7.13 Preoperative frontal photograph of a primary left unilateral complete cleft lip and palate (*left*). Intraoperative frontal view of the same patient (*center*). Postoperative photograph of the same patient after Alonso's personal modification of Millard repair (*right*)

7.7 Mohler Technique

7.7.1 Preoperative Marking

Preoperative marking is performed with methylene blue. Magnifying lens for better identification and precise marking of anatomical landmarks is routinely used. The lowest point of Cupid's bow is marked as point 1, and point 2 corresponds to the contralateral philtral column's lowest point at the white roll and point 3 corresponds to the replication of the distance 1–2. For a 4-month-old patient, the distance between the points 1 and 2 usually measures 3 mm, thereby forming Cupid's bow, which measures 6 mm (distance between points 2 and 3). Point 4 is the most important of the preoperative marking as it determines the final symmetry of the lip in terms of width and height. It determines the lateral Cupid's bow point.

Point 4 is identified at the end of skin pigmentation area of the white roll, typically 1 mm medially to the point recommended by Cutting[45]; thus smaller amount of tissue is lost. If it is marked too medially in order to avoid losing tissue, one can end up with whistled deformity with inappropriate vermilion volume to reconstruct the median tubercle; otherwise it is marked too laterally that one can end up with a short lip in transverse terms. Noordhoff describes this point as the most medial point where the volume of the dry vermilion is greater. We tend not to replicate the distance from the alar crease to the height of the bow from noncleft side to cleft side as proposed by Cutting, because we believe that one can end up losing important tissue laterally specially in those severe cases with the absence of nasoalveolar molding with a significant discrepancy between the palatine plates. Depending on the surgeon experience the position of this point may vary, as one can anticipate the final position of the lip elements at the end of the surgery. More recently, a small laterally based triangular flap above the cutaneous white roll has been incorporated to the preoperative marking. A quadrangular flap is also marked medially to the lateral segment that is usually based either in the nasal turbinate region or in the alveolus as proposed by Millard. This flap will be rotated inside in the transition of nasal skin and nasal mucosa. The most medial region of this flap will be rotated to be sutured to septal flap and form the floor of the nose. The septal flap is usually not marked and the incision is performed based on the extension of the medial portion of "L" flap on the septum. The floor of the nose cannot be too small as there is a chance for obstruction secondary to scar contraction. We have used the diameter of the oral-tracheal tube as a reference for the diameter of upper airway constructed based on the suture between the "L" flap and "S" flap. Point 5 is marked in the region of the cleft alar base about 1 mm into the nostril. Point 6 is marked in the alar base of noncleft side. The point 7 is a reference of lateral based "L" flap and point 8 is drawn at columellar base (Raposo-do-Amaral 2008; Raposo-Amaral et al. 2012) (Figs. 7.14, 7.15, 7.16, 7.17, 7.18, 7.19, 7.20, 7.21, 7.22, 7.23, and 7.24).

7.7.2 Anthropometric Measurements

After the preoperative marking all points are carefully measured with surgical caliper and recorded in the patient chart.

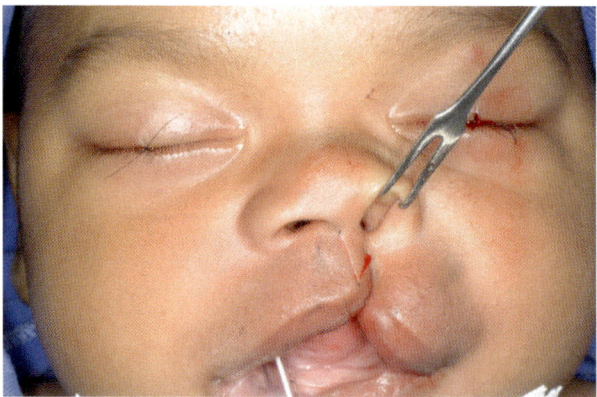

Fig. 7.14 Intraoperative photograph showing a prolabial incision and columella ["C"] flap to elongate the columella in the Mohler technique, using Millard principles

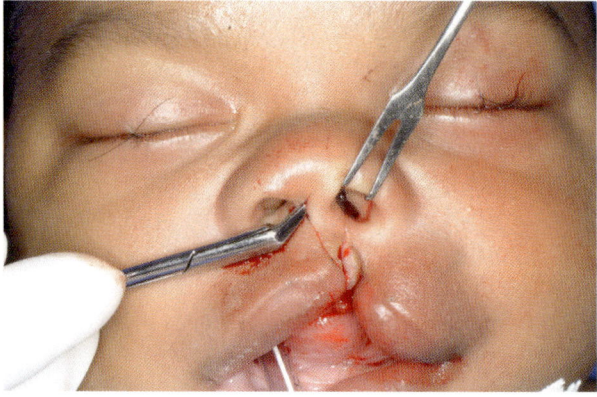

Fig. 7.15 Intraoperative photograph showing nasal undermining using the Converse angulated scissor

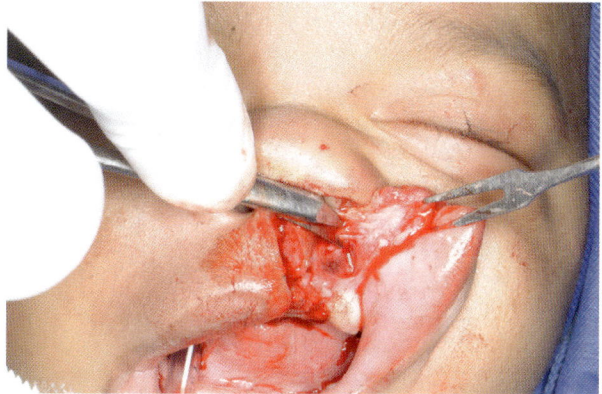

Fig. 7.16 Intraoperative photograph showing the dissection of abnormal nasal muscle fibers attaching the nasal ala to the bony structures of the lateral pyriform aperture. These fibers need to be released to elevate the nasal ala

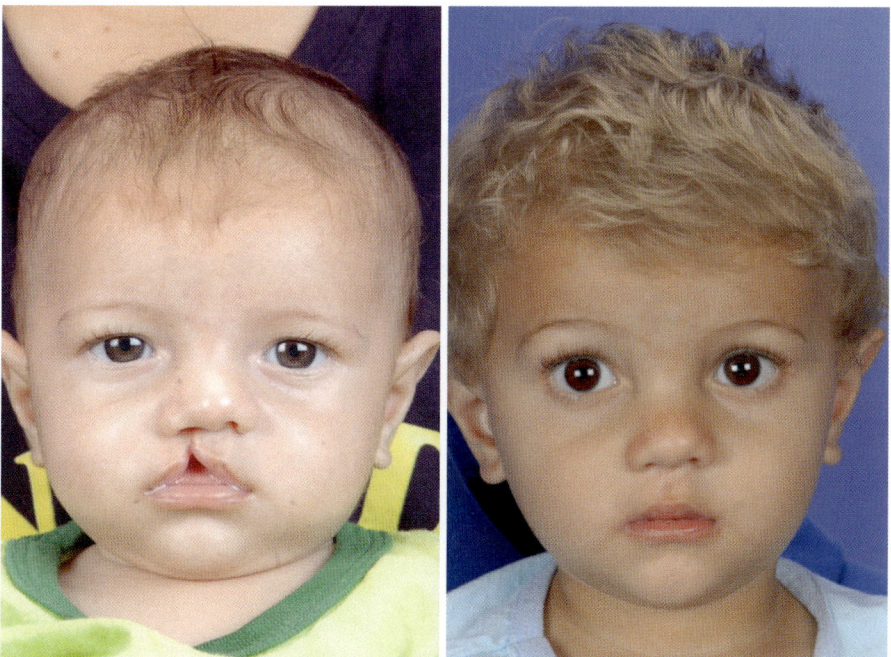

Fig. 7.17 Preoperative and postoperative photograph of right unilateral incomplete cleft lip. Satisfactory nasal symmetry was obtained during the follow-up period (*right*)

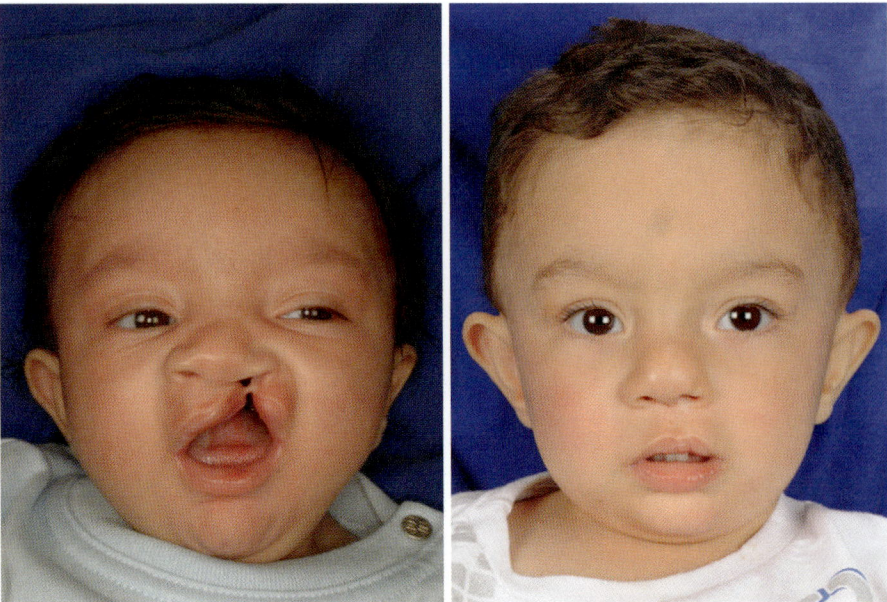

Fig. 7.18 Preoperative photograph of 3-month-old patient with left unilateral complete cleft lip and palate (*left*). Postoperative photograph of the same patient 2 years after cleft lip and nasal repair (*right*)

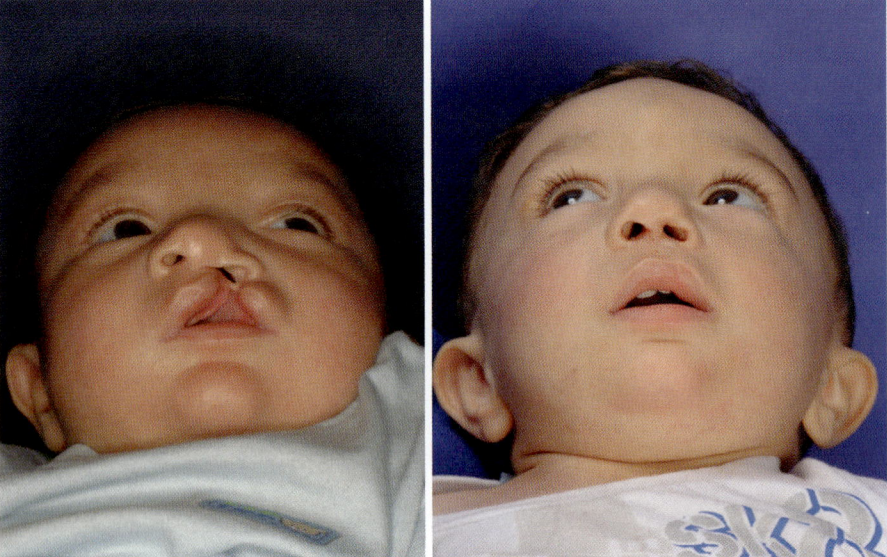

Fig. 7.19 Preoperative basal view of the same patient (*left*). Postoperative basal view of the same patient (*right*)

7 Unilateral Cleft Lip Repair

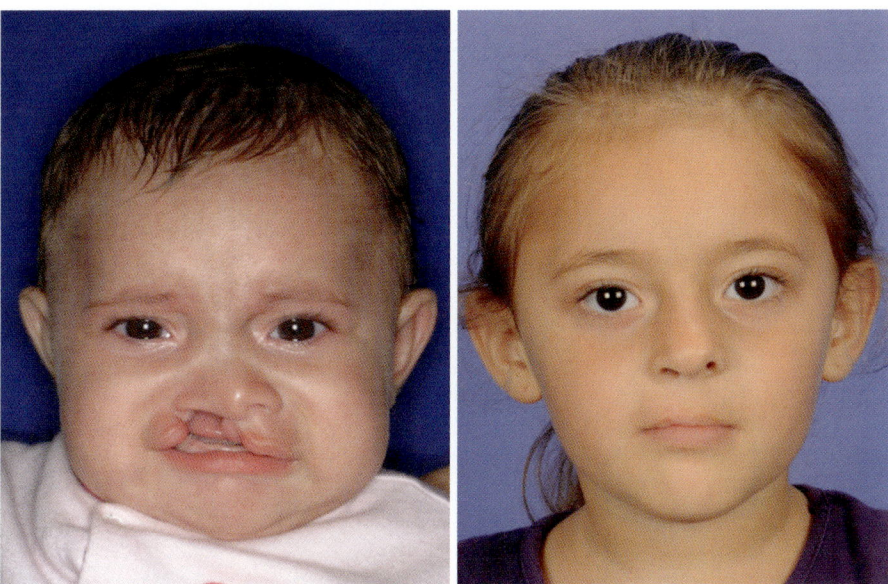

Fig. 7.20 Preoperative photograph of 3-month-old patient with right unilateral complete cleft lip and palate (*left*). Postoperative photograph 3 years after surgery (*right*)

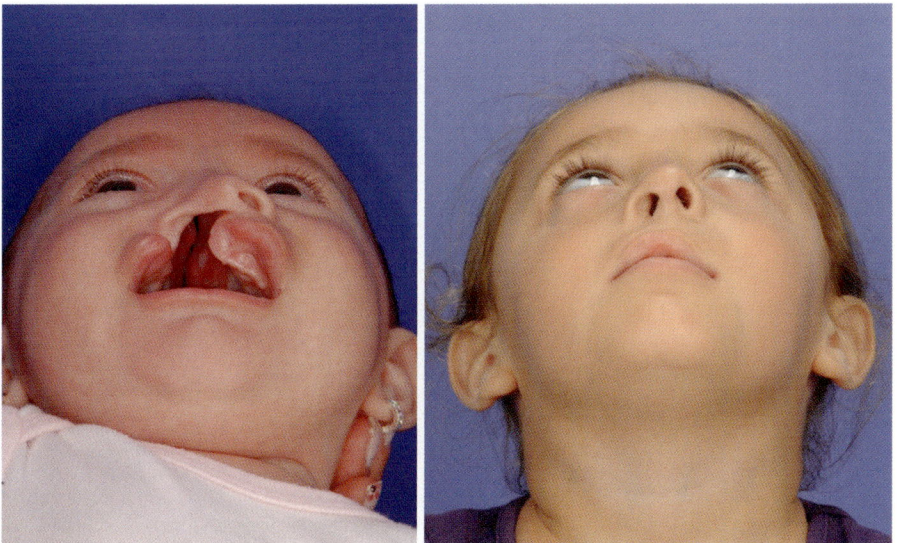

Fig. 7.21 Preoperative basal view of the same patient (*left*). Postoperative basal view of the same patient 3 years after surgery (*right*)

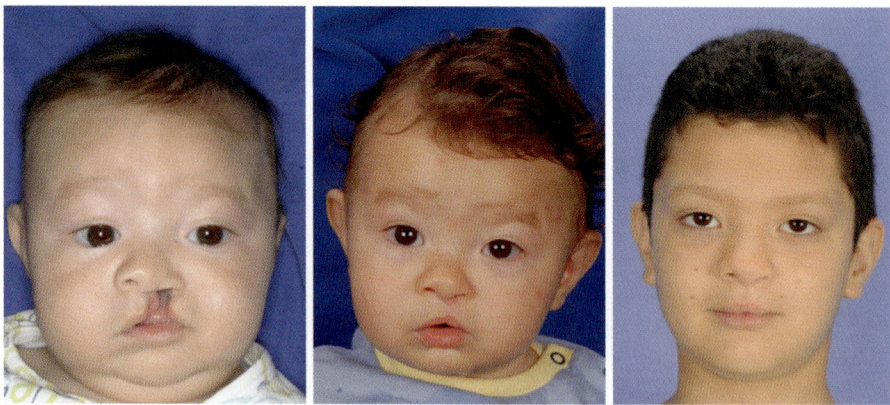

Fig. 7.22 Preoperative (*left*) and postoperative frontal photograph of left unilateral complete cleft lip. Satisfactory nasal symmetry was obtained during the follow-up period (*center*) and after alveolar bone grafting at 7 years of age (*right*)

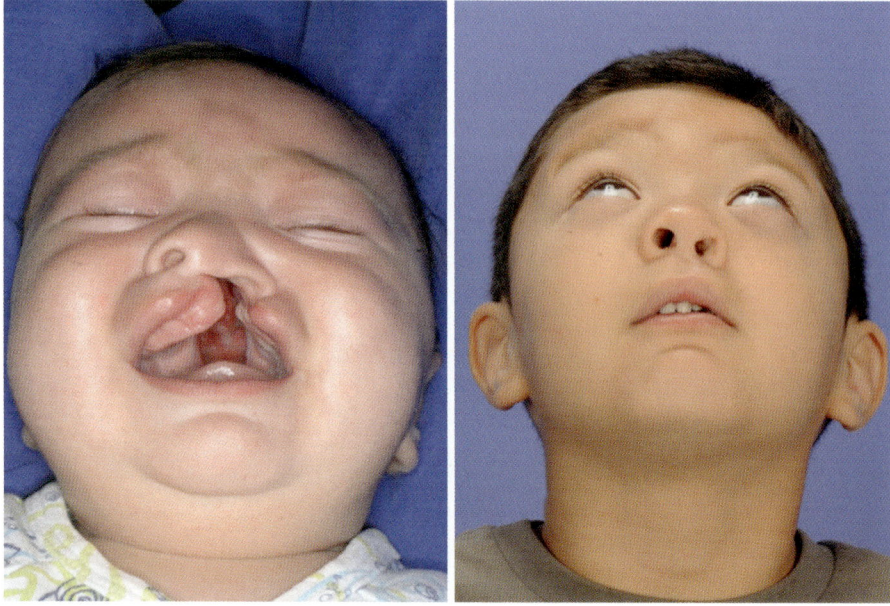

Fig. 7.23 Preoperative (*left*) and postoperative basal photograph of left unilateral complete cleft lip. Satisfactory lip and nasal symmetry was obtained during the follow-up period (*center*) and after alveolar bone grafting at 7 years of age (*right*)

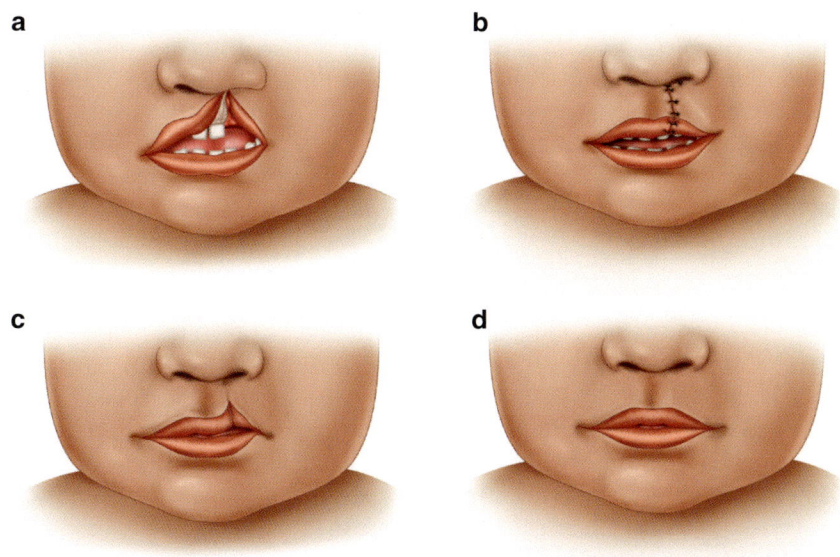

Fig. 7.24 (**a**) Patient with left unilateral complete cleft lip. Illustrative drawings of the physiologic behavior of the straight line scar in the Mohler technique (**b**), after 12 weeks of surgery (**c**) and after a year of surgery (**d**).

7.7.3 Mohler Operative Technique

The surgery starts with the skin incision with number 15 scalpel blade in the pre-marked area in the lip region toward 2 mm in the nasal columella. The columella "C" flap is created (Fig. 7.3). The blade number 11 with a pointed end is positioned in white skin roll in the marking point number 3. A transverse movement is performed generating a slight vermilion excess that can be eventually used at the end of the operation. Upper labial arteries are cauterized with electrocautery level 7 intensity. The small columellar incision is used to offer a skin route for nasal tip dissection. The medial crus of the alar cartilage is freed. The lateral dissection of the lateral crus of the alar cartilage will be completely performed using a lateral access after the elevation of the "L" flap (Fig. 7.5).

The lateral segment of the cleft is incised following the transition of skin and vermilion.

The blade scalpel number 11 is used for a perpendicular cut at point number 4, incising the lip vermilion and carefully following a quadrangular flap (L flap) based on the nasal turbinate. The L flap is completely elevated. The transition of nasal skin and nasal mucosa is incised for the subsequent inset of the L flap. The alar base is completely freed. This route is used for the dissection of lateral alar crus toward the nasal tip and triangular cartilage. Before the rotation of the L flap to nasal vestibule, the gingivobuccal incision is performed lower in the lateral and medial segments. The lateral region is carefully dissected at supraperiosteal plane. We tend to perform a conservative dissection but this decision should be carefully balanced. A wide dissection at this region avoids tension of the lip suture but can cause scarring and maxillar growth restriction. This decision has been empirically based on the severity of the cleft. Medially, the gingivobuccal incision can facilitate downward rotation of the medial segment, and we usually do not undermine the medial segment. When all the structures are freed and completely mobile in all dimensions, the distal portion of the L flap as well as the inner portion are sutured within the nasal mucosa. The septal flap is elevated and the lower portion of L flap is sutured to the S flap creating the floor of the nose. At this time, considering that all nasal structures are freed and floating over the craniofacial skeleton, percutaneous suture at the lateral nasal region is performed to adjust the nasal morphology. We use three sutures at the region of nasal fold, to mold the alar cartilage using as a template the contralateral side and one or two sutures at the tip of nose to allow upward rotation of the medial crus of the alar cartilage. This maneuver aims an overcorrection of the height of cleft nasal tip. However, this goal may be difficult to achieve specially in severe cleft patients with distorted anatomy and significant discrepancy of the palatine shelves, in an anteroposterior and transverse direction. The gingivobuccal incision is advanced and sutured together. The *orbicularis oris* muscle is released both in the medial and lateral segments and the back-cut incision on the base of the columella is performed to allow downward rotation of the medial segment. At this point, the length of the medial segment should have similar dimension of the lateral segment. The first stitch is performed to union the alar base to anterior nasal spine recreating the nostril contour. Then, a series of subsequent stitches are done and at the bottom of the Cupid's bow, where the dermis is also grasped and suture deep at the *orbicularis oris* of the lateral segment. This maneuver tends to recreate the natural depth of this region. Then a double hook is used to lift the cleft nasal tip, allowing the surgeon to identify the excess of the "C" flap. One or two millimeters of excess of "C" flap is trimmed and sutured to the contralateral columellar side. This maneuver lengthens the columella with tissue of "C" flap. The lateral segment is advanced toward the medial segment and the skin is carefully sutured with 5-0 nylon with atraumatic needle. We also use a small triangular flap at the tip of the Cupid's bow in order to decrease secondary elevation of the peak of the bow owing to scar contraction.

The transition of wet vermilion and dry mucosa at the lip region is identified. This point is fundamental in black and Brazilian pardo patients. In white patients this transition is not so evident. These lateral and medial points are approximated to avoid mismatch of lip color. Lip is sutured with absorbable thread.

At the end of the operation, if the nasal tip is not overcorrected in comparison to the contralateral side, additional stitches are performed to elevate the nasal tip, in the same manner as previously described. Either a silicone nasal stents or the orotracheal tube has been used to mold the nostril for 3–6 months after surgery.

The criticism of straight-line closure lies in the potential of scar contraction in postoperative period that may decrease the lip height. We have overcome the criticism about straight-line closure by using some specific maneuvers as follows: hermitic suture of *orbicularis oris* muscle, a small triangular flap at the Cupid's bow peak, implementation of the medial segment lip height that is equal to the contralateral side achieved by the back-cut incision, and small linear incision at the lower medial segment, where the triangular flap is inserted and meticulous skin closure is done by using atraumatic needle and careful removal after 6–7 days of surgery under sedation. We have been using this lip management protocol at SOBRAPAR with pleasing results. In addition, we have shown satisfactory result in incomplete cleft patients, whose lip height does not differ from the normative data, and we also showed that even in major cases with a significant discrepancy between the alveolar arch and without any type of infant presurgical orthopedics, satisfactory lip height has been achieved at 1 year after surgery. Having these data, we can anticipate all the evolution of postoperative lip dynamics to the parents who become aware of the scar contraction in early and late postoperative period, and the need of stitch removal under sedation at operation room. We have been counseling the parents to perform a lip massage at 1 month after surgery. Although there is not a confirmatory positive data about the benefit of postoperative lip massage in the current literature, parents may feel involved in the process and it may generate potential psychological effects until the healing process and scar contraction phenomenon is diminished (Raposo-do-Amaral 2008; Raposo-Amaral et al. 2012; Somensi et al. 2012).

7.7.3.1 Future Perspectives

As was said previously in the beginning of this chapter always new paradigms challenge the surgeons. The news points of discussion are different now, which mainly focus on two concepts of final results: social rehabilitation with final functional and cosmetic result and cost-effectiveness. After these we are back to operative technique and long-term evaluation of facial growth.

We prefer less invasive technique with minimal scars and position the scars in the anatomic landmarks. Fisher's technique (Fisher 2005) is very attractive for unilateral. It is a modern idea based on old straight-line technique concepts but with a very interesting mathematics approach that allows the teaching to be very easy for residents. After 3 years our service starts to adapt the points of Fisher's technique with the previous approach for the nose and the orbicularis oris muscle used as describe above.

The initial results are very interesting because of many reasons but the most important is that the final scar is straight positioned in the philtral crest. There is no scar around the alar base or in the central portion of the columella or in the contralateral philtral column.

The analysis of pros and cons of the technique as we have found include the fact that besides the position of the scar it is very easy to move medially the nasal alar without wide lateral undermining of soft tissue. In the opposite side it is possible to observe some difficulty achieving the final size of the medial part of the upper lip, and some shortness was seen in few cases. If we compare with other techniques too much tissue from the lateral side of the lip is discharged. On the resident's each point of view it is very easy to draw after you learn very precisely the function of which point.

7.7.3.2 Basic Markings

To determine the central points in the columella and also the lateral points in the alar base, philtral crest and white roll in the nonaffected side are the most important steps to learn the size and also the contralateral deformity to be corrected. The rotation of the lateral lip depends on the size of the cleft and lateral position of the alar rim. The medial height of the upper lip in the cleft side will determine the size of the flap that should be drawn on the lateral side of the lip. The described technique by D. Fisher did not touch the nose in the same time, but we always add the maneuver of Skoog's with the elongation of the incision until the intercartilage area. Sutures are always done, after extended dissection in between the two cartilages, lower lateral and upper lateral cartilage. For oral mucosa elongation on medial side of the lip, one medial incision is done in the gingival labial sulcus (Figs. 7.25 and 7.26).

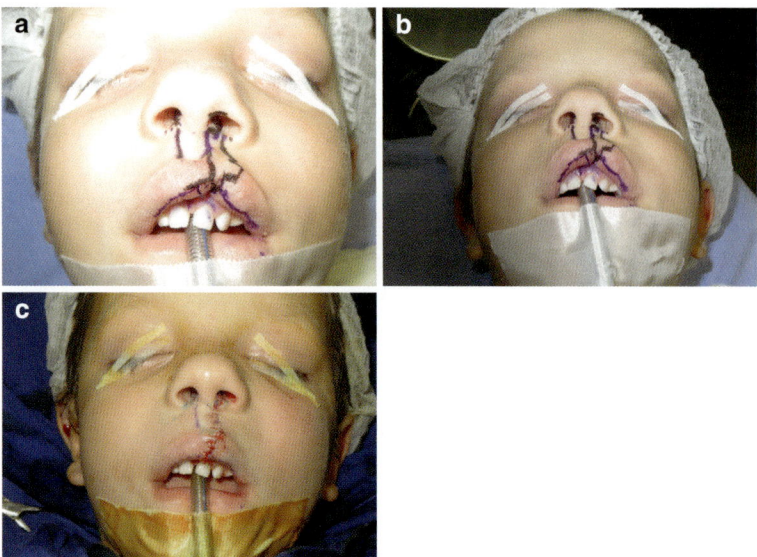

Fig. 7.25 (**a–c**) Intraoperative markings of straight-line technique (Fisher), intraoperative and immediate results showing the final position of the scar

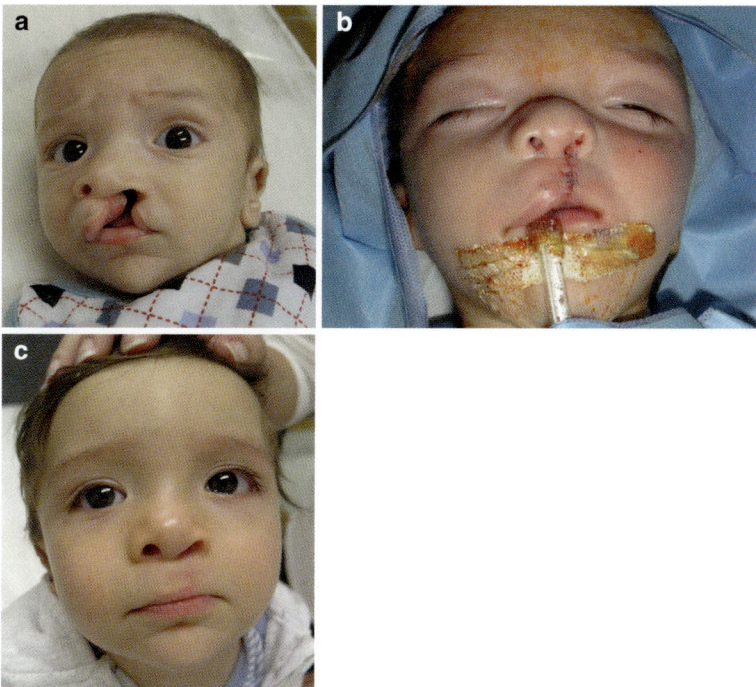

Fig. 7.26 (**a–c**) Wide left cleft pre- and intraoperative straight-line technique associated with rhinoplasty with the postoperative results. Lip scar in the philtral crest

7.8 Summary

There are many techniques developed over the years and straight-line closure was one of them. The principles described by Millard have been used worldwide and serve as a basis to the development of tactics and maneuvers adapted to patients' racial cleft features. The regional characteristics of each patient cohort may change the way cleft surgeon thinks and conducts his/her operation. However, the final goal and endpoint of all surgeons around the world are similar and we believe that the most difficult one is to find consistency in the results and a technique that can be learnt and taught in a standardized manner. Considering that cleft presentation is broad and nonstandardized, maneuvers to consistently achieve a normal face in these population have been described in the literature. In this chapter, Alonso and Raposo-Amaral's experience working in the largest Brazilian centers has been proposed (Figs. 7.27, 7.28 and 7.29).

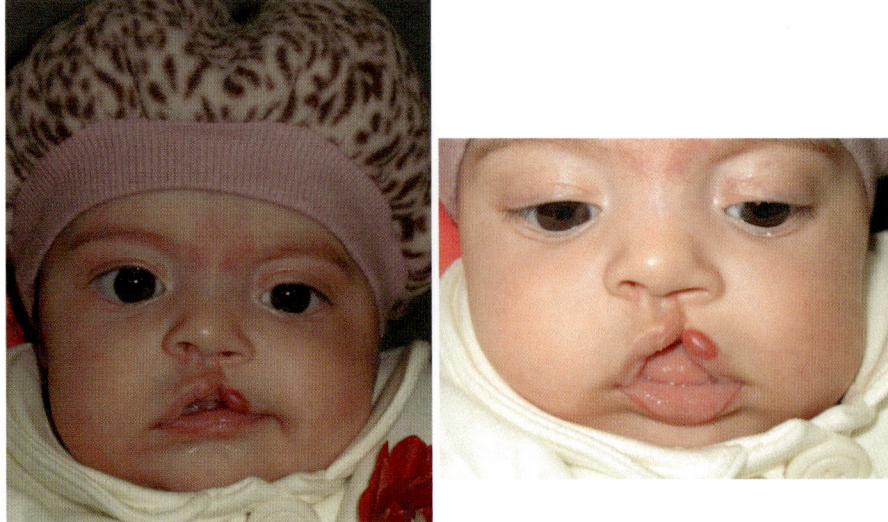

Fig. 7.27 Preoperative photographs of a left unilateral incomplete cleft lip patient with an unusual presentation of a hemangioma on the superior lip and immediate postoperative

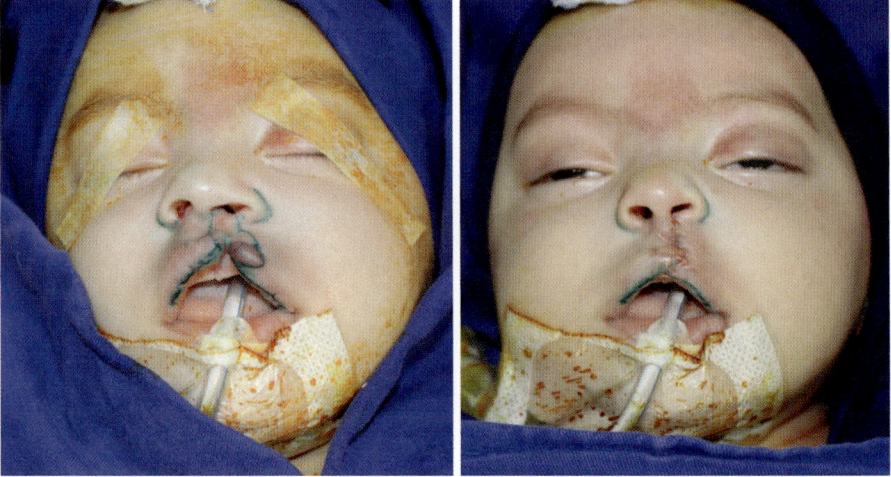

Fig. 7.28 Intraoperative photograph of left unilateral incomplete cleft lip patient with an unusual hemangioma of the superior lip marked using Fisher technique (*left*). Intraoperative photograph of the same patient immediately after surgery (*right*)

7 Unilateral Cleft Lip Repair

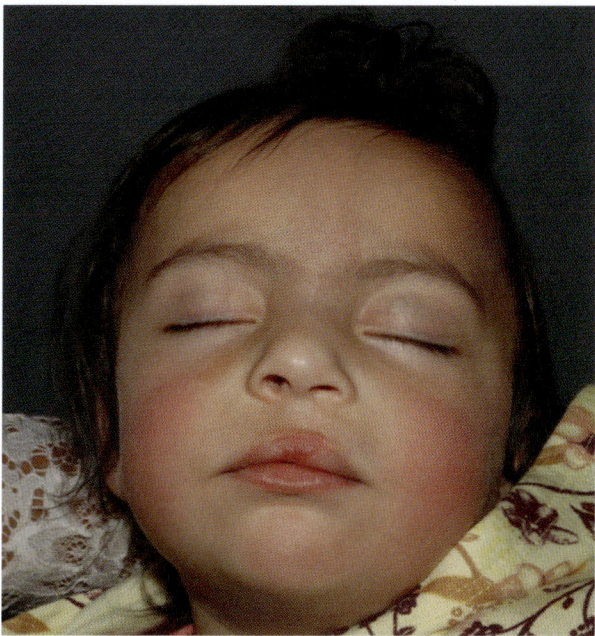

Fig. 7.29 Postoperative photograph of the same patient using Fisher technique

References

Alonso N, Tanikawa DYS, Lima JE, Ferreira MC. Avaliação comparativa e evolutiva dos protocolos de atendimento dos pacientes fissurados. Rev Bras Cir Plást. 2010;25(3):434–8.
Blair VP, Letterman GS. The role of the switched lower lip flap in upper lip restorations. Plast Reconstr Surg. 1950;5(1):1–25.
Blair VP, Robinson RR. Primary closure of harelip. Surg Gynecol Obstet. 1948;86(4):502–4.
Boo CK. An ancient Chinese text on a cleft lip. Plast Reconstr Surg. 1966;38:89–91.
Cardoso AD. A new technique for harelip. Plast Reconstr Surg. 1952;10(2):92–5.
Cutting C. Cleft lip nasal reconstruction. In: Rees T, LaTrenta G, editors. Aesthetic plastic surgery. Philadelphia: Saunders; 1994. p. 497–532.
Cutting CB, Dayan JH. Lip height and lip width after extended Mohler unilateral cleft lip repair. Plast Reconstr Surg. 2003;111:17–23.
Fisher DM. Unilateral cleft lip repair: an anatomical subunit approximation technique. Plast Reconstr Surg. 2005 Jul;116(1):61–71.
Gnudi MT, Wester JP. *The life and times of Gaspare Tagliacozzi. Surgeon of Bologna*.Cópia n0 1403. Los Angeles: Zeitlin & Ver Brugge; 1976.
Hagedorn W. Die operation der Hasenscharte mit Zickzarknaht. Zentralbl Chir. 1892;19:281.

LeMesurier AB. Method of cutting and suturing lip in complete unilateral cleft lip. Plast Reconstr Surg. 1949;4(1):1–12.
Malgaigne JF. Mansesuel de Medicine Operatoire. 7th ed. Paris: Germer Bailliere; 1861.
McComb H. Treatment of the unilateral cleft lip nose. Plast Reconstr Surg. 1975;55:596–601.
Millard DR. Complete unilateral clefts of the lip. Plast Reconstr Surg. 1960;25:595–605.
Millard DR Jr. Cleft Craft. In: The evolution of its surgery, The unilateral deformity, vol. I. Boston: Brown and Company; 1976.
Millard DR Jr. Principalization of plastic surgery. 1st ed. Boston: Brown & Company; 1986.
Millard DR Jr. Saving faces. Autobioghaphy. 1st ed. Fort Lauderdale: Write Stuff Interprise, Inc; 2003.
Millard DR Jr, Morovic CG. Primary unilateral cleft nose correction: a 10-year follow up. PlastReconstSurg. 1998;102:1331–8.
Mirault G. Deux letters sur lóperation du bec-de-lievre considere dans ses divers etats de simplicite et de complication. J Chir (Paris). 1884;2:257.
Mohler L. Unilateral cleft lip repair. Plast Reconstr Surg. 1987;80:511–44.
Mulliken JB, Martinez-Pérez D. The principle of rotation advancement for repair of unilateral complete cleft lip and nasal deformity. Technical variations and analysis of results. Plast Reconstr Surg. 1999;104:1247–60.
Noordhoff MS. Reconstruction of vermilion in unilateral and bilateral cleft lips. Plast Reconstr Surg. 1984;73:52–60.
Paré A. Livres de La Chirurgie. Paris: Jean de Roger; 1964.
Randall P. A triangular flap operation for the primary repair of unilateral clefts of the lip. Plast Reconstr Surg. 1959;23:331–47.
Randall P. Discussion. Growth of cleft lip following a triangular flap repair. Plast Reconstr Surg. 1986;77:238–9.
Raposo-Amaral CE, Giancoli AP, Denadai R, Marques FF, Somensi RS, Raposo-Amaral CA, Alonso N. Lip height improvement during the first year of unilateral complete cleft lip repair using cutting extended Mohler technique. Plast Surg Int. 2012;2012:206481.
Raposo-do-Amaral CE. Prêmio Silvio Zanini ao melhor trabalho da área de Cirurgia Plástica Craniofacial apresentado no 45° Congresso Brasileiro de Cirurgia Plástica da Sociedade Brasileira de Cirurgia Plástica. Brasília; 2008.
Rose W. On harelip and cleft palate. London: Lewis; 1891.
Somensi RS, Giancoli A, Almeida F, Bento DF, Raposo-do-Amaral CA, Buzzo CL, Raposo-do-Amaral CE. Assessment of nasal anthropometric parameters after primary cleft lip repair using the Mohler technique. Rev Bras Cir Plást. 2012;27(1):14–21.
Spina V, Lodovici O. Conservative technique for treatment of unilateral cleft lip. Reconstruction of the midline tubercle of vermillion. Br J Plast Surg. 1960;13:100–17.
Spina V, Psillakis JM, Lapa F, Ferreira MC. Classificação das fissuras lábio palatinas:sugestão de modificação. Rev Hosp Clin Fac Med S Paulo. 1972;27:5–6.
Stal S, Brown RH, Higuera S, et al. Fifty years of the Millard rotation-advancement: looking back and moving forward. Plast Reconstr Surg. 2009;123:1364–77.
Tennison CW. The repair of the unilateral cleft lip by the stencil method. Plast Reconstr Surg. 1952;9(2):115–20.

Thompson JE. An artistic and mathematically accurate method of repairing the defects in cases of harelip. Surg Gynecol Obstet. 1912;14:498–02.

Wong GB, Burvin R, Mulliken JB. Resorbable internal splint: an adjunct to primary correction of unilateral cleft-lip nasal deformity. Plast Reconstr Surg. 2002;110:385–91.

Xu H, Salyer KE, Genecov ER. Primary bilateral one-stage cleft lip/nose repair: 40-year Dallas experience: part I. J Craniofac Surg. 2009;20(Suppl 2):1913–26.

Treatment of Bilateral Cleft Lip and Palate: Protocol for Surgical Treatment

8

Nivaldo Alonso and Julia Amundson

Bilateral cleft lip and palate (BCLP), although representing around 20% of cleft cases (Trindade and Silva Filho 2007), is one of the greatest challenges faced by craniofacial surgeons, well summarized by Dr. James Barrett Brown as "Bilateral cleft lip is twice as difficult to repair as unilateral, and the results are only half as good" (Brown et al. 1947). Bilateral clefts tend to represent the more severe cases of cleft lip and palate, for which reason an in-depth analysis is warranted, with special attention paid to treatment choice (Brown et al. 1947; Semb 1991). The major surgical challenges of treating BLCP stay from the technical difficulty of achieving symmetry of the lips, muscular continuity, lengthening of the columella, nasal projection, and proper positioning of the premaxilla. Of these challenges, nasal asymmetry, malpositioned or projected premaxilla, and prolabium underdevelopment, which are associated with a lack of muscular continuity, are some of the most difficult to overcome (Mulliken 1985; Millard 1977; Spina et al. 1978).

Of course the final result needs much more surgical skill to achieve the final goal of social reintegration of these patients. The dental occlusion and the speech have double attention for obtaining good functional results.

There are several main points of contention and discussion with regard to bilateral cleft repair: first, the time and type of lip repair, and whether to perform a staged or non-staged repair; secondly, the use of preoperative orthopedic devices, whether active or passive; thirdly, premaxilla repositioning; and finally the ideal time for primary rhinoplasty (Bishara and Olin 1972; Bittermann et al. 2016; Liou et al. 2007; Mulliken 2000).

N. Alonso, M.D., Ph.D. (✉)
Divisao de Cirurgia Plastica e Queimaduras, Hospital das Clínicas da Faculdade de Medicina da Universidade de São Paulo, São Paulo, Brazil
e-mail: nivalonso@gmail.com

J. Amundson, B.S.
Miller School of Medicine, University of Miami, Miami, FL 33136, USA
e-mail: jamundson2@gmail.com

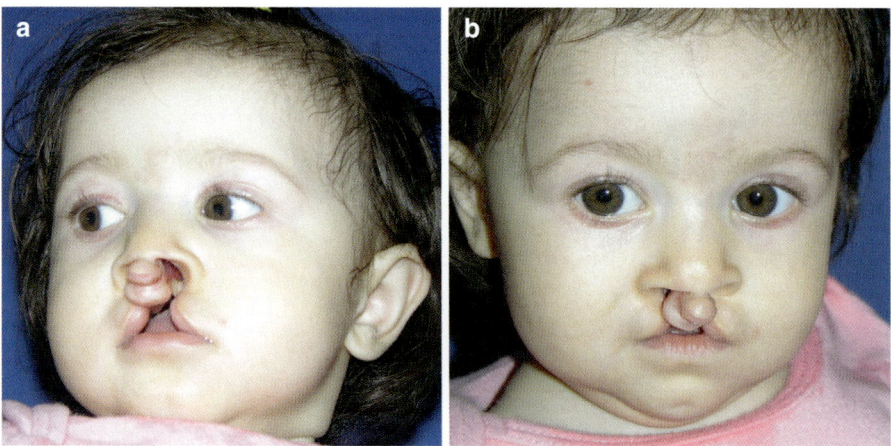

Fig. 8.1 (**a, b**) Protruding premaxilla in a complete bilateral cleft. Frontal and lateral view showing the severe projection of the central part of the lip

Bilateral cleft classification is initially determined by whether the cleft is complete or incomplete as defined by the presence or absence of a cutaneous band that maintains the continuity of the inferior aspect of the nares (Spina et al. 1972; Victor 1931). In the complete bilateral the position of the premaxilla is important, which is either projected or not. Nonprotruding premaxilla has the lip repair, nasal elongation, and muscular repositioning as surgical steps; added to all this the complete has the protruding premaxilla limiting the lip repair and primary rhinoplasty.

Bilateral alveolar clefts result in a premaxilla solely fixed to the vomer bone and freely mobile (Bittermann et al. 2016). The malpositioned premaxilla is, without doubt, the anatomic element that causes the greatest technical difficulty. These bilateral clefts can also be differentiated by the grade of development of the prolabium, without muscle and hypoplastic vermillion dry and wet (Spina 1966) (Figs. 8.1 and 8.2).

The protocol of the craniofacial service at the Hospital das Clínicas, University of São Paulo Medical School, is based on two anatomic aspects of the patient: the position of the premaxilla and the dry vermillion and prolabium development. When there is no projection of the premaxilla, primary queiloplasty is done in one stage. The technique for repair is determined by the second criterion, with a well-developed dry vermillion and prolabium allowing for the principles of Spina's technique, and if either is poorly developed, the principles of Noordhoff's technique modified in the department by the senior author (Spina et al. 1978; Spina 1966; Noordhoff 1986) (Figs. 8.3–8.5).

Principles of Spina's technique are used to avoid disruption of the white line in a well-developed dry vermillion. The technique involves using the lateral soft tissue of the lip to reconstruct the median tubercle whilst maintaining the mucocutaneous

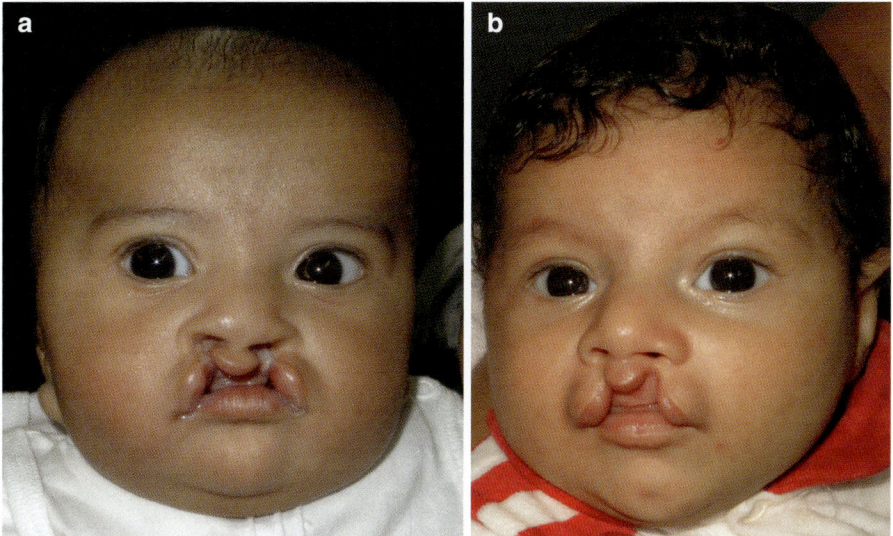

Fig. 8.2 (**a**, **b**) Nonprotruding premaxilla with hypoplastic prolabium in two different patients

vermillion border. Principles of our modified technique allow for proper reconstruction of an underdeveloped white line of the dry vermillion. The entire reconstruction of the medial tubercle and medial dry vermillion is performed using the lateral soft tissue of the lip and the mucocutaneous vermillion border is recreated with the same lateral tissue. The muscular belt is done, and the orbicularis oris is sutured in the midline with nonresorbable suture, two guide stitches close to columella and at the upper transition of vermillion (Fig. 8.6–8.10).

In the case of a projected premaxilla, primary queiloplasty must be undertaken in a staged manner. The first repair, which is typically performed between 3 and 6 months of age, is simply a joining of the cutaneous lip borders to help guide the premaxilla to its proper position during facial growth. This first stage is either unilateral or bilateral, depending on the size of the cleft and what is possible, with larger clefts often not allowing for bilateral approximation of the cutaneous lip borders. If this is the case, the widest cleft is closed first and the second side closed 12 weeks later however, if the pre maxilla is not projected, a single stage queiloplasty is performed (less than 7 mm projected). (Spina 1966). Technique for the staged definitive repair, which typically is performed after palatal closure at 12 months of age, is determined once again by the development of the dry vermillion and the prolabium. Spina's repair is performed when the patient has a well-developed dry vermillion and prolabium and the modified bilateral local technique repair is performed when this is lacking. The original description of Spina technique, the final lip repair was done at the age of 5 years old.

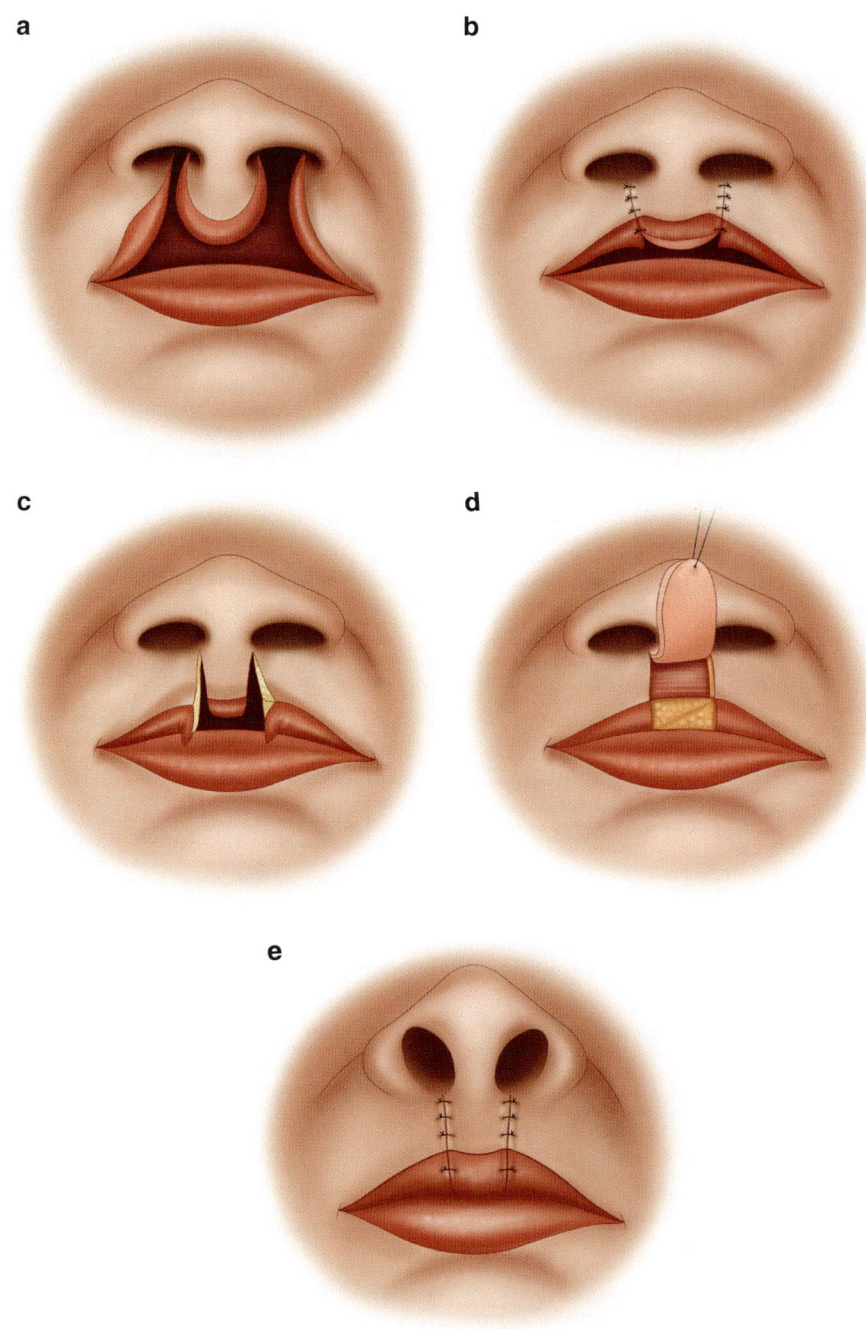

Fig. 8.3 Spina's technique drawings

8 Treatment of Bilateral Cleft Lip and Palate: Protocol for Surgical Treatment

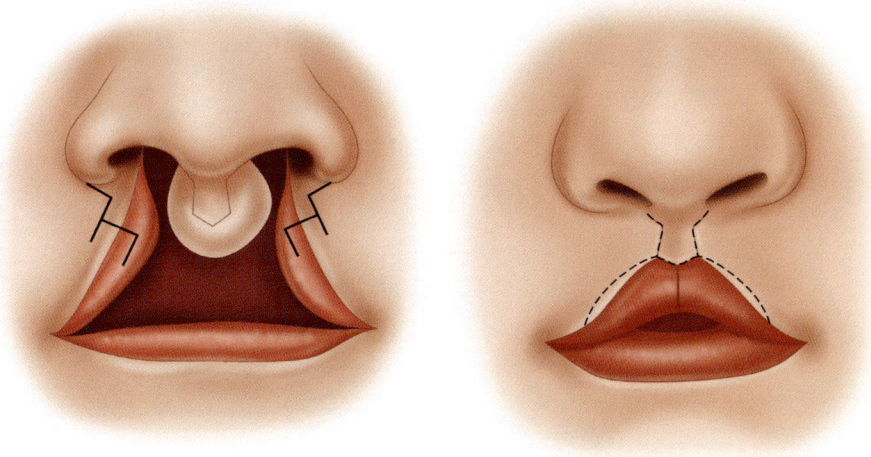

Fig. 8.4 Principles of Noordhoff's technique with some personal modifications

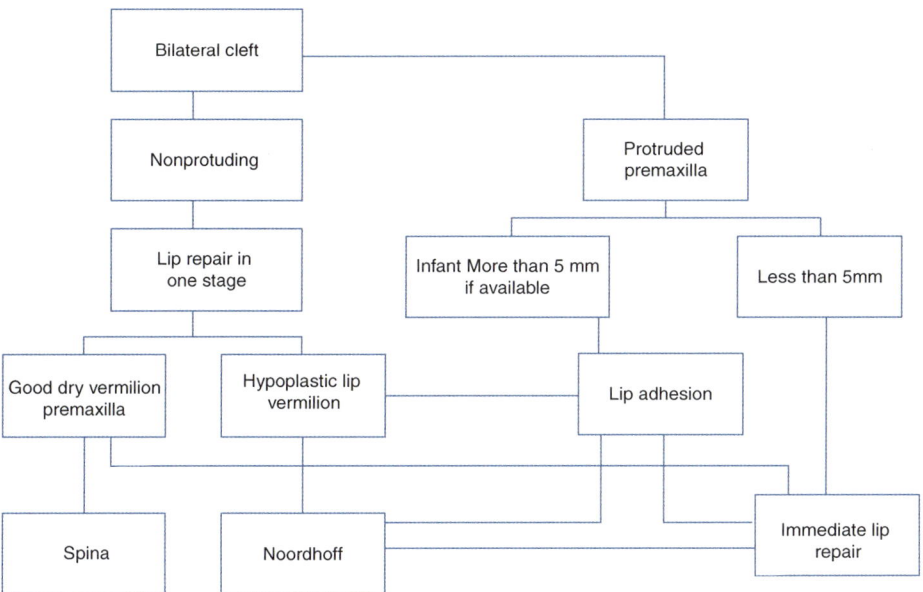

Fig. 8.5 Algorithm of bilateral cleft treatment

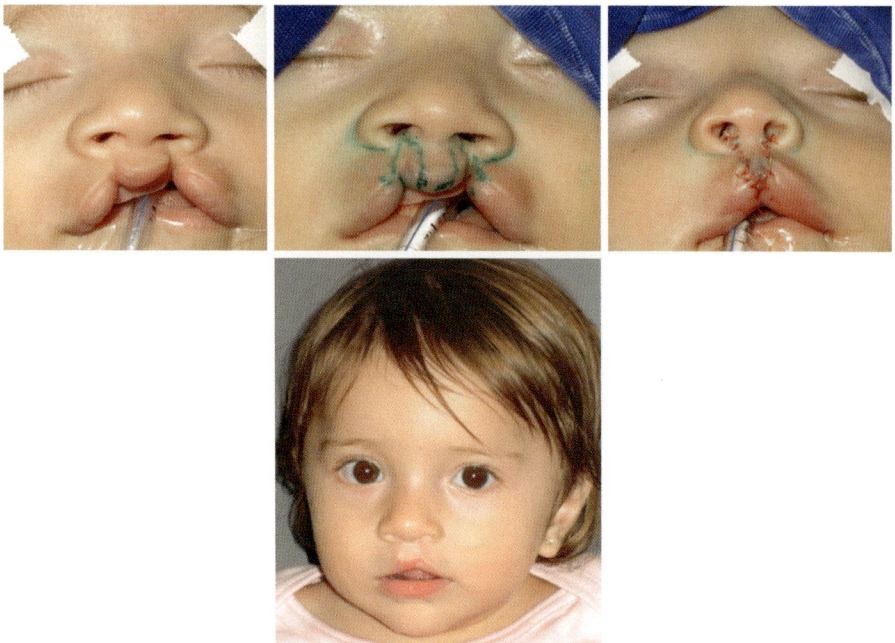

Fig. 8.6 Nonprotruding premaxilla with good dry vermillion Spina's one stage

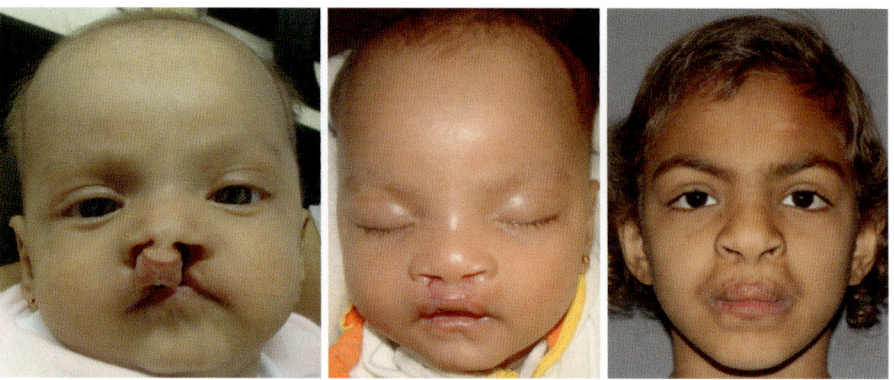

Fig. 8.7 Two-staged premaxilla protruding premaxilla

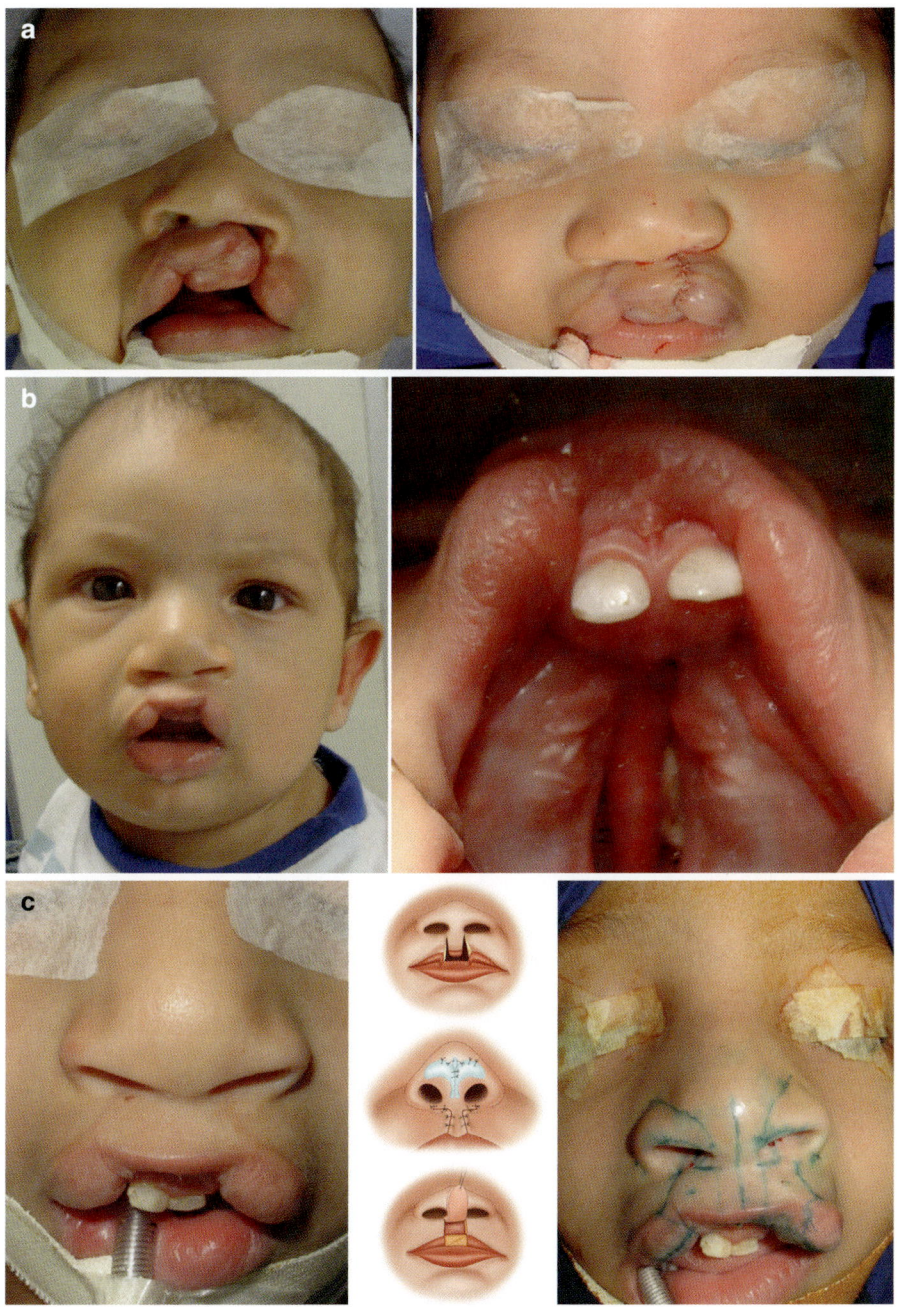

Fig. 8.8 (a–e) (**a**) Spina three stages second-side adhesion, (**b**) premaxilla after lip adhesion, (**c**) Spina definite repair, (**d**) final position of premaxilla after adhesion, (**e**) demarcation of Spina definitive repair

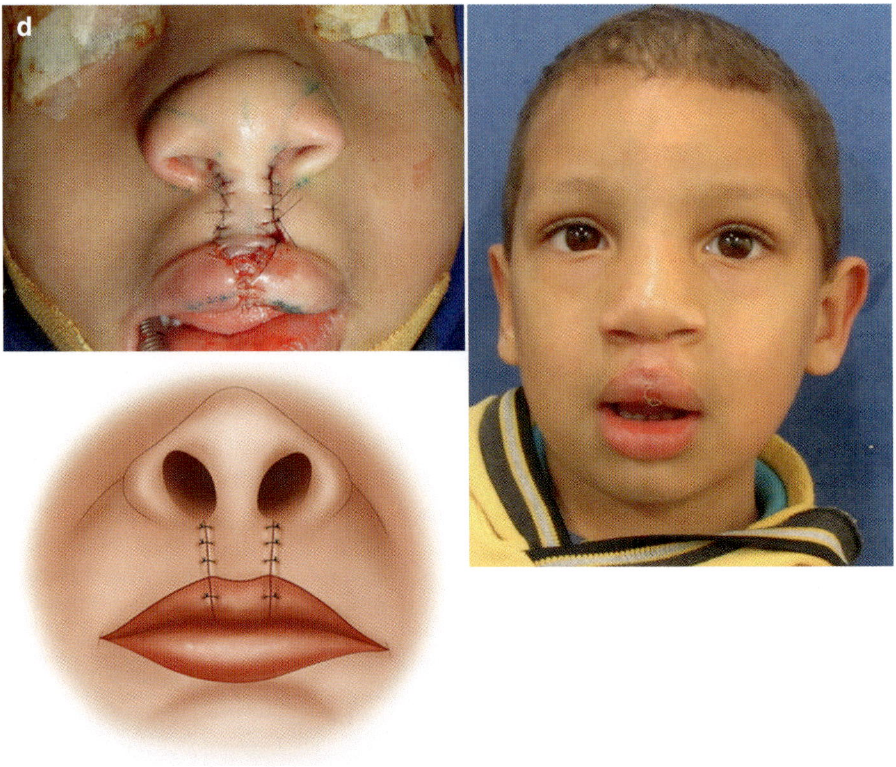

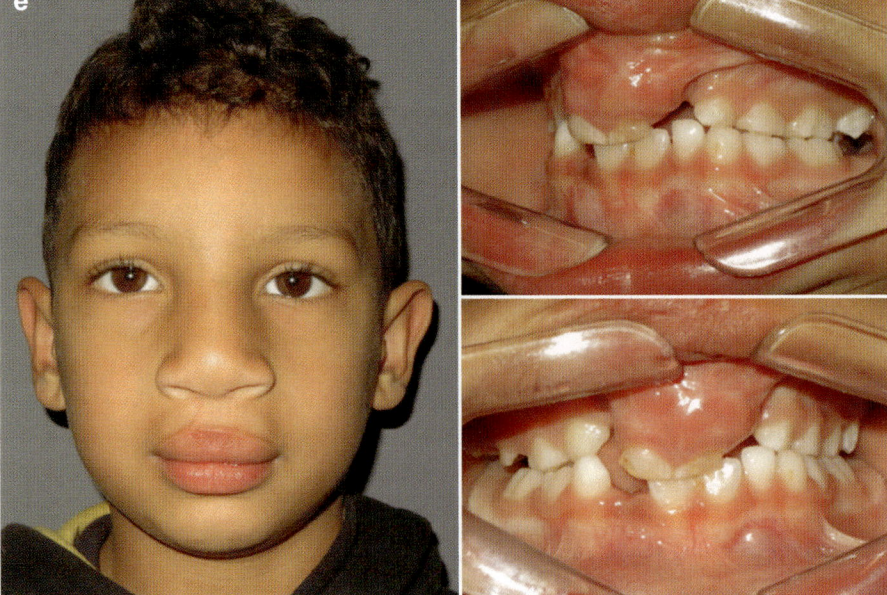

Fig. 8.8 (continued)

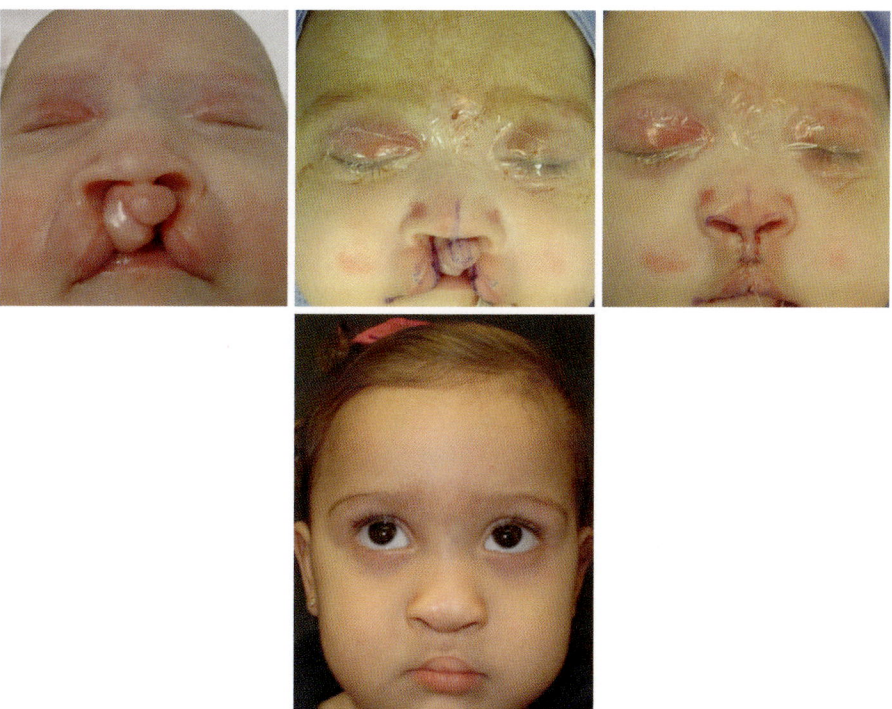

Fig. 8.9 Protruding and asymmetrical pre maxilla hypoplastic vermillion (less than 7 mm) Noordhoff's modification

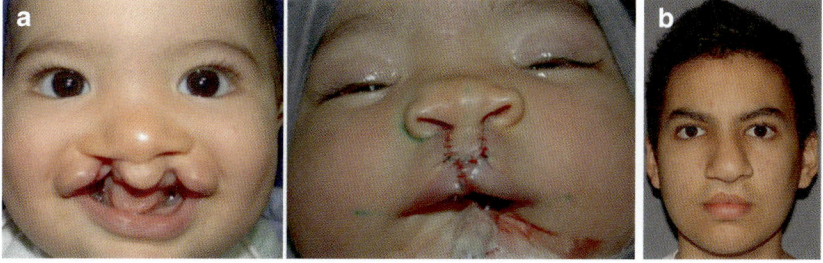

Fig. 8.10 Noordhoff's modification long-term follow-up. (**a**, **b**) Noordhoff's modified one stage with nasal repair pre maxilla non projected

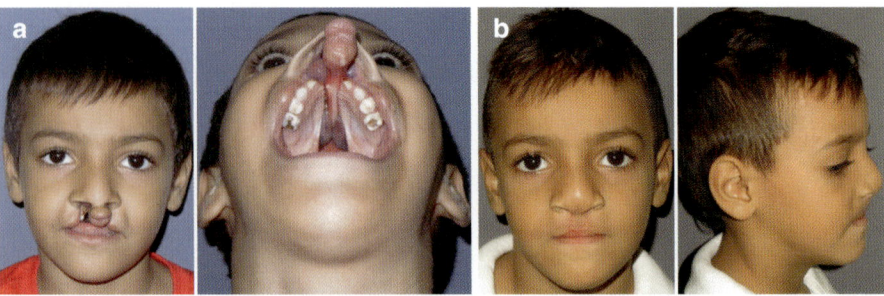

Fig. 8.11 Projected premaxilla nonoperated bilateral cleft patient with repositioning of premaxilla at 6 years old. (**a, b**) A projected premaxilla after lip repair; (**b**) useless external traction after surgical procedure and orthodontic

At the time of primary queiloplasty, if there is a projected premaxilla, it is not possible to perform an adequate primary rhinoplasty. The moment of the primary queiloplasty is, nevertheless, the best moment to reposition the nasal cartilage and elongate the columella (Mulliken 1985, 2000, 2001). Primary rhinoplasty is important for achieving final esthetic results in BCLP patients. Historically, nasal alveolar molds (NAM) were used with the desired outcome of approximating tissues preoperatively (Grayson et al. 1999). Many studies have shown no benefit to the use of preoperative devices compared to controls, besides the fact that in many places this practice is not possible (Semb 1991; Spina et al. 1978; Liou et al. 2007; Mackay 2016). In cases of delayed primary rhinoplasty due to a severe projected premaxilla, current practice is to perform a primary rhinoplasty after repositioning of the premaxilla.

There is much discussion surrounding the ideal age for repositioning of projected premaxilla, which is present in the vast majority (70%) of BCLP patients at our institution (Alonso 2016). Our protocol indicates surgical correction for the pre maxilla between 8 and 10 years of age, at the same moment as performing an alveolar bone graft to fix bony discontinuity of the maxilla. If surgical repositioning is performed prematurely, it often results in significant impingement on facial growth (Bishara and Olin 1972; Bittermann et al. 2016; Padwa et al. 1999). Between the moment of primary queiloplasty and surgical repositioning of the premaxilla, orthopedic devices have often been used to provide nonsurgical repositioning of the premaxilla. The presurgical devices are not used in our protocol; only external compression with tapes and elastics bands can be used. Concerns regarding the use of active orthopedic devices that exert traction on a projected premaxilla include possible restriction of the natural progression of facial growth, and data from reference centers show an increased incidence of orthognathic surgery in BCLP patients who previously used orthopedic devices (Good et al. 2007).

A caveat to the timing of performing surgical correction of excess projection of the premaxilla is delayed presentation of a bilateral cleft patient. If the patient has not yet undergone primary queiloplasty by 6–8 years of age, the temporal indication for surgical repositioning of the premaxilla is as soon as possible with the lip repair. The vomer-premaxillary suture is closed by 6–8 years of age; therefore premaxilla repositioning after this age will not impair facial growth. The primary queiloplasty and premaxilla repositioning will take place at the same time (Bishara and Olin 1972; Padwa et al. 1999). In these cases, there is significant difficulty with respect to primary rhinoplasty, due to extensive local vascularization (Fig. 8.11).

With a large variety of clinical presentations and an array of repair techniques available, even though many improvement was seen still there are several points of contention that often arise with regard to care for BLCP patients. These points of contention are whether queiloplasty should be performed in a staged or non-staged manner, the use of preoperative orthopedic devices, the ideal age for surgical repositioning of a projected premaxilla, and the use of primary rhinoplasty. Evidences are scare as to the best manner in which to answer these questions, and as bilateral cleft patients represent a small percentage of all patients with cleft lip and palate, there has been to date a lack of randomized controlled trials evaluating treatment options. Despite this dearth of evidence, just like care for unilateral cleft, care for bilateral cleft is essential (Bittermann et al. 2016).

References

Alonso N. Evidencias no tratamento de fissuras bilaterais. São Paulo: Congresso da Asociacao Brasileira de Cirurgia Craniomaxilofacial; 2016.
Bishara SE, Olin WH. Surgical repositioning of the premaxilla in complete bilateral cleft lip and palate. Angle Orthod. 1972;42(2):139–47.
Bittermann GK, de Ruiter AP, Janssen NG, Bittermann AJ, van der Molen AM, van Es RJ, et al. Management of the premaxilla in the treatment of bilateral cleft of lip and palate: what can the literature tell us? Clin Oral Investig. 2016;20(2):207–17.
Brown JB, Mc DF, Byars LT. Double clefts of the lip. Surg Gynecol Obstet. 1947;85(1):20–9.
Good PM, Mulliken JB, Padwa BL. Frequency of Le Fort I osteotomy after repaired cleft lip and palate or cleft palate. Cleft Palate Craniofac J. 2007;44(4):396–401.
Grayson BH, Santiago PE, Brecht LE, Cutting CB. Presurgical nasoalveolar molding in infants with cleft lip and palate. Cleft Palate Craniofac J. 1999;36(6):486–98.
Liou EJ, Subramanian M, Chen PK. Progressive changes of columella length and nasal growth after nasoalveolar molding in bilateral cleft patients: a 3-year follow-up study. Plast Reconstr Surg. 2007;119(2):642–8.
Mackay D, editor. Is NAM a scam? Los Angeles: American Society of Plastic Surgery; 2016.
Millard DR Jr. Cleft Craft -The evolution of its surgery II- Bilateral and rare deformities. Boston: Little, Brown & Co; 1977. p. 2964.
Mulliken JB. Principles and techniques of bilateral complete cleft lip repair. Plast Reconstr Surg. 1985;75(4):477–87.
Mulliken JB. Repair of bilateral complete cleft lip and nasal deformity--state of the art. Cleft Palate Craniofac J. 2000;37(4):342–7.
Mulliken JB. Primary repair of bilateral cleft lip and nasal deformity. Plast Reconstr Surg. 2001;108(1):181–94. examination, 95-6
Noordhoff MS. Bilateral cleft lip reconstruction. Plast Reconstr Surg. 1986;78(1):45–54.
Padwa BL, Sonis A, Bagheri S, Mulliken JB. Children with repaired bilateral cleft lip/palate: effect of age at premaxillary osteotomy on facial growth. Plast Reconstr Surg. 1999;104(5):1261–9.

Semb G. A study of facial growth in patients with bilateral cleft lip and palate treated by the Oslo CLP Team. Cleft Palate Craniofac J. 1991;28(1):22–39. discussion 46-8

Spina V. The advantages of two stages in repair of bilateral cleft lip. Cleft Palate J. 1966;3:56–60.

Spina V, Psillakis JM, Lapa FS, Ferreira MC. Classification of cleft lip and cleft palate. Suggested changes. Rev Hosp Clin Fac Med Sao Paulo. 1972;27(1):5–6.

Spina V, Kamakura L, Lapa F. Surgical management of bilateral cleft lip. Ann Plast Surg. 1978;1(5):497–505.

Trindade IEKSF, Silva Filho OG. Fissuras lábiopalatinas: uma abordagem interdisciplinar. 1st ed. São Paulo: Ed Santos; 2007.

Victor V, editor. Division palatine. Paris: Masson; 1931.

Current Management of Bilateral Cleft Lip

9

Cassio Eduardo Raposo-Amaral
and Cesar Augusto Raposo-Amaral

9.1　Introduction

9.1.1　Concept

Bilateral cleft lip has some unique embryological and anatomical characteristics and therefore requires a different therapeutic approach. The deformity is a consequence of fusion failure or lack of mesodermal migration that generates a discontinuation between the nasomedial process and the lateral maxillary process that separate the lip and alveolar arch into three pieces (Pruzansky 1971; Heidbuchel et al. 1998).

The bilateral cleft presents a wide phenotypical spectrum that can be shown as an asymmetric form evolving the lip and maxillary arch in different degrees. Possible manifestations involve the presence of Keith scar, preforamen incisive incomplete or complete, and transforamen incisive, with presence or absence of Simonart band (Spina et al. 1972). The involvement of the lip may similarly occur on cleft sides or be totally uneven, requiring an individualized treatment for each case. The prolabium and premaxilla are shown in the preforamen and transforamen incisive forms.

The prolabium contains the portion corresponding to the philtrum with absence of the *orbicularis muscle* (Khosla et al. 2012). The premaxilla remains connected to the vomer and projected in relation to the maxillary arch. Common nasal alterations seen in the bilateral clefts are the wide alar base with laterally flared nasal valve with malpositioning of the lower lateral cartilage, wide nasal base, short columella, malpositioning of the domes, and bifid nasal tip.

C.E. Raposo-Amaral, M.D., Ph.D. (✉)
Institute of Plastic and Craniofacial Surgery, SOBRAPAR Hospital,
Campinas, São Paulo 13084-880, Brazil

Universidade de São Paulo, São Paulo, Brazil
e-mail: cassioraposo@hotmail.com

C.A. Raposo-Amaral, M.D.
Institute of Plastic and Craniofacial Surgery, SOBRAPAR Hospital, Campinas, São Paulo, Brazil

A particularity of the bilateral clefts that should be emphasized is the symmetry of the deformities and the similarity between the sides of the affected nose. Generally, there is a symmetrical involvement of the alar base. As the lower lateral cartilage is malpositioned and anatomically lower compared to the normal position, it results in reduction of the projection of the nasal tip and columella height. However, the nasal base often remains symmetrical.

The palatine cleft tends to be wider in bilaterals with the narrow palatal shelves and centered vomer. All these characteristics make the rehabilitation of the bilateral cleft lip and palate a major challenge for the cleft team. The plastic surgeon should be aware of the three main variables that are the keystones of the rehabilitation: speech, nasolabial aesthetics, and facial growth.

Aiming to overcome the difficulties and limitations of surgery in a bilateral cleft, a delicate and atraumatic technique, the development of principles to maintain the long-term satisfactory outcome and avoid recurrence as well as the ability to deal with complications are critical (Cutting et al. 1998).

9.1.2 Principles

The modern principles of the bilateral cleft lip repair can be summarized below which description is credited to Mulliken (Mulliken et al. 2003):

- Try to establish symmetry or decrease the asymmetry.
- Realign the alveolar arch especially for those with severely protruding premaxilla using presurgical orthopedics or premaxilla setback.
- Insert the vertical lip scar into the aesthetic lip subunits lines that can possibly mirror a natural philtral column.
- Construct the median tubercle and Cupid's bow using lateral labial elements and mobilize the *orbicularis oris* muscle to the middle, whenever possible.
- Reposition the lower lateral cartilage and refine nasal tip and columella.

Ideally, a successful protocol is based on intelligible speech, satisfactory functional and aesthetic outcome, absence of sequels, and facilitation of the orthodontic treatment with inhibition of major facial growth disturbance. In most cases a minor degree of maxillary retrusion is expectable as a consequence of scar tissue produced by the closure of the lip and palate or both. Some of the trends and techniques used in the bilateral are not a consensus among the cleft teams worldwide, such as whether or not to use a presurgical orthopedics, or surgically manipulate the severely protruded and deviated premaxilla and finally to perform the lip repair in one or two stages. It is important to emphasize our understanding as a craniofacial plastic surgeons that the maxillary retrusion can be predictably corrected by orthognathic surgery either using distraction osteogenesis in younger patients with severe discrepancy between the jaws or by immediate movements at an adult age. Thus, the keystone for patient rehabilitation should be based on the normal speech first, satisfactory nasolabial appearance without the bilateral cleft stigmata, and second and normal facial growth third.

9.1.3 Infant Presurgical Orthopedics

The concept and philosophy of presurgical orthopedics was initially proposed by McNeil in 1954, who developed a device for premaxillary repositioning before surgery (Winters and Hurwitz 1995). Since then there were several modifications as done by the Brazilians Spina and Lapa that utilized elastics to set back the premaxilla in the severe bilateral patients (Lapa and Spina 1969).

During the last five decades of evolution and progress, the infant preoperative orthopedics has significantly changed with the development of molding of the nasoalveolar region and the premaxillary segment. One of these devices of premaxilla setback was developed by Georgidane (Georgiade et al. 1989) and modified by Millard and Latham (Millard and Latham 1990). It consists of acrylic plates fixed to the maxillary shelves and through an elastic system daily activated that can bring the premaxilla back and expand the anterior palatal segments (Millard and Latham 1990).

Cutting and Grayson described a nasoalveolar molding apparatus that consists of a passive plate to reduce the width of cleft and reshape the nasal contour by elevating the nostril and can be adapted to elongate the columella (Grayson and Cutting 2001). Weekly changes and adaptations are necessary to maximize the potential benefits of this passive device.

Bennun and Figueroa proposed a more loosely intraoral plate that takes advantage of the force of the tongue during movements to push upward the nasal nostril through a flexible spring connected to the acrylic plate (Bennun and Figueroa 2006; Bennun and Langsam 2009).

The major advantages of infant presurgical orthopedics has been the alignment of the alveolar arch, facilitation of feeding, improvement of the speech, and modification of nasolabial morphology (Ross and MacNamera 1994; Uzel and Alparslan 2011). In addition, it may have reduced the number of secondary surgeries by generating longitudinal nasal symmetry.

A recent study showed that surgeons rated the severity of the cleft as minimal in patients prepared with NAM in comparison to their controls without NAM preparation, and pointed out that less cleft severity yields the better outcomes (Rubin et al. 2015).

NAM and Latham devices reduced the width of the cleft by bringing back the premaxillary segment and promoting similar objectives. Thus, the NAM could facilitate the closing of the palate shelves and alveolar gaps and allow maxillary stability, absence of oronasal fistulas, and better nasal positioning and labial philtrum format. However, Uzel and Alparslan (Uzel and Alparslan 2011) have found in a systematic review that only 09 studies with high-level evidence showed changes on nasal symmetry after PSO and NAM and only one had a control group. One study by Ross and MacNamera in a bilateral cleft did not identify differences in aesthetics scores between groups with and without PSO (Uzel and Alparslan 2011). Opponents of NAM have implicated its use to additional cost and labor intensiveness (Xu et al. 2009), lack of expansion of the maxillary segment, and inability to align the protruded premaxillary segment to alveolar arch and its complication associated to inflammation of the mucosa and ulceration of the skin when the prolabial band is tight, and eventual airway obstruction. It has been postulated that the NAM therapy does not have any influence on facial growth as other type of active apparatus that may cause facial growth disturbance, maxillary retrusion, and crossbite owing to pressure at an infant age (Ross and MacNamera 1994; Uzel and Alparslan 2011). In addition, the treatment of bilateral cleft has its inherent implication on facial growth, restricting the vertical and anterior dimension of the maxilla. Thus, it can be difficult to determine if the NAM or the surgeries that are responsible for the restriction of facial growth.

As stated by Meara and Abbot, NAM appears to be a promising technique that still requires a high-level evidence to demonstrate its efficacy (Abbott and Meara 2012). The group of Chang Gung University has shown in a controlled clinical trial comparing different groups with or without NAM therapy that the association of NAM and primary surgical therapy yielded the optimal result by approximating the operated anatomy to normal (Chang et al. 2014).

In Brazil very few centers adopted infant presurgical orthopedics technique as it is not covered by our unified health insurance (SUS); on the other hand a majority of centers of North America use some type of presurgical orthopedics (Sitzman et al. 2008).

Thus, further studies may identify the role of facial orthopedics on decreasing the tension of the final cutaneous suture, scar contraction, and lip height deficiency, especially in severe patients with wide clefts. These population are best candidates for NAM therapy or any other type of IPSO.

9.1.4 Surgical Technique

9.1.4.1 Surgical Goals

One of the greatest challenges in correcting a bilateral cleft is to construct a well-defined curvilinear Cupid's bow with emphasis on the midline white roll that is absent in bilateral prolabium. Construction of a philtral dimple and elevated ridges as previously pointed out "can be beyond one's surgical skills" and it may be highly depended on individuals' response to scar formation and contraction (Rogers et al. 2014). The final scar should be symmetrical and simulate the philtrum column bilaterally. The transition of the dry and wet lip vermilion on the lateral side toward the medial side should be smooth with an inconspicuous scar in the midline and without a color or volume mismatch in the midline tubercle. The static and dynamic lip anatomy should look equally satisfactory as the *orbicularis oris muscle* adequately healing determines the ability to move the lips without compromise of pickling and whistling.

The nose should be symmetrical and as close to normal as possible. Common postoperative deformities have been a consequence of severely intrinsic anomaly or mistaken preoperative markings (Losee et al. 2003) or might be a lack of full understanding of the bilateral deformity and current philosophy and principles to be followed as most of the poor results in Brazil come from the nonspecialized centers.

9.1.4.2 Markings

The peak of the Cupid's bow is initially marked, and then two points are marked laterally 3 mm from the first one; thus the width of the philtrum is usually 6–7 mm. The vertical line that simulates the philtrum column is slightly angulated toward 1–2 mm below the columellar line. The base of the prolabium flap is usually narrow to 5 mm of measurement in its width (Fig. 9.1).

The peak of the Cupid's bow is marked laterally, placing the lateral point at the attenuation of the white roll as previously emphasized. Then we marked also a 3 mm straight line (similar distance of half dimension of the philtrum width) in the lateral skin component at 01 mm above the white roll (distance named in our drawing as distance A). This incision will facilitate rotation of the lip vermilion as it will not efface the white roll. If the incision is placed in the white roll there is a tendency to efface the natural curvature of the bow and the continuation of the tiny roll. The lateral prolabium tissue is used for the nasal floor if needed. A small triangular region of skin is deepithelialized as marked in Fig. 9.2.

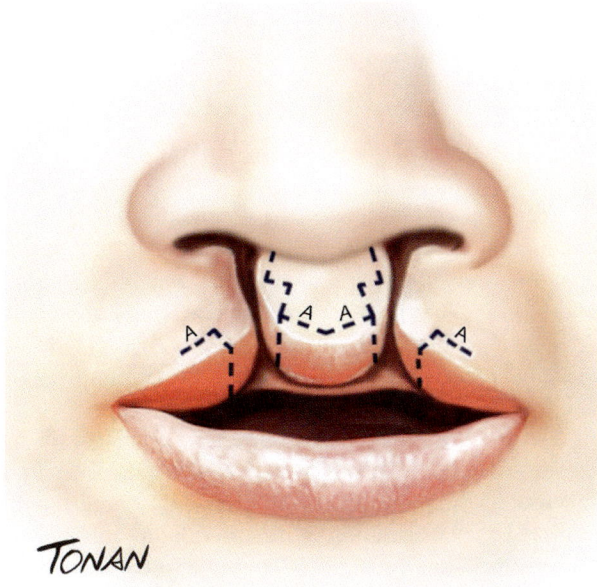

Fig. 9.1 Illustration of the preoperative markings. Note the strip of skin above the white roll marked in a dotted line (letter A). The lateral segments are designed to build the median lip tubercle

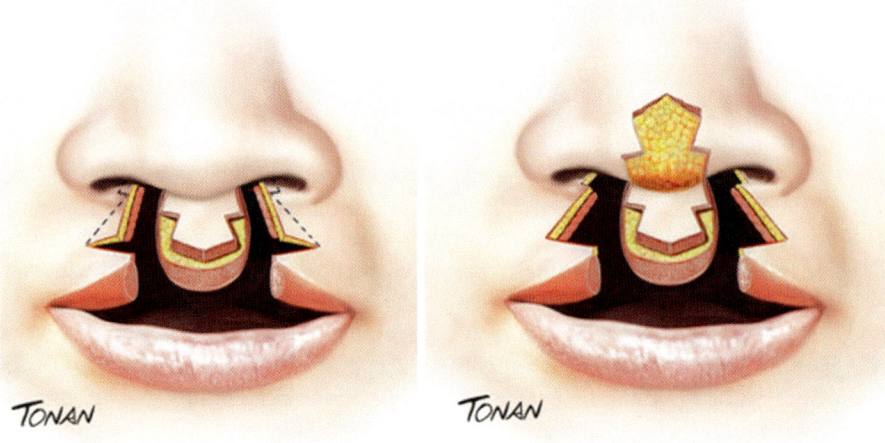

Fig. 9.2 Illustration of the surgical sequence. *Left*: The lateral segments are incised and rotated medially and then the area formed by the most caudal point on the lateral segment and the upper point on the cleft edge (bilateral triangular area) is deepithelialized. This area allows sagittal projection of the philtrum column. *Right*: The philtral flap is elevated toward the columella, and the septal columellar incision is performed

9.1.4.3 Operative Technique

The Cupid's bow peak is initially marked, and then two points are marked laterally, 3 mm from the first one; thus, the width of the philtrum is usually 6 mm. The vertical lines that simulate the philtrum column are slightly angulated toward 1 to 2 mm below the columellar line. The base of the prolabium flap is usually narrow, measuring 4 mm in its width.

The peak of Cupid's bow is marked laterally, placing the lateral point at the attenuation of the white roll, as previously emphasized. Then we also marked a 3 mm straight line (similar distance of one-half the dimension of the prolabium width) in the lateral skin component at 1 mm above the white roll (named distance A in our drawing). This incision will facilitate rotation of the lip vermilion, as it will not efface the white roll. The lateral prolabium tissue is used for the nasal floor, if needed.

The first maneuver usually elevates the prolabium and goes in the direction of the septum-columellar junction that is also cut. This incision is extended to the tip mucosa, as the nasal tip can be exposed for suturing of the medial crura of the alar cartilages after elevation of the prolabium-columellar flap. The remaining prolabium vermilion is used to offer tissue to the gingivobuccal sulcus; therefore, little tissue is trimmed. The lateral incision starts at the transverse incision determined as letter A (Fig. 9.2). This 3 mm incision in the lateral segment (A incision) is performed 1 mm above and parallel to the white roll and rotates it down, toward the midline at the central portion of the lip vermilion. The lateral skin tissue within the lateral vermilion-mucosal flaps is dissected and prepared for a latter rotation forming the central lip bow. The lateral incisions are performed in a triangular fashion

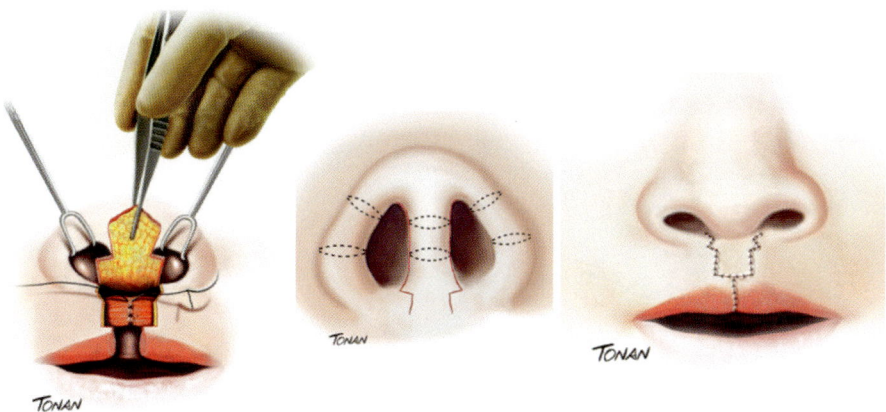

Fig. 9.3 *Left*: The *orbicularis oris* muscle is isolated from the lateral labial segments, and the muscle fibers are directed to the midline to form the central lip. *Center*: Details of the suturing of the medial alar crus and alar cartilage that prevent vestibular webbing. *Right*: Final aspect of the lip repair with well-defined curvilinear Cupid's bow. The strip of skin avoids the scar into the white roll

from the most caudal point on the lateral segment to the upper point on the cleft edge. This area of skin is deepithelialized (Fig. 9.2). The supra-periosteum dissection is accomplished by a gingivobuccal incision. The extension of the dissection is usually dictated by the severity of the cleft, as the most severe clefts require the widest dissection. The floor of the nose can be constructed using the L flap (lateral flap) sutured to the vestibular mucosa and the S flap (nasal septum flap), as previously described for unilateral cleft lip repair (Cutting and Dayan 2003). The two lateral segments are brought together. The *orbicularis oris* muscle is isolated and sutured in the midline. The skin is gently sutured with nylon thread and an atraumatic needle, as we previously described for unilateral clefts, and removed 7 days after surgery under sedation (Raposo-Amaral et al. 2012, 2014) (Fig. 9.3).

9.1.4.4 Premaxillary Setback and Lip Adhesion

Premaxillary setback combined with lip adhesion was performed in all patients with protruded and deviated premaxilla (over 10 mm). The projection of the premaxilla is measured from the lateral segments, alveolar arch and the premaxillary arch. This distance determines the length of bone resection to be performed. The mucosa is incised and undermined toward the septum. The maxillary growth center bulb is identified, and the osteotomy is performed 2 mm caudally of this bulb with a long and small reciprocating saw (Aesculap®). The triangular resection of the cartilaginous septum is performed either with a scissor or a number 11 blade. The bone and septal cartilage are removed (Fig. 9.4, below), and two bony segments are brought together and fixed with one number 0-wire (Ethicon®). This wire is twisted and trimmed and covered by the mucosa sutured with a 4–0 polyglactin suture (Vicryl, Ethicon®) that can be removed during the palatoplasty if needed. The basis of the premaxillary setback was described by Millard (1977). The final lip repair is performed after palate repair and 12–13 months after premaxillary setback and lip adhesion (Fig. 9.5–9.13).

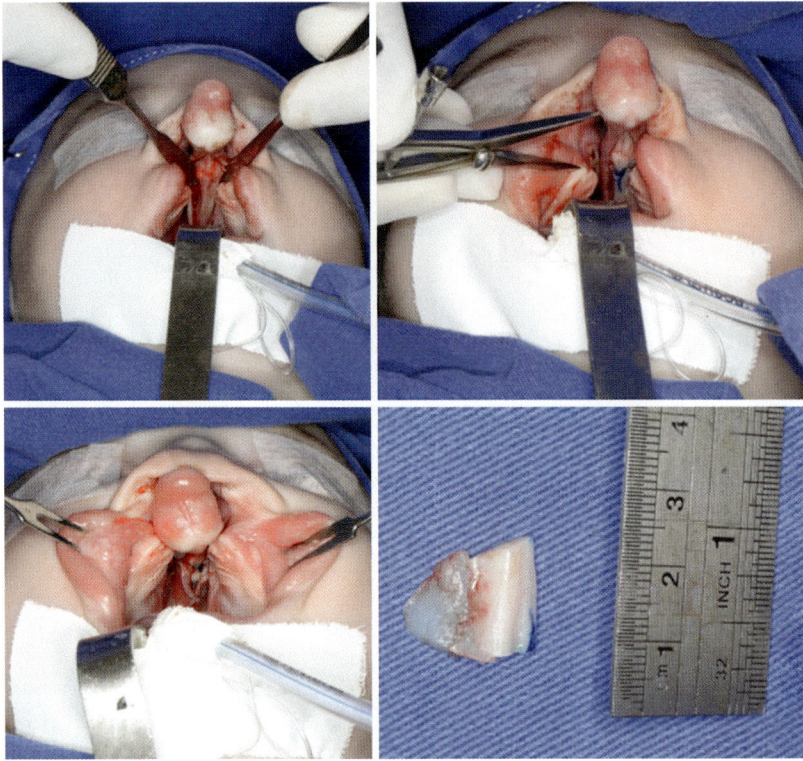

Fig. 9.4 *Left and above*: Photograph of a bilateral patient showing a premaxillary projection of 25 mm. The *methylene blue* marked the amount of resection to be performed to set back the central segment and to fit it into the alveolar arch. *Right and above*: The caliper was used to measure the amount of premaxillary projection. *Left and below*: Photograph of the same patient after the premaxillary setback. The alveolar arch is aligned. Lip adhesion is performed in conjunction with the premaxillary setback and the final lip repair after palate repair. *Right and below*: The osseous cartilaginous resection in a triangular fashion of the vomerine-septal region

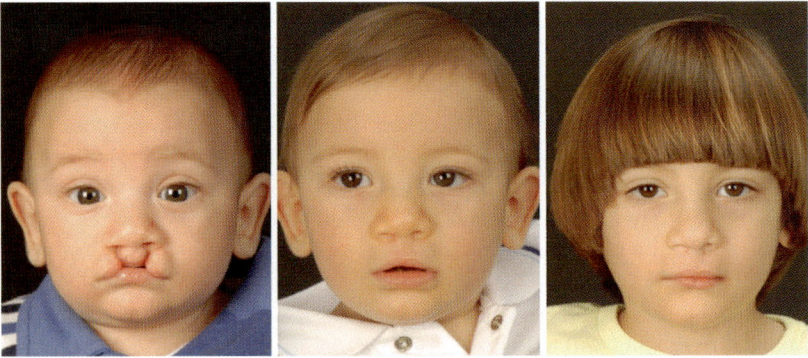

Fig. 9.5 *Left*: Preoperative photograph of a bilateral complete cleft lip and palate patient. *Center*: Postoperative photograph of the same patient at 3 months after surgery. *Right*: Postoperative photograph of the same patient at 2 years after surgery

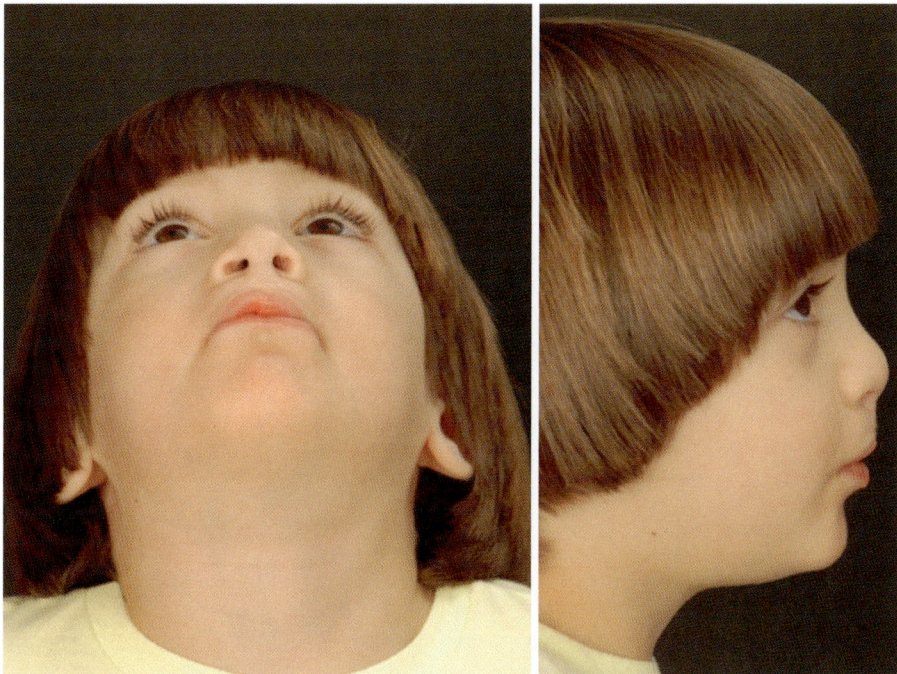

Fig. 9.6 *Left*: Postoperative basal view of the same patient and *Right*, lateral view

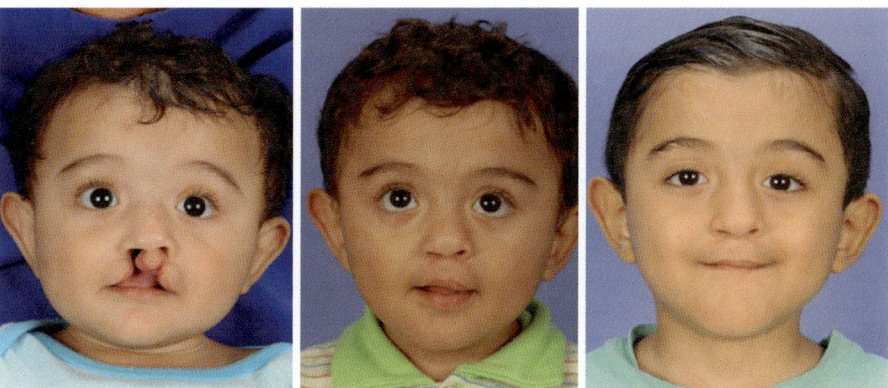

Fig. 9.7 *Left*: Preoperative photograph of an asymmetric bilateral cleft lip and palate patient. *Center*: Postoperative photograph of the same patient at 3 months after surgery. *Right*: Postoperative photograph of the same patient at 2 years after surgery

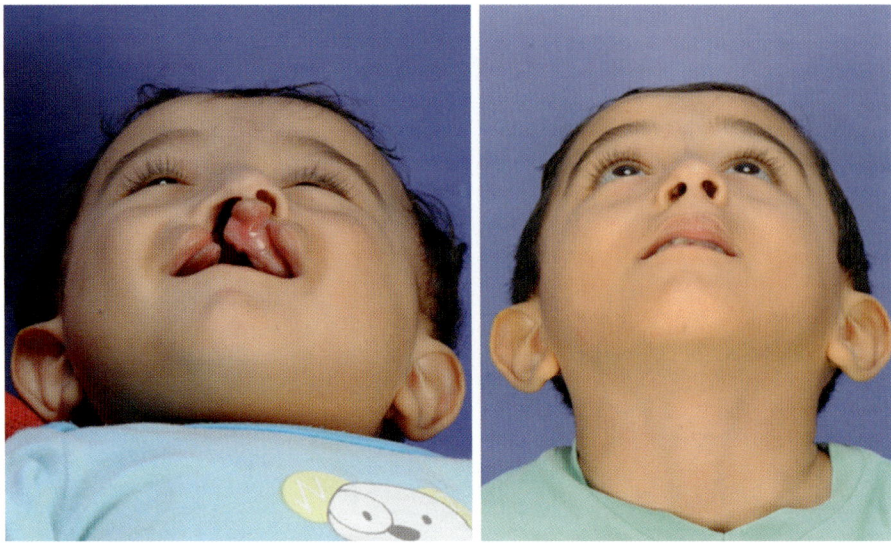

Fig. 9.8 *Left*: Preoperative basal view of the same patient, and *right*, postoperative basal view

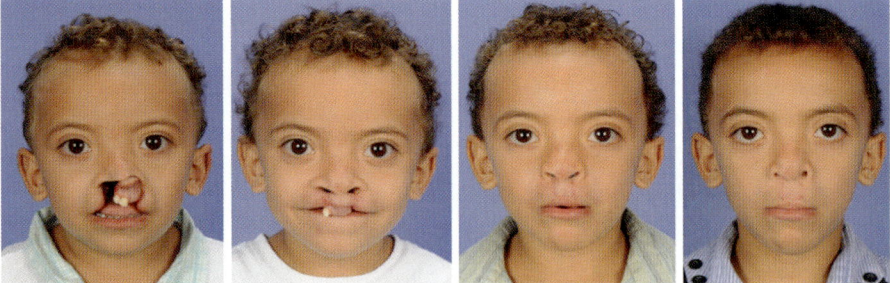

Fig. 9.9 *Left*: Preoperative photograph of a 4-year-old bilateral complete cleft lip and palate patient showing a protruded and deviated premaxilla. *Center*: Postoperative photograph of the same patient at 3 months after surgery. *Right*: Postoperative photograph of the same patient at 2 years after surgery

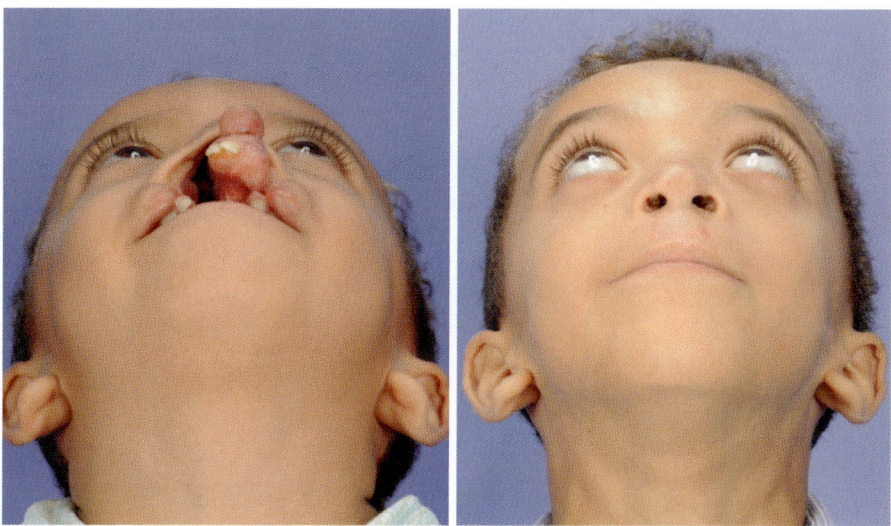

Fig. 9.10 *Left*: Preoperative basal view of the same patient, and *right*, postoperative basal view

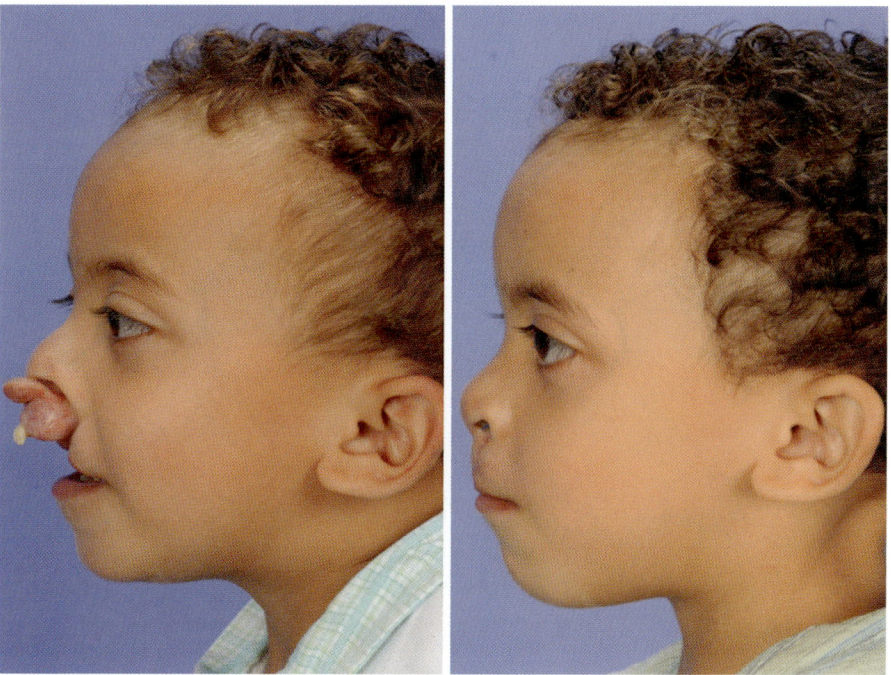

Fig. 9.11 *Left*: Profile view of the same patient, and *right*, postoperative profile view

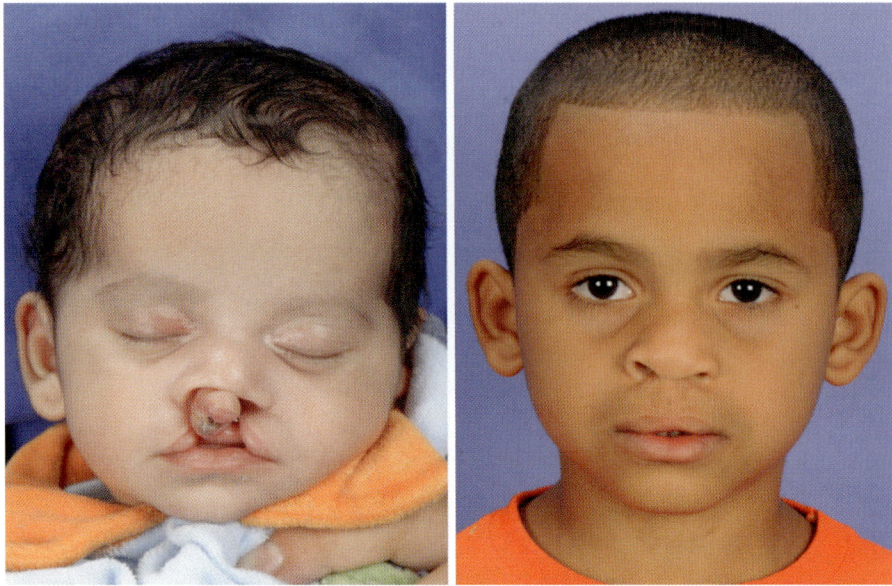

Fig. 9.12 *Left*: Preoperative frontal photograph of a patient with a severely deviated and protruded premaxilla. *Right*: Postoperative frontal photograph after premaxillary setback and lip adhesion and final lip repair

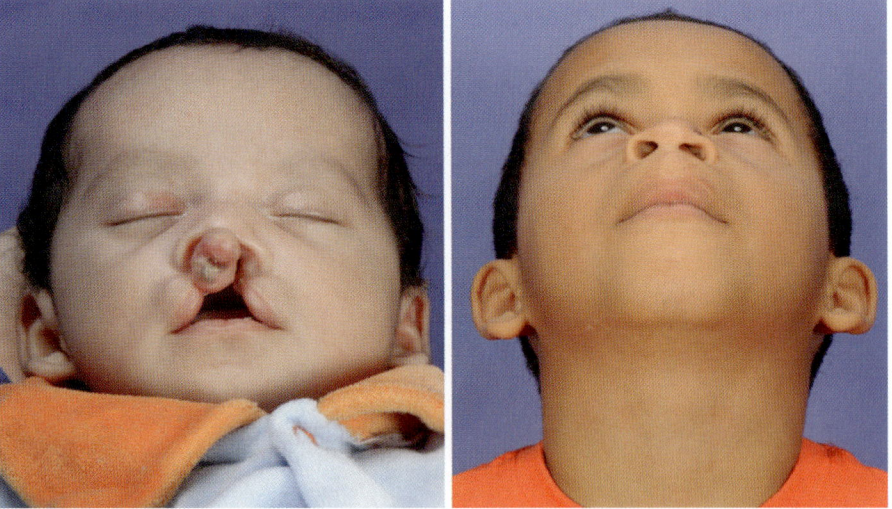

Fig. 9.13 *Left*: Preoperative basal view of the same patient, and *right*, postoperative basal view

9.1.4.5 Controversies

The bilateral cleft lip repair carries controversies. Among the highly important ones are whether to repair the lip in one or two stages or surgically primarily retrude the premaxilla.

Historically, the treatment of the bilateral lip repair was performed in two stages by operating the most severe side first.

Victor Spina in 1964 proposed the method of staging the operations in patients with protruded premaxilla to avoid maxillary growth restriction, probably one of the most used techniques in Brazil to date (Spina 1964). He performed adhesion of one side first, then the other one, and at 3 years of age the definitive repair by using the philtrum mucosa to construct the median tubercle with the lateral segments. Similar principles became popularized worldwide by Manchester (1970). In fact, Spina's main concern was the facial growth by avoiding a tight lip. In this technique the *orbicularis oris* muscle is rarely sutured in the midline and the philtrum width tends to be wider in comparison to lips treated by the modern current techniques. Current trends construct a lip surrounded by a straight-line bilateral scar (one in each side). In addition, old techniques that advocate using the philtrum mucosa to recreate the median tubercle often end up with a color mismatch between the lateral mucosa and philtrum mucosa as well as lip volume discrepancy in the midline known as whistle deformity, a striking stigmata of bilateral cleft. The wide philtrum created by these principles is very difficult to correct in a later stage and has been a wish among patients of our clinic. In addition, Nagase (Nagase et al. 1998) has shown no growth disturbance after *orbicularis oris* muscle repositioning. However, it is our belief that it is dependable on the degree of protrusion of the premaxillary segment.

Millard also described a staged method in which a forked skin flap was primarily banked to improve columella height in a second stage in addition to nasal suspension (Millard 1971). The banked flap has been no longer used by cleft surgeons around the globe as it effaces the natural columellar-lip junction. There is a continuous debate over performing the lip correction in one or two stages. We believe that performing it into a single stage is easier to achieve the final symmetry. Exception to this rule is when the premaxilla is highly protruded and deviated, and then we perform the premaxilla setback and lip adhesion first and then in a second stage perform the lip repair simultaneously addressing the both sides. The setback is reserved either for patients with severely protruded or a deviated premaxilla in 3-month-old child or for primary patients with late presentation.

The key element to achieve the proper fullness of the tubercle is the preoperative markings of the peak of the Cupid's bow. This point should be marked at the point where the white roll started to be attenuated (Xu et al. 2009) that usually coincides with the point proposed by Losee "before the beginning of the vertical attenuation of the lip fullness" (Losee et al. 2003). The long-lasting lip fullness depends on where one places the incision. Two incisions in the lateral segment are critical. The first one is the top of nasal labial junction and at lower margin of the alar base and the second incision should be at 01 mm above the transition toward the lateral segment and allowing skin to be rotated with musculocutaneous flap and allowing the tubercle to be filled by lateral tissue. Considering that the tubercle white roll is missing in the bilateral clefts, it is important that the lateral well-defined white roll rotates downward to be sutured together in the midline. If the incision is placed in the immediate transition of white roll and dry mucosa, the postoperative scar tends to obliterate the natural white roll curvature as it might lose its natural design. However, to accomplish such a maneuver one has to be able to make sure that the premaxilla is aligned into the alveolar arch and not overprotruded. As we in our center do not offer NAM or any type of infant orthopedics, we plan the premaxillary setback in severe patients with protruded and deviated premaxilla, cleft patients with a very short columella (less than 2 mm). This maneuver is done in conjunction with the lip adhesion. The final lip repair is done after the palate repair. The *orbicularis oris* muscle is sutured in the midline whenever possible. The osteotomy is performed behind the growth center bulb to avoid premaxillary growth disturbance. The segments are fixed with wires and enough stability is guaranteed. We understand that the setback is easier to perform when the palate is still open because once it is close the osteotomy lines needed to be done anteriorly, close to the septum jeopardizing the growth center bulb and vascularity of the premaxillary segment.

The muscle dissection on the maxilla can be accomplished subperiosteally or supraperiosteally. There is no evidence for which type of dissection promotes less facial growth disturbance. It is our belief that dissecting over the periosteal plane is easier to mobilize the lateral segments medially.

With regard to nasal approach, we do believe that the tip exposure can be achieved by a minimal extension of the septum columellar incision on the tip mucosa similarly as described by Cutting as a retrograde method (Cutting et al. 1998). The Tajima incision may be an option, but the skin incision and subsequent healing may be subject to parent's complaints. The idea is offering enough room for alar crus harvesting and suturing, allowing tip projection either by a Tajima incision or a retrograde method as described by Cutting. The blood supply of the prolabium is derived from the external branches of the anterior ethmoid arteries as it allows retrograde elevation of the prolabial flap and exposure of the nasal cartilages.

9.2 Summary

We review our approaches to bilateral cleft patients. Based on our national characteristics of our unified health system, we do not work with infant presurgical orthopedics and we tend to approach the lip in one stage following the current modern trends of bilateral cleft lip repair. We use a premaxilla setback in severely deviated and protruded premaxilla. This maneuver facilitates lip closure without tension. We have been using our own SOBRAPAR modification of bilateral cleft lip repair shown in our sequencing drawings. We have been able to avoid the current cleft stigmata often seen in patients whose surgery was not performed in Brazilian cleft centers.

Acknowledgments The authors thank the artist Rodrigo Tonan for the drawings.

References

Abbott MM, Meara JG. Nasoalveolar molding in cleft care: is it efficacious? Plast Reconstr Surg. 2012;130(3):659–66.

Bennun RD, Figueroa AA. Dynamic presurgical nasal remodeling in patients with unilateral and bilateral cleft lip and palate: modification to the original technique. Cleft Palate Craniofac J. 2006;43(6):639–48.

Bennun RD, Langsam AC. Long-term results after using dynamic presurgical nasoalveolar remodeling technique in patients with unilateral and bilateral cleft lips and palates. J Craniofac Surg. 2009;20(Suppl 1):670–4.

Chang CS, Wallace CG, Pai BC, Chiu YT, Hsieh YJ, Chen IJ, et al. Comparison of two nasoalveolar molding techniques in unilateral complete cleft lip patients: a randomized, prospective, single-blind trial to compare nasal outcomes. Plast Reconstr Surg. 2014;134(2):275–82.

Cutting CB, Dayan JH. Lip height and lip width after extended Mohler unilateral cleft lip repair. Plast Reconstr Surg. 2003;111(1):17–23. discussion 4-6

Cutting C, Grayson B, Brecht L, Santiago P, Wood R, Kwon S. Presurgical columellar elongation and primary retrograde nasal reconstruction in one-stage bilateral cleft lip and nose repair. Plast Reconstr Surg. 1998;101(3):630–9.

Georgiade NG, Mason R, Riefkohl R, Georgiade G, Barwick W. Preoperative positioning of the protruding premaxilla in the bilateral cleft lip patient. Plast Reconstr Surg. 1989;83(1):32–40.

Grayson BH, Cutting CB. Presurgical nasoalveolar orthopedic molding in primary correction of the nose, lip, and alveolus of infants born with unilateral and bilateral clefts. Cleft Palate Craniofac J. 2001;38(3):193–8.

Heidbuchel KL, Kuijpers-Jagtman AM, Kramer GJ, Prahl-Andersen B. Maxillary arch dimensions in bilateral cleft lip and palate from birth until four years of age in boys. Cleft Palate Craniofac J. 1998;35(3):233–9.

Khosla RK, McGregor J, Kelley PK, Gruss JS. Contemporary concepts for the bilateral cleft lip and nasal repair. Semin Plast Surg. 2012;26(4):156–63.

Lapa F, Spina V. The use of a passive orthopedic device in the management of uni and bilateral cleft lip and palate. Panminerva Med. 1969;11(1):64–7.

Losee JE, Selber JC, Arkoulakis N, Serletti JM. The cleft lateral lip element: do traditional markings result in secondary deformities? Ann Plast Surg. 2003;50(6):594–600.

Manchester WM. The repair of double cleft lip as part of an integrated program. Plast Reconstr Surg. 1970;45(3):207–16.

Millard DR Jr. Closure of bilateral cleft lip and elongation of columella by two operations in infancy. Plast Reconstr Surg. 1971;47(4):324–31.

Millard DR Jr. Cleft Craft, volume II, bilateral and rare deformities. Boston: Little Brown and co; 1977. p. 41–80.

Millard DR Jr, Latham RA. Improved primary surgical and dental treatment of clefts. Plast Reconstr Surg. 1990;86(5):856–71.

Mulliken JB, Wu JK, Padwa BL. Repair of bilateral cleft lip: review, revisions, and reflections. J Craniofac Surg. 2003;14(5):609–20.

Nagase T, Januszkiewicz JS, Keall HJ, de Geus JJ. The effect of muscle repair on postoperative facial skeletal growth in children with bilateral cleft lip and palate. Scand J Plast Reconstr Surg Hand Surg. 1998;32(4):395–405.

Pruzansky S. The growth of the premaxillary-vomerine complex in complete bilateral cleft lip and palate. Tandlaegebladet. 1971;75(12):1157–69.

Raposo-Amaral CE, Giancolli AP, Denadai R, Marques FF, Somensi RS, Raposo-Amaral CA, et al. Lip height improvement during the first year of unilateral complete cleft lip repair using cutting extended Mohler technique. Plast Surg Int. 2012;2012:206481.

Raposo-Amaral CE, Giancolli AP, Denadai R, Somensi RS, Raposo-Amaral CA. Late cutaneous lip height in unilateral incomplete cleft lip patients does not differ from the normative data. J Craniofac Surg. 2014;25(1):308–13.

Rogers CR, Meara JG, Mulliken JB. The philtrum in cleft lip: review of anatomy and techniques for construction. J Craniofac Surg. 2014;25(1):9–13.

Ross RB, MacNamera MC. Effect of presurgical infant orthopedics on facial esthetics in complete bilateral cleft lip and palate. Cleft Palate Craniofac J. 1994;31(1):68–73.

Rubin MS, Clouston S, Ahmed MM, Lowe KM, Shetye PR, Broder HL, et al. Assessment of presurgical clefts and predicted surgical outcome in patients treated with and without nasoalveolar molding. J Craniofac Surg. 2015;26(1):71–5.

Sitzman TJ, Girotto JA, Marcus JR. Current surgical practices in cleft care: unilateral cleft lip repair. Plast Reconstr Surg. 2008;121(5):261e–70e.

Spina V. Surgery of bilateral harelip: new concept. Preliminary results. Rev Paul Med. 1964;65:248–58.

Spina V, Psillakis JM, Lapa FS, Ferreira MC. Classification of cleft lip and cleft palate. Suggested changes. Rev Hosp Clin Fac Med Sao Paulo. 1972;27(1):5–6.

Uzel A, Alparslan ZN. Long-term effects of presurgical infant orthopedics in patients with cleft lip and palate: a systematic review. Cleft Palate Craniofac J. 2011;48(5):587–95.

Winters JC, Hurwitz DJ. Presurgical orthopedics in the surgical management of unilateral cleft lip and palate. Plast Reconstr Surg. 1995;95(4):755–64.

Xu H, Salyer KE, Genecov ER. Primary bilateral one-stage cleft lip/nose repair: 40-year Dallas experience: part I. J Craniofac Surg. 2009;20(Suppl 2):1913–26.

Cleft Palate: Anatomy and Surgery

10

Nivaldo Alonso, Jonas Eraldo Lima Jr.,
Hagner Lucio de Andrade Lima, and Hillary E. Jenny

10.1 Introduction

In the statement from Charles Down in 1925 it was written that "The repair of palate should be offered before speech is established." Almost 100 years after his principles are still in discussion nowadays; early operation, operation done in several stages, anatomical description, and flexibility and depth of the soft palate should be considered to obtain better results in palatoplasty (Dowd 1925).

Differences between isolated cleft palate and cleft palate associated with cleft lip are notorious, closely related to gender and to other syndromic malformations; isolated cleft palate is another deformity, with very peculiar anatomical problems.

In an effort to reduce the incidence of cleft palate by understanding predisposing conditions, several environmental (use of alcohol in pregnancy, smoking, folic acid deficiency, use of neuroleptics, and others) and genetic (chromosomal anomalies) factors have been extensively studied. Genetics is clearly involved in cleft palate; many genes are candidate for its cause (Brito et al. 2012).

Many years after the first procedures for cleft repair were done still controversy exists on the surgery, age of surgery, and final speech results.

N. Alonso, M.D., Ph.D. (✉)
Divisao de Cirurgia Plastica e Queimaduras, Hospital das Clínicas da Faculdade de Medicina da Universidade de São Paulo, São Paulo, Brazil
e-mail: nivalonso@gmail.com

J.E. Lima Jr., M.D.
Board Certified Brazilian Society of Plastic Surgery, Federal University of Tocantins, Palmas, Tocantins, Brazil

H.L. de Andrade Lima, M.D.
Plastic Surgeon in a Private Clinic, Bauru, São Paulo, Brazil

H.E. Jenny, M.D.
Plastic Surgery Resident in the Program at John Hopkins, Baltimore, MD, USA

10.2 Embryology

The palate is embryologically divided into primary and secondary palate by the incisive foramen. The primary palate develops around the fifth week of gestation from the medial nasal process, originating the upper lip and the upper jaw (including the central incisors), which will merge to the lateral nasal processes, the nose and the lip. The secondary palate begins developing during the 6th week of gestation, and is completely formed by the 12th week. It originates from the maxillar process; the palate lamina migrates medially (previously separated by the superior position of the tongue) and merges anterior-posteriorly (from the incisive foramen to the uvula), forming the hard and soft palates.

There are several theories to explain the origin of cleft lip and palate. It's currently accepted that cleft lip and palate is due to a failure in the migration of neuroectodermal cells, which is responsible for merging the facial processes after ectodermal lysis (RE LJaK 2009).

10.3 Anatomy

To understand cleft palate, it is important to understand the normal palate anatomy. The palate separates the oral and nasal cavities (called the oropharynx and nasopharynx), and is comprised of the soft and hard palate. The hard palate is bony and encloses the anterior portion of the oronasal cavity. This structure maintains the transverse maxillar diameter and connects itself cranially to the vomer, the most caudal segment of the nasal septum. The soft palate contains the most important structures for speech: the levator veli palatini muscles, along with the posterior and lateral pharynx walls, comprise the velopharyngeal sphincter (VPS). The VPS is a valve that separates the oral and nasal cavities in a dynamic way, particularly during deglutition and phonation. It is comprised of the following muscles: levator veli palatini, tensor veli palatini, uvulae, superior pharynx constrictor, palatopharyngeal, palatoglossus and salpingopharyngeal (Fig. 10.1).

The levator veli palatini is considered the most important muscle in the closure of the VPS during speech. It is responsible for the superior-posterior movement of the palate, and, due to its location, passively acts on the Eustachian tube to dislocate the salpingopharyngeal fold. This suggests that the levator veli palatini also accounts for the medial movement of the lateral pharynx walls (Fig. 10.2).

The tensor veli palatini muscle is compound by three functional muscle bundles: medial, lateral, and tensor tympani. The medial and tensor tympani bundles open and close the Eustachian tube during deglutition and other functions. The lateral bundle, which represents the muscle itself, applies tension to the palate. The uvulae muscle extends from the palatal aponeurosis to the uvula mucosa and is thought to increase the muscle volume in the palate's midline, thereby supporting the central part of the pharyngeal sphincter closing.

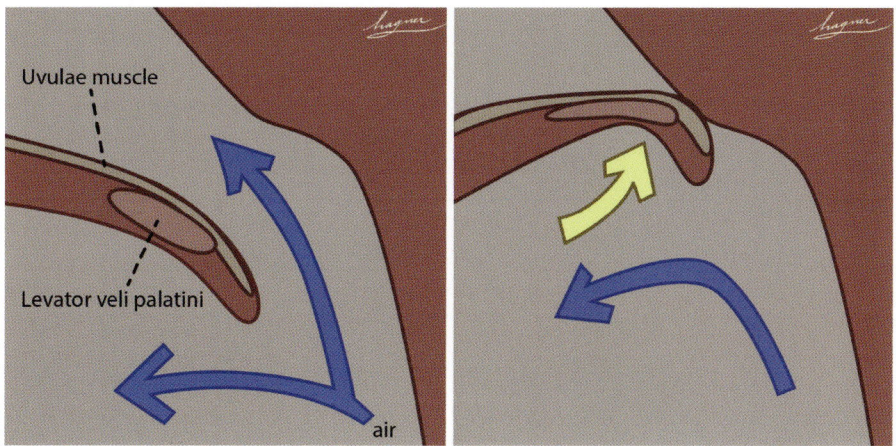

Fig. 10.1 Normal palate movement closing the nasal cavity, detail of the movement of levator and uvulae muscle

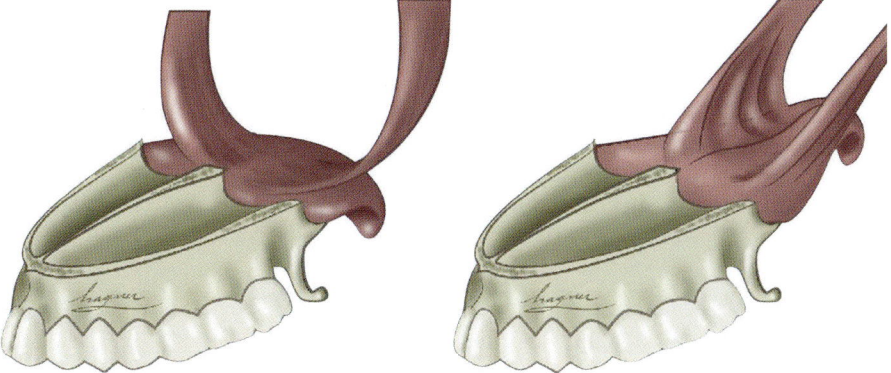

Fig. 10.2 Levator veli palatine action on the soft palate

The superior pharyngeal constrictor narrows the pharynx medially during its contraction by using its posterior (which can form a transverse fold in the posterior-anterior direction, called the Passavant ridge) and lateral walls. However, this muscle is considered the weakest in the pharynx and is divided into four bundles: pterygopharyngeal, buccopharyngeal, myolopharyngeal, and glossopharyngeal. This muscle participates in the compensatory mechanism of VPS closure by acting on the lateral walls.

Two muscles antagonize the levator palatini's superior-posterior movements: the palatopharyngeus and palatoglossus muscles. The palatopharyngeus muscle acts downward and backward to lower the palate, especially during deglutition. The palatoglossus muscle moves the palate downward and forward (Fig. 10.3a, b).

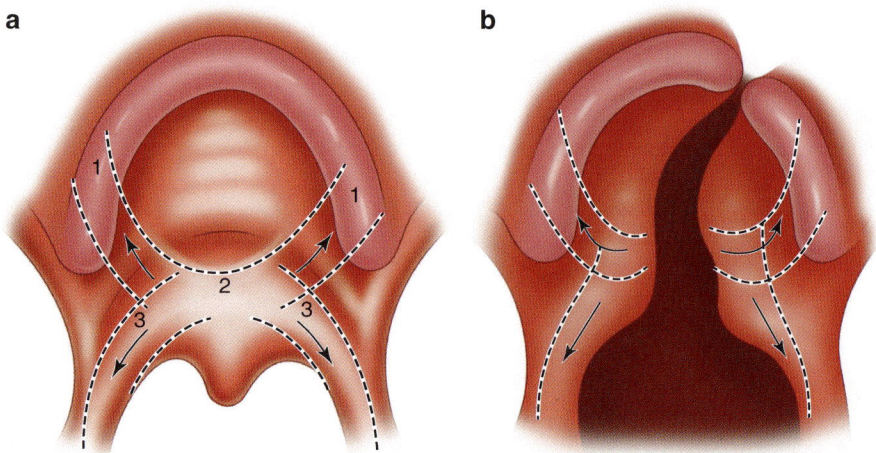

Fig. 10.3 (**a**) Action of the soft palate muscle—synergic action in a normal palate. (**b**) Abnormal traction forward and backward of the muscle in cleft patient

The velopharyngeal sphincter is innervated by the pharyngeal plexus, which contains fibers from the glossopharyngeal and vagus nerves and accessory fibers from the sphenopalatine ganglion. However, there are two exceptions: the tensor veli palatini and the uvular muscles. The first is innervated by the mandibular branch of the trigeminal nerve, and the last by the minor palatine nerve (a branch from the facial nerve) (Kriens 1969a, b, 1970; Shimokawa and Tanaka 2005).

In cleft lip and palate, the insertion of the palatal musculature is anomalous as it is directed anteriorly, towards the hard palate. These muscles are also hypoplastic most of the time. Due to these anomalies, the muscle fibers don't form the muscle bundle needed for the physiologic functioning of the velopharyngeal sphincter. For these reasons, even if the patient had perfect surgery velopharyngeal incompetence could happen.

10.4 Classification

Lip and palate clefts can be classified according to many different criteria, with some based on anatomic parameters and others on more complex aspects such as embryology. Using the incisive foramen as a dividing point between the primary and secondary palate, clefts can be classified as pre-foramen or post-foramen, and incomplete or complete when the cleft extends into the incisive foramen. Clefts involving both the primary and secondary palate are classified as incisive transforaminal clefts. This classification described as Spina's Classification is the most usual in Brazil (Victor 1973) (Fig. 10.4).

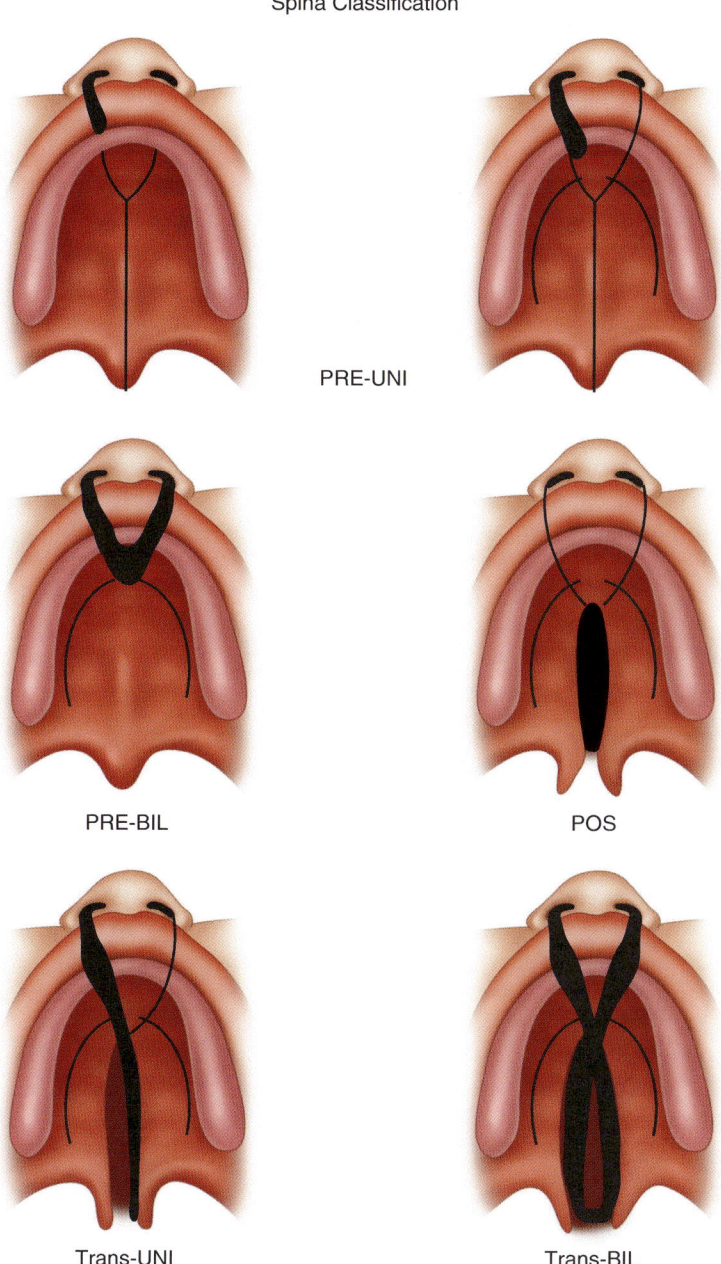

Fig. 10.4 Spina's Classification for cleft lip and palate most used in Brazil

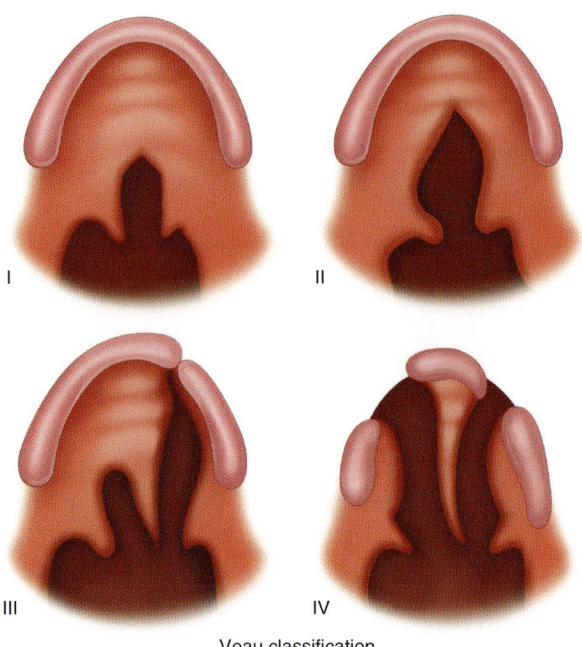

Fig. 10.5 Veau's Classification for cleft lip and palate

Another used classification is the one proposed by Veau, which divides clefts into four types: I, incomplete cleft, in which the cleft only involves the soft palate; II, fissure involving the soft and hard palates, but limited to the secondary palate; III, complete unilateral cleft lip and palate involving both the primary and secondary palate; and IV, complete bilateral cleft (Victor 1931) (Fig. 10.5).

But in both classifications we cannot evaluate precisely the final prognosis of the treatment. For palate cleft the final prognosis could be made based on clinical evaluation and also based on the anatomy of the cleft. If the cleft palate is short and symmetrical or if it is complete or incomplete it could predict the quality of the final speech of the patient.

Submucous palate clefts are characterized by the diastase of the soft palate muscles. As the palatal mucosa remains intact in these cleft, diagnosis is more difficult, as the disorder is often only made apparent around preschool age when the child demonstrates signs of velopharyngeal insufficiency. The presence of a bifid uvula can be indicative of this condition, as well as the presence of a palpable bifid posterior nasal spine. The incidence among the general population could be around 0.02–0.08% with the incidence of velopharyngeal inadequacy among these patients 1–9 (Gosain et al. 1996) (Fig. 10.6).

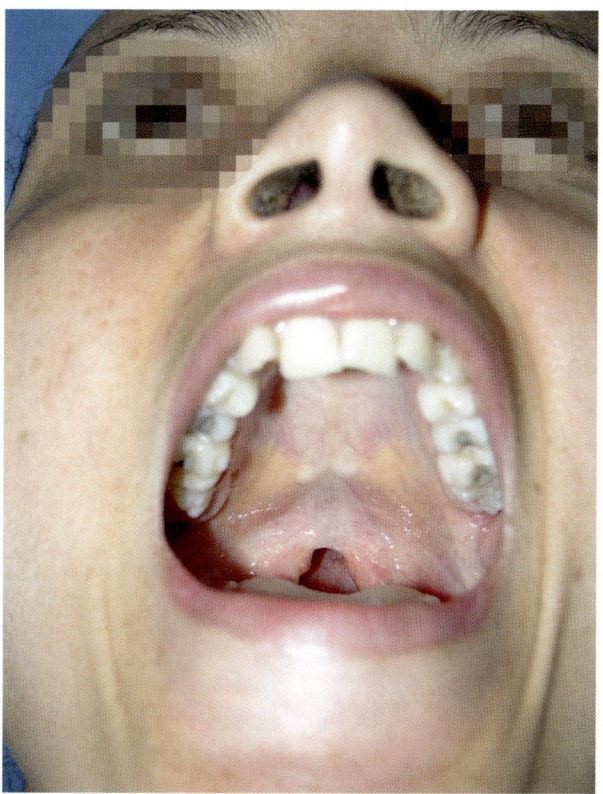

Fig. 10.6 Submucous cleft with bifid posterior nasal spine and abnormal soft palate muscle insertion

10.5 Surgical Treatment

Historically many interesting statements have been made previously about how to fix cleft palate; most of them are procedures and ideal time, but one very interesting statement to start this surgical paragraph is from J. Daniel Subtelny in 1962; in his findings over 10 years of studies of cleft palate growth, he said what is obviously nowadays that "A surgically repaired soft palate can grow adequately if properly repaired"; this statement is still a great challenge for surgeons (Subtelny 1956, 1962).

The treatment of cleft palate has two main goals: anatomical division of the oral and nasal cavities and repair of the soft palate muscles, reconstructing the muscular belt required for proper palate function and velopharyngeal sphincter closure during phonation.

There are several management protocols for patients with cleft lip and palate, where one differs from another with respect to the optimal timing and technique used for defect repair. Better speech results are generally seen in patients operated on early, but these cases show an increased restriction to facial growth; however, the opposite is also true. It is recommended to correct cleft palate prior to the start of vocal articulation to both avoid compensatory articulation disorders and enable the child to develop speech skills with the correct placement of the velopharyngeal sphincter muscles. In this way, less aggressive techniques that cause less scarring retractions on the palate are recommended, to avoid interference in the jaw growth.

Currently, major reference centers for treatment of cleft palate use vomerine flaps to close the anterior palate concurrently with lip repair (between 3 and 6 months), followed by veloplasty around 9–12 months to promote soft palate closure. Other centers choose for early closure of the posterior palate and postpone the anterior palatoplasty for about 3 years, to avoid any restriction on maxillary growth (Semb et al. 2005a).

Many multicentric studies have been done to establish unique protocol but it is still in discussion. Eurocleft, American Cleft, and others show quite a big number of options of treatment but randomized and prospective studies in course could bring us more about these details of palate surgery (Mercado et al. 2011; Shaw et al. 2005; Brattstrom et al. 2005; Hathaway et al. 2011).

Few conclusions from multicentric retrospective studies have shown that primary alveolar bone grafting and Wardill-Kilner palatoplasty are not recommend.

Several techniques are described for palatoplasty. However, many studies have shown that the surgeon's experience and evaluation of each patient's anatomical characteristics when choosing surgical technique are more important factors for achieving good long-term results than the technique itself (Semb et al. 2005a, b; Mercado et al. 2011; Hathaway et al. 2011; Daskalogiannakis et al. 2011; Molsted et al. 2005).

10.6 Hard Palate Approach

Hard palate correction means vomerine flap the only discussion about when is best time for the procedure. Unilateral or bilateral cleft is very difficult to correct the hard palate in late age. So for this reason approach to hard palate at the time of lip repair is our preference. This approach can make the surgery for alveolar bone grafting in future more simple.

10.7 Vomerine Flap

The vomerine flap was first described by Pichler H. in 1926. The technique used nowadays has some modifications and can be made associated to lip repair or isolated (Shi and Losee 2015).

Incision is made on the vomer bone and undermining is done under the periosteum. Another incision on the oral mucosa of the hard palate is done in the opposite side. The two flaps are joined with a type of suture that put two raw areas together. At the end of the surgery a raw area will be left on the medial side of the cleft (Fig. 10.7a, b).

In patients with bilateral cleft lip and palate, trans-incisive foramen type, the significant distance between the palate sections makes primary closure of the nasal plane very difficult. To perform this closure, two mucoperiosteal flaps are needed, created from an

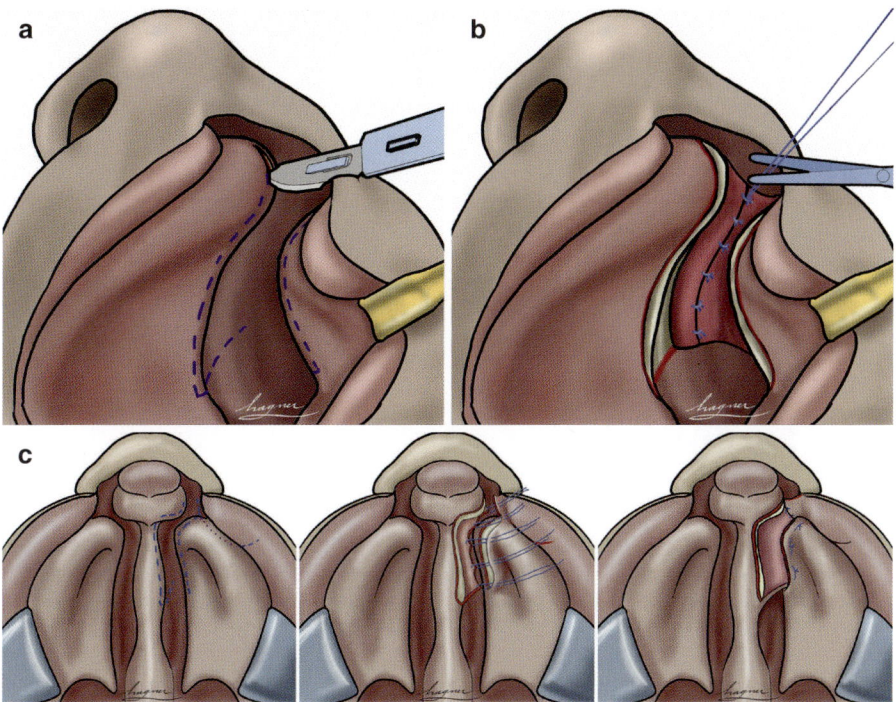

Fig. 10.7 (**a**, **b**) Vomer flap for unilateral cleft. (**a**) Demarcation of the flap. (**b**) Vomer flap sutured to the hard palate mucosa. (**c**) Vomer flap for bilateral cleft

incision on the median line of the vomer mucosa. It is detached to both sides of the cleft, closing their respective nasal mucosa detached from the hard palate remaining. The desnuded vomer area will be then healing by second intention (Fig. 10.7c).

10.8 Von Langenbeck's Technique

Broadly used, the von Langenbeck's technique consists of two relaxing incisions on palate mucosa that begin anteriorly on the hard palate, follow the alveolar margin, and end up posterior to the large alveolar tuberosity very close to the hamulus (Bernhard 1972).

Incisions are made following the borders of the palate cleft, following the boundaries between the nasal and palatal mucosa. Bone retractors are used to lift and detach the mucoperiosteal flaps in the nasal and oral planes under the palate lamina. The main neurovascular pedicle (which contains the great palatal vessels) is conserved, thereby creating a flap with two pedicles. Dissection continues in the soft palate with identification and dissection of palate muscles, repositioning them posteriorly to the nasal and palatal mucosa. The nasal mucosa is then closed and the extended intravelar veloplasty is performed.

Lastly, the palatal mucosa is sutured without tension to avoid complications such as fistulas. This is the objective of the relaxing incisions cited above—they allow the wound to heal by secondary intention (Fig. 10.8).

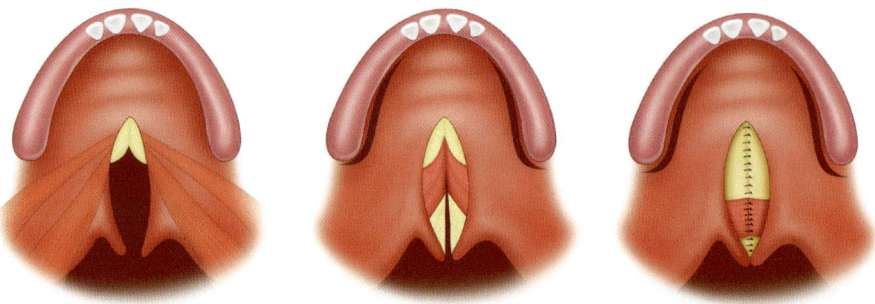

Fig. 10.8 Von Langenbeck's technique with lateral relaxing incision with muscle repositioning

10.9 Soft Palate Approach

10.9.1 Intravelar Veloplasty

Surgical management of soft palate clefts was originally based on simply creating a wound and closing it at midline, without any mobilization of soft palate muscles. One of the first authors to propose the mobilization of these muscles through posterior and medial repositioning was Kriens in 1969. His principles are still followed today, with some variations in the methodology of dissection, isolation of musculature, and retropositioning of the levator muscle (Kriens 1969b). The actual techniques include some details also from those described by Veau and Braithwaite (Victor 1931; Braithwaite 1968).

Generally, muscles adhered posteriorly to palatal shelves are gently released and dissected from the palatal and nasal mucosal planes. This promotes the release of the entire muscle group, which is then sutured medially in the correct position with nonabsorbable sutures. Surgeons currently seek to promote this dissection by identifying these muscles onto the pterygoid bone hamulus, so the mobilization is complete and its position is the most appropriate possible. Sommerlad has demonstrated that the use of a microscope during the dissection and isolation of these muscles, especially the levator veli palatini muscle in all its extension, results in better speech outcomes in postoperative follow-up (Sommerlad 2003a, b).

There is no doubt that nowadays to reposition the muscle of soft palate mainly levator veli palatini muscle is the main goal of the palatoplasty with or without microscope. There is no more place for any technique that does not isolate the muscle (Fig. 10.9a–e).

10.10 Furlow's Technique

This technique is widely used for years by many surgeons as it was believed that the use of Z-plasty promotes an elongation of the palate, in addition to muscle reposition. Flaps in the oral mucosal plane take into account the length of the soft palate and

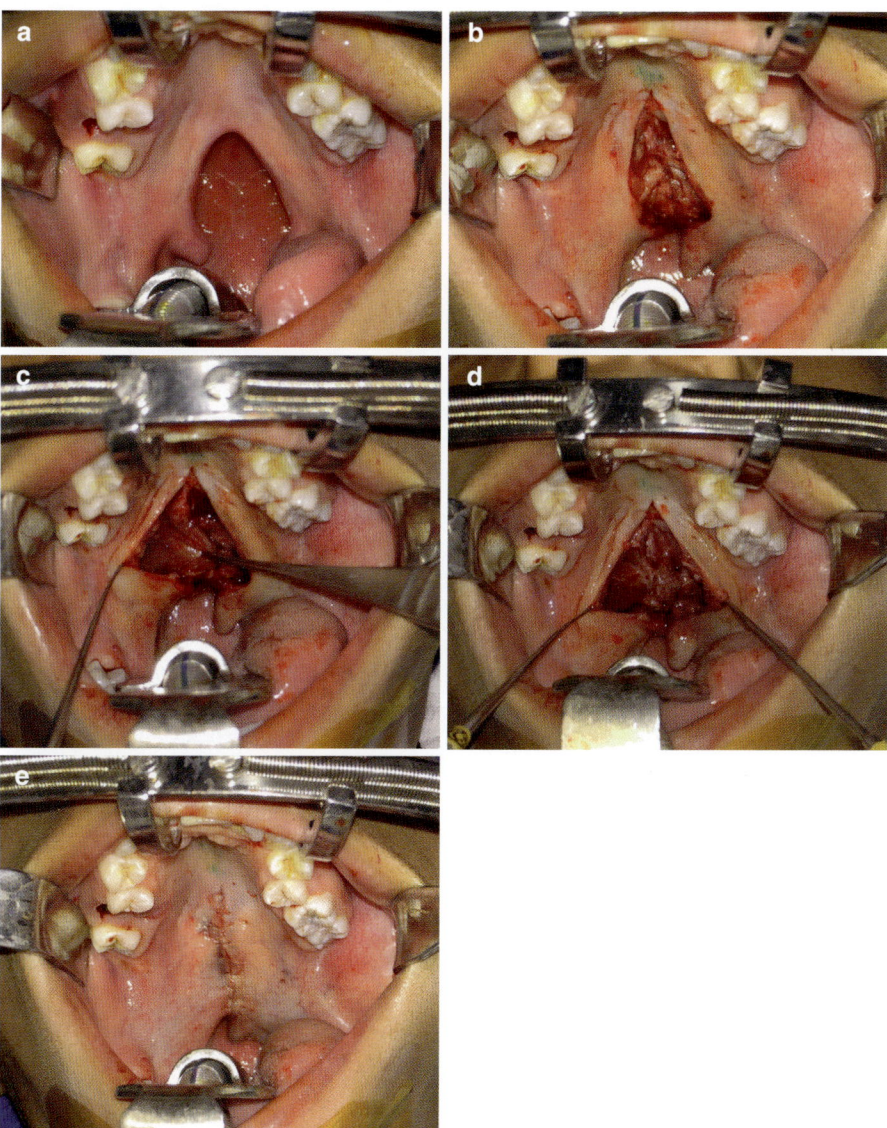

Fig. 10.9 (a–e) (a) Incomplete cleft palate. (b) Incision on the border of the cleft and muscle dissection on the oral side. (c) Isolation of levator veli palatine muscle. (d) Midline and backward repositioning of levator with nonabsorbable suture. (e) Final suture without any relaxing suture

extend into the retroalveolar space. On one side, the flap is lifted together with all the ipsilateral soft palate muscles, leaving the nasal mucosa uncovered; on the other side, palatal mucosa is dissected, leaving the muscles adhered to the nasal mucosa. A new Z-plasty is demarcated in the nasal plane, and after flap transposition, the palatal muscle belt is positioned by overlaying the muscles in the midline (Furlow 1986, 1995).

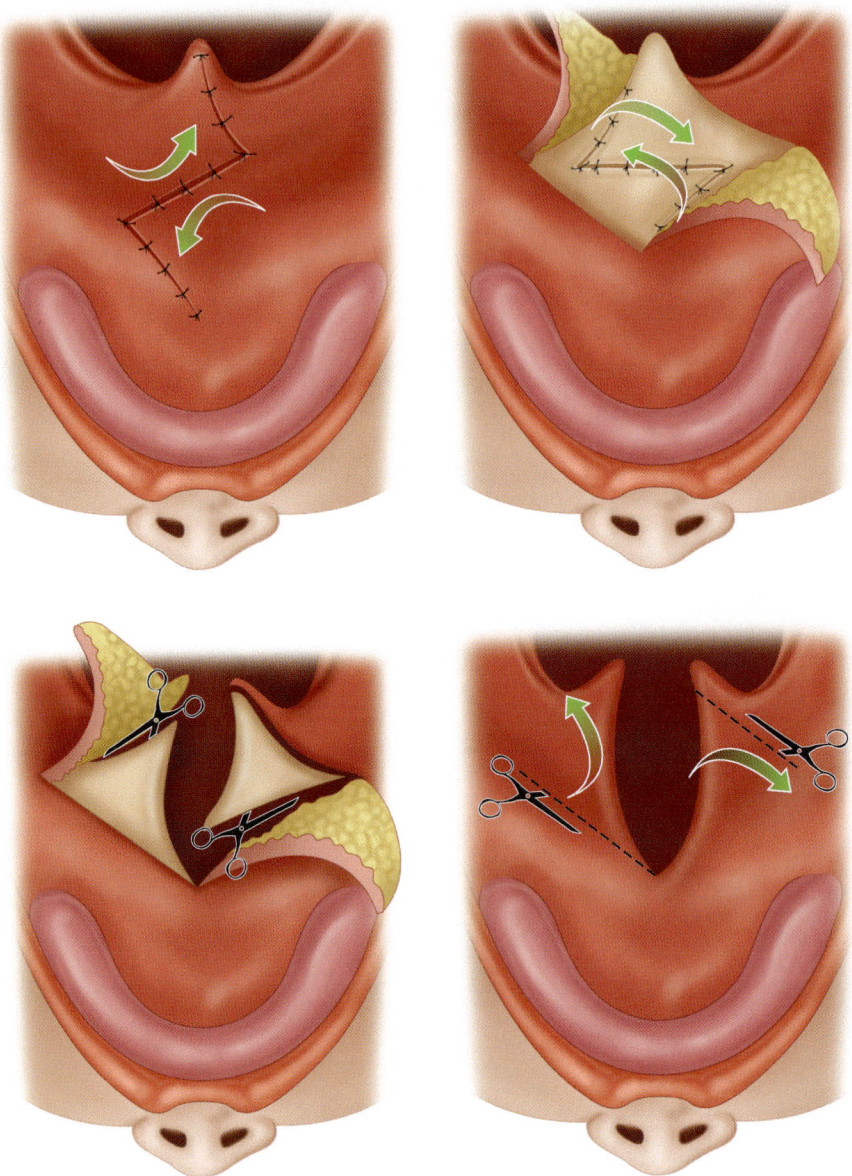

Fig. 10.10 Furlow's technique double Z-palatoplasty

Even though worldwide used Furlow's technique is not an anatomical repositioning technique which means that it is useful for some very special situations but not for all palate correction. Williams et al. showed no differences in a prospective study for primary palatoplasties in unilateral cleft patients between Furlow's and Langenbeck's technique (Williams et al. 2011) (Fig. 10.10).

10.11 Wardill-Kilner (V-Y Pushback)

Initially, Veau described a technique very similar to Von Langenbeck's, with the exception of full liberation of the mucoperiosteal flaps anteriorly, leaving only one, posterior pedicle from the great palatal artery. The association of this technique with the treatment of post-foramen incisive clefts and the format of the anterior flaps allow its closing in V-Y, which gives more lengthening in the soft palate. Nonetheless, this lengthening gain occurs due to an extensive operative wound in the hard palate, which, during healing by secondary intention, can lead to fibrosis and future facial growth restriction (Victor 1931).

Recent discussions about time for the surgery have shown that before 12 months is the best for speech even some authors mention that before 7 months is better. But also one or two stages of palatoplasty could bring some doubts for the impairment of facial growth. The time for speech is before 12 months but two-stage technique for palatoplasty looks better for facial growth (Pereira et al. 2011).

10.12 Complications and Postoperative Care

The most common acute complication of palatoplasty is bleeding, which usually occurs in the first 4 h after the procedure and is generally diffuse (i.e., not involving compromise of a large vessel). Although local tamponade can often control this bleeding, it is sometimes necessary to return to the OR to cauterize bleeding points.

Primary necrosis and flap dehiscence can also occur, especially with inadequate surgical planning. However, respecting the basic principles of flap vascularization during dissection and suturing without tension, minimize the incidence of these complications.

The fistula incidence after primary cleft palate repair is around 8.6% more elevated in cleft lip and palate patient than in isolated cleft palate as shown in a systematic review done in 2014. This study clearly presents that no matter the technique used or the surgeon skills still the morphology of the cleft is important. In this paper isolate cleft had less fistula incidence (5.4%) than cleft lip and palate had 17.9% (Hardwicke et al. 2014).

Many alternative for fistula correction can be used like local flap, buccal flap or even in extended fistula palatal prosthesis could be the option for treatment (Mann et al. 2011).

Even if the palate surgery is done early in life the evaluation of its result on the speech will be seen around 3 years old. Velopharyngeal incompetence could be one of the late complications.

Another point of observation is what is the best time for fistula correction. As was described previously many surgeries on the palate can impair facial growth but also fistulas could disturb the speech. So the best time for fistula correction depends on the size and its effect on the speech. If it is big enough to charge the speech articulation then its early correction is necessary; if not it could be postponed for late correction (Fig. 10.11a–c).

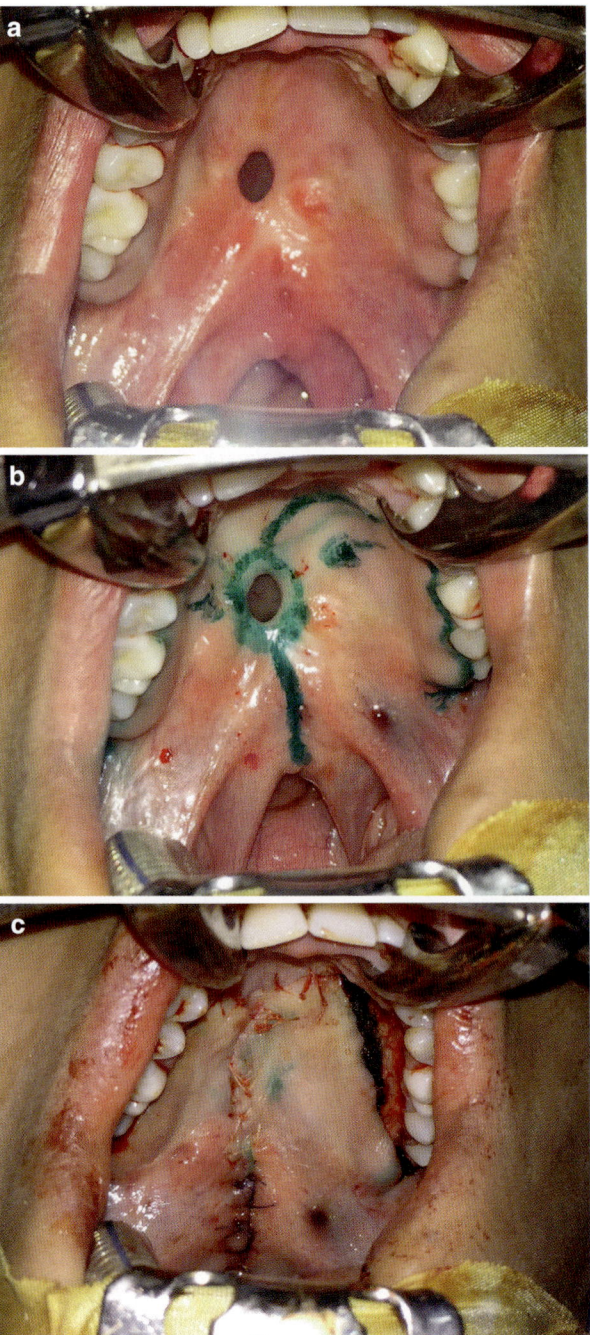

Fig. 10.11 (a–c). (a) Fistula between hard and soft palate. (b) Marking for fistula correction, muscle repositioning, and palate elongation. (c) Final aspect of the surgery

References

Bernhard L. Operation der angeborenen totalen spaltung des harten gaumens nach einer neuen methode. Plast Reconstr Surg. 1972:323–4.
Braithwaite F. The importance of the levator palati muscle in cleft palate closure. Br J Plast Surg. 1968;21:60–2.
Brattstrom VMK, Prahl-Andersen B, Semb G, Shaw W. The Eurocleft Study: intercenter study of treatment outcome in patients with complete cleft lip and palate. Part 2: craniofacial form and nasolabial appearance. Cleft Palate Craniofac J. 2005;42(1):69–77.
Brito LA, Meira JG, Kobayashi GS, Passos-Bueno MR. Genetics and management of the patient with orofacial cleft. Plast Surg Int. 2012;2012:782821.
Daskalogiannakis J, Mercado A, Russell K, Hathaway R, Dugas G, Long RE Jr, et al. The Americleft study: an inter-center study of treatment outcomes for patients with unilateral cleft lip and palate part 3. Analysis of craniofacial form. Cleft Palate Craniofac J. 2011;48(3):252–8.
Dowd CN. The surgical treatment of cleft palate. Ann Surg. 1925;81:573–84.
Furlow LT Jr. Cleft palate repair by double opposing Z-plasty. Plast Reconstr Surg. 1986;78(6):724–38.
Furlow LT Jr. Cleft palate repair by double oppositing Z-plasty. Oper Tech Plast Reconstr Surg. 1995;2(4):223–32.
Gosain AK, Conley SF, Marks S, Larson DL. Submucous cleft palate: diagnostic methods and outcomes of surgical treatment. Plast Reconstr Surg. 1996;97(7):1497–509.
Hardwicke JT, Landini G, Richard BM. Fistula incidence after primary cleft palate repair: a systematic review of the literature. Plast Reconstr Surg. 2014;134(4):618e–27e.
Hathaway R, Daskalogiannakis J, Mercado A, Russell K, Long RE Jr, Cohen M, et al. The Americleft study: an inter-center study of treatment outcomes for patients with unilateral cleft lip and palate part 2. Dental arch relationships. Cleft Palate Craniofac J. 2011;48(3):244–51.
Kriens OB. Fundamental anatomic findings for an intravelar veloplasty. Plast Reconstr Surg. 1969a;43(1):29–41.
Kriens OB. An anatomical approach to veloplasty. Plast Reconstr Surg. 1969b;43(1):29–41.
Kriens OB. Fundamental anatomic findings for an intravelar veloplasty. Cleft Palate J. 1970;7:27–36.
Mann RJ, Neaman KC, Armstrong SD, Ebner B, Bajnrauh R, Naum S. The double-opposing buccal flap procedure for palatal lengthening. Plast Reconstr Surg. 2011;127(6):2413–8.
Mercado AR, Russell K, Hathaway R, Deskalogiannakis J, Sadek H, Long RE, Cohen M, Semb G, Shaw W. The Americancleft Study: an inter-center study of treatment outcomes for patients with unilateral cleft lip and palate. Part 4. Nasolabial aesthetics. Cleft Palate Craniofac J. 2011;48(3):259–64.
Molsted KB, Kozelj V, Prahl-Anderson B, Shaw W, Semb W. The Eurocleft Study: intercenter study of treatment outcome in patients with complete cleft lip and palate. Part 3: dental arch relationships. Cleft Palate Craniofac J. 2005;42(1):78–82.
Pereira RMR, Melo EMC, Coutinho SB, Vale DM, Siqueira N, Alonso N. Avaliação do crescimento craniofacial em portadores de fissuras labiopaltinas submetidos a palatoplastia em dois tempos cirurgicos. Revista Brasileira de Cirurgia Plastica. 2011;26:624–30.
RE LJaK. Comprehensive cleft care. 1st ed. New York: Mc Graw Hill; 2009.
Semb G, Brattström V, Molsted K, Prahl-Andersen B, Shaw WC. The Eurocleft study: intercenter study of treatment outcome in patients with complete cleft lip and palat. Part 1: introduction and treatment experience. Cleft Palate Craniofac J. 2005a;42(1):64–8.
Semb GB, Brattström V, Molsted K, Prahl-Andersen B, Zuurbier P, Nichola Rumsey BA, Shaw WC. The Eurocleft Study: Study of treatment outcome in patients with complete cleft lip and palate. Part 4: relationship among treatment outcome, patient/parent satisfaction, and burden of care. Cleft Palate Craniofac J. 2005b;42(1):83–92.

Shaw WB, Kozelj V, Molsted K, Prahl-Andersen B, Roberts CT, Semb G. The Eurocleft Study: study of treatment outcome in patients with complete cleft lip and palate. Part 5. Cleft Palate Craniofac J. 2005;42(1):93–8.

Shi B, Losee JE. The impact of cleft lip and palate repair on maxillofacial growth. Int J Oral Sci. 2015;7(1):14–7.

Shimokawa TYS, Tanaka S. Nerve supply to the soft palate muscles with special references to the distribution of the lesser palatine nerve. Cleft Palate Craniofac J. 2005;42(5):495–500.

Sommerlad BC. The use of the operating microscope for cleft palate repair and pharyngoplasty. Plast Reconstr Surg. 2003a;112(6):1540–1.

Sommerlad BC. A technique for cleft palate repair. Plast Reconstr Surg. 2003b;112(6):1542–8.

Subtelny JD. A cephalometric study of the growth of the soft palate. Plast Reconstr Surg. 1956;19(1):49–62.

Subtelny JD. A review of cleft palate growth studies reported. Plast Reconstr Surg. 1962;30(1):56–67.

Victor V, editor. Division palatine. Paris: Masson; 1931.

Victor S. A proposed modification for the classification of cleft lip and cleft palate. Cleft Palate J. 1973;110:251.

Williams WN, Seagle MB, Pegoraro-Krook MI, Souza TV, Garla L, Silva ML, et al. Prospective clinical trial comparing outcome measures between Furlow and von Langenbeck Palatoplasties for UCLP. Ann Plast Surg. 2011;66(2):154–63.

Buccinator Myomucosal Flap in Cleft Palate Repair: The SOBRAPAR Hospital Experience

11

Rafael Denadai, Cassio Eduardo Raposo-Amaral, and Cesar Augusto Raposo-Amaral

11.1 Buccinator Myomucosal Flap

In 1989, Bozola et al. (1989) published the first anatomic description of a posterior buccinator myomucosal flap based on the buccal branch of the internal maxillary artery. Different types and technical modifications of the buccinator myomucosal flap have been described reflecting its versatility for numerous reconstructive applications (Bozola et al. 1989; Vaira et al. 2017; Jowett et al. 2017; Ayad and Xie 2015; Rahpeyma and Khajehahmadi 2015a, 2013; Franco et al. 2014; Massarelli et al. 2013; Zhao et al. 1999; Pribaz et al. 1992; Carstens et al. 1991). Based on a dense vascular network between the facial artery and the internal maxillary artery there are variations as the posteriorly based flap (buccal branch of the internal maxillary artery, which enters its lateral aspect just anterior to the pterygomandibular raphe), the superiorly and antero-inferiorly based flaps with direct (facial artery musculomucosal [FAMM] flap) or retrograde flow (reverse-flow facial artery buccinator flap), and the island flap (a vascular island variant of FAMM flap, in which the facial artery and vein are skeletonized) (Bozola et al. 1989; Vaira et al. 2017; Jowett et al. 2017; Ayad and Xie 2015; Rahpeyma and Khajehahmadi 2015a, 2013; Franco et al. 2014; Massarelli et al. 2013; Zhao et al. 1999; Pribaz et al. 1992; Carstens et al. 1991).

The buccinator myomucosal flap offers thin, mobile, well-vascularized, and sensitive tissue in accordance with the principle of replacing "like with like" (Bozola et al. 1989; Vaira et al. 2017; Jowett et al. 2017; Ayad and Xie 2015; Rahpeyma and Khajehahmadi 2015a, 2013; Franco et al. 2014; Massarelli et al. 2013; Zhao et al.

R. Denadai, M.D. (✉) • C.A. Raposo-Amaral, M.D.
Institute of Plastic and Craniofacial Surgery, SOBRAPAR Hospital, Campinas, São Paulo, Brazil
e-mail: denadai.rafael@hotmail.com

C.E. Raposo-Amaral, M.D., Ph.D.
Institute of Plastic and Craniofacial Surgery, SOBRAPAR Hospital,
Campinas, São Paulo 13084-880, Brazil

Universidade de São Paulo, São Paulo, Brazil

1999; Pribaz et al. 1992; Carstens et al. 1991). In addition, donor-site morbidity (e.g., mouth opening, oral commissure symmetry, inner vestibule restoration, and cheek mucosal lining) associated with this flap has been demonstrated to be low (Rahpeyma and Khajehahmadi 2016; Ferrari et al. 2011). Therefore, reconstructions based on the buccinator myomucosal flap should be part of the surgical armamentarium of plastic surgeons treating patients with intra-oral deformities, including congenital (e.g., cleft palate) and non-congenital (e.g., neoplastic or posttraumatic) intra-oral defects (Bozola et al. 1989; Vaira et al. 2017; Jowett et al. 2017; Ayad and Xie 2015; Rahpeyma and Khajehahmadi 2015a, 2013; Franco et al. 2014; Massarelli et al. 2013; Zhao et al. 1999; Pribaz et al. 1992; Carstens et al. 1991).

Particularly in cleft care, the buccinator myomucosal flaps have been adopted in primary cleft palate repair (Mann et al. 2017; Yang et al. 2013; Jackson et al. 2004, 1983; Jagannathan and Dixit 2004; Chen and Zhong 2003; Mann and Fisher 1997; Nakakita et al. 1991; Freedlander and Jackson 1989; Maeda et al. 1987; Kaplan 1975; Mukherji 1969; Ecker 1960), palatal cleft fistula repair (Sohail et al. 2016; Rahpeyma and Khajehahmadi 2015b; Kobayashi et al. 2014; Fang et al. 2014; Shetty et al. 2013; Khanna and Dagum 2012; Abdel-Aziz 2008; Lahiri and Richard 2007; Ashtiani et al. 2005), and velopharyngeal insufficiency treatment (Logjes et al. 2017; Dias et al. 2016; Lee and Alizadeh 2016; Ahl et al. 2016; Varghese et al. 2015; Abdaly et al. 2015; Hens et al. 2013; Mann et al. 2011; Robertson et al. 2008; Hill et al. 2004; Raposo-do-Amaral 2013). In this chapter, we present the SOBRAPAR Hospital experience in the application of the buccinator myomucosal flaps in the surgical management of selected cleft palate patients, emphasizing our therapeutic algorithms.

11.2 The Multidisciplinary SOBRAPAR Hospital Team

The main therapeutic endpoint of the comprehensive and standardized cleft palate management at the SOBRAPAR Hospital has been the speech development and outcomes, while the midfacial growth has been a secondary level of importance (further arguments on our rational and concepts can be found in another chapter ["An overview of protocols and outcomes in cleft care"] of this book). All cleft palate patients have regular feeding, hearing, speech, and psychological evaluations by the multidisciplinary SOBRAPAR Hospital team (speech-language pathologists, otolaryngologists, psychologists, social workers, and plastic surgeons), starting in the first consultation at our center (regardless of age at presentation) and often continuing into adulthood according to the individual needs.

In summary, psychologists prepared and followed all patients for better compliance with prolonged speech therapy, nasopharyngoscopy examinations, and surgical interventions. Orthodontists have performed the necessary corrections according to the stage of development of patients' dental arches. Intensive speech therapy has been initiated for all patients 1 month after cleft palate surgery to learn how to use the new anatomical situation properly. All repaired cleft palate patients have been screened for velopharyngeal insufficiency (associated or not with hearing loss and/or palatal fistula) by the speech-language pathologist team using specific recommendations (Alfwaress et al. 2015; Fitzsimons 2014; Henningsson et al. 2008). Patients determined to have velopharyngeal insufficiency have been evaluated with nasopharyngoscopy (i.e., the orientation of the *levator veli palatine* musculature, and the velopharyngeal gap size and patterns) performed by a trained plastic surgeon with the speech-language pathology team in attendance (this is possible from the age of 3 years due to the longitudinal and systematic preparation performed by the psychologist team). Obstructive sleep apnea has also been actively screened by taking a thorough preoperative and postoperative patient/family history according to previously validated screening tools (Chung et al. 2016; Fonseca et al. 2016; Johns 1991; Bertolazi et al. 2009; Chiu et al. 2016; Nagappa et al. 2015; Kendzerska et al. 2014; Silva et al. 2011; Vana et al. 2013).

11.3 Surgical Experience at the SOBRAPAR Hospital

Following a visit to the Charles Pinto Cleft Centre at Thrissur's Jubilee Mission Hospital, India, and observation of Dr. Adenwalla (Adenwalla et al. 2005), a renowned cleft surgeon, the buccinator myomucosal flap was incorporated into the surgical arsenal of one of the authors (C.A.R-A). Since 2007, the buccinator myomucosal flap has been a valuable option in the management of selected cleft palate patients (namely primary cleft palate repair, palatal cleft fistula repair, and velopharyngeal insufficiency management) at the SOBRAPAR Hospital. This flap has been our "workhorse flap" in these situations as its pattern can be adapted to each patient's anatomy/defect. As described in the following sections, the flap is planned preoperatively or intraoperatively according to the "cut-as-you-go" principle.

11.3.1 Surgical Technique

Firstly, the palatal defects were defined. As in cleft palate fistula repair the apparent defect may not reflect the actual tissue loss; the exact "true" tissue defects were designed with resection tissue distorted by tension, scar, and/or prior fistulae repair. In primary cleft palate repair or velopharyngeal insufficiency management, the defects were created at the transition between the hard and soft palates. Further surgical maneuvers to allow retropositioning of the soft palate without tension were implemented depending on the actual soft palate status (i.e., soft tissue availability and/or magnitude of scar tissue).

After the establishment of the palatal defects, posteriorly based pedicled buccinator myomucosal flaps (Table 11.1) were planned in the midpart of the cheeks, below the opening of the Stensen's ducts; anteriorly, the flaps were designed with a "V" shape few millimeters behind the oral commissures; posteriorly, cranial flap marking is connected to the defect created at the soft palate in primary cleft palate repair or velopharyngeal insufficiency management. The flap width depends directly on the palatal defect created after completed dissection. The specific flap design varies based on the location and size of the defect as well as the arc of rotation. Following incisions of flap margins, the flap is raised in an anteroposterior direction, including a full thickness of the buccinator muscle. It is important to avoid opening or disturbing the fascia over the buccal fat pad. The flaps were then inserted into the defect.

Table 11.1 Key technical points for the buccinator myomucosal flap procedures

Key technical points	Maneuver
Stensen's duct	Precise location of Stensen's duct adjacent to the superior second molar[a]
Buccopharyngeal fascia	Respect the buccopharyngeal fascia[b] avoiding oral fat pad hernia and facial nerve terminal branch lesion
Pedicle	Preserve the buccal artery pedicle[c] Pivot the flap at the base of the pedicle and inset into the retromolar trigone and palate avoiding great tensions/torsion of the pedicle when positioning the flap Avoid any secondary lesion during the postoperative follow-up[d]

[a]Some have catheterized the duct; and we only respect anatomical boundaries
[b]Buccopharyngeal fascia separates the buccal fat pad from the buccinator muscle
[c]Some have adopted Doppler to locate the artery prior to the incision; and we use careful soft-tissue dissection with preservation of structures
[d]Some have used the island flap; others have used bite blocks; and we have reinforced the postoperative guidelines to all patients with frequent postoperative visits

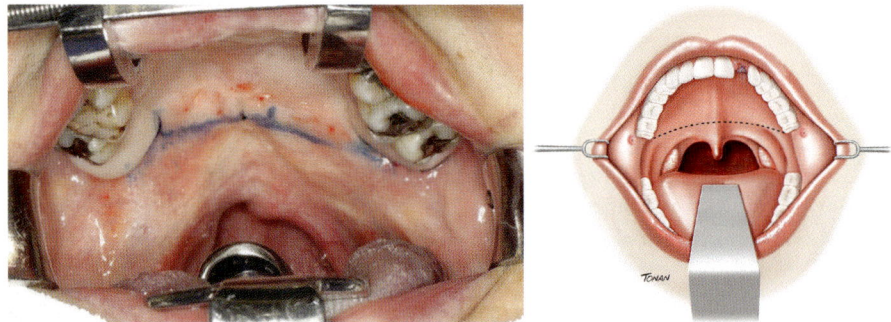

Fig. 11.1 (*Left*) Intraoperative view and (*right*) schematic drawing illustrating the short palate and the surgical marking at the junction of the hard and the soft palates

Ideally and whenever possible, the palatal defects should be repaired with at least a two-layer, tension-free closure. The tissue around the fistula (e.g., marginal fistula hinge flaps) was used in the nasal layer repair according to the availability of healthy tissue. Unilateral or bilateral buccinator myomucosal flaps were used according to the characteristics of palatal defect. Small fistulas were reconstructed with the left-sided flap sutured (4-0 polyglactin 910) with the mucosal surface down into the oral layer. Some large fistulas were managed with bilateral flaps with the ends of the flaps sutured together in the medial portion of the defect. Large fistulas, wide cleft palates, and velopharyngeal insufficiency were managed with bilateral flaps: the left-sided flap was sutured (4-0 polyglactin 910) into the nasal layer with the mucosa facing the nasal lumen, whereas the right-sided flap was sutured with the mucosal surface down into the oral layer. The donor sites were closed (4-0 polyglactin 910) directly, with the exception of the base of the flap. Figures 11.1–11.6 illustrate the application of the bilateral buccinator myomucosal flap for velopharyngeal insufficiency management. Three to six weeks after surgery, the pedicles were divided in the presence of difficulty mastication and/or limitation of mouth opening.

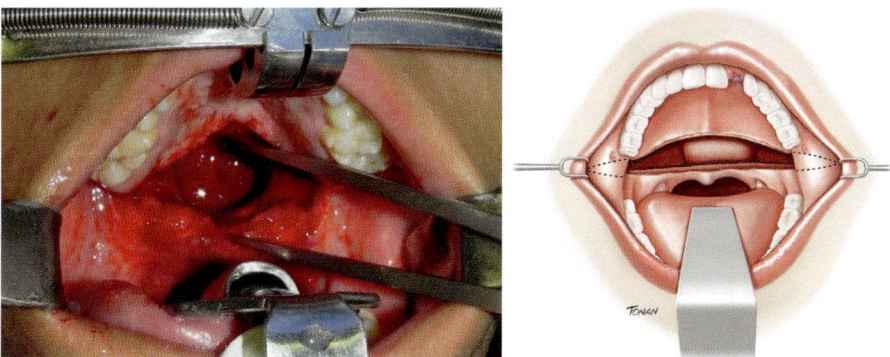

Fig. 11.2 (*Left*) Intraoperative view and (*right*) schematic drawing demonstrating the division of junction of the hard and the soft palates with the detaching of the soft palate and allowing it to move toward the posterior pharyngeal wall, resulting in a surgically created palatal defect

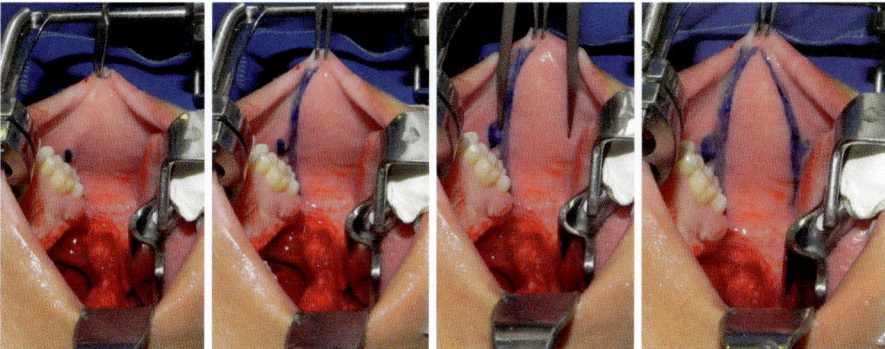

Fig. 11.3 Intraoperative views illustrating the buccinator myomucosal flap marking. The flap was planned in the midpart of the cheek, below the opening of the Stensen's ducts; anteriorly, the flap was designed with a "V" shape few millimeters behind the oral commissures; posteriorly, cranial flap marking is connected to the defect created at the soft palate. Note that the flap width depends directly on the defect created between the soft and hard palates after completed dissection (Fig. 11.3)

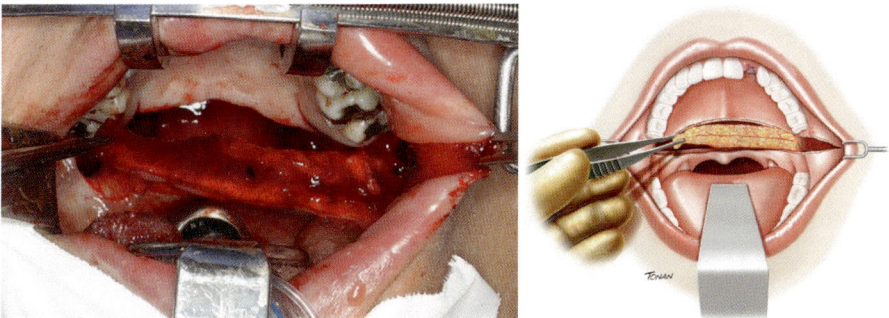

Fig. 11.4 (*Left*) Intraoperative view and (*right*) schematic drawing revealing the left-sided flap inserted into the defect and sutured (4-0 polyglactin 910) into the remaining nasal layer with the flap mucosa facing the nasal lumen

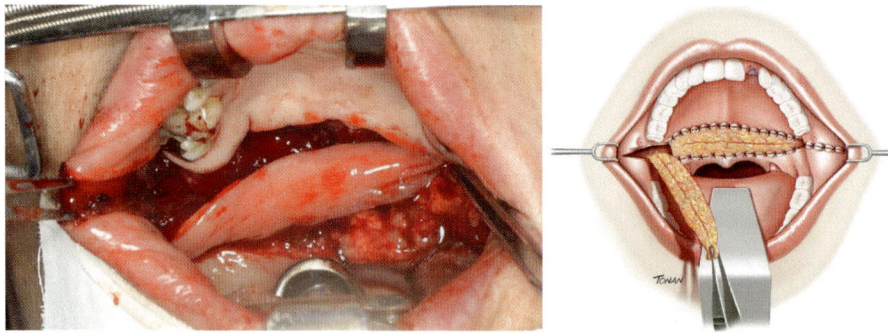

Fig. 11.5 (*Left*) Intraoperative view and (*right*) schematic drawing revealing the right-sided flap inserted into the defect and sutured (4-0 polyglactin 910) into the oral layer with the flap mucosa facing the oral lumen

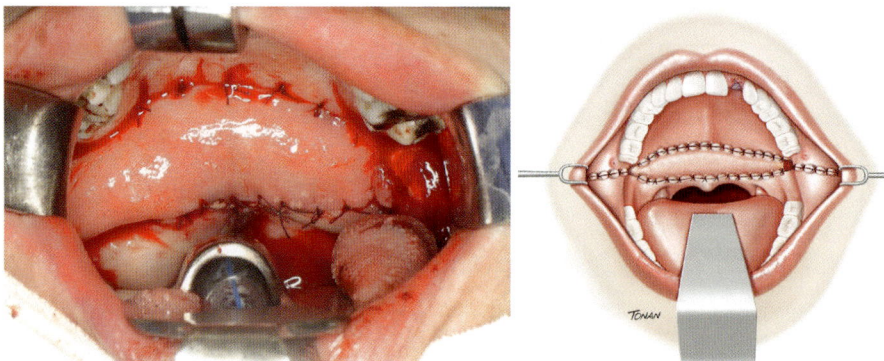

Fig. 11.6 (*Left*) Intraoperative view and (*right*) schematic drawing demonstrating the palatal lengthening by the bilateral buccinator myomucosal flap. The donor sites were closed (4-0 polyglactin 910) directly, with the exception of the base of the left-sided flap. Note that as the cranial demarcations (located caudally to the Stensen's duct) were connected to the defect in the soft palate, the pedicles were positioned at the retromolar trigone after the mobilization and insertion of the flaps.

11.3.2 Primary Cleft Palate Repair

Although different groups (Mann et al. 2017; Yang et al. 2013; Jackson et al. 2004, 1983; Jagannathan and Dixit 2004; Chen and Zhong 2003; Mann and Fisher 1997; Nakakita et al. 1991; Freedlander and Jackson 1989; Maeda et al. 1987; Kaplan 1975; Mukherji 1969; Ecker 1960) have published excellent functional outcomes with the buccinator myomucosal flap in primary cleft palate repair, we prefer not to use this particular flap on primary cleft palate repair of patients treated within the SOBRAPAR cleft palate repair protocol (primary cleft palate repair within 12–18 months of age; additional details can be ascertained in the chapter "An overview of protocols and outcomes in cleft care" of this book). In this group of patients, we prefer to store this surgical alternative as a "lifeboat" flap for future potential needs (e.g., cleft palate fistulae and/or velopharyngeal insufficiency).

In unrepaired cleft palate patients with an advanced age (often adopted patients or from rural and incipient regions in Brazil with low human development index), both cleft width and intraoperative details have been adopted in our surgical rationale (Fig. 11.7).

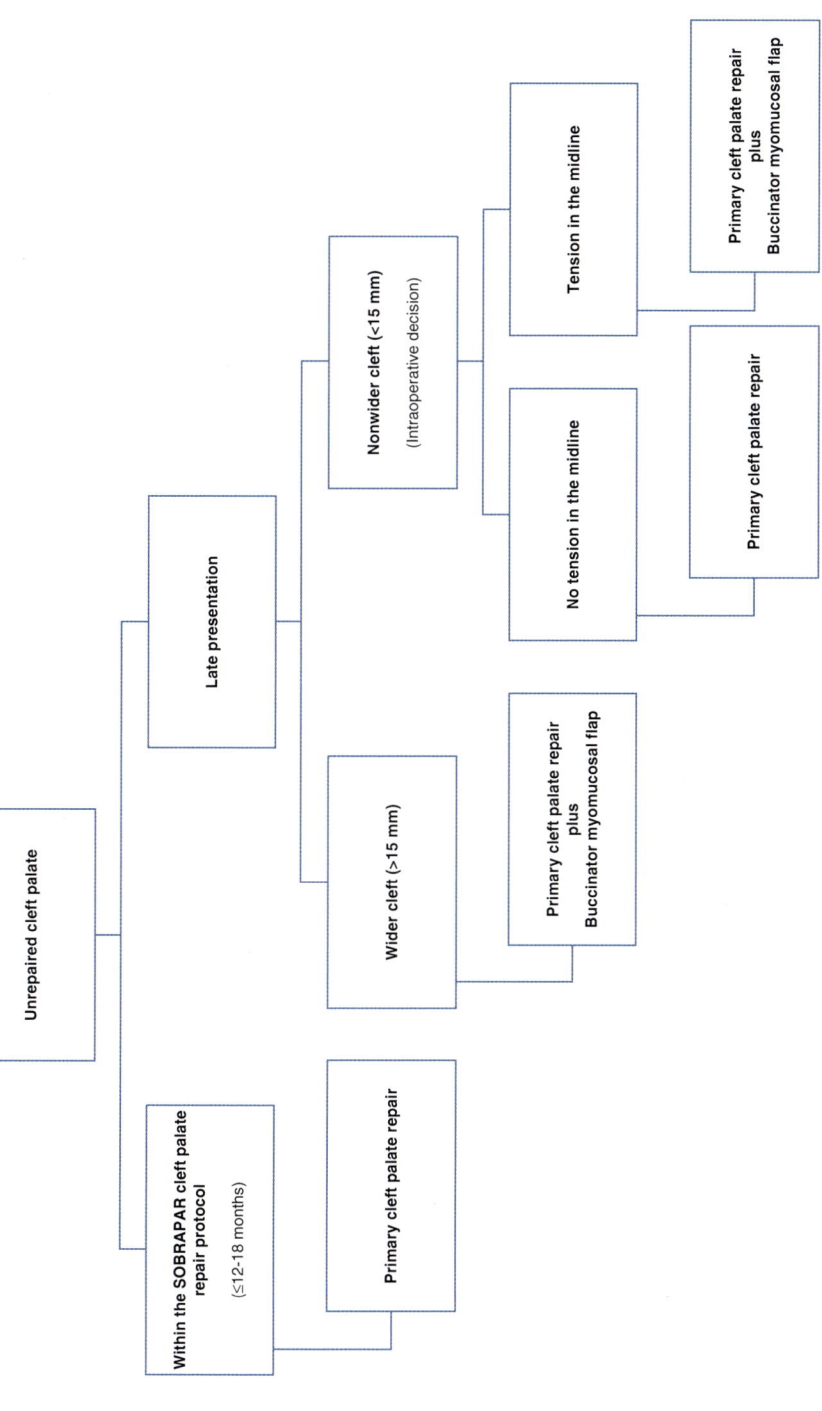

Fig. 11.7 The SOBRAPAR Hospital algorithm for unrepaired cleft palate patients. Our rationale was based on the following criteria: age (early versus late presentation according to the SOBRAPAR protocol for primary cleft palate repair); cleft width (wider [the distance between the medial edges of the hard palate is >1.5 cm] versus nonwider [<1.5 cm] cleft palate); and intraoperative details such as position of the vascular pedicle (i.e., cranially/laterally displaced vascular pedicle limiting the medialization of the mucoperiosteal flaps) and/or tension at the suture line (primarily at the junction of the hard and soft palates)

Patients with wider clefts (the distance between the medial edges of the hard palate is >1.5 cm) (Bardach 1999), with cranially/laterally displaced vascular pedicle limiting the medialization of the mucoperiosteal flaps, and/or tension at the suture line (primarily at the junction of the hard and soft palates) despite additional surgical maneuvers (e.g., skeletonization of the vascular pedicle, mucosal velar relaxing incisions, osteotomy of the bony foramen, and/or breaking of hamulus) have been managed with primary cleft palate repair plus buccinator myomucosal flap. In our experience, mainly adult and/or syndromic patients have been treated with this buccinator myomucosal flap association for lengthening the soft palate and decreasing the chance of postoperative fistulae and/or velopharyngeal insufficiency (Figs. 11.8–11.13).

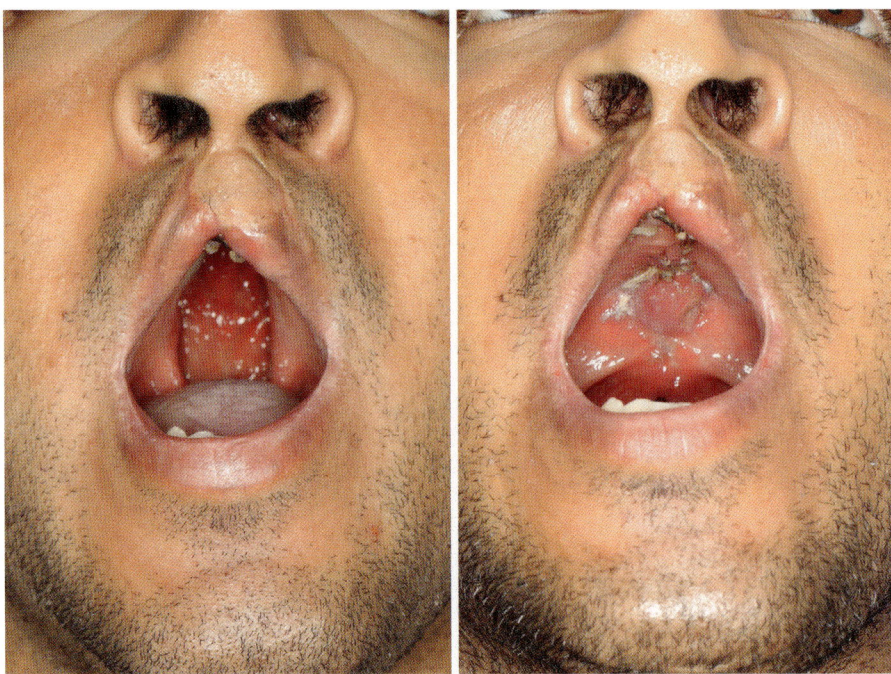

Fig. 11.8 Adult patient with wide unrepaired cleft palate surgically treated with two-flap palatoplasty with intravelar veloplasty plus buccinator myomucosal flap

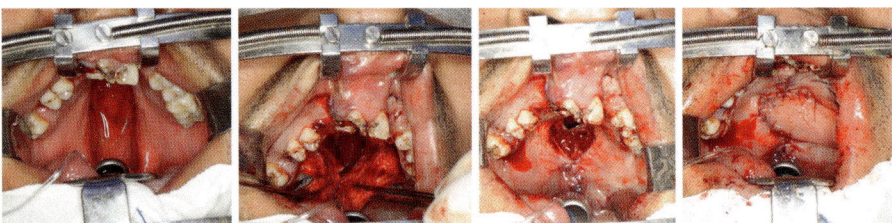

Fig. 11.9 Intraoperative view of the same patient of Fig. 11.8. (*Left*) Wide unrepaired cleft palate. (*Left, center*) Mucoperiosteal flaps elevated and the vascular pedicles oriented cephalically and laterally. (*Right, center*) Mucoperiosteal flaps mobilized and sutured demonstrating a palatal defect at the junction of the hard and soft palates. (*Right*) Left-sided buccinator myomucosal flap inserted into the defect and sutured (4-0 polyglactin 910) with the flap mucosa facing the oral lumen

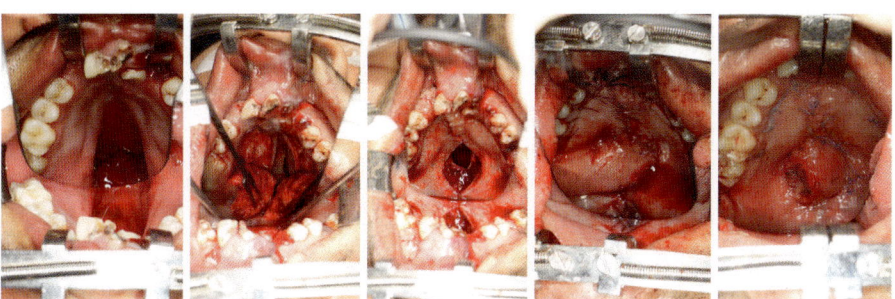

Fig. 11.10 Intraoperative palatal mirror view of the same patient of Figs. 11.8–11.9. (*Left*) Wide unrepaired cleft palate. (*Left, center*) Mucoperiosteal flaps elevated and the vascular pedicles oriented cephalically and laterally. (*Center*) Mucoperiosteal flaps mobilized and sutured showing a palatal defect at the junction of the hard and soft palates. (*Right, center*) Left-sided buccinator myomucosal flap inserted into the defect and sutured (4-0 polyglactin 910) with the flap mucosa facing the oral lumen. (*Right*) Repaired cleft palate after division of pedicle

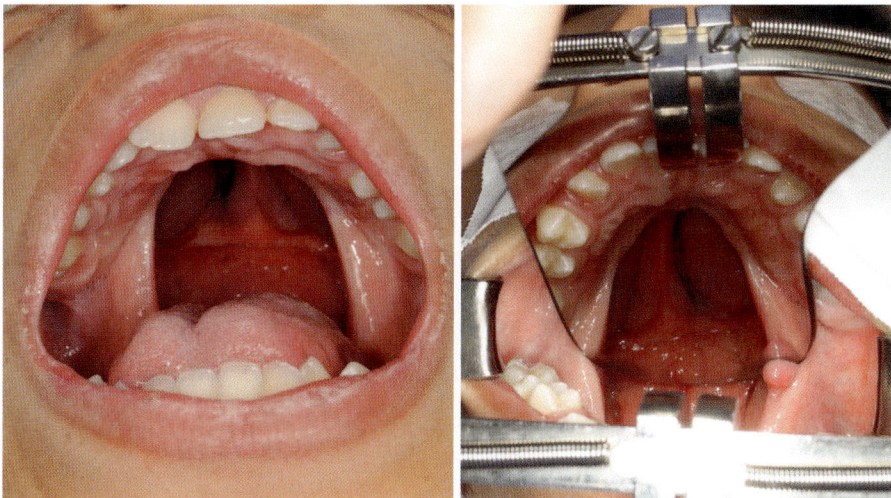

Fig. 11.11 Treacher Collins patient with wide unrepaired cleft palate surgically treated with two-flap palatoplasty with intravelar veloplasty plus buccinator myomucosal flap. (*Left*) Intraoral and (*right*) palatal mirror views

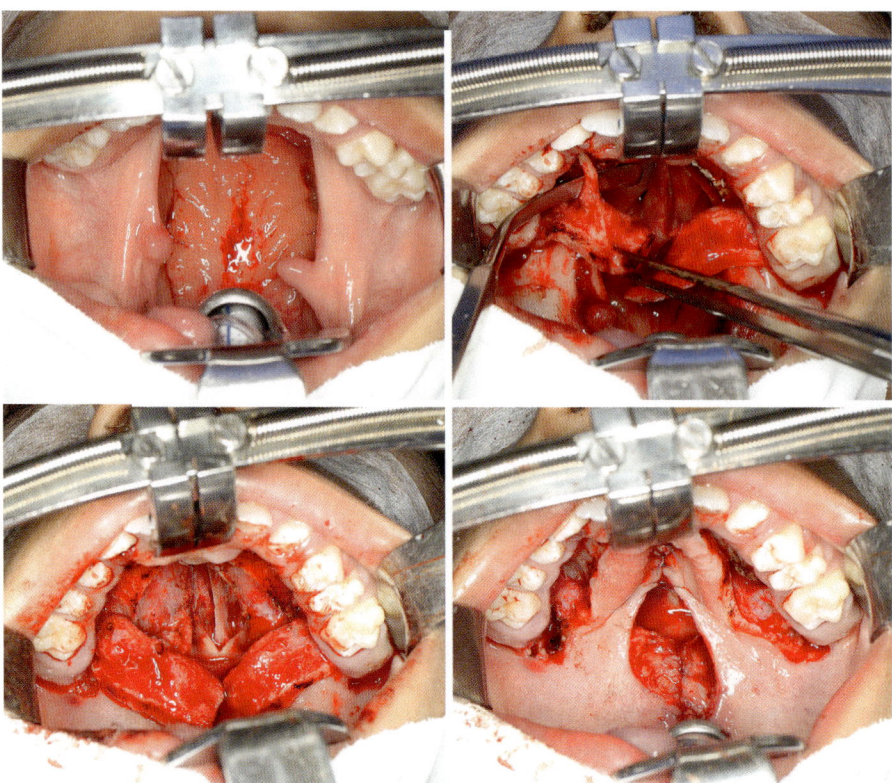

Fig. 11.12 Intraoperative view of the same patient of Fig. 11.11. (*Top*, *left*) Wide unrepaired cleft palate. (*Top*, *right*) Mucoperiosteal flaps elevated and the vascular pedicles oriented cephalically and laterally. (*Bottom*, *left*) Nasal layer reconstructed with vomer flaps. (*Bottom*, *right*) Mobilized and sutured mucoperiosteal flaps with a palatal defect at the junction of the hard and soft palates

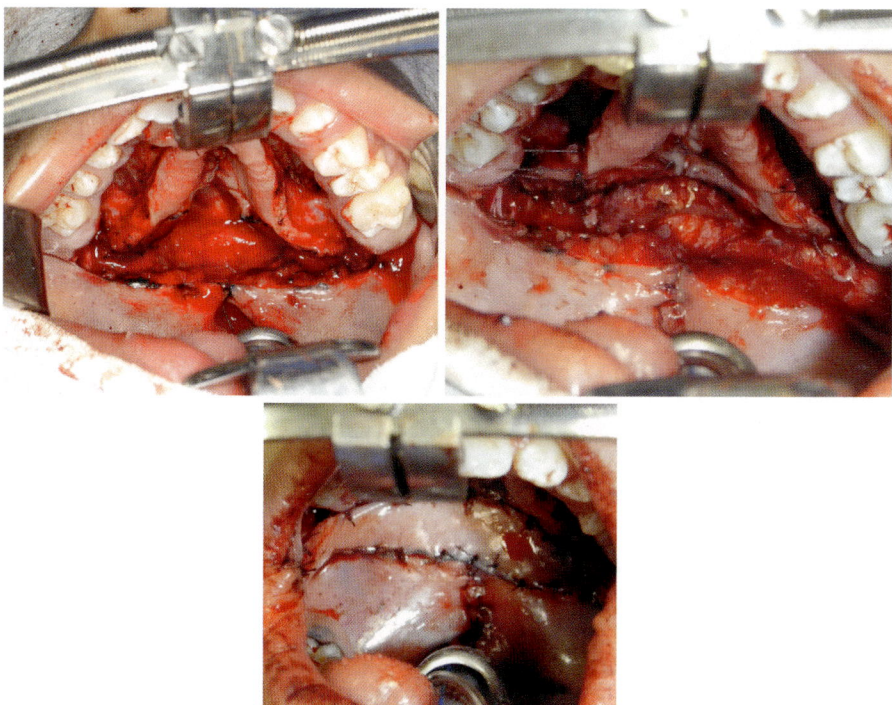

Fig. 11.13 Intraoperative view of the same patient of Figs. 11.11–11.12. (*Top, left*) Division of junction of the hard and the soft palates with the detaching of the soft palate and allowing it to move toward the posterior pharyngeal wall, resulting in a surgically created palatal defect. (*Top, right*) The left-sided buccinator myomucosal flap sutured into the nasal layer with the mucosa facing the nasal lumen. (*Bottom*) The right-sided buccinator myomucosal flap sutured with the mucosal surface down into the oral layer

11.3.3 Cleft Palate Fistulae

Postoperative fistula is an extremely relevant complication of cleft palate surgery (Salimi et al. 2017; Bykowski et al. 2015; Hardwicke et al. 2014). Fistulas may be best characterized by whether they are clinically important leading to nasal air emission, hypernasal resonance, decreased intraoral pressure, regurgitation of fluid and food, and/or halitosis. The Pittsburgh Fistula Classification System (Smith et al. 2007) stratified anatomically the fistulas as follows: fistulas at the uvula, or bifid uvulae (type I); within the soft palate (type II); at the junction of the soft and hard palates (type III); within the hard palate (type IV); at the incisive foramen, or junction of the primary and secondary palates (type V; this designation is reserved for use with Veau type IV clefts); lingual-alveolar (type VI); and labial-alveolar (type VII).

In the cleft literature (Alsalman et al. 2016; Bonanthaya et al. 2016; Habib and Brennan 2016; Mahajan et al. 2014; Rossell-Perry and Arrascue 2012; Murthy 2011; Freda et al. 2010; Sadhu 2009; Diah et al. 2007; Penna et al. 2007; Murrell et al. 2001; Muzaffar et al. 2001; Emory et al. 1997; Cohen et al. 1991; Guerrero-Santos and Fernandez 1973; Jackson 1972; Guerrero Santos and Altamirano 1966; Gart and Gosain 2014; Hopper et al. 2014; Kummer 2014; Seagle et al. 2016; Deren et al. 2005; Perkins et al. 2005; Sie et al. 2005; Sommerlad et al. 2002; Bishop et al. 2014; Abdel-Aziz et al. 2011), different reconstructive options (e.g., local flap with marginal turnover flaps combined with local rotation flaps; revision two-flap palatoplasty; regional flaps from the tongue, pharynx, or buccal areas; and microsurgical free flaps) have been adopted for fistula repair with no evidence-based guidelines completely defined to date. Our therapeutic approach is based on both the SOBRAPAR Hospital experience and the previously published studies (Sohail et al. 2016; Rahpeyma and Khajehahmadi 2015b; Kobayashi et al. 2014; Fang et al. 2014; Shetty et al. 2013; Khanna and Dagum 2012; Abdel-Aziz 2008; Lahiri and Richard 2007; Ashtiani et al. 2005; Alsalman et al. 2016; Bonanthaya et al. 2016; Habib and Brennan 2016; Mahajan et al. 2014; Rossell-Perry and Arrascue 2012; Murthy 2011; Freda et al. 2010; Sadhu 2009; Diah et al. 2007; Penna et al. 2007; Murrell et al. 2001; Muzaffar et al. 2001; Emory et al. 1997; Cohen et al. 1991; Guerrero-Santos and Fernandez 1973; Jackson 1972; Guerrero Santos and Altamirano 1966; Gart and Gosain 2014; Hopper et al. 2014; Kummer 2014; Seagle et al. 2016; Deren et al. 2005; Perkins et al. 2005; Sie et al. 2005; Sommerlad et al. 2002; Bishop et al. 2014; Abdel-Aziz et al. 2011).

Speech-related problems and regurgitation associated with palatal fistulae have been systematically assessed by our cleft multidisciplinary team. From 3 years of age, cleft patients have been evaluated with nasopharyngoscopy examinations to determinate appropriate treatment. A period of observation is appropriate for small, early postoperative fistulae as these may close spontaneously. Asymptomatic fistulas (without nasal regurgitation or speech problems) have been treated conservatively and should be monitored for conversion to symptomatic fistulae (e.g., after orthodontic palatal expansion). Types VI and VII were treated in conjunction with the secondary alveolar bone graft. The SOBRAPAR Hospital algorithm (Fig. 11.14)

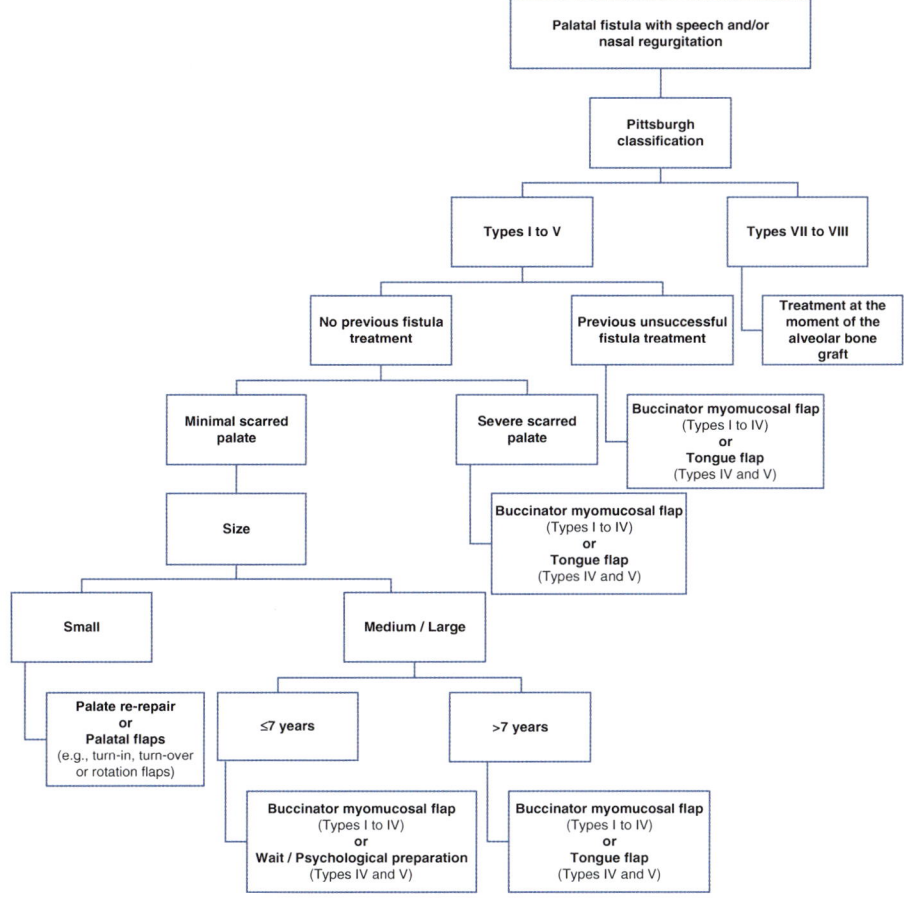

Fig. 11.14 The SOBRAPAR Hospital algorithm for repaired cleft palate patients with palatal fistula. Our rationale was based on the following criteria: asymptomatic (without nasal regurgitation or speech problems) versus symptomatic palatal fistulas; age; previous unsuccessful surgical treatment of fistula (i.e., palate re-repair, local flaps, and/or tongue flap); the quality of the surrounding tissue and the availability of local tissue (i.e., amount of scarring near the fistula); Pittsburgh Fistula Classification System (types I to VII); and size (small [<2 mm], medium [3–5 mm], or large [>5 mm])

for cleft patients with symptomatic palatal fistula was based on the following criteria: age; previous unsuccessful surgical treatment of fistula (i.e., palate re-repair, local flaps, and/or tongue flap); quality of the surrounding tissue and the availability of local tissue (i.e., amount of scarring near the fistula); type (Pittsburgh Fistula Classification System (Smith et al. 2007)); and size of fistula (small [<2 mm], medium [3–5 mm], or large [>5 mm] (Muzaffar et al. 2001)). Patients with fistulas associated with speech impairment should undergo early repair (after performing the nasopharyngoscopic evaluation), whereas the closure of fistulas not associated with speech problems should be delayed, if possible, until completion of

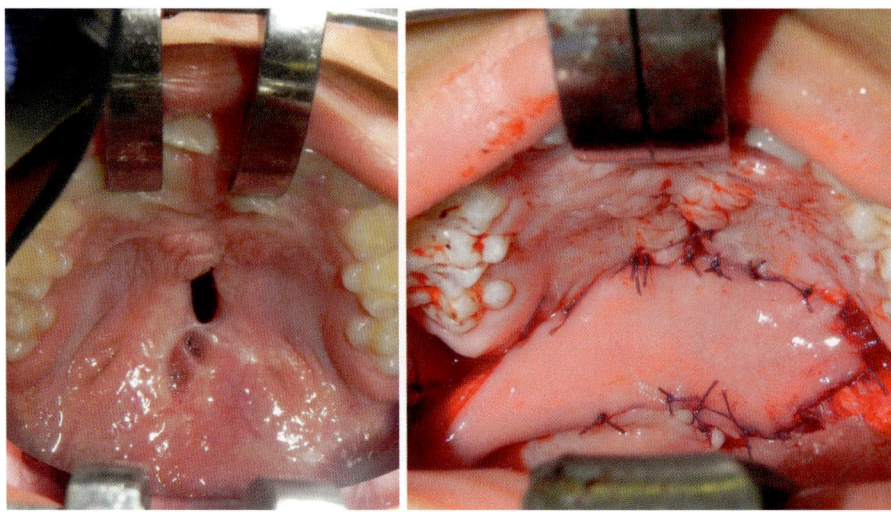

Fig. 11.15 (*Left*) Intraoperative palatal mirror view of cleft patient with palatal fistula and velopharyngeal insufficiency managed with (*right*) the bilateral buccinator myomucosal flap

orthodontic maxillary arch expansion and be combined with secondary alveolar bone grafting. Patients with medium/large fistula, recurrent fistula, or fistula associated with a severely scarred palate (i.e., multiple irregular scars on the palate with hard mucosal consistency and dense fibrotic tissue surrounding the fistula) have been managed with the buccinator myomucosal flap (types I to IV) or tongue flap (types IV and V). Pediatric patients ($\leq$7 years) with medium/large-sized type I–IV fistulas also receive the buccinator myomucosal flap. As pediatric patients ($\leq$ 7 years) with medium/large-sized type IV or V fistulas do not support the first stage of the tongue flap, they have been systematically and longitudinally prepared by the psychology team until psychological maturation to support the palatal reconstruction. The decision about which flap (buccinator myomucosal flap versus tongue flap) should be adopted in type IV fistula reconstructions depends on the specific location of the palatal defect (fistulas closest to the transition between hard palate and soft palate have been treated with the buccinator myomucosal flap, while fistulas closest to the incisive foramen have been treated with the tongue flap). In addition, particularly fistulas at the junction of the soft and hard palates (type III) associated with velopharyngeal insufficiency have been preferentially managed with the buccinator myomucosal flap, regardless of size (Fig. 11.15).

11.3.4 Velopharyngeal Insufficiency

Velopharyngeal insufficiency after primary cleft palate repair remains a relevant challenge in cleft care (Gart and Gosain 2014; Hopper et al. 2014; Kummer 2014). Surgery is the mainstay of treatment of velopharyngeal insufficiency with the goal of creating a functional seal between the nasopharynx and the oropharynx during speech (Gart and Gosain 2014; Hopper et al. 2014; Kummer 2014). Currently, the most commonly adopted surgical interventions are the superiorly based pharyngeal flap, sphincter pharyngoplasty, double-opposing Z-palatoplasty, palatal muscle retropositioning, and posterior pharyngeal wall argumentation, each with their advocates, advantages, and disadvantages (Gart and Gosain 2014; Hopper et al. 2014; Seagle et al. 2016; Deren et al. 2005; Perkins et al. 2005; Sie et al. 2005; Sommerlad et al. 2002; Bishop et al. 2014). Particularly velopharyngeal insufficiency patients with moderate or large velopharyngeal gaps have been successfully managed with the pharyngeal flap or the sphincter pharyngoplasty according to the velopharyngeal closure patterns (Gart and Gosain 2014; Hopper et al. 2014; Abdel-Aziz et al. 2011; Armour et al. 2005). However, these approaches are accompanied by obstructive sleep apnea, snoring, mouth breathing, and/or hyponasality (Collins et al. 2012).

In this context, some cleft groups (Logjes et al. 2017; Dias et al. 2016; Lee and Alizadeh 2016; Ahl et al. 2016; Varghese et al. 2015; Abdaly et al. 2015; Hens et al. 2013; Mann et al. 2011; Robertson et al. 2008; Hill et al. 2004) have adopted the palate lengthening by the buccinator myomucosal flaps to achieve normal velopharyngeal function without causing upper airway obstruction. Although the reported buccinator myomucosal flap outcome-related data are encouraging (Logjes et al. 2017; Dias et al. 2016; Lee and Alizadeh 2016; Ahl et al. 2016; Varghese et al. 2015; Abdaly et al. 2015; Hens et al. 2013; Mann et al. 2011; Robertson et al. 2008; Hill et al. 2004), the speech outcome interpretation is hampered by the variability of studies (Logjes et al. 2017; Dias et al. 2016; Lee and Alizadeh 2016; Ahl et al. 2016; Varghese et al. 2015; Abdaly et al. 2015; Hens et al. 2013; Mann et al. 2011; Robertson et al. 2008; Hill et al. 2004). In addition, potential predictive factors that may influence the speech outcomes were poorly investigated to date (Hens et al. 2013).

Recently, we (Denadai et al. 2017) performed a prospective study with 53 consecutive nonsyndromic patients with repaired cleft palate (±cleft lip) who underwent the bilateral buccinator myomucosal flap according to the SOBRAPAR Hospital algorithm (Figs. 11.16–11.18). Our algorithm for repaired cleft palate patients with velopharyngeal insufficiency was based on the following criteria: previous unsuccessful surgical treatment of velopharyngeal insufficiency; amount of scarring at the junction between the hard palate and the soft palate; and *levator veli palatini* musculature orientation and velopharyngeal gap size. The buccinators myomucosal flaps were indicated regardless of velopharyngeal closure pattern. In addition, patients with prior sphincter pharyngoplasty or pharyngeal flap were not considered in our surgical protocol as this is an additional and specific arm of VPI management (Katzel et al. 2016). Further details about the SOBRAPAR Hospital algorithm for repaired cleft palate patients with velopharyngeal insufficiency can be found in another chapter ("Surgical Management of Velopharyngeal Insufficiency: The SOBRAPAR Hospital Algorithm") of this book.

We assessed the surgical outcomes for velopharyngeal insufficiency by blind analysis of pre- and postoperative high-quality digital audio-video recordings of a well-defined and representative speech sample and velopharyngeal function. As there is

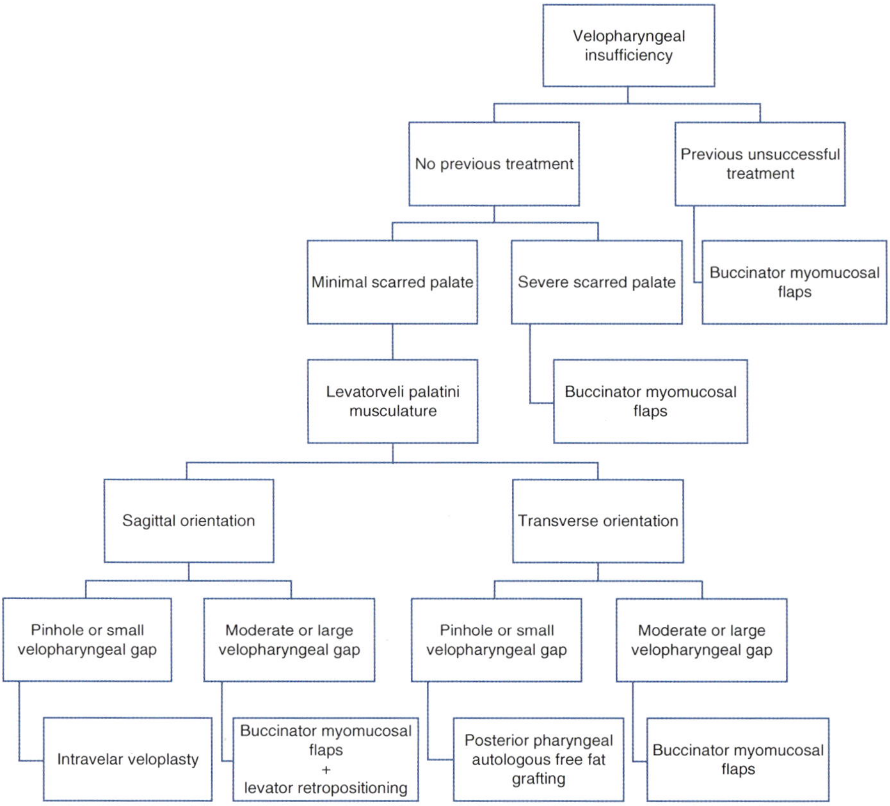

```
                    ┌─────────────────────┐
                    │    Velopharyngeal   │
                    │     insufficiency   │
                    └──────────┬──────────┘
               ┌───────────────┴───────────────┐
    ┌──────────────────────┐         ┌──────────────────────┐
    │  No previous treatment│         │ Previous unsuccessful │
    │                      │         │      treatment        │
    └──────────┬───────────┘         └──────────┬───────────┘
         ┌─────┴──────┐                         │
┌────────────────┐ ┌────────────────┐ ┌────────────────────┐
│ Minimal scarred│ │ Severe scarred │ │ Buccinator myomucosal│
│    palate      │ │     palate     │ │       flaps         │
└────────┬───────┘ └────────┬───────┘ └────────────────────┘
         │                  │
┌────────────────┐ ┌────────────────────┐
│ Levatorveli    │ │ Buccinator myomucosal│
│ palatini       │ │       flaps         │
│ musculature    │ │                     │
└────────┬───────┘ └────────────────────┘
    ┌────┴────┐
┌─────────────┐ ┌─────────────┐
│  Sagittal   │ │  Transverse │
│ orientation │ │ orientation │
└──────┬──────┘ └──────┬──────┘
```

Fig. 11.16 The SOBRAPAR Hospital algorithm for repaired cleft palate patients with velopharyngeal insufficiency. Our rationale was based on the following criteria: previous unsuccessful surgical treatment of velopharyngeal insufficiency (i.e., posterior pharyngeal free fat grafting, palatal muscle retropositioning, or double-opposing Z-palatoplasty); amount of scarring at the junction between the hard palate and the soft palate by oroscopy; and *levator veli palatini* musculature orientation (sagittal or horizontal) and velopharyngeal gap size (pinhole, small, moderate, or large) during maximal closure on phonation by nasopharyngoscopic examination

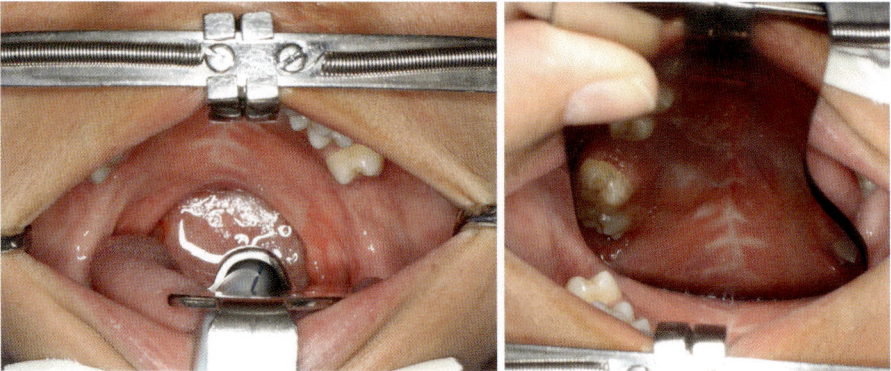

Fig. 11.17 Intraoral and palatal mirror views demonstrating a short, severely scarred palate

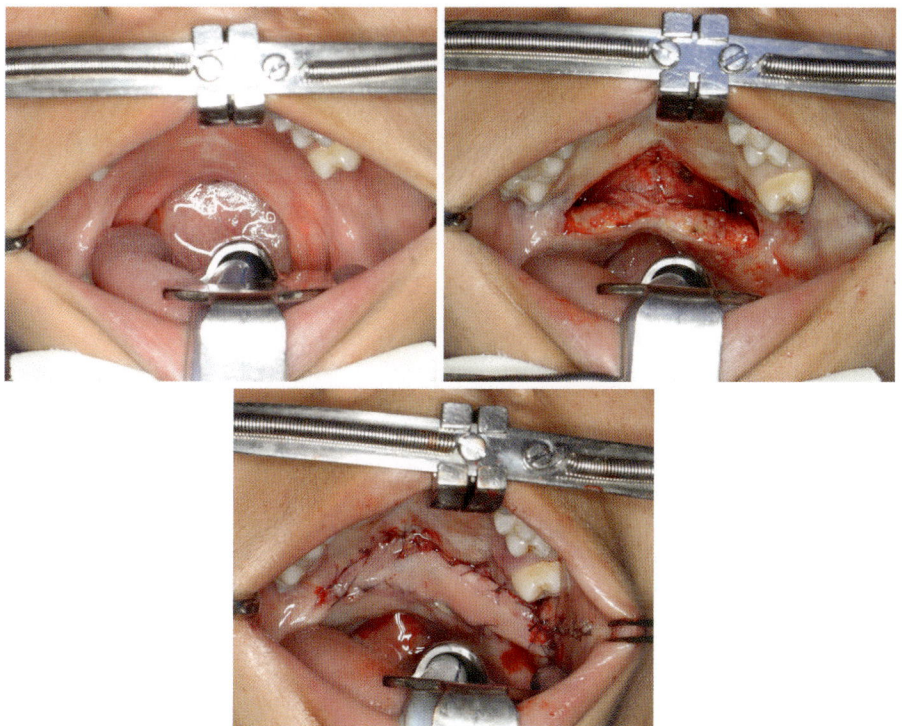

Fig. 11.18 Intraoperative view of the same patient of Fig. 11.17. (*Top, left*) The short palate. (*Top, right*) The division of junction of the hard and the soft palates with the detaching of the soft palate and allowing it to move toward the posterior pharyngeal wall. (*Bottom*) The palatal lengthening by the bilateral buccinator myomucosal flap

currently no standardized scale for perceptual speech assessment, we adopted previously published (Deren et al. 2005; Park et al. 2016; Wermker et al. 2014; Ma et al. 2013; Sullivan et al. 2010; Lam et al. 2007) perceptual rating method with categorical judgments to assess three structurally correctable variables. Speech outcomes were based on hypernasality, audible nasal air emission, intraoral pressure, and hyponasality scores (Henningsson et al. 2008; Deren et al. 2005; Park et al. 2016; Wermker et al. 2014; Ma et al. 2013; Sullivan et al. 2010). Overall velopharyngeal competence was graded as normal, borderline competent, borderline insufficient, or insufficient (Park et al. 2016; Sullivan et al. 2010; Lam et al. 2007), and successful or unsuccessful speech outcome was defined at 15 months postoperatively. In addition, we adopted the nasopharyngoscopy (Pigott 1969; Pigott et al. 1969) because it is superior to videofluoroscopy in finding the location of a velopharyngeal gap, confirming the size of the opening, and to evaluate the orientation of the *levator veli palatini* (Lam et al. 2006*)*. Although it has been found that nasopharyngoscopy and videofluoroscopy are not in perfect agreement when applied to the same patient (Shprintzen and Golding-Kushner 1989), we are in favor of using nasopharyngoscopy alone as thinner fiber-optic endoscopes can be adopted without discomfort to pediatric cases and it could be performed in an office setting without a radiologist and fluoroscopic equipment.

Our sample was mainly composed by older patients (including adults) with scarred palate (previous successful treatment of the palatal fistula and prior unsuccessful attempts to correct the velopharyngeal insufficiency) and with preoperative overall velopharyngeal function classified as insufficient and preoperative moderate-to-large velopharyngeal gap sizes. After 15 months of follow-up, complete velopharyngeal closure was obtained in 77.4% of patients (41 of 53 patients) and successful speech outcome in 84.9% (45 patients). All surgically treated patients showed different grades of reduction in velopharyngeal active gap size and improvement in hypernasality, audible nasal air emission, and intraoral pressure, but it was unsatisfactory in 15.1% patients (eight patients) who needed additional velopharyngeal insufficiency surgery, namely posterior pharyngeal free fat grafting, as they presented with pinhole or small velopharyngeal gaps. In the velopharyngeal insufficiency literature, the success speech rates with the buccinator myomucosal flaps have been reported between 48 and 93% (Logjes et al. 2017; Dias et al. 2016; Lee and Alizadeh 2016; Ahl et al. 2016; Varghese et al. 2015; Abdaly et al. 2015; Hens et al. 2013; Mann et al. 2011; Robertson et al. 2008; Hill et al. 2004).

In this context, with the movement to tailor the velopharyngeal insufficiency surgical management to the individual patient's needs (Sie et al. 2005; Armour et al. 2005; Sullivan et al. 2010; Yamaguchi et al. 2016), it is useful to have predictors of speech outcomes to counsel patients/parents and to plan for further speech rehabilitation after the specific operation (Sie et al. 2005; Armour et al. 2005; Setabutr et al. 2015; McComb et al. 2011). However, such important predictors have been sparsely tested in the buccinator myomucosal flap reports (Hens et al. 2013). Hens et al. (2013) demonstrated that none of the potential prognostic factors (male, age >7 years, previous velopharyngeal insufficiency surgery, syndromic diagnosis, surgical learning curve, and no simultaneous levator retropositioning) was able to influence the poor outcome (need for revision surgery) after the buccinator myomucosal flap procedures; these results were probably due to the small sample size (Hens et al. 2013). In a further branch of our data, we therefore were interested in determining which variables were most likely to influence successful speech outcomes in repaired cleft palate patients undergoing the bilateral buccinator myomucosal flap for velopharyngeal insufficiency management, instead of failure. We hypothesize that preoperative velopharyngeal closure pattern does not affect speech outcomes. Bivariate and multivariate logistic regression analyses were performed to identify independent variables with a significant association with successful speech outcome (dependent variable). The sample size estimate was 28 patients ($\alpha = 0.05$, two-sided; $\beta = 0.13$). Interestingly, although a larger cohort ($n = 53$) has been analyzed, we did not identify significant (all $p > 0.05$) predictors of success (Table 11.2). Nevertheless, some of the tested variables should be discussed because they underlie our current protocol until further investigations expand or confront our data.

The mean age of our patients is significantly older than the recommended age for velopharyngeal insufficiency surgical management, as interventions in patients aged 4–12 years seem to be related with better speech outcomes (Deren et al. 2005; Perkins et al. 2005; Sie et al. 2005; Sommerlad et al. 2002; Sullivan et al. 2010; Fukushiro and Trindade 2011). Previous buccinator myomucosal flap experiences

Table 11.2 Bivariate and multivariate analyses of the possible independent predictors of successful speech outcome

Independent variables	Successful speech outcome		
	Bivariate analysis	Multivariate analysis	
	p-value	Coefficient	p-value
Constant	–	382.48	0.993
Gender	0.409	120.69	0.998
Age	0.120	−87.83	0.998
Veau hierarchy	0.304	−69.53	0.999
Previous fistulae surgery	0.803	33.56	0.999
Previous velopharyngeal insufficiency surgery	0.391	64.65	0.999
Preoperative velopharyngeal closure pattern	0.231	16.31	0.999
Preoperative velopharyngeal gap size	0.282	105.42	0.999
Surgical learning curve	0.276	−8.97	1.000
Simultaneous intravelar veloplasty	0.340	77.98	0.999
Buccinator pedicle divided	0.954	−147.76	0.998
Complications	0.139	−130.06	0.999

– Not applied
Study performed according to the SOBRAPAR Hospital algorithm for repaired cleft palate patients ($n = 53$) with velopharyngeal insufficiency

(Logjes et al. 2017; Dias et al. 2016; Lee and Alizadeh 2016; Ahl et al. 2016; Varghese et al. 2015; Abdaly et al. 2015; Hens et al. 2013; Mann et al. 2011; Robertson et al. 2008; Hill et al. 2004) were mainly composed by pediatric patients with velopharyngeal insufficiency. In our report, 24 of 53 patients (45.3%) were aged 18 years or older. Our data are therefore complementary to those previously presented (Logjes et al. 2017; Dias et al. 2016; Lee and Alizadeh 2016; Ahl et al. 2016; Varghese et al. 2015; Abdaly et al. 2015; Hens et al. 2013; Mann et al. 2011; Robertson et al. 2008; Hill et al. 2004) as the bilateral buccinator myomucosal flap was effective in the surgical management of older patients (including adults). The increased age of our sample reflects the reality of velopharyngeal insufficiency surgical treatment in our and other cleft centers (Setabutr et al. 2015; Follmar et al. 2015; Carlson et al. 2016). Older patients with unrepaired cleft palate or repaired cleft palate with velopharyngeal insufficiency (often adopted patients or from rural and incipient regions with low human development index) have been lately referred to us as we act as a reference cleft center in our country (Raposo-Amaral and Raposo-Amaral 2012; Denadai et al. 2015a, b).

Further important aspect in surgical management of velopharyngeal insufficiency is the anatomical status of the velopharyngeal sphincter as the surgical protocols have been based on the selection of one or more surgical techniques according to the preoperative instrumental characterization of the velopharyngeal closure size and pattern (Gart and Gosain 2014; Hopper et al. 2014; Seagle et al. 2016; Abdel-Aziz et al. 2011; Armour et al. 2005; Sullivan et al. 2010; Yamaguchi et al. 2016). In general, most patients with moderate or large velopharyngeal gaps have been treated with sphincter pharyngoplasty or pharyngeal flap (Gart and Gosain 2014; Hopper et al. 2014; Seagle et al. 2016; Abdel-Aziz et al. 2011; Armour et al. 2005;

Sullivan et al. 2010; Yamaguchi et al. 2016). A detailed analysis of previous buccinator myomucosal flap studies (Logjes et al. 2017; Dias et al. 2016; Lee and Alizadeh 2016; Ahl et al. 2016; Varghese et al. 2015; Abdaly et al. 2015; Hens et al. 2013; Mann et al. 2011; Robertson et al. 2008; Hill et al. 2004) reveals a lack of standardized data regarding pre- and postoperative velopharyngeal gap sizes and patterns. Although extrapolation of this limited data (Logjes et al. 2017; Dias et al. 2016; Lee and Alizadeh 2016; Ahl et al. 2016; Varghese et al. 2015; Abdaly et al. 2015; Hens et al. 2013; Mann et al. 2011; Robertson et al. 2008; Hill et al. 2004) can culminate in argument that the buccinator myomucosal flap is a safe and reliable means of achieving soft palate lengthening in patients with varying degrees of velopharyngeal gaps, we believe that a detailed analysis should be carried out to statistically determine if the velopharyngeal closure size and/or patterns can interfere with the speech outcomes, exactly as has been assessed in other therapeutic approaches (Armour et al. 2005).

In favor of our initial hypothesis, we demonstrated similar successful speech outcomes in preoperative coronal or noncoronal velopharyngeal closure patterns. We also presented that the preoperative velopharyngeal gap size (moderate versus large) does not influence the surgical success. We believe that the present study, along with standardized assessment of the results, provides additional information for the broad field of knowledge of surgical outcomes of velopharyngeal insufficiency in cleft patients. Now, there is scientific support to adopt the bilateral buccinator myomucosal flap in repaired cleft palate patients with moderate or large velopharyngeal gaps, regardless of the velopharyngeal closure pattern.

Moreover, our findings reinforce advantages of the buccinator myomucosal flaps previously described (Logjes et al. 2017; Dias et al. 2016; Lee and Alizadeh 2016; Ahl et al. 2016; Varghese et al. 2015; Abdaly et al. 2015; Hens et al. 2013; Mann et al. 2011; Robertson et al. 2008; Hill et al. 2004; Raposo-do-Amaral 2013). This flap can be performed as a single velopharyngeal insufficiency treatment, but when it fails, it is possible to combine it with posterior pharyngeal fat grafting. In addition, the buccinator myomucosal flaps can be applied in a broad spectrum of velopharyngeal insufficiency patients because aspects such as the number and/or types of cleft palate surgeries previously performed and/or the amount of palatal scarring are not limiting factors. In fact, the palatal lengthening with the interposition of the buccinator myomucosal flaps, a highly vascularized, elastic, and malleable tissue, breaks the functional restriction imposed by the large amount of scar tissue in a poor vascularized area (Hens et al. 2013). This characteristic becomes extremely relevant in the setting of our and previous cohorts (Hens et al. 2013) composed by velopharyngeal insufficiency patients with multiple previous palatal surgeries (i.e., primary cleft palate repair, previous successful fistula repair, and unsuccessful velopharyngeal insufficiency correction) than cohorts formed by velopharyngeal insufficiency patients who underwent only primary cleft palate repair (Deren et al. 2005; Sommerlad et al. 2002; Sullivan et al. 2010). On the other hand, the indication of posteriorly based pedicled buccinator myomucosal flaps is limited in situations where there are doubts about the integrity of the buccinator muscle, buccal artery, or their branches and/or the availability of nonscarred myomucosal tissue (e.g., in patients with prior intraoral cheek scar secondary, for example, to bimaxillary orthognathic surgery).

Previous reports (Logjes et al. 2017; Dias et al. 2016; Lee and Alizadeh 2016; Ahl et al. 2016; Varghese et al. 2015; Abdaly et al. 2015; Hens et al. 2013; Mann et al. 2011; Robertson et al. 2008; Hill et al. 2004; Raposo-do-Amaral 2013) have also highlighted that the buccinator myomucosal flap is more "anatomical and physiological" than the sphincter pharyngoplasty and pharyngeal flap, because if the palate is anatomically short, it is lengthened with no permanent pharyngeal cushion or bridge. We and some groups adopted the bilateral buccinator myomucosal flap for restoration of the nasal and oral layers, while others use only the unilateral buccinator myomucosal flap for oral layer reconstruction (Logjes et al. 2017; Dias et al. 2016; Lee and Alizadeh 2016; Ahl et al. 2016; Varghese et al. 2015; Abdaly et al. 2015; Hens et al. 2013; Mann et al. 2011; Robertson et al. 2008; Hill et al. 2004; Raposo-do-Amaral 2013). Although using unilateral flap can be based on the "lifeboat" plastic surgical principle, we and others (Hill et al. 2004) believe that the absence of the nasal layer reconstruction can result in soft-tissue contraction. If a raw area in the nasal lining heals secondarily, the flap applied in the oral layer reconstruction may theoretically result in sagittal shortening of the palate. This anatomic change is strongly supported by our and others' (Ahl et al. 2016; Hens et al. 2013; Mann et al. 2011) significant and persistent improvement in late postoperative speech scores. However, there are mixed evidence (Freedlander and Jackson 1989; Hens et al. 2013) on the maintaining of its size over the long term, especially if the unilateral flaps are used.

This probably "anatomical and physiological theory" is also evidenced by the absence of postoperative hyponasality and/or obstructive airway complaints reported in our and previous series (Logjes et al. 2017; Dias et al. 2016; Lee and Alizadeh 2016; Ahl et al. 2016; Varghese et al. 2015; Abdaly et al. 2015; Hens et al. 2013; Mann et al. 2011; Robertson et al. 2008; Hill et al. 2004; Raposo-do-Amaral 2013). We screened obstructive sleep apnea preoperatively and postoperatively with the previously validated Brazilian-Portuguese versions of the STOP-Bang questionnaire and the Epworth Sleepiness Scale (Chung et al. 2016; Fonseca et al. 2016; Johns 1991; Bertolazi et al. 2009; Chiu et al. 2016; Nagappa et al. 2015; Kendzerska et al. 2014; Silva et al. 2011; Vana et al. 2013). We only scored 0–1 and 0–7 in the STOP-BANG questionnaire and Epworth Sleepiness Scale, respectively. As our patients presented with low risk for obstructive sleep apnea preoperatively and postoperatively, polysomnography was not routinely performed for the diagnosis of obstructive sleep apnea. This rationale has been adopted in other velopharyngeal insufficiency reports (Ahl et al. 2016; Abdaly et al. 2015; Hens et al. 2013; Mann et al. 2011; Hill et al. 2004; Yamaguchi et al. 2016) and also established in some questionnaires and clinical models for screening obstructive sleep apnea (Chung et al. 2016; Fonseca et al. 2016; Johns 1991; Bertolazi et al. 2009; Chiu et al. 2016; Nagappa et al. 2015; Kendzerska et al. 2014; Silva et al. 2011; Vana et al. 2013).

In our previously published cohort, there were 11 (20.8%) surgical related complications: three (27.3%) partial dehiscence at the junction of the hard and soft palates, which healed spontaneously; three (27.3%) mouth opening limitations resolved with the division of the pedicles; two (18.2%) donor-site hematomas surgically drained; two (18.2%) partial tip necrosis of the oral flaps, which healed spontaneously; and one (9%) fistula at the junction of the hard and soft palates successfully treated with tongue flap after the end of data collection. Our complication rate (20.8%) is similar to the previously described trends (8–31%) (Logjes et al. 2017; Dias et al. 2016; Lee and Alizadeh 2016; Ahl et al. 2016; Varghese et al. 2015; Abdaly et al. 2015; Hens et al. 2013; Mann et al. 2011; Robertson et al. 2008; Hill et al. 2004; Raposo-do-Amaral 2013). All complications occurred at the beginning of the surgeon (C.A.R-A) learning curve (2010–2012 period), as also described by another surgeon (Mann et al. 2011) who demonstrated a reduction in complication rates with increase in the experience with the flap. In addition, some groups (Ahl et al. 2016; Hens et al. 2013; Mann et al. 2011) have changed the buccinator myomucosal flap design (e.g., pedicles placed at the retromolar trigone or islanded flaps) or the postoperative care (e.g., use of bite blocks) to reduce the potential blood supply-related complications (e.g., biting of the pedicles). In our flap design for velopharyngeal insufficiency management, as the cranial demarcations (located caudally to the Stensen's duct) were connected to the defect in the soft palate, the pedicles were positioned at the retromolar trigone after the mobilization of the flaps. As there were no specific technical changes in the surgeries performed in the overall analyzed period, we believe that the progressive acquisition of experience with this flap (i.e., meticulous dissections of the palatal and flap tissues and more detailed postoperative guidelines for the patients) was sufficient to maintain the low rate of complications in the last 2 years analyzed. However, as no comparative analysis was performed to test the effectiveness of described modifications to date (Logjes et al. 2017; Dias et al. 2016; Lee and Alizadeh 2016; Ahl et al. 2016; Varghese et al. 2015; Abdaly et al. 2015; Hens et al. 2013; Mann et al. 2011; Robertson et al. 2008; Hill et al. 2004; Raposo-do-Amaral 2013), future comparative studies are needed to assess if any particular surgical refinement presents superior outcomes.

11.4 Summary

The authors report the SOBRAPAR experience with the buccinator myomucosal flaps in cleft palate repair, including the management of primary cleft palate, palatal cleft fistulae, and persistent velopharyngeal insufficiency.

References

Abdaly H, Omranyfard M, Ardekany MR, Babaei K. Buccinator flap as a method for palatal fistula and VPI management. Adv Biomed Res. 2015;4:135.

Abdel-Aziz M. The use of buccal flap in the closure of posterior post-palatoplasty fistula. Int J Pediatr Otorhinolaryngol. 2008;72:1657–61.

Abdel-Aziz M, El-Hoshy H, Ghandour H. Treatment of velopharyngeal insufficiency after cleft palate repair depending on the velopharyngeal closure pattern. J Craniofac Surg. 2011;22:813–7.

Adenwalla HS, Narayanan PV, Rajshree CJ. The history and evolution of cleft surgery in India. Indian J Plast Surg. 2005;38:188–91.

Ahl R, Harding-Bell A, Wharton L, Jordan A, Hall P. The Buccinator mucomuscular flap: an in-depth analysis and evaluation of its role in the management of velopharyngeal dysfunction. Cleft Palate Craniofac J. 2016;53:e177–84.

Alfwaress FS, Khwaileh FA, Khamaiseh ZA. The speech language Pathologist's role in the Cleft lip and palate team. J Craniofac Surg. 2015;26:1439–42.

Alsalman AK, Algadiem EA, Alwabari MS, Almugarrab FJ. Single-layer Closure with tongue flap for palatal fistula in Cleft palate patients. Plast Reconstr Surg Glob Open. 2016;4:e852.

Armour A, Fischbach S, Klaiman P, Fisher DM. Does velopharyngeal closure pattern affect the success of pharyngeal flap pharyngoplasty? Plast Reconstr Surg. 2005;115:45–52.

Ashtiani AK, Emami SA, Rasti M. Closure of complicated palatal fistula with facial artery musculomucosal flap. Plast Reconstr Surg. 2005;116:381–6. discussion 387–388

Ayad T, Xie L. Facial artery musculomucosal flap in head and neck reconstruction: a systematic review. Head Neck. 2015;37:1375–86.

Bardach J, editor. Atlas of craniofacial and Cleft surgery, vol. 2. Philadelphia: Lippincott Raven; 1999.

Bertolazi AN, Fagondes SC, Holff LS, Pedro VD, Menna Barreto SS, Johns MW. Portuguese-language version of the Epworth sleepiness scale. Validation for use in Brazil. J Bras Pneumol. 2009;35:877–83.

Bishop A, Hong P, Bezuhly M. Autologous fat grafting for the treatment of velopharyngeal insufficiency: state of the art. J Plast Reconstr Aesthet Surg. 2014;67:1–8.

Bonanthaya K, Shetty P, Sharma A, Ahlawat J, Passi D, Singh M. Treatment modalities for surgical management of anterior palatal fistula: comparison of various techniques, their outcomes, and the factors governing treatment plan: a retrospective study. Natl J Maxillofac Surg. 2016;7:148–52.

Bozola AR, Gasques JA, Carriquiry CE, Cardoso de Oliveira M. The buccinator musculomucosal flap: anatomic study and clinical application. Plast Reconstr Surg. 1989;84:250–7.

Bykowski MR, Naran S, Winger DG, Losee JE. The rate of Oronasal fistula following primary Cleft palate surgery: a meta-analysis. Cleft Palate Craniofac J. 2015;52:e81–7.

Carlson LC, Hatcher KW, Tomberg L, Kabetu C, Ayala R, Vander Burg R. Inequitable access to timely Cleft palate surgery in low- and middle-income countries. World J Surg. 2016;40:1047–52.

Carstens MH, Stofman GM, Sotereanos GC, Hurwitz DJ. A new approach for repair of oro-antral-nasal fistulae. The anteriorly based buccinator myomucosal island flap. J Craniomaxillofac Surg. 1991;19:64–70.

Chen GF, Zhong LP. A bilateral musculomucosal buccal flap method for cleft palate surgery. J Oral Maxillofac Surg. 2003;61:1399–404.

Chiu HY, Chen PY, Chuang LP, Chen NH, Tu YK, Hsieh YJ, Wang YC, Guilleminault C. Diagnostic accuracy of the Berlin questionnaire, STOP-BANG, STOP, and Epworth sleepiness scale in detecting obstructive sleep apnea: a bivariate meta-analysis. Sleep Med Rev. 2016; doi:10.1016/j.smrv.2016.10.004. [Epub ahead of print]

Chung F, Abdullah HR, Liao P. STOP-bang questionnaire: a practical approach to screen for obstructive sleep apnea. Chest. 2016;149:631–8.

Cohen SR, Kalinowski J, LaRossa D, Randall P. Cleft palate fistulas: a multivariate statistical analysis of prevalence, etiology, and surgical management. Plast Reconstr Surg. 1991;87:1041–7.

Collins J, Cheung K, Farrokhyar F, Strumas N. Pharyngeal flap versus sphincter pharyngoplasty for the treatment of velopharyngeal insufficiency: a meta-analysis. J Plast Reconstr Aesthet Surg. 2012;65:864–8.

Denadai R, Samartine Junior H, Denadai R, Raposo-Amaral CE. The public recognizes plastic surgeons as leading experts in the treatment of congenital cleft and craniofacial anomalies. J Craniofac Surg. 2015a;26:e684–9.

Denadai R, Muraro CA, Raposo-Amaral CE. Residents' perceptions of plastic surgeons as craniofacial surgery specialists. J Craniofac Surg. 2015b;26:2334–8.

Denadai R, Sabbag A, Raposo-Amaral CE, Filho JC, Nagae MH, Raposo-Amaral CA. Bilateral buccinator myomucosal flap outcomes in nonsyndromic patients with repaired cleft palate and velopharyngeal insufficiency. J Plast Reconstr Aesthet Surg. 2017;70:1598–1607.

Deren O, Ayhan M, Tuncel A, Görgü M, Altuntaş A, Kutlay R, Erdoğan B. The correction of velopharyngeal insufficiency by Furlow palatoplasty in patients older than 3 years undergoing Veau-Wardill-Kilner palatoplasty: a prospective clinical study. Plast Reconstr Surg. 2005;116:85–93.

Diah E, Lo LJ, Yun C, Wang R, Wahyuni LK, Chen YR. Cleft oronasal fistula: a review of treatment results and a surgical management algorithm proposal. Chung Gang Med J. 2007;30:529–37.

Dias DK, Fernando PD, Dissanayake RD. Improvement of quality of speech in patients with velo-pharyngeal insufficiency corrected using a buccinator myomucosal flap. Ceylon Med J. 2016;61:130–4.

Ecker HA. The use of the buccal flap in cleft palate repair. Plast Reconstr Surg Transplant Bull. 1960;25:235–9.

Emory RE, Clay RP, Bite U, Jackson IT. Fistula formation and repair after palatal closure: an institutional perspective. Plast Reconstr Surg. 1997;99:1535–8.

Fang L, Yang M, Wang C, Ma T, Zhao Z, Yin N, Wei L, Yin J. A clinical study of various buccinator musculomucosal flaps for palatal fistulae closure after cleft palate surgery. J Craniofac Surg. 2014;25:e197–202.

Ferrari S, Ferri A, Bianchi B, Copelli C, Boni P, Sesenna E. Donor site morbidity using the buccinator myomucosal island flap. Oral Surg Oral Med Oral Pathol Oral Radiol Endod. 2011;111:306–11.

Fitzsimons DA. International confederation for cleft lip and palate and related craniofacial anomalies task force report: speech assessment. Cleft Palate Craniofac J. 2014;51:e138–45.

Follmar KE, Yuan N, Pendleton CS, Dorafshar AH, Kolk CV, Redett RJ 3rd. Velopharyngeal insufficiency rates after delayed cleft palate repair: lessons learned from internationally adopted patients. Ann Plast Surg. 2015;75:302–5.

Fonseca LB, Silveira EA, Lima NM, Rabahi MF. STOP-bang questionnaire: translation to Portuguese and cross-cultural adaptation for use in Brazil. J Bras Pneumol. 2016;42:266–72.

Franco D, Rocha D, Arnaut M Jr, Freitas R, Alonso N. Versatility of the buccinator myomucosal flap in atypical palate reconstructions. J Craniomaxillofac Surg. 2014;42:1310–4.

Freda N, Rauso R, Curinga G, Clemente M, Gherardini G. Easy closure of anterior palatal fistula with local flaps. J Craniofac Surg. 2010;21:229–32.

Freedlander E, Jackson IT. The fate of buccal mucosal flaps in primary palatal repair. Cleft Palate J. 1989;26:110–2. discussion 112–113

Fukushiro AP, Trindade IE. Nasometric and aerodynamic outcome analysis of pharyngeal flap surgery for the management of velopharyngeal insufficiency. J Craniofac Surg. 2011;22:1647–51.

Gart MS, Gosain AK. Surgical management of velopharyngeal insufficiency. Clin Plast Surg. 2014;41:253–70.

Guerrero Santos J, Altamirano JT. The use of lingual flaps in repair of fistulae of the hard palate. Plast Reconstr Surg. 1966;38:123.

Guerrero-Santos J, Fernandez JM. Further experience with tongue flap in cleft palate repair. Cleft Palate J. 1973;10:192–202.

Habib AS, Brennan PA. The Deepithelialized dorsal tongue flap for reconstruction of anterior palatal fistulae: literature review and presentation of our experience in Egypt. Cleft Palate Craniofac J. 2016;53:589–96.

Hardwicke JT, Landini G, Richard BM. Fistula incidence after primary cleft palate repair: a systematic review of the literature. Plast Reconstr Surg. 2014;134:618e–27e.

Henningsson G, Kuehn DP, Sell D, Sweeney T, Trost-Cardamone JE, Whitehill TL, Speech Parameters Group. Universal parameters for reporting speech outcomes in individuals with cleft palate. Cleft Palate Craniofac J. 2008;45:1–17.

Hens G, Sell D, Pinkstone M, Birch MJ, Hay N, Sommerlad BC, Kangesu L. Palate lengthening by buccinator myomucosal flaps for velopharyngeal insufficiency. Cleft Palate Craniofac J. 2013;50:e84–91.

Hill C, Hayden C, Riaz M, Leonard AG. Buccinator sandwich pushback: a new technique for treatment of secondary velopharyngeal incompetence. Cleft Palate Craniofac J. 2004;41:230–7.

Hopper RA, Tse R, Smartt J, Swanson J, Kinter S. Cleft palate repair and velopharyngeal dysfunction. Plast Reconstr Surg. 2014;133:852e–64e.

Jackson IT. Closure of secondary palatal fistulae with intraoral tissue and bone grafting. Brit J Plast Surg. 1972;25:73.

Jackson IT, McLennan G, Scheker LR. Primary veloplasty or primary palatoplasty: some preliminary findings. Plast Reconstr Surg. 1983;72:153–7.

Jackson IT, Moreira-Gonzalez AA, Rogers A, Beal BJ. The buccal flap--a useful technique in cleft palate repair? Cleft Palate Craniofac J. 2004;41:144–51.

Jagannathan M, Dixit V. Palatal lengthening following use of buccal myomucosal flap in primary palatoplasty-real or apparent? A study of physical variables. Eur J Plast Surg. 2004;26:414–8.

Johns MW. A new method for measuring daytime sleepiness: the Epworth sleepiness scale. Sleep. 1991;14:540–5.

Jowett N, Hadlock TA, Sela E, Toth M, Knecht R, Lörincz BB. Facial mimetic, cosmetic, and functional standardized assessment of the facial artery musculomucosal (FAMM) flap. Auris Nasus Larynx. 2017;44:220–6.

Kaplan EN. Soft palate repair by levator muscle reconstruction and a buccal mucosal flap. Plast Reconstr Surg. 1975;56:129–36.

Katzel EB, Shakir S, Naran S, MacIsaac Z, Camison L, Greives M, Goldstein JA, Grunwaldt LJ, Ford MD, Losee JE. Speech outcomes after clinically indicated posterior pharyngeal flap takedown. Ann Plast Surg. 2016;77:420–4.

Kendzerska TB, Smith PM, Brignardello-Petersen R, Leung RS, Tomlinson GA. Evaluation of the measurement properties of the Epworth sleepiness scale: a systematic review. Sleep Med Rev. 2014;18:321–31.

Khanna S, Dagum AB. Waltzing a facial artery musculomucosal flap to salvage a recurrent palatal fistula. Cleft Palate Craniofac J. 2012;49:750–2.

Kobayashi S, Fukawa T, Hirakawa T, Maegawa J. The folded buccal musculomucosal flap for large palatal fistulae in cleft palate. Plast Reconstr Surg Glob Open. 2014;2:e112.

Kummer AW. Speech evaluation for patients with cleft palate. Clin Plast Surg. 2014;41:241–51.

Lahiri A, Richard B. Superiorly based facial artery musculomucosal flap for large anterior palatal fistulae in clefts. Cleft Palate Craniofac J. 2007;44:523–7.

Lam DJ, Starr JR, Perkins JA, Lewis CW, Eblen LE, Dunlap J, Sie KC. A comparison of nasendoscopy and multiview videofluoroscopy in assessing velopharyngeal insufficiency. Otolaryngol Head Neck Surg. 2006;134:394–402.

Lam E, Hundert S, Wilkes GH. Lateral pharyngeal wall and velar movement and tailoring velopharyngeal surgery: determinants of velopharyngeal incompetence resolution in patients with cleft palate. Plast Reconstr Surg. 2007;120:495–505.

Lee JY, Alizadeh K. Spacer facial artery musculomucosal flap: simultaneous closure of oronasal fistulas and palatal lengthening. Plast Reconstr Surg. 2016;137:240–3.

Logjes RJ, van den Aardweg MT, Blezer MM, van der Heul AM, Breugem CC. Velopharyngeal insufficiency treated with levator muscle repositioning and unilateral myomucosal buccinator flap. J Craniomaxillofac Surg. 2017;45:1–7.

Ma L, Shi B, Li Y, Zheng Q. Velopharyngeal function assessment in patients with cleft palate: perceptual speech assessment versus nasopharyngoscopy. J Craniofac Surg. 2013;24:1229–31.

Maeda K, Ojimi H, Utsugi R, Ando S. A T-shape musculomucosal buccal flap method for cleft palate surgery. Plast Reconstr Surg. 1987;79:888–96.

Mahajan RK, Chhajlani R, Ghildiyal HC. Role of tongue flap in palatal fistula repair: a series of 41 cases. Indian J Plast Surg. 2014;47:210–5.

Mann RJ, Fisher DM. Bilateral buccal flaps with double opposing Z-plasty for wider palatal clefts. Plast Reconstr Surg. 1997;100:1139–43.

Mann RJ, Neaman KC, Armstrong SD, Ebner B, Bajnrauh R, Naum S. The double-opposing buccal flap procedure for palatal lengthening. Plast Reconstr Surg. 2011;127:2413–8.

Mann RJ, Martin MD, Eichhorn MG, Neaman KC, Sierzant CG, Polley JW, Girotto JA. The double opposing Z-Plasty plus or minus Buccal flap approach for repair of Cleft palate: a review of 505 consecutive cases. Plast Reconstr Surg. 2017;139:735e–44e.

Massarelli O, Baj A, Gobbi R, Soma D, Marelli S, De Riu G, Tullio A, Giannì AB. Cheek mucosa: a versatile donor site of myomucosal flaps. Technical and functional considerations. Head Neck. 2013;35:109–17.

McComb RW, Marrinan EM, Nuss RC, Labrie RA, Mulliken JB, Padwa BL. Predictors of velopharyngeal insufficiency after le fort I maxillary advancement in patients with cleft palate. J Oral Maxillofac Surg. 2011;69:2226–32.

Mukherji MM. Cheek flap for short palates. Cleft Palate J. 1969;6:415–20.

Murrell GL, Requena R, Karakla DW. Oronasal fistula repair with three layers. Plast Reconstr Surg. 2001;107:143–7.

Murthy J. Descriptive study of management of palatal fistula in one hundred and ninety-four cleft individuals. Indian J Plast Surg. 2011;44:41–6.

Muzaffar AR, Byrd HS, Rohrich RJ, Johns DF, LeBlanc D, Beran SJ, Anderson C, Papaioannou AA. Incidence of cleft palate fistula: an institutional experience with two-stage palatal repair. Plast Reconstr Surg. 2001;108:1515–8.

Nagappa M, Liao P, Wong J, Auckley D, Ramachandran SK, Memtsoudis S, Mokhlesi B, Chung F. Validation of the STOP-bang questionnaire as a screening tool for obstructive sleep apnea among different populations: a systematic review and meta-analysis. PLoS One. 2015;10:e0143697.

Nakakita N, Maeda K, Ojimi H, Utsugi R, Maekawa J. The modified buccal musculomucosal flap method for cleft palate surgery. Plast Reconstr Surg. 1991;88:421–6.

Park SW, Oh TS, Koh KS. Repeat double-opposing Z-Plasty for the Management of Persistent Velopharyngeal Insufficiency. Ann Plast Surg. 2016;77:626–9.

Penna V, Bannasch H, Stark GB. The turbinate flap for oronasal fistula closure. Ann Plast Surg. 2007;59:679–81.

Perkins JA, Lewis CW, Gruss JS, Eblen LE, Sie KC. Furlow palatoplasty for management of velopharyngeal insufficiency: a prospective study of 148 consecutive patients. Plast Reconstr Surg. 2005;116:72–80. discussion 81–84

Pigott RW. The nasendoscopic appearance of the normal palatopharyngeal valve. Plast Reconstr Surg. 1969;43:19–24.

Pigott RW, Bensen JF, White FD. Nasendoscopy in the diagnosis of velopharyngeal incompetence. Plast Reconstr Surg. 1969;43:141–7.

Pribaz J, Stephens W, Crespo L, Gifford G. A new intraoral flap: Facial artery musculomucosal (FAMM) flap. Plast Reconstr Surg. 1992;90:421–9.

Rahpeyma A, Khajehahmadi S. Buccinator-based myomucosal flaps in intraoral reconstruction: a review and new classification. Natl J Maxillofac Surg. 2013;4:25–32.

Rahpeyma A, Khajehahmadi S. Inferiorly based buccinator myomucosal island flap in oral and pharyngeal reconstruction. Four techniques to increase its application. Int J Surg Case Rep. 2015a;14:58–62.

Rahpeyma A, Khajehahmadi S. Closure of huge palatal fistula in an adult patient with isolated cleft palate: a technical note. Plast Reconstr Surg Glob Open. 2015b;3:e306.

Rahpeyma A, Khajehahmadi S. Donor site morbidity in buccinator-based myomucosal flaps: a retrospective study. Asian J Surg. 2016;40(3):210–4. doi:10.1016/j.asjsur.2015.10.010. [Epub ahead of print]

Raposo-Amaral CE, Raposo-Amaral CA. Changing face of cleft care: specialized centers in developing countries. J Craniofac Surg. 2012;23:206–9.

Raposo-do-Amaral CA. Bilateral buccinator myomucosal flap for the treatment of velopharyngeal insufficiency: preliminary results. Rev Bras Cir Plást. 2013;28:455–661.

Robertson AG, McKeown DJ, Bello-Rojas G, Chang YJ, Rogers A, Beal BJ, Blake M, Jackson IT. Use of buccal myomucosal flap in secondary cleft palate repair. Plast Reconstr Surg. 2008;122:910–7.

Rossell-Perry P, Arrascue HM. The nasal artery musculomucosal cutaneous flap in difficult palatal fistula closure. Craniomaxillofac Trauma Reconstr. 2012;5:175–84.

Sadhu P. Oronasal fistula in cleft palate surgery. Indian J Plast Surg. 2009;42(Suppl):S123–8.

Salimi N, Aleksejūnienė J, Yen EH, Loo AY. Fistula in Cleft lip and palate patients-a systematic scoping review. Ann Plast Surg. 2017;78:91–102.

Seagle MB, Williams WN, Dixon-Wood V. Treatment of velopharyngeal insufficiency: fifteen-year experience at the University of Florida. Ann Plast Surg. 2016;76:285–7.

Setabutr D, Roth CT, Nolen DD, Cervenka B, Sykes JM, Senders CW, Tollefson TT. Revision rates and speech outcomes following pharyngeal flap surgery for velopharyngeal insufficiency. JAMA Facial Plast Surg. 2015;17:197–201.

Shetty R, Lamba S, Gupta AK. Role of facial artery musculomucosal flap in large and recurrent palatal fistulae. Cleft Palate Craniofac J. 2013;50:730–3.

Shprintzen RJ, Golding-Kushner K. Evaluation of velopharyngeal insufficiency. Otolaryngol Clin N Am. 1989;22:519–36.

Sie KC, Tampakopoulou DA, Sorom J, Gruss JS, Eblen LE. Results with Furlow palatoplasty in management of velopharyngeal insufficiency. Plast Reconstr Surg. 2005;108:17–25. discussion 26–29

Silva GE, Vana KD, Goodwin JL, Sherrill DL, Quan SF. Identification of patients with sleep disordered breathing: comparing the four-variable screening tool, STOP, STOP-bang, and Epworth sleepiness scales. J Clin Sleep Med. 2011;7:467–72.

Smith DM, Vecchione L, Jiang S, Ford M, Deleyiannis FW, Haralam MA, Naran S, Worrall CI, Dudas JR, Afifi AM, Marazita ML, Losee JE. The Pittsburgh fistula classification system: a standardized scheme for the description of palatal fistulas. Cleft Palate Craniofac J. 2007;44:590–4.

Sohail M, Bashir MM, Khan FA, Ashraf N. Comparison of clinical outcome of facial artery Myomucosal flap and tongue flap for Closure of large anterior palatal fistulas. J Craniofac Surg. 2016;27:1465–8.

Sommerlad BC, Mehendale FV, Birch MJ, Sell D, Hattee C, Harland K. Palate re-repair revisited. Cleft Palate Craniofac J. 2002;39:295–307.

Sullivan SR, Marrinan EM, Mulliken JB. Pharyngeal flap outcomes in nonsyndromic children with repaired cleft palate and velopharyngeal insufficiency. Plast Reconstr Surg. 2010;125:290–8.

Vaira LA, Massarelli O, Gobbi R, Soma D, Dell'aversana Orabona G, Piombino P, De Riu G. Evaluation of discriminative sensibility in patient with buccinators myomucosal flap oral cavity reconstructions. Eur J Plast Surg. 2017; doi:10.1007/s00238-017-1277-z.

Vana KD, Silva GE, Goldberg R. Predictive abilities of the STOP-bang and Epworth sleepiness scale in identifying sleep clinic patients at high risk for obstructive sleep apnea. Res Nurs Health. 2013;36:84–94.

Varghese D, Datta S, Varghese A. Use of buccal myomucosal flap for palatal lengthening in cleft palate patient: experience of 20 cases. Contemp Clin Dent. 2015;6:S36–40.

Wermker K, Lünenbürger H, Joos U, Kleinheinz J, Jung S. Results of speech improvement following simultaneous push-back together with velopharyngeal flap surgery in cleft palate patients. J Craniomaxillofac Surg. 2014;42:525–30.

Yamaguchi K, Lonic D, Lee CH, Wang SH, Yun C, Lo LJ. A treatment protocol for velopharyngeal insufficiency and the outcome. Plast Reconstr Surg. 2016;138:290e–9e.

Yang Z, Liu L, Fan J, Chen W, Fu S, Yin Z. Use of the buccinator musculomucosal flap for bone coverage in primary cleft palate repair. Aesthet Plast Surg. 2013;37:1171–5.

Zhao Z, Li S, Yan Y, Li Y, Yang M, Mu L, Huang W, Liu Y, Zhai H, Jin J, Ma X. New buccinator myomucosal island flap: anatomic study and clinical application. Plast Reconstr Surg. 1999;104:55–64.

Velopharyngeal Insufficiency: Etiopathology and Treatment

12

Nivaldo Alonso, Jonas Eraldo Lima Jr., and Hillary E. Jenny

12.1 Introduction

The human voice is the sound produced by the passage of air across the vocal folds, and it is used for many functions, including speech. In turn, speech is defined as the process of making a sound with a coherent meaning according to the linguistic convention of any language. For the full execution of this function, a complex process must occur that depends on many variables, including the proper closure of the velopharyngeal sphincter (VPS) in the articulation of oral phonemes (Garcia 1854; Skolnick and McCall 1973).

The closure of the velopharyngeal ring, which is bounded by the palate and lateral and posterior pharyngeal walls, is necessary to promote either partial or total separation of the oral and nasal cavities during breathing, blowing, swallowing, sucking, vomiting, and emitting oral and nasal phonemes. With the complete separation of these cavities, the sound produced by the larynx from the passage of the airstream can be directed into the oral cavity with the intraoral pressure required to appropriately produce oral phonemes (Skolnick 1969) (Fig. 12.1).

However, when you have a cleft in the palate the closing does not occur properly, and this airflow escapes into the nasal cavity, generating two speech signals that are considered primary components of velopharyngeal incompetence: hypernasality (voice production with increased nasal resonance) and nasal air escape (Fig. 12.2).

N. Alonso, M.D., Ph.D. (✉)
Divisao de Cirurgia Plastica e Queimaduras, Hospital das Clínicas da Faculdade de Medicina da Universidade de São Paulo, Sao Paulo, Brazil
e-mail: nivalonso@gmail.com

J.E. Lima Jr., M.D.
Board Certified Brazilian Society of Plastic Surgery, Federal University of Tocantins, Palmas, Tocantins, Brazil

H.E. Jenny, M.D.
Plastic Surgery Resident in the Program at John Hopkins, Baltimore, MD, USA

© Springer International Publishing AG 2018
N. Alonso, C.E. Raposo-Amaral (eds.), *Cleft Lip and Palate Treatment*,
https://doi.org/10.1007/978-3-319-63290-2_12

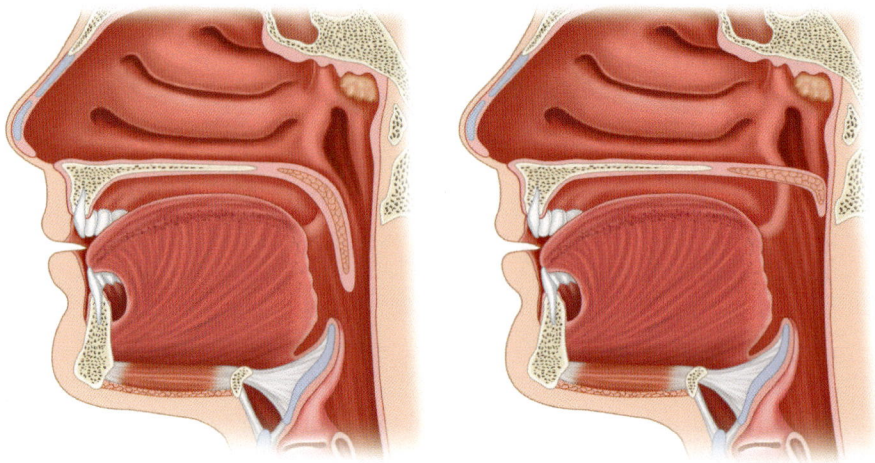

Fig. 12.1 Closure of velopharyngeal ring in a normal speech

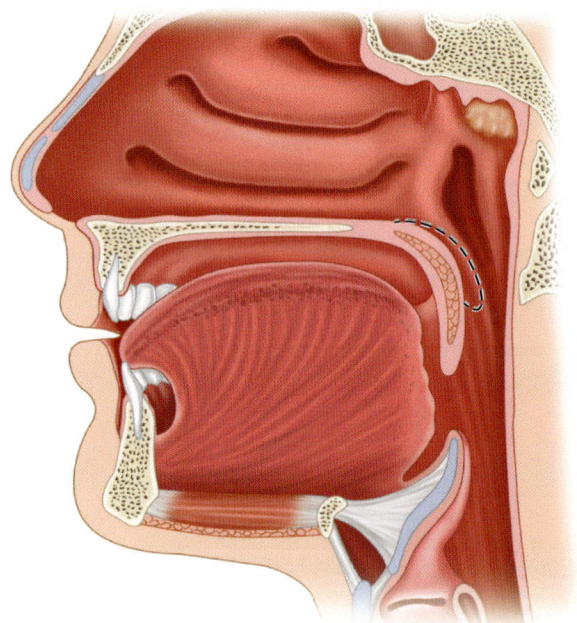

Fig. 12.2 Velopharyngeal insufficiency

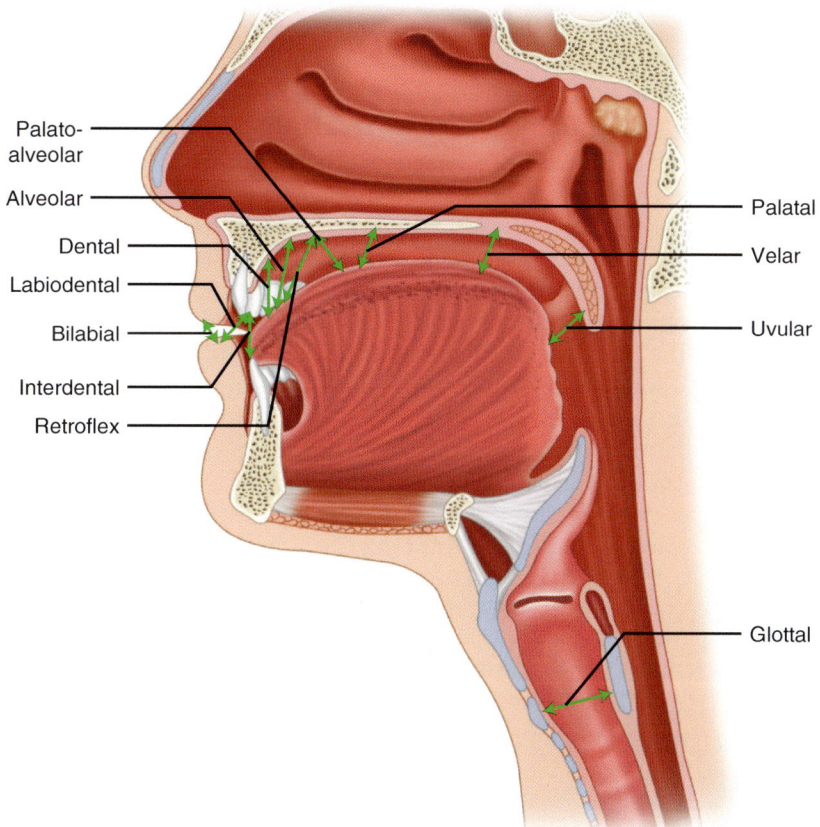

Fig. 12.3 Points of compensatory articulatory disorders in the oral cavity

Thus, cleft patients, many times, are forced to develop compensatory mechanisms for the articulation of phonemes that should be produced. This phenomenon is a minor component of velopharyngeal insufficiency (VPI), and is called compensatory articulation disorder (CAD) (Pamplona et al. 1999, 2005, 2014) (Fig. 12.3).

In individuals with cleft lip and palate, the anatomy and physiology of the VPS are changed, which can lead to VPI. Cleft type can be an additional determining factor in the pathogenesis of VPI, for patients with cleft lip and palate seem to have a higher incidence of this disorder than patients with isolated cleft palate.

12.2 Physiology of the Velopharyngeal Sphincter (VPS)

The closing of VPS is an extremely complex mechanism that has been studied extensively, with widely divergent opinions among researchers (Skolnick et al. 1973).

Initially, it was believed that the closure of this region is only due to movement of the soft palate closing against the posterior wall of the pharynx during swallowing; it was later reported that the same type of movement also occurred during speech (Braithwaite 1968; Boorman and Sommerlad 1985).

With further study, however, it was observed that the soft palate is not solely responsible for the closing of the sphincter: the posterior wall also moves during sphincter closure and forms a prominence (Passavant's ridge) that comes against the palate and pharyngeal sidewalls to perform medial displacement. Although some authors consider the side and back walls of the sphincter as a single functional unit, in fact, the back of the VPS contains two distinct parts of the upper pharyngeal constrictor muscle separated by salpingopharyngeal folds (Casey and Emrich 1988). The velopharyngeal closure is an important part of the speech, for this correct emission of many phonemes requires oral airflow and oral resonance for intelligible speech.

The soft palate contributes to the VPS closure through its displacement upwards and backwards, increasing its length to pass from the rest position to the functional position of the speech. This palatal elongation is followed by two velar movements: sealing and coupling. Sealing occurs as the creation of a very strong seal, usually between the three anterior sections and the back of the soft palate. Coupling is marked by changes in the space between the oral and nasal cavities, causing changes in the acoustic resonance during the emission of the oral and nasal phonemes. The levator muscle exerts a force up and back, while the palatopharyngeal and palatoglossus muscles exert antagonistic forces, promoting a dynamic interaction resulting in balance (Braithwaite 1968).

The posterior section of the lateral pharyngeal walls moves medially by joint action of the superior pharyngeal constrictor muscle and the levator veli palatini muscle, with different closing patterns at the various levels of pharynx.

As previously mentioned, the posterior wall can form Passavant's ridge during sphincter closure. This prominence varies in shape, direction, location within the pharynx, and degree of projection. In some patients, the ridge is located such that it does not contribute to the closure of the VPS, and may even be absent in around 30% of the population.

The closing of the VPS varies individually, with four main closing patterns: coronal or transverse (most common), sagittal, circular, and circular using or not Passavant's ridge; the latter pattern can be either normal or pathological (Fig. 12.4a, b).

All of these aspects must be considered in a clinical assessment in conjunction with imaging to perform an accurate diagnosis of VPI and decide upon the most appropriate treatment and postoperative follow-up.

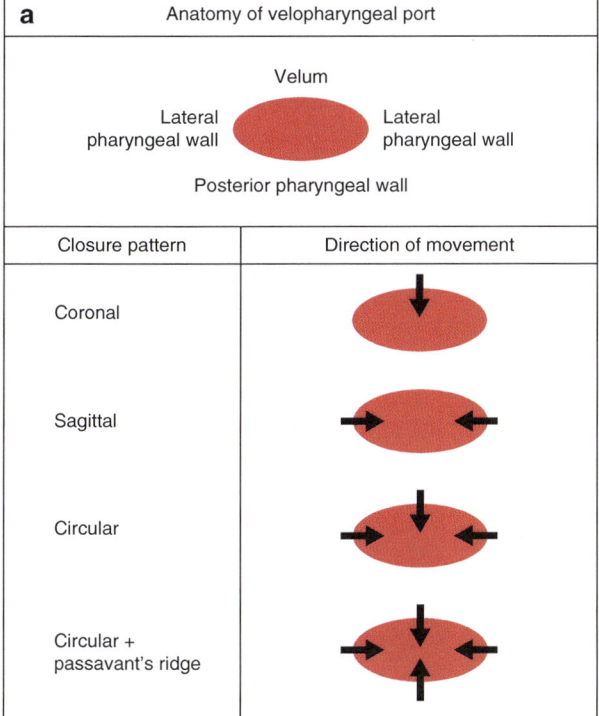

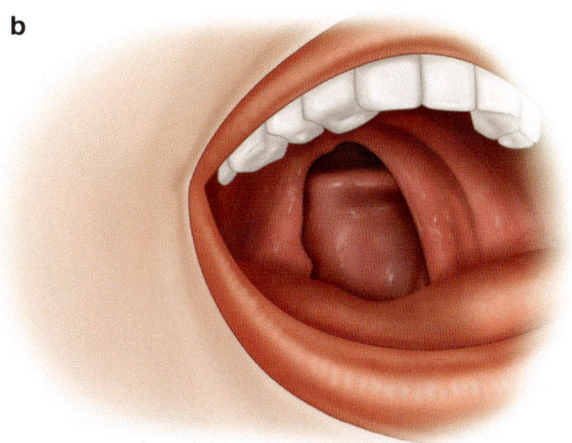

Fig. 12.4 (**a**) Types of velopharyngeal ring closure. (**b**) Passavant's ridge

12.3 Diagnosis

First thing to say is that the diagnosis of velopharyngeal insufficiency is always done by the physician in the multidisciplinary clinical consultation (Fig. 12.5a, b).

A good clinical assessment should be performed whenever possible, with the help of a specialized speech therapy team. Initially, the two main signs of velopharyngeal insufficiency are evaluated: hypernasality, assessed through the resonance test (cul de sac), and nasal escape, assessed through the mirror test. The secondary component of velopharyngeal insufficiency, compensatory articulation disorder, should also be evaluated, noting that the following are the most commonly identified types: glottal stops, pharyngeal fricatives and plosives, posterior nasal fricatives, and velar fricatives.

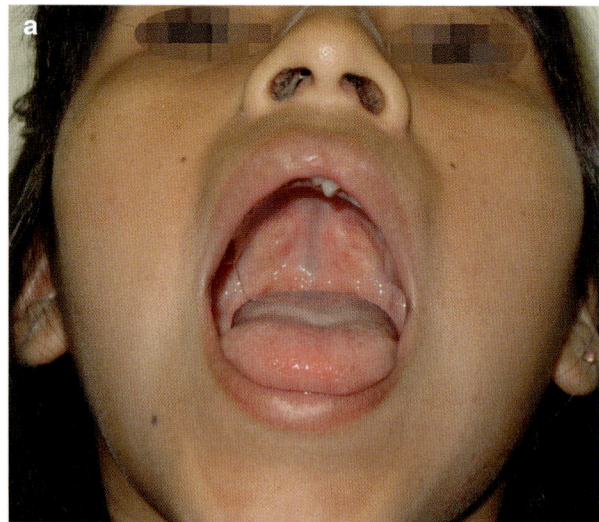

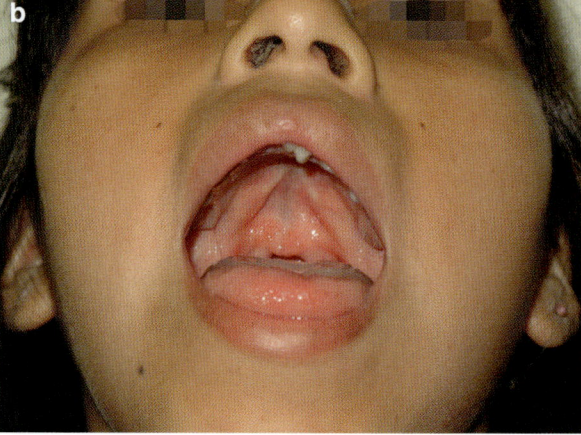

Fig. 12.5 (**a**) Patient with hypernasality and submucous cleft. (**b**) Anomalous insertion of palate muscles during the dynamic exam

A very detailed physical exam should then be carried out, observing the facial movements associated with speech, the movements of the nasal wings (external nasal valve), and the presence of dental occlusive changes (these mainly occur in cases of major jaw retrusion preventing an adequate lip seal, thereby permitting air passage, in which case the patient should also be evaluated for alveolar fistulas). A detailed assessment of the oral cavity should also be performed, including the hard and soft palates: look for the presence of fistulas and fibrosis; measure the anteroposterior diameter, transverse jaw, and palate length; observe the mobility of the soft palate and the symmetry of movement; identify the insertion of the muscles of the soft palate; check for tonsil and adenoid hypertrophy; and observe the movements of the side wall and posterior walls when present.

After this thorough evaluation, additional imaging studies are needed to measure the closing failures and more accurately demonstrate the changes that are preventing proper closure of the VPS. This will help aid therapeutic planning. Several complementary radiological examinations can be used, including simple static radiography, through radiography, cineradiography, xeroradiography, computed tomography, magnetic resonance imaging, and dynamic radiological images, such as videofluoroscopy.

Videofluoroscopy was considered a good method of imaging because it allows a dynamic analysis of the VPS. Although it has the disadvantage of subjecting patients to radiation, this allows both the study of the palate and posterior pharyngeal wall during speech and a complete anteroposterior exam, allowing visualization of the lateral walls of the pharynx.

Nasoendoscopy is an optical fiber endoscopic evaluation method that allows visualization of the nasal cavity, pharynx, and larynx with dynamic images. This technology is widely used for visualization of both the anatomical structures that comprise the VPS and its function, as it allows observation of the movement patterns of the soft palate and lateral and posterior pharyngeal walls during sphincter closing. It is an excellent dynamic assessment, and it is the most widely used diagnostic tool, in conjunction with clinical evaluation, to study velopharyngeal incompetence, assist in the choice of treatment, monitor after surgical procedures, and follow up long-term cases (Pegoraro-Krook et al. 2008).

12.4 Surgical Treatment

The surgical treatment is based on the clinical examination of the palate and the nasoendoscopy observation in our service.

Surgical treatment of VPI aims to improve the primary components of this framework: hypernasality and nasal escape. As the VPS mechanism is very complex, its treatment is similarly intricate. There are several different protocols of care for patients with cleft lip and palate in different reference centers. Each center has technical and clinical preferences, as well as a preference for the age at which this procedure must be performed.

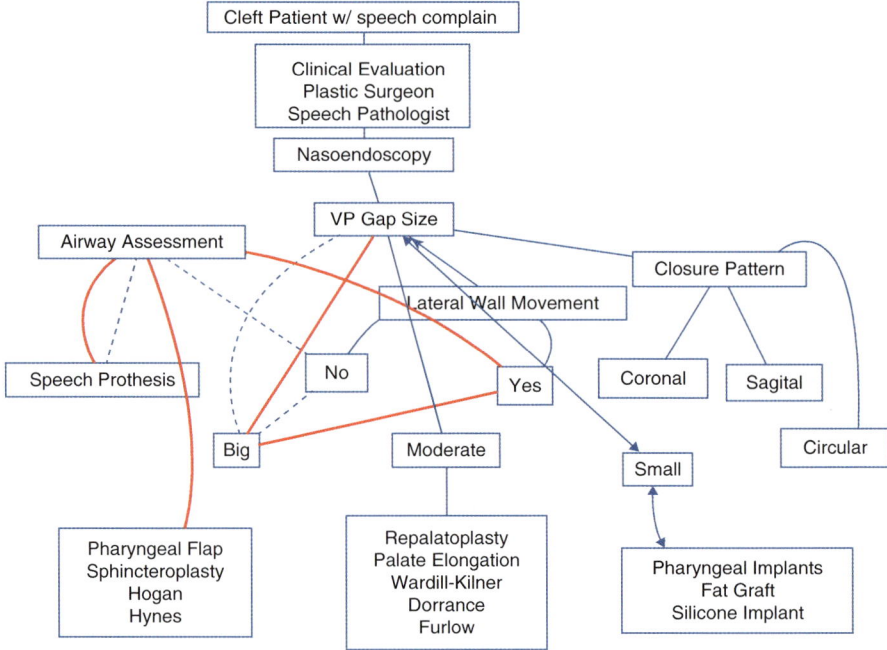

Fig. 12.6 Algorithm for VPI correction

In general, it is believed that the ideal age is about 5 years, at which time the child has developed enough speech for a proper assessment, but the patient is young enough that it is still easier to reverse compensatory articulation disorders through speech therapy than it is with adults. In the latter, the presence of these compensatory mechanisms limits a good prognosis for treatment, making rehabilitation more difficult and prolonged.

There are several techniques for the surgical treatment of VPI, which can be assembled into different groups. The choice of technique will depend on the individual assessment of each case, observing the patient's clinical status, the movement of the structures that form the VPS, and the gap size formed during speech between the soft palate and the posterior pharyngeal wall (Fig. 12.6).

12.5 Repositioning Back of Muscle Palate Lift (Repalatoplasty)

For many years, surgical correction in patients with cleft palate was limited to simple suture of the borders in the median plane without the addition of intravelar veloplasty, i.e. mobilization and posteriorization of the soft palate muscles, especially the levator veli palatini. Thus, even a palate of adequate length would not move properly to promote closure of the VPS.

For this reason, a detailed evaluation of the patient should be conducted, taking into account both the length of the palate and its mobility. This will include evaluation of the insertion of the muscles, as well as checking for the presence of a small closure failure that is correctable without the need for techniques to increase the rear wall length, as described later.

This procedure involves subjecting the patient to a "new" palatoplasty or repalatoplasty in which all structures—particularly the palate muscles, including the levator muscle of the soft palate—are dissected and identified. In this approach, an extended intravelar veloplasty is performed, posteriorly displacing the muscles that were attached to the hard palate border.

12.6 Small Gap in the Velopharyngeal Ring

12.6.1 Techniques of Palate Retropositioning (Push-Back)

Some palatal push-back techniques were described, such as the technique described by Veau-Wardill-Kilner and the Furlow technique (Furlow 1986; Victor 1931; Wardill 1937). They both attempt to promote a greater palate length through mobilization of the hard palate. Thus, these techniques are used in patients who have an inadequate palate length with normal mobility, and a moderate VPS closure failure.

Another technique that promotes this palate elongation is the technique described by Dorrance, in which a "U"-shaped incision is used. This incision extends from the retromolar area of one side to the other, following the alveolar arch, about 3 mm below the implantation of teeth. After the detachment of the hard palate mucosal flap in a subperiosteal plane, a release of the nasal mucosa in the horizontal direction at the junction of the hard and soft palate is achieved. This enables posteriorization of the palate and its muscles, after identification and isolation of the vascular pedicle formed around the greater palatine artery. As in the other techniques previously described, the recalcitrant wounds will heal by secondary intention, causing fibrosis. This fibrosis may subsequently promote growth restriction of the median third. The open area of the nasal plane can also suffer from scar contraction during healing, which may in turn be responsible for the loss of palatal elasticity (Dorrance 1972).

12.6.2 Posterior Wall Pharynx Lengthening (Augmentation)

These procedures are performed in cases where the palate has an acceptable length and mobility, but it is not able to promote the complete closure of the VPS, leading to a small, persistent gap. Thus, these techniques promote an anteroposterior increase in the posterior pharyngeal wall where it should meet the soft palate, leading to complete occlusion of the velopharyngeal ring. After criterious evaluation of the nasoendoscopy small gap could be solved by augmentation of the posterior

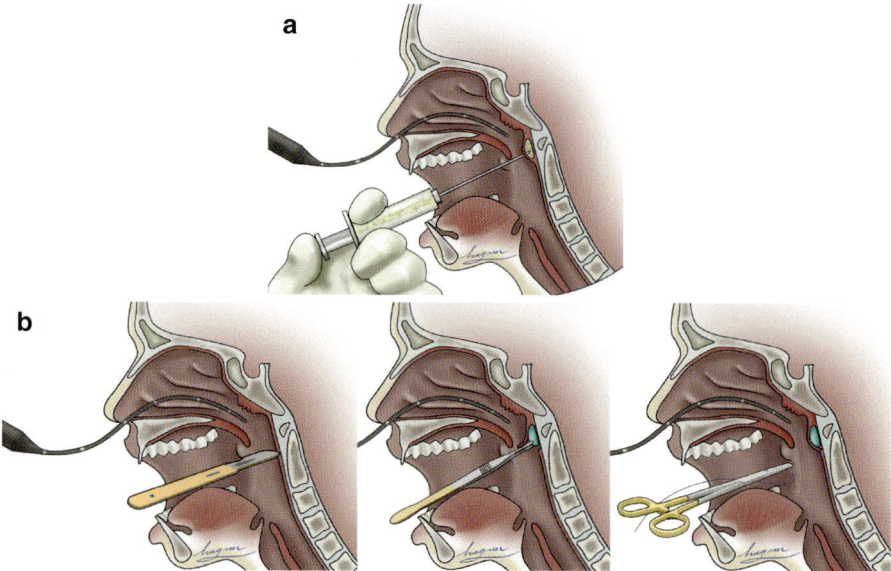

Fig. 12.7 (**a**, **b**) Posterior pharynx wall augmentation for small gap in the VPI. (**a**) Fat graft injection. (**b**) Alloplastic material for augmentation

wall of the pharynx, more recently with autologous fat graft injection and also with other solid materials like Silicone block and Teflon (Wolford et al. 1989; Cantarella et al. 2012) (Fig. 12.7a, b).

12.6.3 Moderate and Great Gap in the Velopharyngeal Ring

12.6.3.1 Sphincteroplasty

When we are faced with a big gap the functioning of the lateral wall plus the size of the gap are the parameters to study to decide the best correction for VPI.

Good movement of lateral walls is the best indication in big gap for pharyngeal flaps, lateral (sphincteroplasty) or medial (pharyngeal flap).

Pharyngoplasty, as first described by Hynes in 1950, is a technique that involves the use of two vertical myomucosal flaps (pharyngeal side and posterior wall mucosa and salpingopharyngeus muscle) superior pedicle sutured horizontally from each other by muscle transposition at 90°, providing a lift to the posterior pharyngeal wall. Hynes later modified his technique to include the salpingopharyngeal and palatopharyngeal muscles and part of the upper pharyngeal constrictor (Moss et al. 1987). Other changes were also described by Orticochea (1968), who suggested performing suturing of the flaps at a lower level than suggested by Hynes; this modification would provide a dynamic sphincter to close velar area. This technique is very well known actually as sphincteroplasty (Orticochea 1968).

Sphincteroplasty is when the ends of the myomucosal flaps are joined together after transposition, rather than suturing the entire flaps together. This maneuver creates a central opening between the flaps and the posterior pharyngeal wall and is supposed to be dynamic. Despite its name, this technique does not create a sphincter itself, but rather further lengthens the posterior pharyngeal wall (Orticochea 1968; Jackson 1983).

12.6.3.2 Pharyngeal Flaps

In patients with a short palate, no apparent mobility, a great VPS closing deficit, and preserved medial mobility of the lateral pharyngeal walls, the pharyngeal flap is a surgical treatment option. Pharyngeal flaps are myomucosal flaps (mucosa of the posterior pharyngeal wall and fibers of the superior constrictor muscle of the pharynx) with a superior or an inferior pedicle, which unites the posterior pharyngeal wall to the soft palate in the center of the velopharyngeal ring, keeping two side holes to allow the passage of the air column. To prevent nasal escape and hypernasality, medial movement of the lateral pharyngeal walls occludes these side holes.

It is extremely important to individually assess each case through nasoendoscopy to analyze the gap size and the side wall mobility to define the flap's display and width. It should be wider in cases where the mobilization is not so evident, and narrower with larger deficits in cases with good mobility.

In extremely huge gap in the VP ring our option could be to go for palatal prosthesis first, and then after a very intense speech therapy, another nasoendoscopy could decide the size of the pharyngeal flap. This option is also considered to adults over 30 years old with complains on night apnea.

Overall, both the upper and lower pedicle flaps are myomucosal. The width of the flaps, which is determined by the needs of each patient, is usually two-thirds of the total width of the posterior pharyngeal wall, and the size of the pharyngeal flap is based on the nasoendoscopic evaluation by the surgeon, dissected superficially to the prevertebral fascia. There is no place nowadays for inferiorly based pharyngeal flap because of the position it can reach, not so high, to close the velopharyngeal ring.

The soft palate is incised and dissected, and the palatal mucosa and muscles of the soft palate and nasal mucosa are identified. The latter is dissected to generate a flap that allows partial coverage of the raw surface of the pharyngeal flap. The pharyngeal flap is then sutured onto the palatal mucosa of the soft palate. For the most caudal position of the flap, the holes are placed in a region where the lateral wall does not move effectively. Placing the holes in this area can cause treatment failure, making the superior pedicle flap a more viable option.

The dissection of the superior pedicle flap is similar to the inferior pedicle, but differs in the marking of its limits. The base of the flap is demarcated from the first cervical vertebra position, and the flap is dissected to reach the uppermost anatomic level. Its length is also calculated with the intention that its end will reach the soft palate. The soft palate is opened the midline, and the nasal portion is incised towards the lateral pharyngeal wall. This creates a flap that will be able to completely cover the wound portion of the pharyngeal flap to prevent scar retractions that would otherwise lead to changes in the flap's size and width. The holes are marked using a 14 port tube introduced through the nostril so that they remain a standard size on both sides. The lateral pharyngeal wall is sutured to the flap edge, avoiding areas that could later cause stenosis of this hole. Sutures join the flap to the oral mucosa of the soft palate, covering the caudal portion with nasal mucosa and leaving the flap donor area to heal by secondary intention (Hogan 1973) (Figs. 12.8a, b and 12.9a–e).

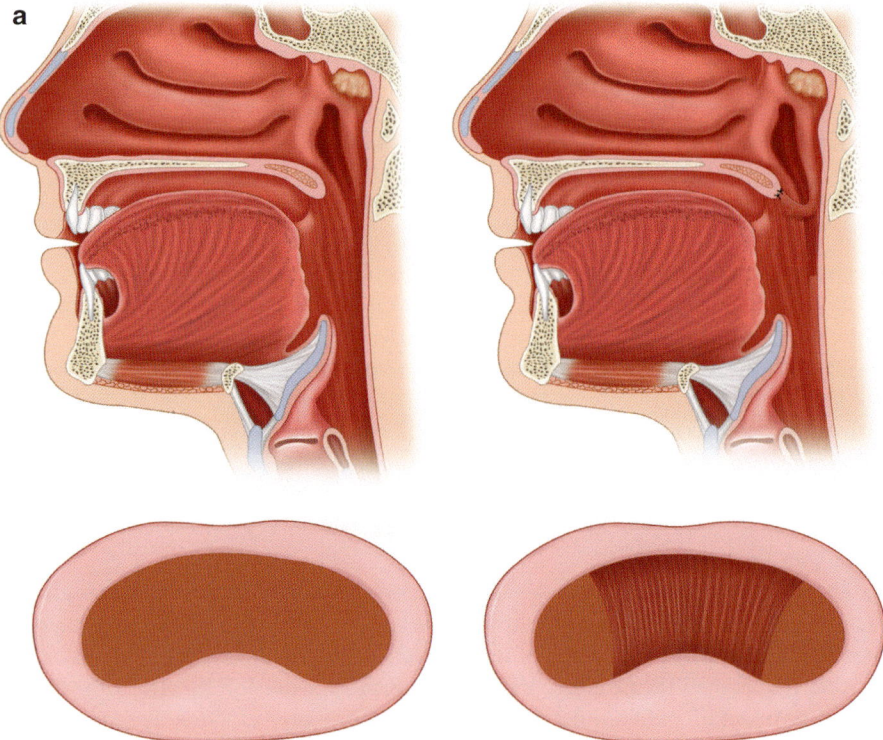

Fig. 12.8 (a, b) Pharyngeal flap for severe VPI Hogan's technique

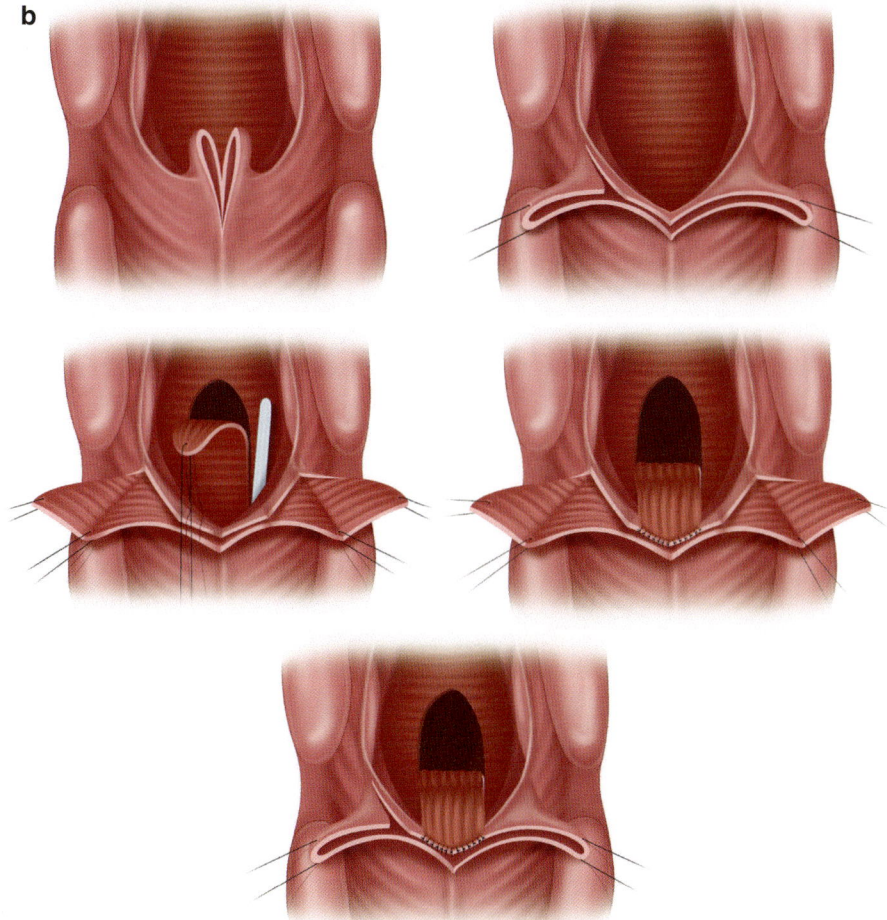

Fig. 12.8 (continued)

No significant differences were found on the evaluation of the final speech when comparison was made between sphincteroplasty and pharyngeal flaps for treatment of velopharyngeal insufficiency (Abyholm et al. 2005).

After surgery, patients may notice a change in breathing pattern, and several centers have studied the incidence of sleep-disordered breathing (SDB) after general pharyngoplasty or sphincteroplasty (Ettinger et al. 2012). SDB is due to obstruction of the velopharyngeal sphincter preventing the passage of the air column; even partial obstruction can lead to SDB. Research has shown that patients with cleft lip and palate have preexisting anatomical changes that

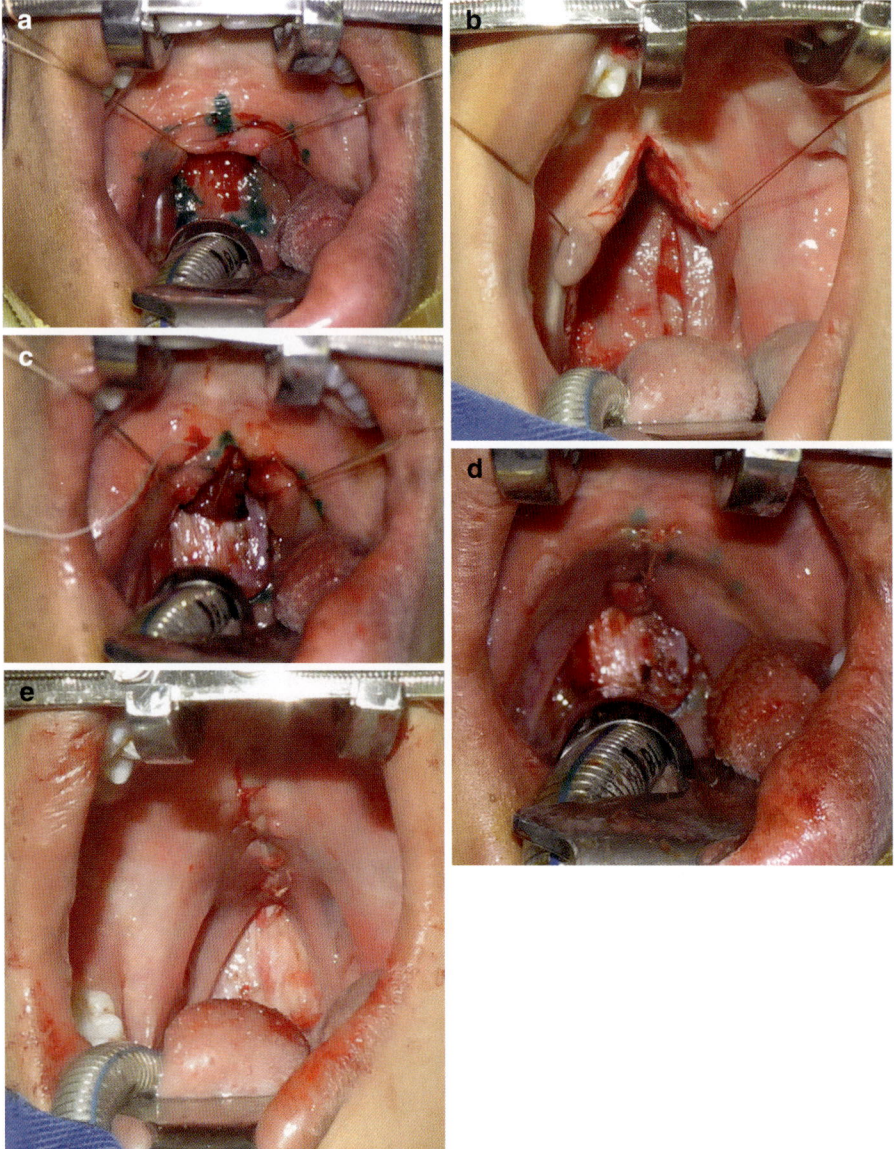

Fig. 12.9 (**a, b, c, d**)—Clinical case of Hogan's technique. (**a**) High position of the flap's base elevation of the soft palate. (**b**) Midline soft palate incision for exposition of the posterior pharynx wall. (**c**) Pharyngeal wall flap elevation. (**d**) Donor site left without suture. (**e**) Final aspect of pharyngeal flap superior pedicle

favor the presence of SDBs such as apnea or hypopnea and in some patients surgeries attempting to correct the VPI can exacerbate these disorders (Liao et al. 2002, 2004).

The planning of the position of the pharyngeal flap is very important on the evaluation of nasal airway obstruction and the speech final result. The flap must be positioned in the exact point of the closure of the VP ring (Lima Junior et al. 2012).

Recent study showed no differences between two different techniques for palate closure that means many other factors can influence the incidence of VPI (Ferreira et al. 2015).

The important statement about VPI is quality of life; good speech is referred as the most asked improvement for adult cleft patients (Raposo-Amaral et al. 2011).

References

Abyholm F, D'Antonio L, Davidson Ward SL, Kjoll L, Saeed M, Shaw W, et al. Pharyngeal flap and sphincterplasty for velopharyngeal insufficiency have equal outcome at 1 year postoperatively: results of a randomized trial. Cleft Palate Craniofac J. 2005;42(5):501–11.

Boorman JG, Sommerlad BC. Levator palati and palatal dimples- their anatomy, relationship and clinical significance. Br J Plast Surg. 1985;38:326–32.

Braithwaite F. The importance of the levator palati muscle in cleft palate closure. Br J Plast Surg. 1968;21:60–2.

Cantarella G, Mazzola RF, Mantovani M, Mazzola IC, Baracca G, Pignataro L. Fat injections for the treatment of velopharyngeal insufficiency. J Craniofac Surg. 2012;23(3):634–7.

Casey DM, Emrich LJ. Passavant ridge in patients with soft palatectomy. Cleft Palate Craniofac J. 1988;25(1):72–7.

Dorrance G. The Classic Reprint: Lengthening the soft palate in cleft palate operations. Plast Reconstr Surg. 1972;50(3):275–9.

Ettinger RE, Oppenheimer AJ, Lau D, Hassan F, Newman MH, Buchman SR, et al. Obstructive sleep apnea after dynamic sphincter pharyngoplasty. J Craniofac Surg. 2012;23(7 Suppl 1):1974–6.

Ferreira GZ, Dutka Jde C, Whitaker ME, Souza OM, Marino VC, Pegoraro-Krook MI. Nasoendoscopic findings after primary palatal surgery: can the Furlow technique result in a smaller velopharyngeal gap? Codas. 2015;27(4):365–71.

Furlow LT Jr. Cleft palate repair by double opposing Z-plasty. Plast Reconstr Surg. 1986;78(6):724–38.

Garcia M. Observations on the human voice. Proc R Soc Lond. 1854;7:399–410.

Hogan VM. A Clarification of the Surgical Goals in Cleft Palate Speech and the Introduction of the Lateral Port Control Pharyngeal Flap. Cleft Palate Craniofac J. 1973;10:331–45.

Jackson I. A Review of 236 Cleft Palate Patients Treated with Dynamic Muscle Sphincter. Plast Reconstr Surg. 1983;71:187–8.

Liao YF, Chuang ML, Chen PK, Chen NH, Yun C, Huang CS. Incidence and severity of obstructive sleep apnea following pharyngeal flap surgery in patients with cleft palate. Cleft Palate Craniofac J. 2002;39(3):312–6.

Liao YF, Noordhoff MS, Huang CS, Chen PK, Chen NH, Yun C, et al. Comparison of obstructive sleep apnea syndrome in children with cleft palate following Furlow palatoplasty or pharyngeal flap for velopharyngeal insufficiency. Cleft Palate Craniofac J. 2004;41(2):152–6.

Lima Junior JE, Tanikawa DY, Rocha DL, Alonso N. Pharyngoplasty applied to velopharyngeal insufficiency: efficacy versus morbidity. Plast Reconstr Surg. 2012;129(6):1015e–7e.

Moss ALH, Pigott RW, Albery EH. Hynes pharyngoplasty revisited. Plast Reconstr Surg. 1987;79(3):346–52.

Orticochea M. Construction of A Dynamic Muscle Sphincter in Cleft Palates. Plast Reconstr Surg. 1968;41(4):323–7.

Pamplona C, Ysunza A, Espinoza J. A comparative trial for two modalities of speech interventions for compensatory articulations for cleft palate children: phonalogic approach versus articulatory approach. Int J Pediatr Otorrinolaryngol. 1999;49:21–6.

Pamplona C, Ysunza A, Patino C, Ramirez E, Drucker M, Mazon JJ. Speech summer camp for treating articulation disorders in cleft palate patients. Int J Pediatr Otorhinolaryngol. 2005;69(3):351–9.

Pamplona MC, Ysunza A, Morales S. Strategies for treating compensatory articulation in patients with cleft palate. Int J Biomed Sci. 2014;10(1):43–51.

Pegoraro-Krook MI, Dutka-Souza JCR, Marino VCC. Nasoendoscopy of Velopharynx before and during diagnostic therapy. J Appl Oral Sci. 2008;16(3):181–8.

Raposo-Amaral CE, Kuczynsski E, Alonso N. Quality of life among children with cleft lips and palates: a critical review of measurements instruments. Revista Brasileira de Cirurgia Plastica. 2011;26(4):639–44.

Skolnick ML. Video velopharyngography in patients with nasal speech with emphasis on lateral pharyngeal motion in velopharyngeal closure. Radiology. 1969;93(4):774.

Skolnick ML, McCall GN. A radiographic technique for demontrating the causes of persistent nasality in patients with pharyngeal flaps. Br J Plast Surg. 1973;26(1):12–5.

Skolnick ML, McCall GN, Barnes M. The sphincteric mechanism of velopharyngeal closure. Cleft Palate J. 1973;10:286–305.

Victor V, editor. Division Palatine. Paris France: Masson; 1931.

Wardill W. Technique of Operation for Cleft Palate. Br J Surg. 1937;25:117.

Wolford LM, Oelschlaeger M, Deal R. Proplast as a Pharyngeal Wall Implant to Correct Velopharyngeal Insufficiency. Cleft Palate J. 1989;26(2):119–28.

Surgical Management of Velopharyngeal Insufficiency: The SOBRAPAR Hospital Algorithm

13

Rafael Denadai, Cassio Eduardo Raposo-Amaral, Anelise Sabbag, and Cesar Augusto Raposo-Amaral

13.1 Velopharyngeal Insufficiency

Velopharyngeal insufficiency (VPI) is defined as an incomplete closure of the velopharynx, a functional port composed of a complex group of structures that act together to control airflow through the nose and mouth by elevation of the soft palate and constriction of both the lateral and posterior pharyngeal walls (Kummer 2014; Hopper et al. 2014; Gart and Gosain 2014; Woo 2012; Fisher and Sommerlad 2011; Smith and Guyette 2004). VPI most commonly manifests as nasal resonance, improper audible nasal air emission, and a decrease in intra-oral air pressure during the production of oral speech sounds (Kummer 2014; Hopper et al. 2014; Gart and Gosain 2014; Woo 2012; Fisher and Sommerlad 2011; Smith and Guyette 2004). These patients will also frequently develop maladaptive articulations to compensate for their speech difficulties (Kummer 2014; Hopper et al. 2014; Gart and Gosain 2014; Woo 2012; Fisher and Sommerlad 2011; Smith and Guyette 2004).

The most common cause of VPI is patients with repaired cleft palate as the soft palate may be too short (or "insufficient") to permit adequate velopharyngeal closure. Palatal scar tissue and/or aberrant insertion of the *levator veli palatini* muscles can also decrease the mobility of the velum. Palatal fistulas can also lead to abnormal intraoral air escape (Kummer 2014; Hopper et al. 2014; Gart and Gosain 2014; Woo 2012; Fisher and Sommerlad 2011; Smith and Guyette 2004). It has been demonstrated that VPI after cleft palate repair can severely and significantly affect

---

R. Denadai, M.D. (✉) • A. Sabbag, S.L.P • C.A. Raposo-Amaral, M.D.
Institute of Plastic and Craniofacial Surgery, SOBRAPAR Hospital,
Campinas, São Paulo, Brazil
e-mail: denadai.rafael@hotmail.com

C.E. Raposo-Amaral, M.D., Ph.D.
Institute of Plastic and Craniofacial Surgery, SOBRAPAR Hospital,
Campinas, São Paulo 13084-880, Brazil

Universidade de São Paulo, São Paulo, Brazil

© Springer International Publishing AG 2018
N. Alonso, C.E. Raposo-Amaral (eds.), *Cleft Lip and Palate Treatment*,
https://doi.org/10.1007/978-3-319-63290-2_13

both the patient's and the family's quality of life (Barr et al. 2007; Boseley and Hartnick 2004; Skirko et al. 2015; Lee et al. 2017).

Surgery is the mainstay of treatment of VPI with the goal of creating a functional seal between the nasopharynx and the oropharynx during speech (Kummer 2014; Hopper et al. 2014; Gart and Gosain 2014; Woo 2012; Fisher and Sommerlad 2011; Smith and Guyette 2004). In this chapter, we present the experience of the SOBRAPAR Hospital in the implementation of a therapeutic algorithm for the surgical management of selected patients with repaired cleft palate and VPI.

13.2 The Multidisciplinary SOBRAPAR Hospital Team

The multidisciplinary SOBRAPAR Hospital team has the speech outcomes as the main therapeutic endpoint of the cleft palate management (further arguments on our rationale and concepts can be found in another chapter ["An overview of protocols and outcomes in cleft care"] of this book). In this comprehensive and standardized cleft palate care, social workers, psychologists, speech-language pathologists, otolaryngologists, and plastic surgeons have deployed essential roles.

Social workers automatically contacted all patients and families to avoid being lost to follow-up appointments as there are some cleft patients and parents with low socioeconomic and intellectual status and living far from our center and who can have difficulty to maintain longitudinal follow-up. We are a nationally referred hospital for the treatment of cleft lip and palate patients from all regions of Brazil, including rural and underprivileged areas, and most of them have demonstrating lack of adherence because of low levels of understanding and education compromising the strict pre- and postoperative follow-up. In addition, psychologists prepared and followed all patients for better compliance with prolonged follow-up. Psychologists also prepared cleft patients for nasopharyngoscopy as it may be an awkward and uncomfortable procedure and consequently younger patients may have difficulty with cooperating with the speech sample during the examination. A simulation of the procedure (e.g., environment, objects, professionals, and speech samples) in a repetitive and playful way has aided in this preparation. Parents have actively participated in the whole process, complementing the simulated training at home.

Speech-language pathologists and otolaryngologists have systematically performed otological and audiological investigations and then treated middle-ear problems and hearing loss (>25 dB [hearing loss in decibels]) according to individual needs. Intensive speech therapy has been initiated for all patients 1 month after cleft palate surgery to learn how to use the new anatomical situation properly and to address compensatory misarticulations. Parents have been trained to deliver speech therapy to cleft palate children as it was previously shown that this early therapy results in improved speech accuracy with fewer compensatory misarticulations (Scherer et al. 2008).

All repaired cleft palate patients have been screened for velopharyngeal insufficiency (associated or not with hearing loss and/or palatal fistula) by the speech-language pathologist team using specific recommendations (namely, thorough patient history, physical examination, perceptual speech evaluation, and instrumental anatomical assessment of velopharyngeal closure) (Fig. 13.1) (Alfwaress et al. 2015; Fitzsimons 2014; Henningsson et al. 2008). Obstructive sleep apnea has also been actively screened

HOSPITAL SOBRAPAR CRÂNIO E FACE

SOBRAPAR - Sociedade Brasileira de Pesquisa e Assistência para Reabilitação Craniofacial

Data ____/____/____

DVD Nº ________

AVALIAÇÃO DA FUNÇÃO VELOFARÍNGEA - NASOFIBROSCOPIA

Data e tipo da última cirurgia: ________

Objetivo deste exame: ________

Nome: ________ Prontuário: ________

DN: ____/____/____ Idade: ________ Tipo de Anomalia: ________

Posição do paciente durante o exame ________

Condição atual do palato: ( ) íntegro ( ) aberto ( ) operado ( ) com fístula ( ) submucosa
( ) outros ________

Permeabilidade das narinas ao espelho: D ( ) permeável ( ) parcialmente obstruída ( ) obstruída
E ( ) permeável ( ) parcialmente obstruída ( ) obstruída

Escape de ar nasal ao espelho de Glatzel:

Sopro:	( ) +	( ) -	( ) unilateral à__	( ) bilateral
Sonora nasal: /m/	( ) +	( ) -	( ) unilateral à__	( ) bilateral
Plosivos isolados: /p/ -/t/	( ) +	( ) -	( ) unilateral à__	( ) bilateral
Fricativos isolados: /f/-/v/-/s/	( ) +	( ) -	( ) unilateral à__	( ) bilateral
Velar: /k/-/g/	( ) +	( ) -	( ) unilateral à__	( ) bilateral
Vocábulos: /ka/ /ga/	( ) +	( ) -	( ) unilateral à__	( ) bilateral
Vocábulos: /fa/-/sa/-	( ) +	( ) -	( ) unilateral à__	( ) bilateral

RESSONÂNCIA (Julgamento Perceptivo Auditivo)

a) Avaliador I

( ) equilíbrio oronosal
( ) hipernasalidade: ( ) leve ( ) moderada ( ) severa
( ) hiponasalidade: ( ) leve ( ) moderada ( ) severa

b) Avaliador II

( ) equilíbrio oronasal
( ) hipernasalidade: ( ) leve ( ) moderada ( ) severa
( ) hiponasalidade: ( ) leve ( ) moderada ( ) severa

c) Avaliador III

( ) equilíbrio oronasal
( ) hipernasalidade: ( ) leve ( ) moderada ( ) severa
( ) hiponasalidade: ( ) leve ( ) moderada ( ) severa

Fibroscópio na narina: ( ) D ( ) E ( ) Não colaborou para o exame
No meato: ( ) médio ( ) inferior

SOBRAPAR - Sociedade Brasileira de Pesquisa e Assistência para Reabilitação Craniofacial
Av. Adopho Lutz, 100 - Cidade Universitária - CP 6028 - CEP 13083-880 - Campinas - SP - Brasil
Fone: 55 19 3749 9700 Fax: 55 19 3289 5380 sobrapar@sobrapar.org.br www.sobrapar.org.br 1

Fig. 13.1 Portuguese version of the SOBRAPAR Hospital protocol for flexible nasoendoscopic evaluation of velopharyngeal insufficiency. It was adapted from a previously published protocol (Di Ninno CQ, Guedes ZC, Sabbag A, Jesus MS. Avaliação da função velofaríngea—Nasofibroscopia. In: Jesus MS, Di Ninno CQ. Fissura labiopalatina: fundamentos para prática fonoaudiológica. São Paulo: Editora Roca, 2009. p. 242–3)

HOSPITAL SOBRAPAR
CRÂNIO E FACE
SOBRAPAR - Sociedade Brasileira de Pesquisa e Assistência para Reabilitação Craniofacial

AVALIAÇÃO DA FUNÇÃO VELOFARÍNGEA - NASOFIBROSCOPIA

Marcar com "+" escape e "-" fechamento

Paciente repete o próprio nome
Contar de 1 a 10

Sopro:	/s/	/a/:	/i/:
/p/:	papai:	Papai pediu pipoca.	
/t/:	tatu:	O tatu saiu da toca.	
/k/:	caqui:	O caqui caiu.	
/f/:	fifa:	A foto ficou feia.	
/s/:	saci:	O saci saiu cedo.	
/ch/:	xuxa:	Chico chupa xupeta.	
/m/:	mamãe:	Mamãe comeu mamão.	

Mobilidade de palato mole: ( ) ausente ( ) pobre ( ) moderada ( ) boa

Mobilidade de paredes laterais: ( ) ausente ( ) pobre ( ) moderada ( ) boa

Fechamento velo-adenoideano: ( ) ausente ( ) presente

Gap predominante: ( ) ausente ( ) puntiforme ( ) pequeno ( ) médio ( ) grande
( ) coronal ( ) sagital ( ) circular ( ) circular com Passavant
Medida _____

Piora da FVF com maior complexidade da fala: ( ) + ( ) -
Melhora da FVF com treino articulatório: ( ) + ( ) -

Articulação: ( ) normal ( ) fraca pressão I.O. ( ) subs. compensatória _____
( ) art. compensatória _____ ( ) distorção _____ ( ) golpe de glote
( ) distúrbio articulatório _____ ( ) mímica nasal ( ) fricativos faríngeos _____
( ) outros _____

Características da PPVV: _____

Achados ORL: _____

Observações: _____

Conclusão: classificar como insuficiente ou incompetente: _____

Conduta: _____

Exame realizado por: Dr. _____

Fonoaudiólogo: _____

SOBRAPAR - Sociedade Brasileira de Pesquisa e Assistência para Reabilitação Craniofacial
Av. Adopho Lutz, 100 - Cidade Universitária - CP 6028 - CEP 13083-880 - Campinas - SP - Brasil
Fone: 55 19 3749 9700 Fax: 55 19 3289 5380 sobrapar@sobrapar.org.br www.sobrapar.org.br

Fig. 13.1 (continued)

by taking a thorough preoperative and postoperative patient/family history according to previously validated screening tools (Chung et al. 2016; Fonseca et al. 2016; Johns 1991; Bertolazi et al. 2009). Patients determined to have velopharyngeal insufficiency (associated or not with hearing loss and/or palatal fistula) have been evaluated with nasopharyngoscopy performed by a trained plastic surgeon with the speech-language pathology team in attendance. Based on the described psychological approach, we have performed nasopharyngoscopy in patients as young as 3 years of age. The orientation (sagittal or horizontal) of the *levator veli palatini* musculature, the velopharyngeal closure patterns (coronal, sagittal, or circular, with or without the presence of a Passavant ridge), the velopharyngeal gap size (complete velopharyngeal closure, pinhole, small, moderate, or large) during maximal closure on phonation, and the presence of pulsations in the lateral pharyngeal walls have been characterized. All nasopharyngoscopy examinations have been prospectively recorded (composed of both video and audio data) for later review by the multidisciplinary team (it plays a critical role in the decision-making process for treatment) and for scientific purposes.

13.3 The SOBRAPAR HOSPITAL Algorithm

Our therapeutic rationale for VPI management was based on the surgical experience and outcomes accumulated over the past 38 years as detailed in the sequence. Acting as a national reference for the treatment of cleft patients (Raposo-Amaral and Raposo-Amaral 2012; Denadai et al. 2015a, b), we have received a broad spectrum of patients with VPI. Some cleft patients have previously been treated according to different surgical protocols, besides several cleft palate patients who have been treated at random, without any standardized protocol. Many cleft patients present with previously unsuccessful surgical management of VPI, primarily posterior pharyngeal free fat grafting, palatal muscle retropositioning, or double-opposing Z-palatoplasty. Another part of the cleft patients present with the repaired palate, but the palatal musculature remains oriented in a nonanatomical way. Patients with cleft palates with a large amount of scar tissue have also been routinely evaluated. Another relevant aspect is the experience accumulated with different surgical interventions. Although there are well-established outcomes with several surgical alternatives including the superiorly based pharyngeal flap and the sphincter pharyngoplasty (Yamaguchi et al. 2016; Ekin et al. 2017; Rogers et al. 2016; Seagle et al. 2016; Abdel-Aziz et al. 2011; Armour et al. 2005; Wermker et al. 2014; Sullivan et al. 2010; Lam et al. 2007; Setabutr et al. 2015; Samoy et al. 2015; Abyholm et al. 2005), our historical experience with the superiorly based pharyngeal flap has not been convincing as many patients presented postoperative obstructive sleep apnea in addition to unsatisfactory speech outcomes. We therefore abandoned this surgical approach as a modified protocol has been established. In addition, as our speech and complication data have been intermittently and critically assessed, we redirect our protocol accordingly.

The present algorithm was then more recently established with the ultimate purpose to include a greater number of repaired cleft palate patients with VPI who have been assisted in our institution and to balance efficacy (competent velopharyngeal closure) and complication. It is in accordance to the movement to tailor the VPI surgical management to the individual patient's needs (Yamaguchi et al. 2016; Abdel-Aziz et al. 2011; Armour et al. 2005). The SOBRAPAR Hospital algorithm (Fig. 13.2) for repaired cleft palate patients with VPI was based on the following criteria: previous unsuccessful surgical treatment of velopharyngeal insufficiency (i.e., posterior pharyngeal free fat grafting, palatal muscle retropositioning, or double-opposing Z-palatoplasty); amount of scarring at the junction between the hard palate and the soft palate by oroscopy; and *levator veli palatini* musculature

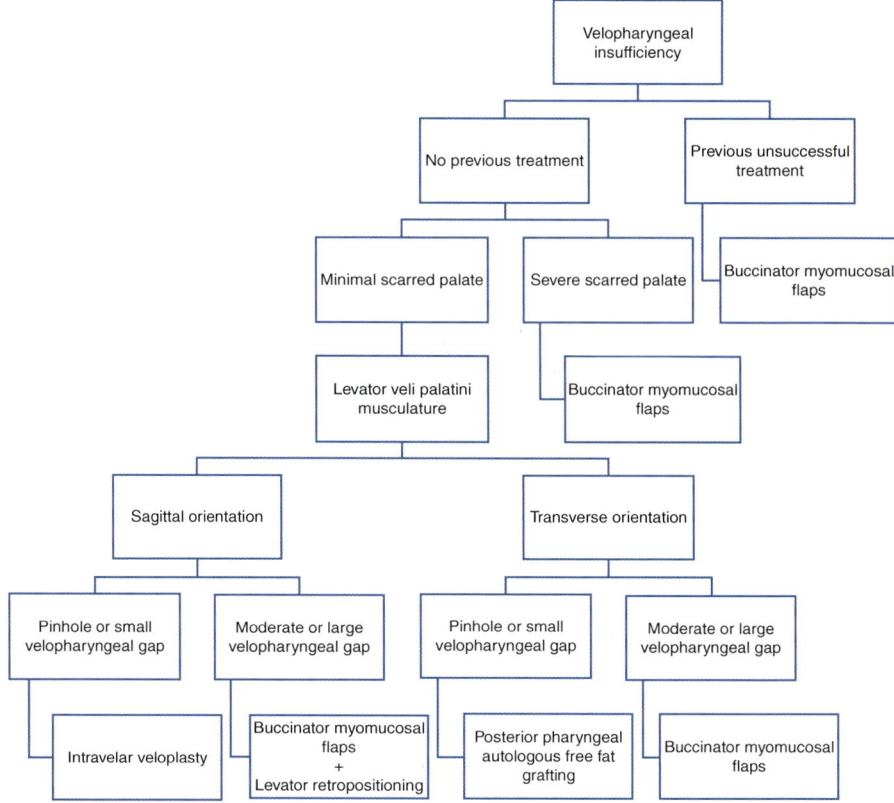

Fig. 13.2 The SOBRAPAR Hospital algorithm for repaired cleft palate patients with velopharyngeal insufficiency. Our rationale was based on the following criteria: previous unsuccessful surgical treatment of velopharyngeal insufficiency (i.e., posterior pharyngeal free fat grafting, palatal muscle retropositioning, or double-opposing Z-palatoplasty); amount of scarring at the junction between the hard palate and the soft palate by oroscopy; and *levator veli palatini* musculature orientation (sagittal or horizontal) and velopharyngeal gap size (pinhole, small, moderate, or large) during maximal closure on phonation by nasopharyngoscopic examination

orientation (sagittal or horizontal) and velopharyngeal gap size by nasopharyngoscopic examination.

In the cleft literature, there are different therapeutic algorithms for the treatment of VPI following cleft palate repair (Hopper et al. 2014; Gart and Gosain 2014; Woo 2012; Fisher and Sommerlad 2011; Yamaguchi et al. 2016; Seagle et al. 2016; Abdel-Aziz et al. 2011; Armour et al. 2005; Sullivan et al. 2010). However, the algorithms involve multiple procedures with inconsistent screenings, indications and/or outcomes, and lack of homogenous cohort, evidence, and/or large data support. In addition, no consensus exists regarding the best reported algorithm as none of the algorithms is completely ideal for treating the broad spectrum of VPI presentation both effectively and safely. A more simplified algorithm adopting double-opposing Z-palatoplasty and pharyngeal flap was recently published (Yamaguchi et al. 2016). Our algorithm is also simplified as it requires only a detailed evaluation for the establishment of patient status (thorough patient history, intraoral examination, and nasopharyngoscopy) and then one of only three surgical procedures (palate re-repair with intravelar veloplasty, posterior pharyngeal autologous free fat grafting, or bilateral buccinator myomucosal flap) is indicated. Age, severity of structurally correctable variables (i.e., hypernasality, nasal air emission, and intraoral pressure), velopharyngeal closure pattern, and/or videofluoroscopy have not been relevant or essential in patient stratification for inclusion in our algorithm. As palatal fistulas can lead to abnormal intraoral air escape, patients with palatal fistula and VPI have been treated according to other protocols (further details can be found in another chapter ["Buccinator Myomucosal Flaps in Cleft Palate Repair: The SOBRAPAR Hospital Experience"] of this book). In addition, patients with prior sphincter pharyngoplasty or pharyngeal flap were not considered in our surgical protocol as we believe that this subgroup of patients should be treated in a different way (Katzel et al. 2016). Palatal lift prosthesis is rarely recommended for patients who are poor surgical candidates (e.g., comorbidities) and/or for patients who opt to avoid surgery.

13.4 Surgical Techniques

Different surgical interventions (e.g., superiorly based pharyngeal flap, sphincter pharyngoplasty, double-opposing Z-palatoplasty, palatal muscle retropositioning, posterior pharyngeal wall argumentation, and buccinator myomucosal flap) have been adopted for treatment of VPI, each with their advocates, advantages, and disadvantages (Hopper et al. 2014; Gart and Gosain 2014; Woo 2012; Fisher and Sommerlad 2011; Yamaguchi et al. 2016; Ekin et al. 2017; Rogers et al. 2016; Seagle et al. 2016; Abdel-Aziz et al. 2011; Armour et al. 2005; Wermker et al. 2014; Sullivan et al. 2010; Lam et al. 2007; Setabutr et al. 2015; Samoy et al. 2015; Abyholm et al. 2005; Katzel et al. 2016; Collins et al. 2012; Park et al. 2016; Pet et al. 2015; Wójcicki and Wójcicka 2010; Deren et al. 2005; Perkins et al. 2005; Sie et al. 2005). Despite the increasing number of studies addressing VPI (Yamaguchi et al. 2016; Ekin et al. 2017; Rogers et al. 2016; Seagle et al. 2016; Abdel-Aziz et al. 2011; Armour et al. 2005; Wermker et al. 2014; Sullivan et al. 2010; Lam et al. 2007; Setabutr et al. 2015; Samoy et al. 2015; Abyholm et al. 2005; Katzel et al. 2016; Collins et al. 2012; Park et al. 2016; Pet et al. 2015; Wójcicki and Wójcicka 2010; Deren et al. 2005; Perkins et al. 2005; Sie et al. 2005), little evidence exists suggesting whether a procedure is superior to the other in each specific clinical scenario and there are no evidence-based guidelines for the choice of optimal surgical technique completely defined to date.

As described in the previous subheading, our therapeutic rationale was tailored to the patient's specific need and dependent on what is found in the preoperative assessment and was also based on the weighting between efficacy and morbidity. In summary, pharyngeal flap and sphincter pharyngoplasty have variable success rates and have been associated with obstructive sleep apnea (Collins et al. 2012), especially in our own experience. Double-opposing Z-palatoplasty is another alternative that presents excellent results (Park et al. 2016; Pet et al. 2015; Wójcicki and Wójcicka 2010; Deren et al. 2005; Perkins et al. 2005; Sie et al. 2005), but it is not completely applicable to our spectrum of patients mainly because aspects such as the number and/or types of cleft palate surgeries previously performed and/or the amount of palatal scarring are limiting factors. Alternatively, there is a growing

Table 13.1 Additional speech surgery for unsuccessful speech outcome with the three procedures (palate re-repair with intravelar veloplasty, posterior pharyngeal autologous free fat grafting, or bilateral buccinator myomucosal flap) adopted in the SOBRAPAR Hospital algorithm for repaired cleft palate patients with velopharyngeal insufficiency

Repaired cleft palate patients with VPI	Primary surgery for VPI (unsuccessful speech outcome)	Additional speech surgery
Minimal scarred palate, sagittal orientation of *levator veli palatini* musculature, and pinhole or small velopharyngeal gap	Palate re-repair with intravelar veloplasty	Posterior pharyngeal fat grafting[a] or bilateral buccinator myomucosal flap[b,c]
Minimal scarred palate, transverse orientation of *levator veli palatini* musculature, and pinhole or small velopharyngeal gap	Posterior pharyngeal fat grafting[a]	Posterior pharyngeal fat grafting[a] or bilateral buccinator myomucosal flap[c]
Several previous unsuccessful VPI treatments, severed scarred palate, and/or moderate or severe velopharyngeal gap	Bilateral buccinator myomucosal flap[b]	Posterior pharyngeal fat grafting[a]

VPI velopharyngeal insufficiency
[a]A second posterior pharyngeal fat grafting procedure can be performed as there is an extremely variable retention rate
[b]Bilateral buccinator myomucosal flap plus intravelar veloplasty, if there is sagittal orientation of *levator veli palatini* musculature
[c]The indication of posteriorly based pedicled buccinator myomucosal flap is limited in situations where there are doubts about the integrity of the buccinator muscle, buccal artery, or their branches and/or the availability of nonscarred myomucosal tissue (e.g., in patients with prior intraoral cheek scar secondary, for example, to bimaxillary orthognathic surgery)

body of literature describing satisfactory results with the techniques adopted in our algorithm, namely palate re-repair with intravelar veloplasty (Sommerlad et al. 2002, 1994; Mehendale et al. 2004; Raposo do Amaral et al. 2009), posterior pharyngeal autologous free fat grafting (Dinsever Eliküçük et al. 2017; Mazzola et al. 2015; Piotet et al. 2015; Bishop et al. 2014; Filip et al. 2013, 2011; Lau et al. 2013; Cantarella et al. 2012; Leboulanger et al. 2011), and buccinator myomucosal flap (Denadai et al. 2017a; Logjes et al. 2017; Dias et al. 2016; Lee and Alizadeh 2016; Ahl et al. 2016; Varghese et al. 2015; Abdaly et al. 2015; Hens et al. 2013; Mann et al. 2011; Robertson et al. 2008; Hill et al. 2004; Raposo-do-Amaral 2013). It is important to point out that the results are directly connected with the appropriate and careful selection of the patients. In addition, these surgical alternatives can be performed as a single VPI treatment (i.e., successful speech outcome), but when it fails (i.e., unsuccessful speech outcome), it is possible to make an exchange between the adopted techniques. For example, if there is unsuccessful speech outcome after the posterior pharyngeal fat grafting it is possible to perform a secondary posterior pharyngeal fat grafting or a bilateral buccinator myomucosal flap (Table 13.1).

13.4.1 Palate Re-repair with Intravelar Veloplasty

The concept of palatal re-repair has largely been advocated by Sommerlad et al. (2002, 1994), (Mehendale et al. 2004) for the secondary correction of VPI in cleft patients who demonstrated anterior insertion of the *levator veli palatini* muscles.

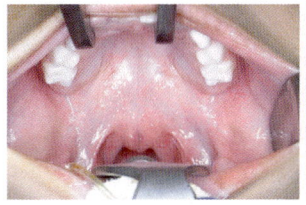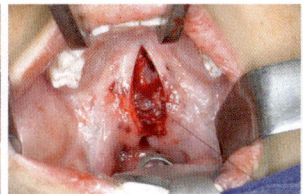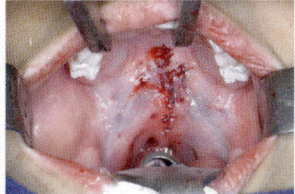

Fig. 13.3 (*Left*) Intraoral view of a repaired cleft palate with incomplete mobilization of the muscle. (*Center*) Intraoral view demonstrating velar muscles after radical dissection, mobilization, retropositioning, and suturing, with intact nasal layer. (*Right*) Intraoral view after oral layer closure (4-0 polyglactin 910)

We have performed a modified palatal re-repair with radical intravelar veloplasty according to principles described by Cutting et al. (1995) and Sommerland et al. (2002, 1994), (Mehendale et al. 2004) in a subgroup of repaired cleft palate patients with VPI, minimal scarred palate, sagittal orientation of *levator veli palatini* musculature (i.e., with no previous muscle repair or incomplete mobilization of the muscle), and pinhole or small velopharyngeal gap (Fig. 13.2; Table 13.1).

After palatal infiltration of local anesthesia (lidocaine 0.05% plus adrenaline 1:100.000), oral mucosal of the soft palate was initially divided at the midline and oral mucosal flaps were then raised. Velar muscles were carefully manipulated with sharp and delicate surgical tools. It involves a radical dissection, mobilization, retropositioning, and suturing (4-0 polyglactin 910 or 4-0 nylon with an atraumatic needle) of the velar muscles. The nasal mucosa was maintained intact and the oral mucosa was closed with vertical mattress stitches (4-0 polyglactin 910) (Fig. 13.3).

13.4.2 Posterior Pharyngeal Autologous Free Fat Grafting

Passavant (1879) described an unsuccessful surgical management of VPI by the posterior pharyngeal wall augmentation utilizing adjacent soft tissues in 1879. Since then, a myriad of autogenous and allogenous materials (e.g., cartilage, fat, fascia, acellular dermis, polytetrafluoroethylene, calcium hydroxyapatite, among others) have been adopted for the posterior pharyngeal wall augmentation (Lypka et al. 2010; Denny et al. 1993; Blocksma 1963; Lewy et al. 1965; Wolford et al. 1989). We have historically been in favor of autogenous tissue in all craniofacial and cleft reconstructions as the allogenous materials have potential problems like infection, exposure, migration, and extrusion. Autologous free fat grafting has been criticized because of a high variability in retention rate (Denadai et al. 2017b). However, the autologous free fat grafting can be repeated according to the individual needs (i.e., until the appropriate final volume is obtained). Therefore, repaired cleft palate patients with VPI, minimal scarred palate, transverse orientation of *levator veli palatini* musculature, and pinhole or small velopharyngeal gap have been managed with posterior pharyngeal autologous free fat grafting (Fig. 13.2; Table 13.1). A thoughtful history-taking, physical examination (including intraoral and pharyngeal examination), and nasopharyngoscopy were performed to exclude any signs of velocardiofacial syndrome and/or other cardiac anomalies in order to assess the possibility of medialized carotid arteries.

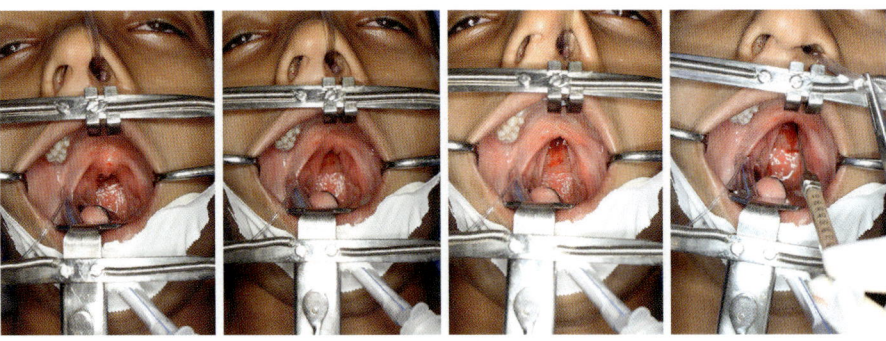

Fig. 13.4 (*Left* and *center*) Intraoperative view showing a catheter passed transnasally to retract the uvula and to expose the posterior pharyngeal wall prior to autologous free fat grafting. (*Right*) Intraoperative view of posterior pharyngeal fat grafting under direct visualization using a slightly curved-gauge one-holed cannula with blunt tip connected to a 1-mL syringe

The details of our fat harvest and preparation were previously reported (Denadai et al. 2017b, 2016; Raposo-Amaral et al. 2013) and it is in accordance with the Coleman technique (Coleman 2004). Under general anesthesia, through 3 mm incisions, 1 mL of a mixed solution (0.5% lidocaine with 1:200.000 of epinephrine in lactated Ringer's solution) per cubic centimeter of fat tissue to be harvested was distributed into the donor sites using a blunt multi-holed cannula. The abdominal region was the donor site for fat harvesting in all cases; in some thinner children, medial thigh was also used. Fat tissue was harvested with a 10-mL syringe attached to a 3-mm two-holed harvesting cannula with a blunt tip; gently pulling back on the plunger of syringe provided a light negative pressure while the cannula was advanced and retracted through the harvested site. The syringe was then centrifuged for 3 min at 3000 rpm to separate the viable from the nonviable components. The middle layer, predominantly fat tissue, was transferred to 1-mL syringes. A shoulder roll was then placed, as necessary, for neck extension. Posterior pharyngeal injection was done transorally with a Dingman mouth gag and a catheter passed transnasally to retract the uvula, exposing the posterior pharyngeal wall and adenoid pad (if present) (Fig. 13.4). Using a slightly curved 17–20-gauge one-holed cannula with blunt tip, fat was injected into the posterior pharyngeal wall in multiple passes (i.e., multipoint and multilayer fat placements according to velopharyngeal gap pattern) through the submucosal and submuscular planes, taking care to remain above the prevertebral fascia. The required volume and location (medially and/or laterally) were determined based on preoperative nasopharyngoscopy findings.

13.4.3 Bilateral Buccinator Myomucosal Flap

Since the first description of the buccinator myomucosal flaps for the VPI treatment by Hill et al. (2004), the cleft groups (Denadai et al. 2017a; Logjes et al.

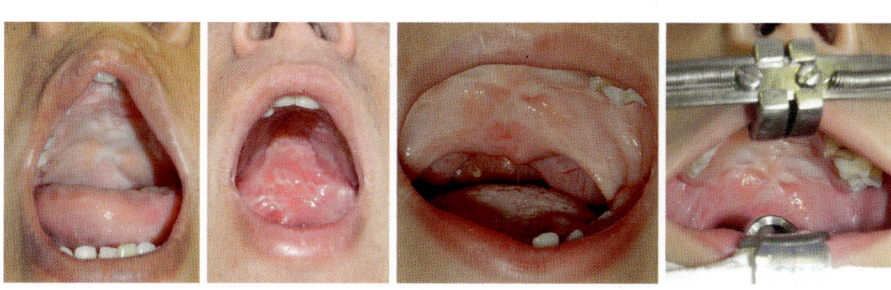

Fig. 13.5 Intraoral views illustrating the clinical examples of severely scarred palates

2017; Dias et al. 2016; Lee and Alizadeh 2016; Ahl et al. 2016; Varghese et al. 2015; Abdaly et al. 2015; Hens et al. 2013; Mann et al. 2011; Robertson et al. 2008; Hill et al. 2004; Raposo-do-Amaral 2013) have treated mixed samples (e.g., nonrepaired palatal fistula, mild-to-severe hypernasality, and/or small-to-large velopharyngeal gap sizes) with unilateral or bilateral buccinator myomucosal flap. We adopted the bilateral buccinator myomucosal flap in repaired cleft palate patients with VPI, several previous unsuccessful VPI treatments, severed scarred palate (Fig. 13.5), and/or moderate or severe velopharyngeal gap (Fig. 13.2; Table 13.1).

After palatal infiltration of local anesthesia (lidocaine 0.05% plus adrenaline 1:100.000), the junction of the hard and the soft palates was divided, resulting in a surgically created palatal defect which was reconstructed with the bilateral buccinator myomucosal flap. Simultaneous levator retropositioning was performed according to the described protocol. Posteriorly based pedicled buccinator myomucosal flaps were then planned in the midpart of the cheeks, below the opening of the Stensen's ducts; anteriorly, the flaps were designed with a "V" shape few millimeters behind the oral commissures; posteriorly, cranial flap marking is connected to the defect created at the soft palate in primary cleft palate repair or velopharyngeal insufficiency management. The flap width depends directly on the palatal defect created after completed dissection. Following incisions of flap margins, the flap was raised in an anteroposterior direction, including a full thickness of the buccinator muscle. It is important to avoid opening or disturbing the fascia over the buccal fat pad. The flaps were then inserted into the defect. Ideally, the palatal defects should be repaired with a two-layer, tension-free closure adopting bilateral flaps: the left-sided flap was sutured (4-0 polyglactin 910) into the nasal layer with the mucosa facing the nasal lumen, whereas the right-sided flap was sutured with the mucosal surface down into the oral layer. The donor sites were closed (4-0 polyglactin 910) directly, with the exception of the base of the flap (Figs. 13.6, 13.7 and 13.8). Three to six weeks after surgery, the pedicles were divided in the presence of difficulty mastication and/or limitation of mouth opening. Further details about the buccinator myomucosal flap can be found in another chapter ("Buccinator Myomucosal Flaps in Cleft Palate Repair: The SOBRAPAR Hospital Experience") of this book.

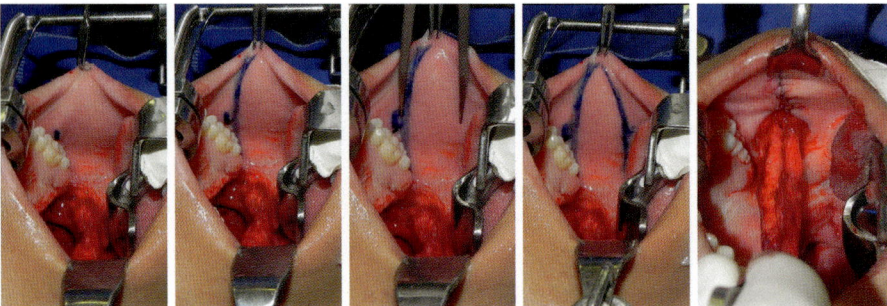

Fig. 13.6 Intraoperative views illustrating the left-sided buccinator myomucosal flap marking. The flap was planned in the midpart of the cheek, below the opening of the Stensen's ducts. Anteriorly, the flap was designed with a "V" shape few millimeters behind the oral commissure. Posteriorly, cranial flap marking is connected to the defect created at the soft palate. The flap width was defined according to the transposition of the measurement of the defect created between the soft and hard palates after completed dissection. The donor site was closed (4-0 polyglactin 910) directly, with the exception of the base of the flap

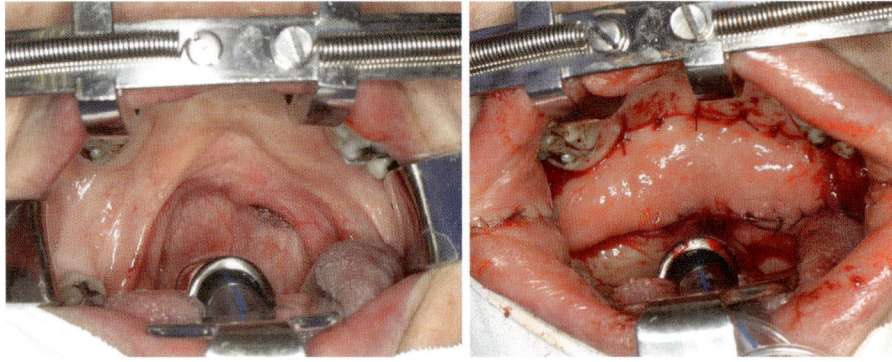

Fig. 13.7 (*Left*) Intraoperative view showing the short palate. (*Right*) Intraoperative view demonstrating the palatal lengthening by the bilateral buccinator myomucosal flap

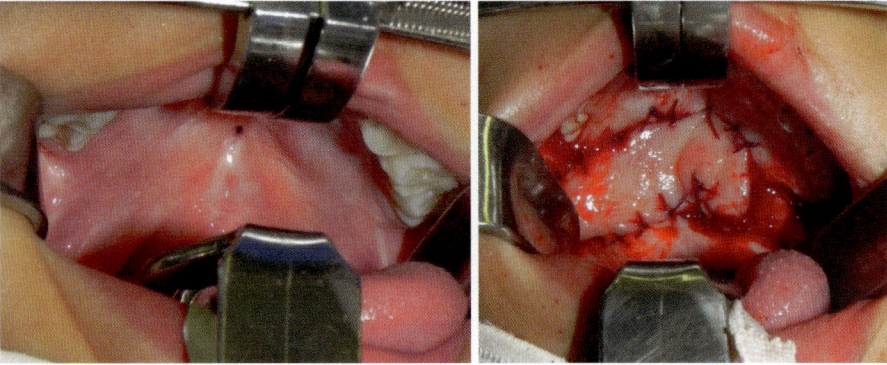

Fig. 13.8 (*Left*) Intraoperative view of a cleft patient with palatal fistula and velopharyngeal insufficiency surgically treated with (*right*) the bilateral buccinator myomucosal flap

13.5 Summary

The authors report the SOBRAPAR experience with the surgical management of velopharyngeal insufficiency in repaired cleft palate patients. The SOBRAPAR Hospital algorithm and the adopted surgical procedures (palate re-repair with intravelar veloplasty, posterior pharyngeal autologous free fat grafting, and bilateral buccinator myomucosal flap) were also included.

References

Abdaly H, Omranyfard M, Ardekany MR, Babaei K. Buccinator flap as a method for palatal fistula and VPI management. Adv Biomed Res. 2015;4:135.

Abdel-Aziz M, El-Hoshy H, Ghandour H. Treatment of velopharyngeal insufficiency after cleft palate repair depending on the velopharyngeal closure pattern. J Craniofac Surg. 2011;22:813–7.

Abyholm F, D'Antonio L, Davidson Ward SL, Kjøll L, Saeed M, Shaw W, Sloan G, Whitby D, Worhington H, Wyatt R, VPI Surgical Group. Pharyngeal flap and sphincterplasty for velopharyngeal insufficiency have equal outcome at 1 year postoperatively: results of a randomized trial. Cleft Palate Craniofac J. 2005;42(5):501–11.

Ahl R, Harding-Bell A, Wharton L, Jordan A, Hall P. The Buccinator mucomuscular flap: an in-depth analysis and evaluation of its role in the management of velopharyngeal dysfunction. Cleft Palate Craniofac J. 2016;53:e177–84.

Alfwaress FS, Khwaileh FA, Khamaiseh ZA. The speech language Pathologist's role in the Cleft lip and palate team. J Craniofac Surg. 2015;26:1439–42.

Armour A, Fischbach S, Klaiman P, Fisher DM. Does velopharyngeal closure pattern affect the success of pharyngeal flap pharyngoplasty? Plast Reconstr Surg. 2005;115:45–52.

Barr L, Thibeault SL, Muntz H, et al. Quality of life in children with velopharyngeal insufficiency. Arch Otolaryngol Head Neck Surg. 2007;133:224–9.

Bertolazi AN, Fagondes SC, Holff LS, Pedro VD, Menna Barreto SS, Johns MW. Portuguese-language version of the Epworth sleepiness scale. Validation for use in Brazil. J Bras Pneumol. 2009;35:877–83.

Bishop A, Hong P, Bezuhly M. Autologous fat grafting for the treatment of velopharyngeal insufficiency: state of the art. J Plast Reconstr Aesthet Surg. 2014;67:1–8.

Blocksma R. Correction of velopharyngeal insufficiency by Silastic pharyngeal implant. Plast Reconstr Surg. 1963;31:268–74.

Boseley ME, Hartnick CJ. Assessing the outcome of surgery to correct velopharyngeal insufficiency with the pediatric voice outcomes survey. Int J Pediatr Otorhinolaryngol. 2004;68:1429–33.

Cantarella G, Mazzola RF, Mantovani M, Mazzola IC, Baracca G, Pignataro L. Fat injections for the treatment of velopharyngeal insufficiency. J Craniofac Surg. 2012;23(3):634–7.

Chung F, Abdullah HR, Liao P. STOP-bang questionnaire: a practical approach to screen for obstructive sleep apnea. Chest. 2016;149:631–8.

Coleman SR. Structural fat grafting. St. Louis, Mo: Quality Medical; 2004. p. 30–175.

Collins J, Cheung K, Farrokhyar F, Strumas N. Pharyngeal flap versus sphincter pharyngoplasty for the treatment of velopharyngeal insufficiency: a meta-analysis. J Plast Reconstr Aesthet Surg. 2012;65:864–8.

Cutting C, Rosenbaum J, Rovati L. The technique of muscle repair in the cleft soft palate. Oper Tech Plast Reconstr Surg. 1995;2:215–22.

Denadai R, Samartine Junior H, Denadai R, Raposo-Amaral CE. The public recognizes plastic surgeons as leading experts in the treatment of congenital Cleft and craniofacial anomalies. J Craniofac Surg. 2015a;26:e684–9.

Denadai R, Muraro CA, Raposo-Amaral CE. Residents' perceptions of plastic surgeons as craniofacial surgery specialists. J Craniofac Surg. 2015b;26:2334–8.

Denadai R, Raposo-Amaral CA, Buzzo CL, Raposo-Amaral CE. Isolated Autologous free fat grafting for Management of Facial Contour Asymmetry in a subset of growing patients with craniofacial Microsomia. Ann Plast Surg. 2016;76:288–94.

Denadai R, Sabbag A, Raposo-Amaral CE, Filho JC, Nagae MH, Raposo-Amaral CA. Bilateral buccinator myomucosal flap outcomes in nonsyndromic patients with repaired cleft palate and velopharyngeal insufficiency. J Plast Reconstr Aesthet Surg. 2017;70:1598–1607.

Denadai R, Raposo-Amaral CA, Pinho AS, Lameiro TM, Buzzo CL, Raposo-Amaral CE. Predictors of Autologous free fat graft retention in the Management of Craniofacial Contour Deformities. Plast Reconstr Surg. 2017;140:50e–60e.

Denny AD, Marks SM, Oliff-Carneol S. Correction of velopharyngeal insufficiency by pharyngeal augmentation using autologous cartilage: a preliminary report. Cleft Palate Craniofac J. 1993;30:46–54.

Deren O, Ayhan M, Tuncel A, Görgü M, Altuntaş A, Kutlay R, Erdoğan B. The correction of velopharyngeal insufficiency by Furlow palatoplasty in patients older than 3 years undergoing Veau-Wardill-Kilner palatoplasty: a prospective clinical study. Plast Reconstr Surg. 2005;116:85–93.

Dias DK, Fernando PD, Dissanayake RD. Improvement of quality of speech in patients with velo-pharyngeal insufficiency corrected using a buccinator myomucosal flap. Ceylon Med J. 2016;61:130–4.

Dinsever Eliküçük Ç, Kulak Kayıkcı ME, Esen Aydınlı F, Çalış M, Özgür FF, Öztürk M, Günaydın RÖ. Investigation of the speech results of posterior pharyngeal wall augmentation with fat grafting for treatment of velopharyngeal insufficiency. J Craniomaxillofac Surg. 2017;45(6):891–6.

Ekin O, Calis M, Kulak Kayikci ME, Icen M, Gunaydin RO, Ozgur F. Modified superior-based pharyngeal flap is effective in treatment of Velopharyngeal insufficiency regardless of the preoperative closure pattern. J Craniofac Surg. 2017;28(2):413–7.

Filip C, Matzen M, Aagenæs I, Aukner R, Kjøll L, Høgevold HE, Abyholm F, Tønseth K. Speech and magnetic resonance imaging results following autologous fat transplantation to the velopharynx in patients withvelopharyngeal insufficiency. Cleft Palate Craniofac J. 2011;48(6):708–16.

Filip C, Matzen M, Aagenæs I, Aukner R, Kjøll L, Høgevold HE, Tønseth K. Autologous fat transplantation to the velopharynx for treating persistent velopharyngeal insufficiency of mild degree secondary to overt or submucous cleft palate. J Plast Reconstr Aesthet Surg. 2013;66(3):337–44.

Fisher DM, Sommerlad BC. Cleft lip, cleft palate, and velopharyngeal insufficiency. Plast Reconstr Surg. 2011;128:342e–60e.

Fitzsimons DA. International confederation for cleft lip and palate and related craniofacial anomalies task force report: speech assessment. Cleft Palate Craniofac J. 2014;51:e138–45.

Fonseca LB, Silveira EA, Lima NM, Rabahi MF. STOP-bang questionnaire: translation to Portuguese and cross-cultural adaptation for use in Brazil. J Bras Pneumol. 2016;42:266–72.

Gart MS, Gosain AK. Surgical management of velopharyngeal insufficiency. Clin Plast Surg. 2014;41:253–70.

Henningsson G, Kuehn DP, Sell D, Sweeney T, Trost-Cardamone JE, Whitehill TL, Speech Parameters Group. Universal parameters for reporting speech outcomes in individuals with cleft palate. Cleft Palate Craniofac J. 2008;45:1–17.

Hens G, Sell D, Pinkstone M, Birch MJ, Hay N, Sommerlad BC, Kangesu L. Palate lengthening by buccinator myomucosal flaps for velopharyngeal insufficiency. Cleft Palate Craniofac J. 2013;50:e84–91.

Hill C, Hayden C, Riaz M, Leonard AG. Buccinator sandwich pushback: a new technique for treatment of secondary velopharyngeal incompetence. Cleft Palate Craniofac J. 2004;41:230–7.

Hopper RA, Tse R, Smartt J, Swanson J, Kinter S. Cleft palate repair and velopharyngeal dysfunction. Plast Reconstr Surg. 2014;133:852e–64e.

Johns MW. A new method for measuring daytime sleepiness: the Epworth sleepiness scale. Sleep. 1991;14:540–5.

Katzel EB, Shakir S, Naran S, MacIsaac Z, Camison L, Greives M, Goldstein JA, Grunwaldt LJ, Ford MD, Losee JE. Speech outcomes after clinically indicated posterior pharyngeal flap takedown. Ann Plast Surg. 2016;77:420–4.

Kummer AW. Speech evaluation for patients with cleft palate. Clin Plast Surg. 2014;41:241–51.

Lam E, Hundert S, Wilkes GH. Lateral pharyngeal wall and velar movement and tailoring velopharyngeal surgery: determinants of velopharyngeal incompetence resolution in patients with cleft palate. Plast Reconstr Surg. 2007;120:495–505.

Lau D, Oppenheimer AJ, Buchman SR, Berger M, Kasten SJ. Posterior pharyngeal fat grafting for velopharyngeal insufficiency. Cleft Palate Craniofac J. 2013;50(1):51–8.

Leboulanger N, Blanchard M, Denoyelle F, Glynn F, Charrier JB, Roger G, Monteil JP, Garabedian EN. Autologous fat transfer in velopharyngeal insufficiency: indications and results of a 25 procedures series. Int J Pediatr Otorhinolaryngol. 2011;75(11):1404–7.

Lee JY, Alizadeh K. Spacer facial artery musculomucosal flap: simultaneous closure of oronasal fistulas and palatal lengthening. Plast Reconstr Surg. 2016;137:240–3.

Lee A, Gibbon FE, Spivey K. Children's attitudes toward peers with unintelligible speech associated with Cleft lip and/or palate. Cleft Palate Craniofac J. 2017;54(3):262–8.

Lewy R, Cole R, Wepman J. Teflon injection in the correction of velopharyngeal insufficiency. Ann Otol Rhinol Laryngol. 1965;74(3):874–9.

Logjes RJ, van den Aardweg MT, Blezer MM, van der Heul AM, Breugem CC. Velopharyngeal insufficiency treated with levator muscle repositioning and unilateral myomucosal buccinator flap. J Craniomaxillofac Surg. 2017;45:1–7.

Lypka M, Bidros R, Rizvi M, Gaon M, Rubenstein A, Fox D, Cronin E. Posterior pharyngeal augmentation in the treatment of velopharyngeal insufficiency: a 40-year experience. Ann Plast Surg. 2010;65(1):48–51.

Mann RJ, Neaman KC, Armstrong SD, Ebner B, Bajnrauh R, Naum S. The double-opposing buccal flap procedure for palatal lengthening. Plast Reconstr Surg. 2011;127:2413–8.

Mazzola RF, Cantarella G, Mazzola IC. Regenerative approach to Velopharyngeal incompetence with fat grafting. Clin Plast Surg. 2015;42(3):365–74.

Mehendale FV, Birch MJ, Birkett L, Sell D, Sommerlad BC. Surgical management of velopharyngeal incompetence in velocardiofacial syndrome. Cleft Palate Craniofac J. 2004;41:124–35.

Park SW, Oh TS, Koh KS. Repeat double-opposing Z-Plasty for the Management of Persistent Velopharyngeal Insufficiency. Ann Plast Surg. 2016;77:626–9.

Passavant G. Über die Verbesserung der Sprache nach der Uranoplastik. Deutch Geselschaft Chirurgie. 1879;23:771–80.

Perkins JA, Lewis CW, Gruss JS, Eblen LE, Sie KC. Furlow palatoplasty for management of velopharyngeal insufficiency: a prospective study of 148 consecutive patients. Plast Reconstr Surg. 2005;116:72–80. discussion 81–84

Pet MA, Marty-Grames L, Blount-Stahl M, Saltzman BS, Molter DW, Woo AS. The Furlow palatoplasty for velopharyngeal dysfunction: velopharyngeal changes, speech improvements, and where they intersect. Cleft Palate Craniofac J. 2015;52(1):12–22.

Piotet E, Beguin C, Broome M, Iglesias K, Olivier F, Leuchter I, Zbinden C, Hohlfeld J, de Buys RA, Schweizer V, Pasche P. Rhinopharyngeal autologous fat injection for treatment of velopharyngeal insufficiency in patients with cleft palate. Eur Arch Otorhinolaryngol. 2015;272(5):1277–85.

Raposo do Amaral CA, Sabbag A, Ferreira LA, Almeida AB, Buzzo CL, Raposo do Amaral CE. Dissecção radical da musculatura do véu palatino em casos secundários de pacientes fissurados. Rev Bras Cir Plást. 2009;24:432–6.

Raposo-Amaral CE, Raposo-Amaral CA. Changing face of cleft care: specialized centers in developing countries. J Craniofac Surg. 2012;23:206–9.

Raposo-Amaral CE, Denadai R, Camargo DN, Artioli TO, Gelmini Y, Buzzo CL, Raposo-Amaral CA. Parry-Romberg syndrome: severity of the deformity does not correlate with quality of life. Aesthet Plast Surg. 2013;37:792–801.

Raposo-do-Amaral CA. Bilateral buccinator myomucosal flap for the treatment of velopharyngeal insufficiency: preliminary results. Rev Bras Cir Plást. 2013;28:455–661.

Robertson AG, McKeown DJ, Bello-Rojas G, Chang YJ, Rogers A, Beal BJ, Blake M, Jackson IT. Use of buccal myomucosal flap in secondary cleft palate repair. Plast Reconstr Surg. 2008;122:910–7.

Rogers C, Konofaos P, Wallace RD. Superiorly based pharyngeal flap for the surgical treatment of Velopharyngeal insufficiency and speech outcomes. J Craniofac Surg. 2016;27(7):1746–9.

Samoy K, Hens G, Verdonck A, Schoenaers J, Dormaar T, Breuls M, Vander Poorten V. Surgery for velopharyngeal insufficiency: the outcomes of the university hospitals Leuven. Int J Pediatr Otorhinolaryngol. 2015;79:2213–20.

Scherer NJ, D'Antonio LL, McGahey H. Early intervention for speech impairment in children with cleft palate. Cleft Palate Craniofac J. 2008;45:18–31.

Seagle MB, Williams WN, Dixon-Wood V. Treatment of velopharyngeal insufficiency: fifteen-year experience at the University of Florida. Ann Plast Surg. 2016;76:285–7.

Setabutr D, Roth CT, Nolen DD, Cervenka B, Sykes JM, Senders CW, Tollefson TT. Revision rates and speech outcomes following pharyngeal flap surgery for velopharyngeal insufficiency. JAMA Facial Plast Surg. 2015;17:197–201.

Sie KC, Tampakopoulou DA, Sorom J, Gruss JS, Eblen LE. Results with Furlow palatoplasty in management of velopharyngeal insufficiency. Plast Reconstr Surg. 2005;108:17–25. discussion 26–29

Skirko JR, Weaver EM, Perkins JA, Kinter S, Eblen L, Martina J, Sie KC. Change in quality of life with velopharyngeal insufficiency surgery. Otolaryngol Head Neck Surg. 2015;153:857–64.

Smith B, Guyette TW. Evaluation of cleft palate speech. Clin Plast Surg. 2004;31:251–60.

Sommerlad BC, Henley M, Birch M, Harland K, Moiemen N, Boorman JG. Cleft palate re-repair—a clinical and radiographic study of 32 consecutive cases. Br J Plast Surg. 1994;47(6):406–10.

Sommerlad BC, Mehendale FV, Birch MJ, Sell D, Hattee C, Harland K. Palate re-repair revisited. Cleft Palate Craniofac J. 2002;39:295–307.

Sullivan SR, Marrinan EM, Mulliken JB. Pharyngeal flap outcomes in nonsyndromic children with repaired cleft palate and velopharyngeal insufficiency. Plast Reconstr Surg. 2010;125:290–8.

Varghese D, Datta S, Varghese A. Use of buccal myomucosal flap for palatal lengthening in cleft palate patient: experience of 20 cases. Contemp Clin Dent. 2015;6:S36–40.

Wermker K, Lünenbürger H, Joos U, Kleinheinz J, Jung S. Results of speech improvement following simultaneous push-back together with velopharyngeal flap surgery in cleft palate patients. J Craniomaxillofac Surg. 2014;42:525–30.

Wójcicki P, Wójcicka G. Prospective evaluation of the outcome of velopharyngeal insufficiency therapy after simultaneous double z-plasty and sphincter pharyngoplasty. Folia Phoniatr Logop. 2010;62(6):271–7.

Wolford LM, Oelschlaeger M, Deal R. Proplast as a pharyngeal wall implant to correct velopharyngeal insufficiency. Cleft Palate J. 1989;26(2):119–26. discussion 126-8

Woo AS. Velopharyngeal dysfunction. Semin Plast Surg. 2012 Nov;26(4):170–7.

Yamaguchi K, Lonic D, Lee CH, Wang SH, Yun C, Lo LJ. A treatment protocol for velopharyngeal insufficiency and the outcome. Plast Reconstr Surg. 2016;138:290e–9e.

Speech Therapy in Cleft Patients

14

Laura Davison Mangilli and Anelise Sabbag

14.1 Introduction—Speech and the Myofunctional Orofacial System

The objective of the speech therapist is prevention, guidance, rehabilitation, and reduction of complications resulting from changes in the myofunctional orofacial system (SMO) (ASHA 2001; Ibayashi et al. 2008; Namura et al. 2008; Castro-Sanchez et al. 2011). These changes include specific conditions or behaviors that could negatively impact the posture and appearance of organs belonging to this system and its functions—breathing, sucking, swallowing, chewing, and speech (Felício and Ferreira 2008; Felício et al. 2010).

Speech therapy for the patient with a cleft lip and palate involves activities far beyond the correction of compensatory articulation changes, common to this population during childhood and adulthood, since the cleft lip and/or palate can compromise different functions such as suction, chewing, swallowing, breathing, hearing, and speech (Johns et al. 2003; Nahai et al. 2005; Hortis-Dzierzbicka et al. 2012; Schuster et al. 2012).

L.D. Mangilli, Ph.D. (✉)
Faculdade de Ceilândia, University of Brasilia, Brasilia, Brazil
e-mail: lauramangilli@usp.br

A. Sabbag, S.L.P.
Institute of Plastic and Craniofacial Surgery, SOBRAPAR Hospital, Campinas, São Paulo, Brazil

14.1.1 Cleft Lip and/or Palate and Its Relations to the Myofunctional Orofacial Functions

14.1.1.1 Sucking, Swallowing, and Breathing

Anatomophysiologic Functions
Suction plays a key role in supplying the nutritional needs during the first months of a baby's life, who has no anatomical development, and sensory and motor swallowing, another natural way of obtaining food (Felício 2009).

After suction, swallowing occurs (Douglas 2002). The swallowing reflex is triggered by fluid accumulation in the oral cavity, and begins to show maturity at around 4 months of life (Felício 2009). The establishment of respiratory function depends on the diameter of the nostrils, nasal cavity, and pharynx, so the passage of air to the lungs is possible. To maintain this diameter, satisfactory anatomy is necessary with proper functionality of all elements involved, as well as the supporting muscles of the head (base of skull, jaw, and tongue) (Altmann 2000; Douglas 2002; Bertier and Trindade 2007).

Functions and Types of Clefts
Malformations in the oral cavity can cause problems with sucking and swallowing. The type and size of cleft are generally related to the degree of difficulty experienced by the child. Isolated unilateral involvement of the lip can lead to some difficulty, while a bilateral lip and cleft palate lead to much more difficulty in carrying out effective sucking (Miller and Kummer 2004).

In the case of an isolated cleft palate, there is adequate grip of the breast, but there is difficulty in generating negative intraoral pressure due to the communication between the oral and nasal cavities through the cleft. The combined cleft lip and palate is considered the most harmful interference to suction, since it leads to difficulties in grasping the nipple/areola as well as difficulty in generating intraoral pressure. However, in clinical practice we see that there are no immutable rules for successful breastfeeding. Breathing is a vital function whether it is nasal or oral (Douglas 2002; Felício 2009). Due to facial anatomic changes, a large number of individuals with a cleft lip and palate present with oral breathing, associated with poor growth of the midface and poor jaw development. This leads to a compensated position of the tongue and lips.

The speech therapists should be in harmony with the other teams due to anatomic conditions and the schedule of surgical treatment.

14.1.1.2 Chew

Anatomophysiology of the Function
Chewing is the initial stage of the digestive process, which begins in the mouth. Muscle of the tongue and face, especially the buccinator and the orbicularis oris, plays a key role in chewing process.

The intensity of the masticatory force, number of chewing strokes, distribution of food by mouth, and occlusal and dental status may influence the chewing function (Douglas 2002).

Function and Types of Clefts

Primary and secondary surgical correction of cleft lip and/or palate can lead to jaw growth deficiencies, with subsequent impairment of the bone (Capelozza Filho et al. 1996). The presence of an anterior crossbite, absence of teeth in the alveolar region of the cleft, or premaxilla projection in bilateral clefts can interfere with chewing.

14.1.1.3 Speech

Anatomophysiology

To accomplish a normal speech, aspects such as organization and planning of the motor act are fundamental and are related to hearing and neuromuscular integrity, as well as coordinated action between the respiratory muscles and vocal cords along with lips, tongue, jaw, and soft palate. Minor changes in one of these actions could compromise the oral communication (Genaro et al. 2007, 2009; Prandini et al. 2011).

It can make a description of speech sounds by phonetic, which encompasses both the articulation and acoustic aspects. The Brazilian-Portuguese has 7 oral vowels, 5 nasal vowels, consonant 19 headphones, and 2 glides (Pinho 2009). The distinction between oral and nasal vowels is related to the action of velopharynx (Pinho 2009; Prandini et al. 2011).

Function and Types of Clefts

In cases of cleft lip and palate, alterations of velopharyngeal function, as well as the palate anatomy (oronasal fistula, dental-altered occlusion), can directly or indirectly lead to symptoms that impair speech intelligibility, such as hypernasality, nasal air emission, weak intraoral pressure, and compensatory articulations. These symptoms may be developed by the individual to compensate for the inability to create pressure in the oral cavity (Smith and Kuehn 2007; Kummer 2004a; Prandini et al. 2011; Hortis-Dzierzbicka et al. 2012; Schuster et al. 2012).

Hypernasality, the most characteristic symptom of velopharyngeal insufficiency (VPI), corresponds to excessive nasal resonance during the production of oral speech sounds (Kummer 2004a, c; Schuster et al. 2012). The nasal air emission is present when there is air outflow through the nasal cavity during speech production. This emission may or may not be audible, the former being much more damaging to speech intelligibility (Kummer 2004a, c; Genaro et al. 2009; Peterson-Falzone et al. 2006; Schuster et al. 2012).

The weak intraoral air pressure during the production of oral speech sounds reduces sound discrimination traits and damages the speech intelligibility (Warren et al. 1981, 1984; Schuster et al. 2012). The patient may develop CAD in response to inadequate intraoral air pressure. These are considered as indirect effects of VPI, since they are derived from articulatory compensations to low intraoral air pressure (Kummer 2004a; Peterson-Falzone et al. 2006; Schuster et al. 2012).

There are other changes in speech that can be considered secondary to the presence of lip and/or cleft palate. These are the changes in the articulation point, due to secondary anatomic and occlusal problems, which can lead to omissions and distortions in sound production (Altmann 2000).

14.2 Speech Therapy—Cleft Lip and Palate Clinic

14.2.1 Guidance in Cases of Intrauterine Diagnosis

With the use of ultrasound in routine obstetric diagnosis, prenatal diagnosis of facial anomalies is more common (Bunduki et al. 2001). The nose and the lip are possible to be identified on ultrasound from the 15th week of gestation, and the palate between the 28th and 33rd weeks. With the availability of this technology, there is an increased demand for clarification and guidance on the craniofacial and functional changes related to cleft lip and palate, as well as treatment options.

When changes suggestive of cleft lip and palate are identified during the prenatal care of a pregnant woman, she should be referred to multidisciplinary specialized services. The speech therapist can advise on the possible implications of cleft lip and palate on the feeding and speech of her baby as well as the possibilities for speech therapy interventions and treatments throughout the child's life.

14.2.2 Orientation and Guidance for Parents (Sabbag, 2009)

Initial interview:

- Collect patient information regarding the general conditions of pregnancy and childbirth, family history, history of global development, eating habits, oral habits, and speech and language development.
- Guidance on infant feeding process (positioning and care for the prevention of common respiratory and ear infections), in addition to other factors contributing to the maintenance of the mother-child bond.

14.2.3 Evaluation

14.2.3.1 Evaluation for Neonates with Craniofacial Anomalies
- Classification of the cleft.
- Evaluation of myofunctional conditions of breathing, sucking, and swallowing.
- Adaptation to feed the child with special bottles, cups, and spoons to be used in the pre- and/or postsurgical lip repair and palatoplasty.
- Hearing exams as screening and early diagnosis of hearing loss, in order to detect and treat these changes that can negatively influence the acquisition of speech and language.

14.2.3.2 Evaluation and Treatment of Patients After 7 Months of Age
Stimulation, attention, and concentration in activities that promote development of oral motor system, ability of language stimulation, and stimulation of phoneme production compatible with the affected anatomical structure of the orofacial complex.

- Periodic audiologic tests in order to monitor the hearing thresholds and tympanometry in order to monitor the middle-ear function.
- Myofunctional therapy, articulation training programs, techniques for airflow direction.
- Periodic assessment of the speech with the team.

Children with cleft lip and palate are at risk for delays in language development and speech acquisition, since factors such as hearing loss or unfavorable domestic environment may lead to changes in language development (Kummer 2004a, b, c).

Periodic clinical assessment of communication skills is essential for early diagnosis of possible changes. The use of standardized protocols for language evaluation will allow the analysis and monitoring of cognitive development, communication skills, and global understanding of the child ability.

14.2.4 Language/Speech

14.2.4.1 Orientation Stimulation

An environment that promotes stimulating experiences is important in language development. According to Kummer (2004c), during the first 5 years of life, the child has the highest neuronal ability to develop language. For children with a cleft lip and palate it is no different. Parents and caregivers should be instructed to promote conditions that are conducive to language development, even prior to the first surgical procedures to correct the lip and palate.

Occlusion of the nostrils is a temporary strategy, while closing the fissure or the VPD has not yet occurred (Pegoraro-Krook et al. 2009). The palatoplasty should be performed between around 12 months of age—the age at which the child begins the production of his or her first words. Therefore it is essential that the velopharyngeal mechanism structures are in good working order, in an attempt to prevent the development of compensatory articulation, which, if already learned, will be eliminated through speech therapy.

14.2.5 Evaluation of the Speech

To understand what occurs during the production of sounds, it is necessary to evaluate the anatomical structures that participate in this function. Thus, an orofacial myofunctional evaluation should be performed, taking into account the following aspects (Capelozza Filho et al. 1996; Smith and Kuehn 2007; Genaro et al. 2007, 2009; Felício and Ferreira 2008; Silva et al. 2008; Felício et al. 2010).

- Lips—Teeth—Tongue—Soft and Hard Palate—Pharyngeal Walls

The perceptual evaluation of speech is considered the main indicator of the burden of the symptoms resulting from velopharyngeal dysfunction (VPD); thus it is an essential part of the clinical diagnosis (Genaro et al. 2007, 2009; Lee et al. 2009;

Prandini et al. 2011). This evaluation identifies changes, measures intensity, and evaluates the effectiveness of the treatments performed, although subjectively (Dotevall et al. 2002; Smith and Kuehn 2007; Prandini et al. 2011; Schuster et al. 2012).

The speech sample that is used should contain counting numbers, and directed speech, repetition, or reading words and simple sentences containing different phonemes in the initial and medial position of the word (e.g., Dad asked popcorn [in Portuguese "papai pediu pipoca"], the Saci left early [in Portuguese o Saci saiu cedo]). During all sounds that can be stored in the media file for later comparison and control, there should be the articulation of each phoneme, to identify the presence of articulatory errors, distortions, or phonological simplifications. It should also analyze the presence of audible nasal air emission, nasal snoring, poor intraoral pressure, and facial movements that may indicate in velopharyngeal closure. In addition, the speech pathologist should evaluate the spontaneous speech and moment of less articulatory control to identify and characterize the speech.

According to Shprintzen (1995), perceptual evaluation is the main determinant of the change in nasality, and the findings are essential in planning the treatment strategy. Hypernasality is the most common type of change of resonance in patients with a cleft lip and palate, especially those with VPD. However, it is often accompanied by the occurrence of hyponasality (insufficient involvement of the nasal cavity during production of nasal phonemes, as [m] and [n]) or even hyponasality associated with hypernasality caused by nasal obstruction (Genaro et al. 2009).

Over the years, the literature (Barbosa 2011; Schuster et al. 2012) reports concerns about improving the perceptual evaluation in order to make it less susceptible to subjective errors. Thus, we suggest the adoption of scores or criteria to represent the judgment of the speech pathologist. The scale absent—mild—moderate and severe for the classification of hypernasality, hyponasality, and speech intelligibility has been used by our groups.

To complement the perceptual evaluation of speech, more proper resonance, additional tests may also be used (Altmann 2000; Trindade et al. 2005; Peterson-Falzone et al. 2006; Genaro et al. 2007, 2009):

The judgment of speech intelligibility is the analysis of speech as a whole, or whether or not the listener can understand the message content of the patient.

14.2.5.1 Instrumental Assessment of Velopharyngeal Function

As recommended by the American Cleft Palate Association—ACPA (2009), the assessment of surgical outcomes for correcting VPI must involve at least one of the following instrumental methods: nasopharyngeal endoscopy, videofluoroscopy, nasometry, or pressure-flow techniques.

We use the nasopharyngeal endoscopy to diagnose VPI and to evaluate the surgical outcome. All tests are performed by a plastic surgeon with experience in clef palate, who evaluates the anatomical aspects, and a speech pathologist, who evaluates the functional aspects of the velopharyngeal mechanism. This is then correlated with the findings of the clinical evaluation of speech and velopharyngeal function.

Because it is a more invasive method, the examination takes place after the age of 3 and 6 months.

The examination is saved electronically for further evaluation, comparison, and control results after anatomical evaluation by a physician.

14.2.5.2 Treatment

One of the main goals of speech therapy in this age group is to direct the airflow through the oral cavity and adjust the mode of articulation, enabling the correct production of oral phonemes (Altmann 2000; Peterson-Falzone et al. 2006; Pegoraro-Krook et al. 2009). The therapy should preferably be initiated after the completion of surgery to ensure adequate velopharyngeal closure. However, it can also (and in some cases must) be performed before the surgery to better evaluate the potential velopharyngeal closure pattern from the correct articulation of oral speech phonemes (Golding-Kushner 2001). In all cases, it is essential that the goal of therapy is very clear and well defined.

In speech therapy for hypernasality, weak intraoral pressure, and nasal snoring, the effectiveness of reparative surgery for velopharyngeal insufficiency must be assessed with clinical and instrumental evaluations. Speech therapy for adequate velopharyngeal closure occurs from the recruitment of the velopharyngeal muscles during oral speech production (Golding-Kushner 2001; Peterson-Falzone et al. 2006; Pegoraro-Krook et al. 2009). The therapist should use strategies that stimulate the perception of intraoral pressure during production of oral phonemes, in the same order as described for the correction of articulatory disorders of isolated phonemes, syllables, words, phrase, and automatic and spontaneous speech.

14.2.6 Socialization

Speech is the primary means of interpersonal communication in our society. We express our feelings and thoughts in a harmonious manner with speech, vocal characteristics, and facial and body expressions (Pinho 2009).

A cleft lip and palate lead to two common stigmas: aesthetics and speech. A face with scars and asymmetries can bring the patient a high degree of dissatisfaction, and speech marked by excessive nasality and the articulatory disorders can lead to excessive shyness and isolation from the environment that they live in (Minervino-Pereira 2005; Sharma et al. 2012).

Additionally, the child who is already acquiring oral language, excessive shyness, or insecurity in relating with others can have a loss of intelligibility much more significantly than excessive nasality (Golding-Kushner 2001; Peterson-Falzone et al. 2006).

Thus, psychosocial care is essential for effective rehabilitation. The interdisciplinary team must be attentive to all stages of development, from birth to adulthood, so together with the family we can successfully reach complete rehabilitation (Graciano et al. 2007).

References

Altmann EBC. Fissuras labiopalatinas. 4th ed. Carapicuíba: Pró-Fono; 2000.
American Cleft Palate-Craniofacial Association. Parameters for evaluation and treatment of patients with cleft lip/palate or other craniofacial anomalies – revised edition [homepage on the Internet]. Chapel Hill: American Cleft Palate-Craniofacial Association. 2009. Disponível em: http://www.acpa-cpf.org/uploads/site/Parameters_Rev_2009.pdf. Accessed 5 Jan 2013.
American Speech-Language-Hearing Association. Roles of speech and language pathologists in swallowing and feeding disorders: technical report. ASHA. 2001. http://www.asha.org/NR/rdonlyres/B8DE1480-C7B4-4383-A1F6-5829E9CB0CF5/0/v3TRRolesSLPSwallowingFeeding.pdf.
Barbosa DA. Resultados de fala e de função velofaríngea do retalho faríngeo e da veloplastia intravelar na correção da insuficiência velofaríngea: estudo comparativo. Dissertação [mestrado]. Bauru; 2011. p 129.
Bertier CE, Trindade IEK. Deformidades nasais: avaliação e tratamento cirúrgico. In: Trindade IEK, Silva Filho OG, editors. Fissuras labiopalatinas: uma abordagem interdisciplinar. São Paulo: Santos; 2007. p. 87–107.
Bunduki V, Ruano R, Sapienza AD, Hanaoka BY, Zugaib M. Diagnóstico Pré-Natal de Fenda Labial e Palatina: Experiência de 40 Casos. Rev Bras Ginecol Obstet. 2001;23(9):561–6.
Capelozza Filho L, Normando AD, Silva Filho OG. Isolated influences of operated and unoperated male adults with UCLP. Cleft Palate J. 1996;33(1):51–6.
Castro-Sanchez AM, Mataran-Penarrocha GA, Arroyo-Morales M, Saavedra-Hernandez M, Fernandez-Sola C, Moreno-Lorenzo C. Effects of myofascial release techniques on pain, physical function, and postural stability in patients with fibromyalgia: a randomized controlled trial. Clin Rehabil. 2011;25(9):800–13.
Dotevall H, Lohmander-Agerskov A, Ejnell H, Bake B. Perceptual evaluation of speech and velopharyngeal function in children with and without cleft palate and the relationship to nasal airflow patterns. Cleft Palate Craniofac J. 2002;39(4):409–24.
Douglas CR. Tratado de Fisiologia aplicado à fonoaudiologia. São Paulo: Robe Editorial; 2002.
Felício CMF. Desenvolvimento normal das funções estomatognáticas. In: Fernandes FDM, Mendes BCA, Navas ALPGP, editors. Tratado de Fonoaudiologia. São Paulo: Roca; 2009. p. 10–27.
Felício CM, Ferreira CLP. Protocolo of orofacial myofunctional evaluation with scores. Int J Pediatr Otorhinolaryngol. 2008;72(3):367–75.
Felício CM, Folha GA, Ferreira CL, Medeiros AP. Expanded protocol of orofacial myofunctional evaluation with scores: validity and reliability. Int J Pediatr Otorhinolaryngol. 2010;74(11):1230–9.
Genaro KF, Fukushiro AP, Suguimoto MLFCP. Avaliação e tratamento dos distúrbios da fala. In: Trindade IEK, Silva Filho OG, editors. Fissuras labiopalatinas: uma abordagem interdisciplinar. São Paulo: Santos; 2007. p. 109–22.
Genaro KF, Yamashita RP, Trindade IEK. Avaliação clínica e instrumental na fissura labiopalatina. In: Fernandes FDM, Mendes BCA, Navas ALPGP, editors. Tratado de Fonoaudiologia. São Paulo: Roca; 2009. p. 488–503.
Golding-Kushner KJ. Therapy techniques for cleft palate speech and related disorders. San Diego: Singular Thomson Learning; 2001.
Graciano MIG, Tavano LD, Bachega MI. Aspectos psicossociais da reabilitação. In: Trindade IEK, Silva Filho OG (org). Fissuras labiopalatinas: uma abordagem interdisciplinar. São Paulo: Santos: 311–333, 2007.
Hortis-Dzierzbicka M, Radkowska E, Fudalej P. Speech outcomes in 10-year-old children with complete unilateral cleft lip and palate after one-stage lip and palate repair in the first year of life. J Plast Reconstr Aesthet Surg. 2012;65:175–81.
Ibayashi H, Fujino Y, Pham TM, Matsuda S. Intervention Study of exercise program for oral function in healthy elderly people. Tohoku J Exp Med. 2008;215:237–45.
Johns DF, Rohrich RJ, Awada M. Velopharyngeal incompetence: a guide for clinical evaluation. Plast Reconstr Surg. 2003;112(7):1890–7.

Kummer AW. Resonance disorders and velopharyngeal dysfunction (VPD). In: Kummer AW, editor. Cleft palate and craniofacial anomalies. San Diego: Singular Thomson Learning; 2004a. p. 176–213.

Kummer AW. Developmental aspects: language, cognition, and phonology. In: Kummer AW, editor. Cleft palate and craniofacial anomalies. San Diego: Singular Thomson Learning; 2004b. p. 129–44.

Kummer AW. Prosthetic managment. In: Kummer AW, editor. Cleft palate and craniofacial anomalies: Effects on speech and resonance. New York: Thomson Delmar Learning; 2004c.

Lee A, Whitehill TL, Ciocca V. Effect of listener training on perceptual judgement of hypernasality. Clin Linguist Phon. 2009;23(5):319–34.

Miller CK, Kummer AW. Feeding problems of infants with cleft lip/alate or craniofacial anomalies. In: Kummer AW, editor. Cleft palate and craniofacial anomalies. San Diego: Singular Thomson Learning; 2004. p. 103–27.

Minervino-Pereira ACM. O processo de enfrentamento vivido por pais de indivíduos com fissure labiopalatina, nas diferentes fases do tratamento. Tese[doutorado]. Bauru; 2005. p 143.

Nahai FR, Williams JK, Thomas J. The management of cleft lip and palate: pathways for treatment and longitudinal assessment. Sem Plast Surg. 2005;19(4):275–85.

Namura M, Motoyoshi M, Namura Y, Shimizu N. The effects of PNF training on the facial profile. J Oral Sci. 2008;50:45–51.

Pegoraro-Krook MI, Dutka-Souza MCR, Magalhaes LCT, Feniman MR. Intervenção fonoaudiológica na fissura palatina. In: Fernandes FDM, Mendes BCA, Navas ALPGP, editors. Tratado de Fonoaudiologia. São Paulo: Roca; 2009. p. 504–12.

Peterson-Falzone SJ, Trost-Cardamone JE, Karnell MP, Hardin-Jones M. The clinican's guide to treating cleft palate speech. St. Louis: Mosby; 2006. p. 17–39.

Pinho SMR. Fisiologia da Fonação. In: Fernandes FDM, Mendes BCA, Navas ALPGP, editors. Tratado de Fonoaudiologia. São Paulo: Roca; 2009. p. 45–51.

Prandini EL, Pegoraro-Krook MI, Dutka JCR, Marino VCC. Occurrence of consonant production errors in liquid phonemes in children with operated cleft lip and palate. J Appl Oral Sci. 2011;19(6):579–85.

Schuster M, Maier A, Bocklet T, Nkenke E, Holst A, Eysholdt U, Stelzle F. Automatically evaluated degree of intelligibility of children with different cleft type from preschool and elementary school measured by automatic speech recognition. Int J Pediatr Otorhinolaryngol. 2012;76:362–9.

Sharma VP, Bella H, Cadier MM, Pigott RW, Goodacre TEE, Richard BM. Outcomes in facial aesthetics in cleft lip and palate surgery: a systematic review. J Plast Reconstr Aesthet Surg. 2012;65:1233–45.

Shprintzen RJ. Instrumental assessment of velopharyngeal valving. In: Shprintzen RJ, Bardach J, editors. Cleft palate speech management: a multidisciplinary approach. St. Louis: Mosby; 1995. p. 221–56.

Silva DP, Dornelles S, Paniagua LM, Costa SS, Collares MVM. Aspectos Patofisiológicos do Esfíncter Velofaríngeo nas Fissuras Palatinas. Int Arch Otorhinolaryngol. 2008;12(3):426–35.

Smith BE, Kuehn DP. Speech Evaluation of Velopharyngeal Dysfunction. J Craniofac Surg. 2007;18(2):251–61.

Trindade IEK, Genaro KF, Yamashita RP, Miguel HC, Fukushiro AP. Proposal for velopharyngeal function rating in a speech perceptual assessment. Pro-Fono. 2005;17(2):259–62.

Warren DW, Hall DJ, Davis J. Oral port constriction and pressure airflow relationships during sibilant productions. Folia Phoniatr. 1981;33:380–94.

Warren DW, Allen GD, King HA. Physiological and perceptual effects of induced anterior open bite. Folia Phoniatr. 1984;36:164–73.

Robin Sequence

15

Nivaldo Alonso, Cristiano Tonello, Ilza Lazarini Marques, Arturo Frick Carpes, Marco Maricevich, and Renata Maricevich

15.1 Definition

Robin sequence (RS) is a congenital condition characterized by micrognathia, glossoptosis, and upper airway obstruction. Consensus was reached that micrognathia is the primary characteristic of RS. Other mandatory diagnostic characteristics include glossoptosis and airway obstruction. Cleft palate is considered a common and additional feature (Breugem and Evans 2016). The incidence of RS in the general population is 1/8500–1/14000 live births (Bush and Williams 1983; Printzlau and Andersen 2004) (Fig. 15.1).

According to Cohen classification (Cohen 1999), there are three distinct groups of RS: RS as a component of a known syndrome; RS associated with an anomaly but without constituting a specific syndrome; and isolated RS, when not associated with other malformations or syndromes. Several syndromes can

---

N. Alonso, M.D., Ph.D. (✉)
Divisao de Cirurgia Plastica e Queimaduras, Hospital das Clínicas da Faculdade de Medicina da Universidade de São Paulo, São Paulo, Brazil
e-mail: nivalonso@gmail.com

C. Tonello, M.D., Ph.D. • I.L. Marques, M.D., Ph.D.
Department of Craniofacial Surgery, Hospital for Rehabilitation of Craniofacial Anomalies, University of São Paulo, São Paulo, Brazil

A.F. Carpes, M.D., Ph.D.
Department of Plastic Surgery, University of São Paulo Hospital, São Paulo, Brazil

M. Maricevich, M.D.
Department of Plastic Surgery, Baylor College of Medicine, Houston, TX, USA

R. Maricevich, M.D.
Department of Plastic Surgery, Texas Children's Hospital – Baylor College of Medicine, Houston, TX, USA

© Springer International Publishing AG 2018
N. Alonso, C.E. Raposo-Amaral (eds.), *Cleft Lip and Palate Treatment*,
https://doi.org/10.1007/978-3-319-63290-2_15

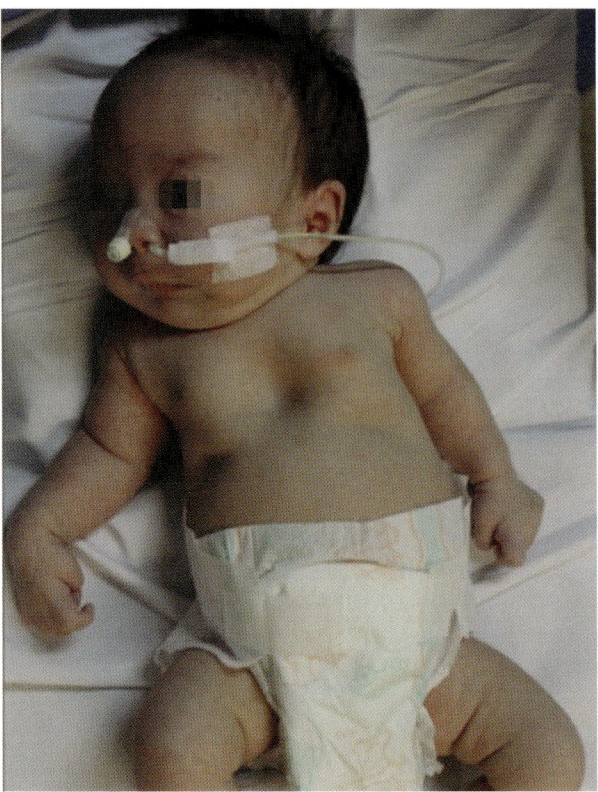

Fig. 15.1 Isolated RS patient (micrognathia and sternal retraction due to respiratory obstruction)

be associated with the RS, the most frequent being Stickler syndrome (Antunes et al. 2012). Other syndromes more frequently associated are velocardiofacial syndrome, fetal alcohol syndrome, Treacher Collins syndrome, and cerebro-costomandibular syndrome (Cohen 1976; Marques et al. 2001; Shprintzen 1992) (Fig. 15.2).

15.2 Etiological Diagnosis

In a sequence, all or most of the anomalies are caused by a primary abnormality. Micrognathia is the hypothesized initiating event in RS and it is a clinical component in several disorders (Breugem and Evans 2016). This way, the great variation of conditions in which the triad appears suggests heterogeneity of the etiological agents (Cohen 1979).

The cause of isolated RS is still unknown; however, patients with isolated RS have a stronger family history of cleft lip and/or palate. Marques et al. (1998) studied 36 infants with isolated RS and found positive family history in 27.7% of cases. In addition, there is an increased incidence in twins when compared to general

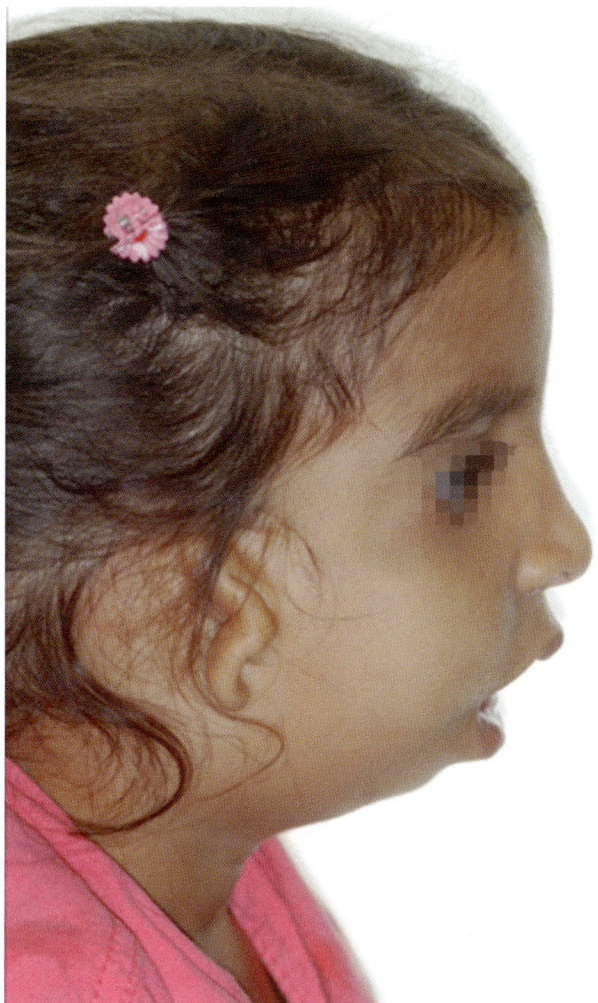

Fig. 15.2 RS associated to Treacher Collins syndrome (severe micrognathia)

population. In the study by Jakobsen et al. (2006), there was a failed attempt to identify causative genes, but it was found that only genes in GAD67 2q31, 11q23-q24 in PVRL1, and SOX9 gene in the 24.3-17q q 25.1 appear to be important. Later in 2007, Jakobsen et al. (2007) studied ten patients with isolated PRS and their findings suggest that this disease can be caused by defect in the SOX9 and KCNJ2 genes, as evidenced by their decreased expressions in the studied patients. The SOX9 gene regulates the growth of collagen during the formation of cartilage and endochondral bone.

For the syndromic patients, the mode of inheritance is particular to each associated syndrome. For example, Stickler syndrome is a connective tissue disorder with autosomal dominant inheritance. The RS plus patient group with associated nonsyndromic anomalies is even more heterogeneous, some of them with genetic abnormalities. RS has been observed in association with congenital hypotonia and skeletal and connective tissue disorders.

15.3 Clinical Presentation

Clinical expression of RS is very heterogeneous, ranging from discrete respiratory distress and mild feeding problems to suffocation and death. The clinical manifestations are more frequent and more severe in the first months of life (Freeman and Manners 1980). It can be apparent shortly after birth or when feeding is initiated. Symptoms of respiratory obstruction are noisy breathing, intercostal retractions, and apnea. Another clinical manifestation is dyspnea, apnea, or very lengthy feeding time. As several factors can contribute to the upper airway obstruction, there may be no correlation between the severity of micrognathia and the severity of respiratory distress and difficulty feeding. Infants with mild degree of mandibular deficiency may show severe respiratory symptoms and dysphagia (Singer and Sidoti 1992).

Some studies have shown that the respiratory and feeding problems are a result of a combination of the abnormal anatomy and factors associated with neuromotor development of pharyngeal and genioglossus muscles (Souza et al. 2003; Marques et al. 2005a).

Respiratory obstruction is multifactorial. It is related to anatomical jaw abnormalities—micrognathia and consequent glossoptosis, with a decrease in effectiveness of the genioglossus muscle to prevent tongue drop, due to its posterior insertion. The respiratory obstruction observed in these patients can be translated by the high prevalence of obstructive sleep apnea syndrome (OSAS) present in RS. Approximately 85% of these patients with less than 1 year present OSAS, with a clear tendency towards greater severity, the younger the child is (Anderson et al. 2011).

Malnutrition is an important contributing factor to the severity of respiratory obstruction because, in the neonatal period and in early childhood, it is associated with delay in neuromuscular development (Marques et al. 2005a).

Feeding difficulties, aspiration, vomiting, and dysphagia are usually secondary to airway obstruction and are worsened by the presence of cleft palate (Lidsky et al. 2008). The obstruction causes difficulties in coordination of sucking, swallowing, and breathing. Glossoptosis doesn't allow anterior position of the tongue and the cleft palate causes less intraoral negative pressure, which is required to create efficient suctioning as well as prevent nasal reflux (Nassar et al. 2006).

Manometry has been used to study the relationship between airway obstruction and difficulty feeding in PRS infants. The negative pharyngeal pressure during breastfeeding increases with continuous suctioning and breathing attempts. A negative pressure greater than 60 mm Hg sucks the tongue, closing the lower pharynx, during attempts to inspiration and suction. It was also reported that the frequent vomiting is due to gastric distension secondary to swallowing of air, during inspiration attempts against the blocked airway (Fletcher et al. 1969). Other studies have shown primary motor dysfunction of upper gastrointestinal tract in infants with RS (Baudon et al. 2002).

The high negative intrathoracic pressure generated during obstructive sleep apnea causes worsening reflux and aspiration in children with obstructive sleep apnea syndrome, which tends to improve with treatment of the respiratory problem.

15.4 Cleft Palate

The abnormal jaw embryological development occurs between the 7th and 11th weeks of gestation, resulting in a high position of the tongue in the nasopharynx, while palatal shelves start their growth towards the midline. An explanation for the presence of cleft palate would be the inability of the tongue to descend, due to lack of mandibular growth, preventing the shelves to fuse (Elliot et al. 1995). There are descriptions of a much higher frequency of U-shaped cleft palate, complete and wide, and this was considered a leading cause of delay in the morphogenesis of the swallowing and mastication musculature and impairment of mandibular growth and worst respiratory impairment (Marques et al. 1998) (Fig. 15.3).

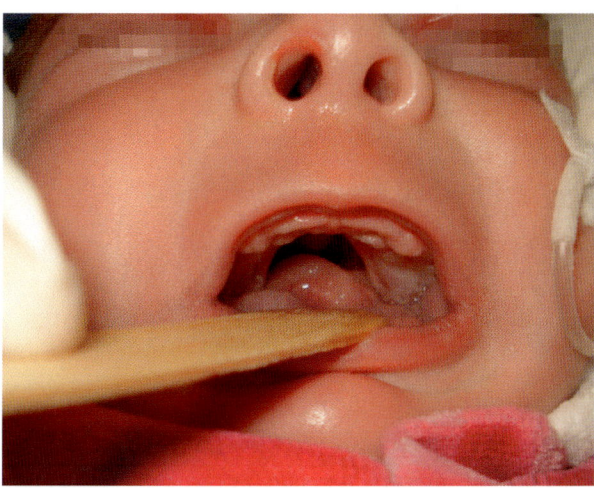

Fig. 15.3 "U"-shaped cleft palate and glossoptosis associated in RS newborn

15.5 Diagnosis

The diagnostic process begins with identification of clinical findings present in RS and classification of the severity of symptoms. The anatomy and function of orofacial structures can contribute to making the diagnosis but do not correlate with severity of symptoms.

It is important to consider that the diagnosis of micrognathia, initiating event of RS, is subjective as glossoptosis. It can be difficult to judge the severity of tongue base airway obstruction and a possibility of multilevel obstruction associated. Signs of upper airway obstruction can be intermittent and are more likely to be present when the infant is asleep. The initial assessment of the clinical features and severity of respiratory distress is important and has practical implications (Breugem and Evans 2016). Therefore, a multidisciplinary team must evaluate suspicious cases of RS and thorough investigation should take place.

15.5.1 Prenatal Diagnosis

Prenatal recognition of suspected RS allows planning and immediate intervention at birth and prevention of life-threatening situation. The main ultrasonographic findings are polyhydramnios, micrognathia, and glossoptosis.

Polyhydramnios is considered because it may be associated to swallowing difficulties. It is observed in approximately 65% of fetuses with micrognathia (Bromley and Benacerraf 1994). Since micrognathia is associated with several syndromes and malformations, it should not be the only finding taken into consideration (Bronshtein et al. 2005; Izumi et al. 2012; Luedders et al. 2011). Glossoptosis is more closely associated with prenatal diagnosis. The ultrasonographic analysis should be dynamic and diagnosis is made when the tongue is positioned posteriorly during most of the examination, approximately 20–30 min, and is not observed anterior to the inferior alveolar margin at any time (Bronshtein et al. 2005).

15.5.2 Physical Examination

The observation of the clinical triad of RS is usually made in the first days of life. Gestational age and birth weight are no different from normal patients and do not vary depending on the severity of cases. At birth, the micrognathia is the most evident feature in patients with RS. It is characterized by a small and/or retropositioned jaw, with increased overjet. The facial profile is convex due to lack of projection of the lower third. The nasolabial angle and maxillary position are normal (Fig. 15.7).

Intraoral examination reveals tongue base collapse, especially when the baby is in supine position. Cleft palate is present in 90% of cases, 75% of cases being wide and complete and 25% of them narrow or incomplete, "V" shaped (Marques et al. 1998; Spina et al. 1972).

Some children with RS are robust and strong, while others may present with significant hypotonia (due to associated neurological impairment) or severe cyanosis (due to cardiac structural changes) (Abadie et al. 2002). Newborns may present with minimal respiratory distress at birth while others have significant airway obstruction, with nasal flaring, cyanosis, stridor, and subcostal retraction. Suspecting the diagnosis of PRS, it is important to identify eventual other associated anomalies and syndromes.

15.5.3 Pulse Oximetry

Continuous pulse oximetry has been used as a tool to assess severity of respiratory distress and sometimes is the only available tool to evaluate pediatric respiratory impairment in settings with limited resources. However, obstruction, central or mixed, and sleep fragmentation are not always associated with decreased oxygen saturation.

Intermittent oxygen desaturation during sleep in children is highly suggestive of the presence of sleep disturbance and it is a good indicative to which of them will require polysomnography. The examination must be continuous for at least 6 h of sleep and a drop of 4% or more is considered desaturation. A set of desaturation happens when there are more desaturation episodes in a period of 10–30 min. The pulse oximetry should be considered positive when there are three or more sets of desaturation and at least three readings below 90% (Brouillette et al. 2000).

15.5.4 Polysomnography

This test allows for evaluation of early respiratory variables, confirming the clinical suspicion of respiratory sleeping disturbances in children, in order to guide any necessary clinical treatment or to justify appropriate surgical intervention (Freed et al. 1988) (Fig. 15.4).

The polysomnogram (PSG) assesses quality of sleep, has excellent reproducibility, and documents the presence of snoring and respiratory events (obstructive sleep apnea, central and mixed, hypopneas, and airflow restriction), oxygen saturation, and patient movements. The PSG distinguishes obstructive from central apnea or epileptic activity in children with neurological diseases (Society 1999). Ideally, the test is performed overnight, but polysomnography during daytime for at least 2 h shows acceptable sensitivity and specificity.

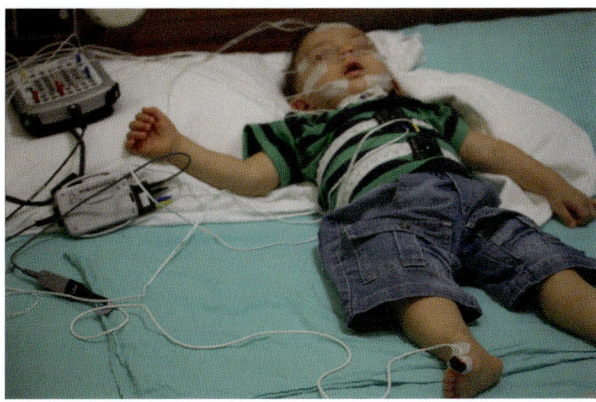

Fig. 15.4 Polysomnography exam in RS to evaluate respiratory disorders

15.5.5 Endoscopic Airway Evaluation

Clinical presentation alone is not sufficient to predict the evolution of airway obstruction in PRS patients. It is important to elucidate the cause to appropriately treat it. The nasopharyngeal endoscopy is the best tool for the visualization of airway in order to detect structural abnormalities (de Sousa et al. 2003).

Glossoptosis is usually the main cause for airway obstruction, but other structures can abnormally function (Fig. 15.5).

The endoscopic examination is subjective and does not evaluate the patient during rest or sleep. Many authors have shown that there is no correlation between clinical severity and isolated glossoptosis. The existence of tonsillar hypertrophy, shape and position of the epiglottis and arytenoids, aspect of the cartilaginous framework, mobility of vocal folds, pharyngeal hypotonia, and nasal atresia must be evaluated. The thorough analysis increases the test sensitivity and specificity. Laryngomalacia is the main cause of stridor in babies.

Respiratory obstruction in PRS is not always caused by glossoptosis. Multilevel obstruction could be associated to glossoptosis and contribute to respiratory distress. Nasopharyngoscopy studies in patients with craniofacial anomalies and obstructive sleep apnea, including RS (Sher et al. 1986; Sher 1992), demonstrated besides laryngomalacia, vocal fold disorder, other types of obstruction. Type 1: the obstruction is due to tongue drop, which rests on posterior pharynx, below the soft palate; type 2: the tongue moves posteriorly and compresses, partially or totally, the soft palate against the posterior wall of the pharynx; type 3: the lateral pharyngeal walls move medially, causing airway obstruction; and type 4: there is a sphincteric constriction of the pharynx in all directions. The tongue doesn't participate in obstruction of types 3 and 4.

The diagnosis of airway obstruction sites is important to direct the treatment modality.

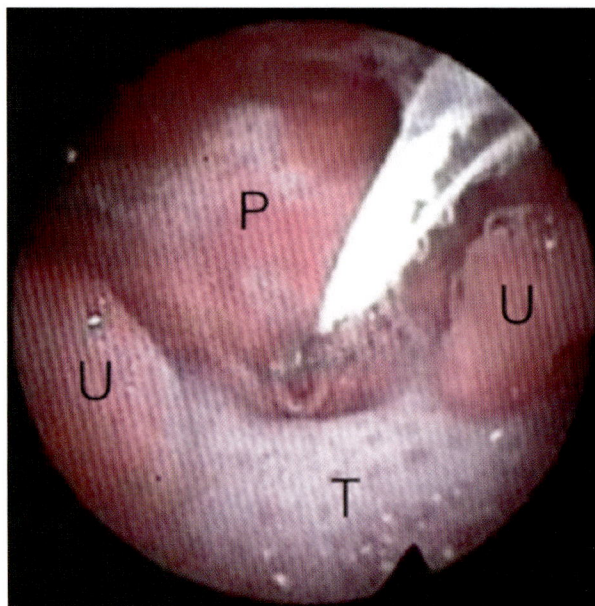

Fig. 15.5 Glossoptosis evaluated by endoscopic superior airway. The base of the tongue is pushing the epiglottis. (T: tongue, U: uvula, P: pharyngeal posterior wall)

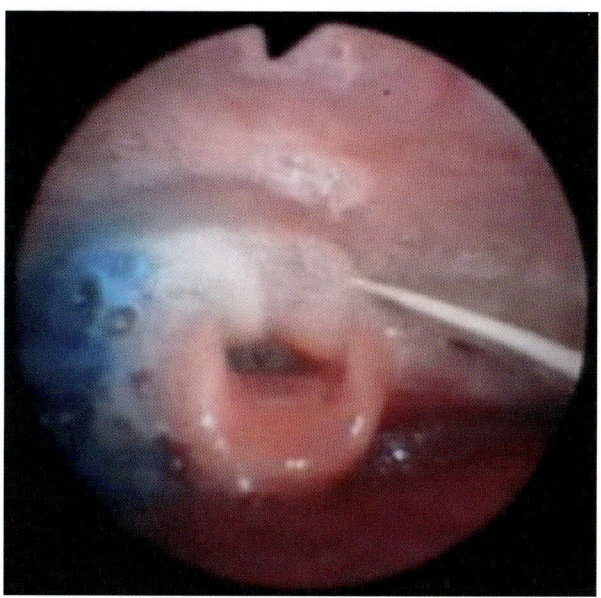

Fig. 15.6 Tracheal aspiration of colored saliva during swallowing endoscopy

15.5.6 Swallowing Studies

Endoscopy is also helpful to evaluate oropharyngeal dysphagia. It is a simple and safe tool, even in infants. It is extremely important before starting diet by mouth, since it evaluates for aspiration risk. When there is reflux of milk through the nasopharyngeal airway and/or delay in swallowing as well as presence of residual milk in the epiglottis, vocal folds or trachea are findings of possible aspiration (Macedo 2000) (Fig. 15.6).

Barium swallow study is another adjunct in evaluating unsynchronized tongue and esophageal movement. It is also considered abnormal when there is evidence of more than 1-s pharyngeal phase of swallowing and penetration of barium in the laryngeal vestibule above the vocal folds or trachea.

All RS patients present some degree of tongue movement abnormality and studies have shown more than 66% presenting penetration of contrast in laryngeal vestibule and 50% presenting residual material in pharyngeal recess during the first months of life (Monasterio et al. 2004).

15.5.7 Genetic Analysis

If there is a suspicion for RS, genetic evaluation should be obtained. Family history of cleft palate may be present in 27% of cases of isolated RS (Marques et al. 1998), but other authors have pointed out that there is no genetic relevant factor in this disease (Edwards and Newall 1985).

There is increased prevalence of prenatal exposure to teratogenic agents and chromosomal abnormalities in patients with RS (Izumi et al. 2012).

It is difficult to make the genetic diagnosis during the neonatal period and usually requires long-term follow-up. The facial features of specific syndromes are usually absent at this early stage and become more obvious with development. Similarly, specific medical characteristics to each syndrome usually develop after the neonatal period.

Stickler syndrome is the genetic diagnosis most commonly associated with PRS, 11 to 18% (Evans et al. 2011). It is an autosomal dominant disease. There is associated hypoplastic midface, flat nasal bridge (Marques et al. 1998), in addition to ocular abnormalities, such as severe myopia, retinal detachment and glaucoma, conductive or neurosensory hearing loss, and joint hypermobility leading to early osteoarthritis (Antunes et al. 2012). Such clinical characteristics are very suggestive of the diagnosis, but molecular analysis is required for confirmation since other syndromes may have similar phenotype. Mutations in the genes COL2A1, COL1A1, COL1A2, or COL9A1 are present in 75% of cases of SS cases. Due to visual and auditory irreversible implications, every child must have an early assessment, no later than 6 months of life (Antunes et al. 2012) (Fig. 15.7).

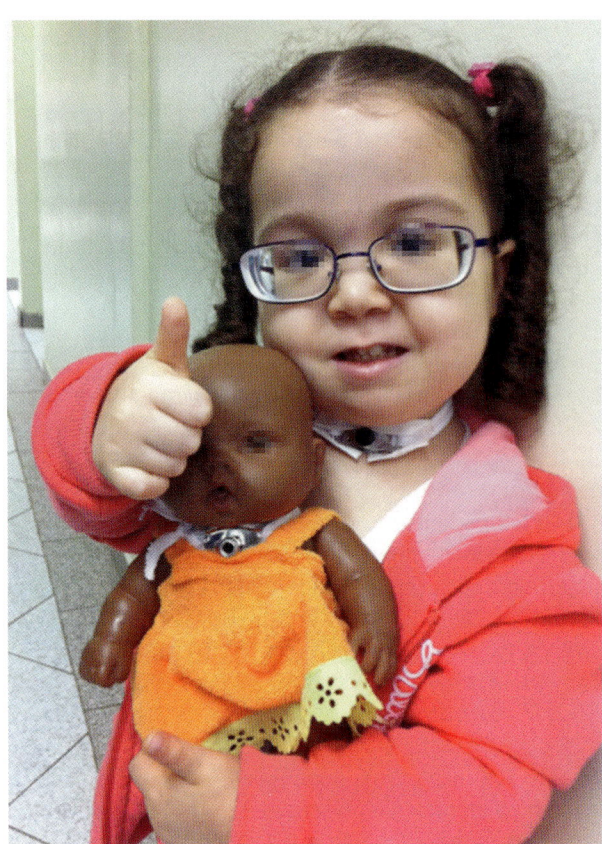

Fig. 15.7 RS and Stickler syndrome

Fig. 15.8 RS and velocardiofacial syndrome

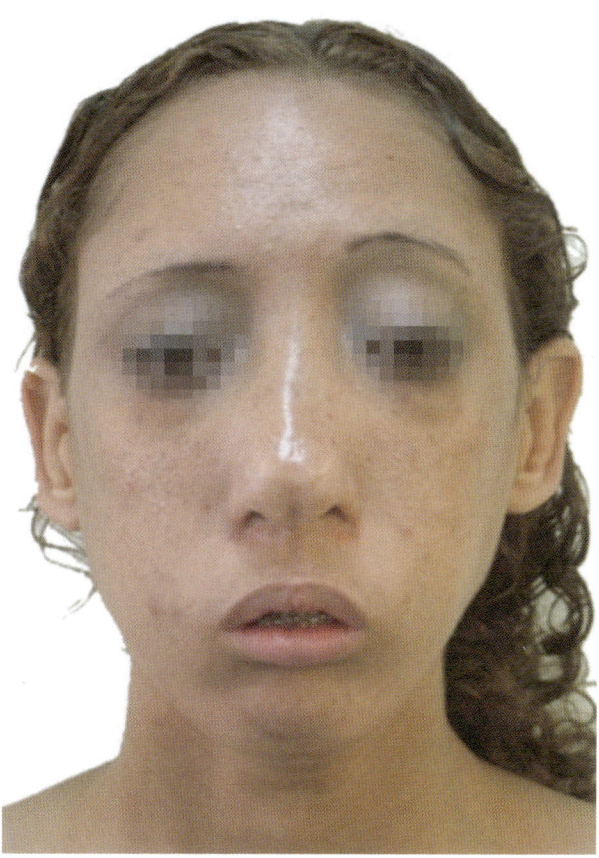

The second most frequent genetic association is velocardiofacial syndrome (Fig. 15.7), present in about 3% of cases (Marques et al. 1998). These patients present with long face due to vertical maxillary excess, prominent nose with wide dorsum and narrow ala base, thin upper lip, narrow palpebral fissures, low-set, malformed ears with long abundance, and microcephaly. Velopharyngeal insufficiency and neuropsychomotor development delay appear in 100% of cases, and cardiac changes in 82%. Deletion of chromosome 22q 11.2 confirms the diagnosis (Izumi et al. 2012) (Fig. 15.8).

15.5.8 Computed Tomography

Computed tomography (CT) is an important asset in difficult differential diagnosis and also for operative planning. The mandible is small and the deficiency is mainly limited to the mandibular body, with an obtuse gonial angle (Rogers et al. 2009). The posterior mandible height is significantly shorter in syndromic PRS patients

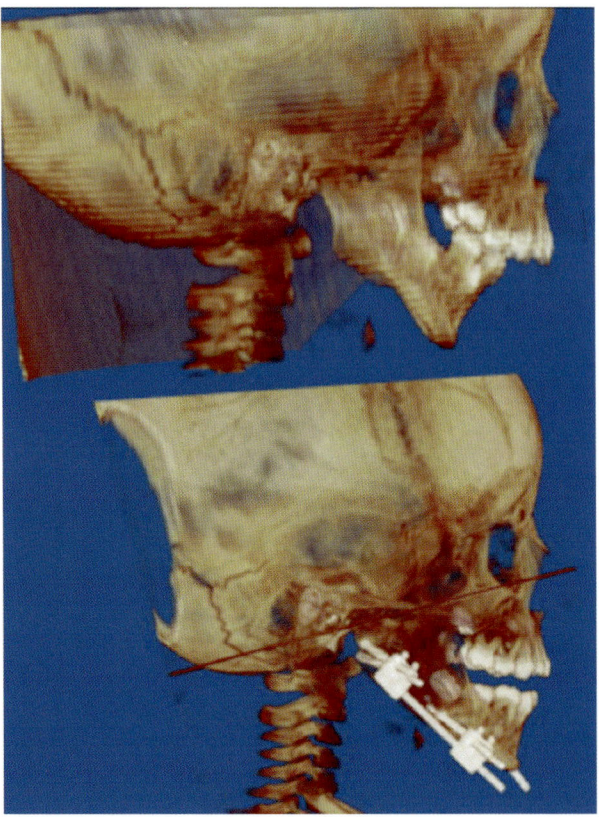

Fig. 15.9 3-dimensional reconstruction of CT scan pre- and postoperatively (MDO)

when compared to isolated cases (Glander and Cisneros 1992). Temporomandibular joint ankylosis or hypoplasia can be the cause of micrognathia. Other malformations, such as mandibular, zygomatic, craniosynostosis, cranial base, and ear, can also be identified with CT use. It is also very helpful in determining the osteotomy and vector for distraction osteogenesis (Chung et al. 2012; Alonso and Freitas 2002) (Fig. 15.9).

15.5.9 24-h Esophageal pH Testing

Gastroesophageal reflux disease (GERD) is present in up to 35% of RS patients and poses increased risk for respiratory events, recurrent pneumonia, ear infections, swallowing problems, and growth delay (Vandenplas et al. 1991). The esophageal pH monitoring should be performed in the inpatient setting after the first month of life and be repeated every 2 months if needed.

15.6 Treatment

The priority in the treatment of RS infants must be the maintenance of a patent airway as early as possible (Breugem and Evans 2016). Maintaining the airway permeability in these patients besides the correction of respiratory impairment and improvement of the alimentary difficulty could be obtained in the same time (Marques et al. 2005).

Airway obstruction in RS does depend not only on the anatomical abnormality of the mandible and/or the position of the tongue, but also on the intrinsic activity of the parapharyngeal muscles. This activity depends on individual maturation during the neonatal period. The degree of neuromuscular dysfunction and the speed of maturation of this function vary among patients and play an important role in the recovery of airway permeability (Marques et al. 2005; Sher 1992).

Another very important aspect to consider is the different evolution observed in patients with isolated SR and the form associated with syndromes.

While conservative treatment of airway obstruction in children with RS is possible and strongly recommended when it is possible, in syndromic conditions these options more frequently fail.

Some modalities of treatment for airway obstruction, surgical and nonsurgical, have been described; however, a consensus about the best approach is still unclear in our current literature.

15.6.1 Prone Position

The prone position could be effective for infants with mild airway obstruction. It facilitates breathing and prevents aspiration of saliva and food due to the cervical hyperextension and gravity position of the tongue. Prone position is not as effective for moderate and severe cases.

15.6.2 Nasopharyngeal Intubation

The nasopharyngeal airway (NPA) is a simple method to provide a patent airway and consists of introduction of a silicone cannula through the nostril showing excellent results specially in isolated RS patients. The cannula diameter measures 3–3.5 mm, and is introduced 7–8 cm passed the nostril, reaching the pharynx. The remaining of the external cannula is trimmed to leave approximately 1 cm outside. The location of the cannula internally remains at the level of the epiglottis (Marques et al. 2001).

NPA prevents the development of high negative pressure, the level of the posterior pharynx during inspiration, suction, and swallowing, improving the airway obstruction caused by the tongue drop. Moreover, the NPA is hollow and allows airflow through it (Fig. 15.10).

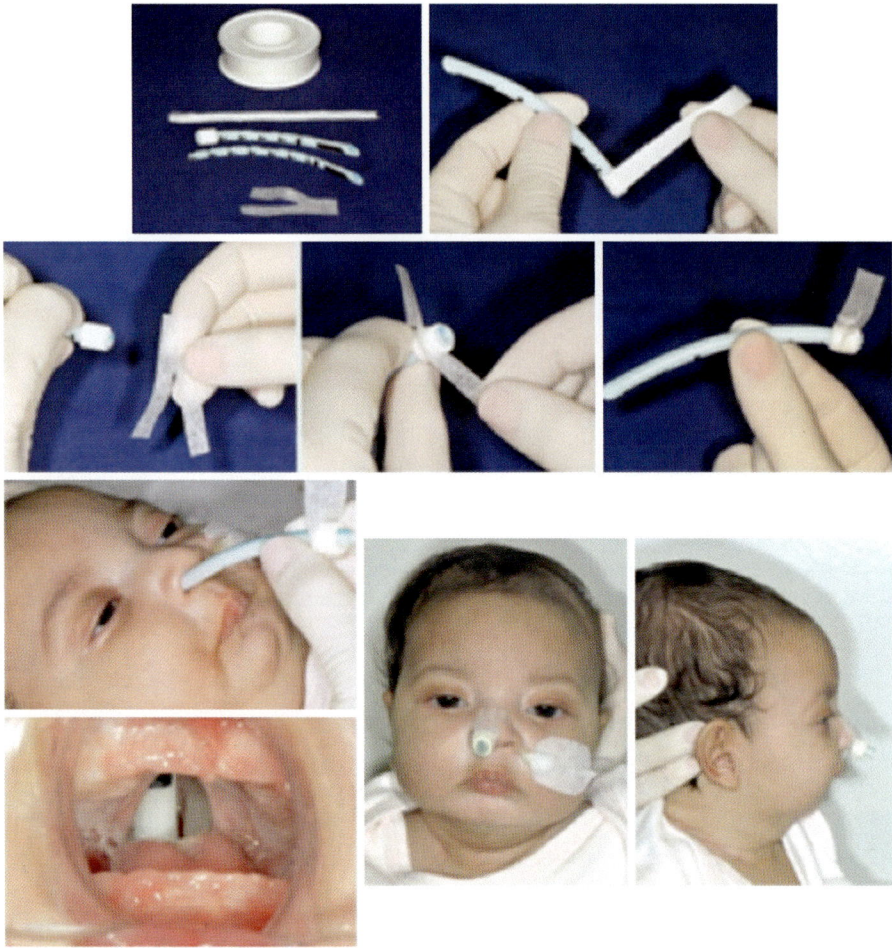

Fig. 15.10 RS patient treated with nasopharyngeal intubation

15.6.3 Glossopexy

In general, glossopexy consists of anchoring the tongue to the lower lip anteriorly and from the base of the tongue to the mandible. This allows the tongue to be anteriorized and respiratory obstruction to be replaced instead of the tracheostomy (Argamaso 1992).

Adhesion is maintained throughout the first year of life and is usually reversed at the time of palatoplasty, which occurs around 12 months of age.

Although the success rate with the use of this technique is high in selected patients, limiting tongue mobility tends to exacerbate the dysphagia, increasing the

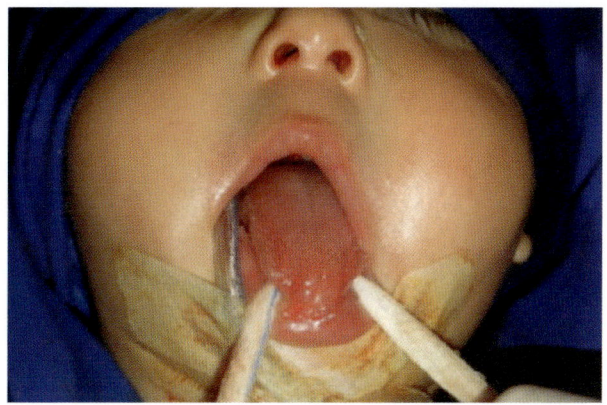

Fig. 15.11 RS patient undergone glossopexy (tongue lip adhesion)

likelihood of requiring a prolonged period of enteral supplementation via the nasogastric tube or gastrostomy (Abramowicz et al. 2012; Scott et al. 2012; Rogers et al. 2011; Evans et al. 2006).

The difficulty in treating dysphagia or even worsening of its symptoms observed after performing the procedure associated with complications such as adhesion dehiscence and pronounced edema of the tongue and oropharynx with a need for postoperative tracheostomy is one of the arguments used by most of the centers that abandoned this technique (Scott et al. 2012; Rogers et al. 2011).

In addition, situations in which the patient presents patterns of respiratory obstruction due to collapse of the pharyngeal walls to nasopharyngoscopy, syndromic diagnosis associated with low birth weight, presence of gastroesophageal reflux, and history of preoperative, among others, presents a high probability of failure with this practice (Marques et al. 2005; Abramowicz et al. 2012; Rogers et al. 2011).

Recent publications, however, have advocated in favor of glossopexy as a treatment of choice for specific groups of patients. The simplicity of the procedure, lower potential for scarring, facial nerve lesion, and dental germs, besides the absence of specialized equipment, are the arguments used by those who advocate their indication, especially when compared to MDO (Abramowicz et al. 2012; Scott et al. 2012; Rogers et al. 2011) (Fig. 15.11).

15.6.4 Mandibular Distraction Osteogenesis

Mandibular distraction osteogenesis (MDO) is characterized as a dynamic process, consisting of the elongation of the facial skeleton and adjacent soft parts, obtained through gradual traction applied to two osteotomized bone surfaces, by means of a mechanical device (Fig. 15.12).

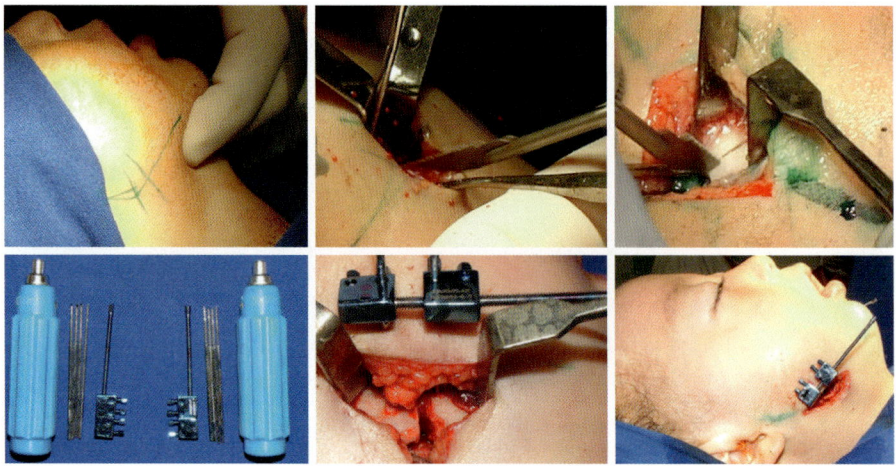

Fig. 15.12 RS patient undergone mandible osteotomy and placement of external devices to mandibular distraction

The MDO represents an alternative method to the traditional upper airway management of RS patients. The mandibular stretching promotes the positioning of the base tongue to a more anterior position, thus allowing the opening of the airway posteriorly. It can be observed that the MDO, when indicated in selected patients, prevents the tracheostomy in patients who did not respond to clinical treatments.

In addition, their results are apparently superior to those obtained with glossopexy, especially with regard to improved swallowing. In this way, this technique allows to avoid, in many cases, the indication of tracheostomy and gastrostomy (Scott et al. 2012; Rogers et al. 2011; Evans et al. 2006).

When compared to tracheostomy, considering the specific indications of each procedure, it presents lower rates of morbidity and mortality in addition to the cost savings of medical and hospital care (Hong et al. 2012).

Success in approximately 90% of cases can be observed when MDO is indicated in selected patients. However, as with other procedures, especially glossopexy, if these patients were adequately treated by specialized teams with gastroesophageal reflux control, use of feeding techniques and use of nasopharyngeal cannula, sometimes surgical indications would be unnecessary (Marques et al. 1998b, 2001, 2005; Scott et al. 2012).

Thus, possibly the best indication for MDO is reserved for cases in which glossoptosis is identified as a main cause of respiratory obstruction in patients with SR, preferably nonsyndromic, who do not respond to the different clinical measures employed and in those situations where we desire decannulation (Fig. 15.13).

Negative points related to MDO are mainly due to complications inherent to the procedure, besides aspects such as the cost of distractors and few services and surgeons being able to perform this procedure. The limitations on the results obtained

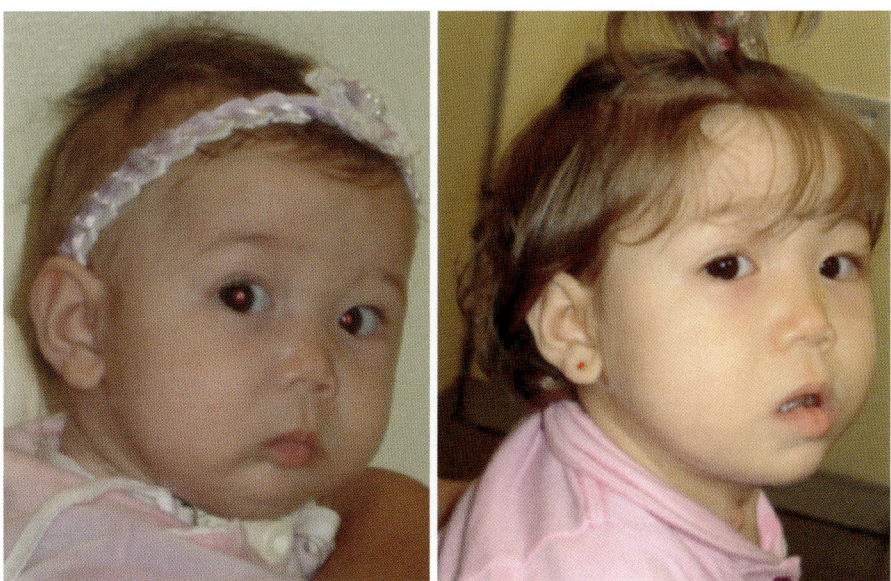

Fig. 15.13 RS patient previously MDO to decannulation and 2-year follow-up MDO

in patients with syndromic SR and those with respiratory obstruction due to collapsed upper airways resemble those of glossopexia. In these cases the tracheostomy appears as the technique of choice (Scott et al. 2012; Jarrahy 2012).

15.6.5 Tracheostomy

Upper airway obstruction treatment protocols usually reserve to tracheostomy, the last indication, or those situations in which other clinical or surgical procedures fail. Although this happens relatively frequently, it should be remembered that tracheostomy is considered the definitive technique to ensure a stable airway in patients with upper airway obstruction.

In addition, some cases will rarely improve with another technique, especially if the patient is an SR associated with the syndrome and present respiratory obstruction in which glossoptosis is not the main cause of respiratory impairment (Marques et al. 1998b, 2001, 2005; Rogers et al. 2011).

Neurologically compromised children have a risk of airway involvement regardless of glossoptosis. For this reason, addressing the obstruction of the tongue base with different techniques of tracheostomy in children with syndromic SR frequently is not appropriate. These interventions do not address associated factors such as hypotonia, poor coordination, or chronic aspiration. For patients with these comorbidities, the tracheostomy associated with gastrostomy allows an improvement of the respiratory function and maintenance of adequate nutrition (Scott et al. 2012).

Although tracheostomy could be the best indication in some situations, it presents considerable morbidity and mortality rates and requires specific care from the family and the care team. Thirteen some complications associated with tracheostomy, most of them observed in the first postoperative days, account for a mortality rate of approximately 0.7%. Adverse events related to this procedure include sudden airway obstruction by accidental decannulation and mucus impaction, airway infections, bleeding, stoma maintenance problems, tracheal stenosis, and appropriate speech inhibition and swallowing development (Scott et al. 2012; Rogers et al. 2011).

15.7 Dysphagia Treatment

Respiratory compromise leads to difficulty in coordination between suction, swallowing, and breathing. Therefore, clearing the airway obstruction is essential to improve feeding and nutrition. Besides this lack of coordination, glossoptosis also makes it difficult for the anteriorization of the tongue, necessary for adequate suction. The cleft palate causes a lack of negative pressure resulting in inefficient suction, nasal reflux of food, and higher risk of aspiration. Nutrition is usually managed through feeding tubes.

Facilitator techniques of feeding have been developed to stimulate oral feeding on PRS infants after treatment and clearance of the obstructed airway (Nassar et al. 2006; Marques et al. 2010). Gradual daily implementation of these techniques, in a short period of time, can promote oral feeding, as well as the discontinuity of feeding tubes. It consists of encouragement of non-nutritional suction through the use of pacifiers, massage to relax and anteriorize the tongue, manual support of the jaw, soft and long bottle nipples with a 1 mm puncture whole, nipple accurately place on the tongue, position of the child in a symmetrical global position, rhythmic movements of the nipple in the oral cavity, and thickening of the milk (Nassar et al. 2006; Marques et al. 2010).

Besides these techniques, swallowing endoscopies are frequently performed to monitor the risk of aspiration and decide the timing to initiate oral diet, which happens in approximately 2 weeks (Elliot et al. 1995; Marques et al. 2010).

Another strategy that can be used is the administration of a hypercaloric diet for newborns that allows the use of smaller volumes. It consists of formula or breastmilk boosted with 5–8% of glucose polymers, 3–5% of medium-chain triglycerides, and essential fatty acids (Marques et al. 2004).

If the patient is not able to be fed by mouth and requires extended tube feeds, gastrostomy tube may be indicated; this has been reported in up to 60% of patients (Salmen 2011).

Different publications have shown that in those institutions where glossopexy or even tracheostomy is indicated routinely, the number of patients submitted to gastrostomy is much higher when compared to those in which clinical measures or even MDO were indicated. In addition, a large proportion of patients with SR associated with neurological syndrome or neurological impairment will most often require surgical treatment, whereas in isolated form it is rarely needed (Marques et al. 2001, 2005; Scott et al. 2012).

15.8 Cleft Palate Repair

Palatoplasty is usually performed at 12 months of age. However, some conditions should be considered with palatoplasty in patients with SR.

Patients with SR present an increased risk of respiratory compromise in the postoperative period when compared to palatoplasty in patients with isolated palatine fissures.

The respiratory discomfort immediately installed after the procedure is a manifestation observed in some cases. Symptoms usually appear within the first 2 h after surgery, and most manifest within 48 h. Prolonged surgical time, excessive pressure exerted on the base of the tongue by the oral opener, and palate and tongue edema secondary to surgical manipulation associated with a basal micrognath condition are the main causes (Antony and Sloan 2002).

The respiratory discomfort after palatoplasty observed in some previously asymptomatic children results from a compromised but compensated upper airway. Respiratory obstruction may not manifest until the period of palatoplasty.

However, author's studies in progress have showed that immediate respiratory discomfort is limited. Clinical and PSG parameters improve following 6 months up the procedure (Carpes 2011).

References

Abadie V, Morisseau-Durand MP, Beyler C, Manach Y, Couly G. Brainstem dysfunction: a possible neuroembryological pathogenesis of isolated Pierre Robin sequence. Eur J Pediatr. 2002;161(5):275–80.

Abramowicz S, Bacic JD, Mulliken JB, Rogers GF. Validation of the GILLS score for tongue-lip adhesion in Robin sequence patients. J Craniofac Surg. 2012;23(2):382–6.

Alonso N, Freitas RS. Mandibular distraction: comparison between intraoral and extraoral devices. Braz J Craniomaxillofac Surg. 2002;5(2):15–8.

Anderson IC, Sedaghat AR, McGinley BM, et al. Prevalence and severity of obstructive sleep apnea and snoring in infants with Pierre Robin sequence. Cleft Palate Craniofac J. 2011;48(5):614–8.

Antony AK, Sloan GM. Airway obstruction following palatoplasty: analysis of 247 consecutive operations. Cleft Palate Craniofac J. 2002;39(2):145–8.

Antunes RB, Alonso N, Paula RG. Importance of early diagnosis of Stickler syndrome in newborns. J Plast Reconstr Aesthet Surg. 2012;65(8):1029–34.

Argamaso RV. Glossopexy for upper airway obstruction in Robin sequence. Cleft Palate Craniofac J. 1992;29(3):232–8.

Baudon JJ, Renault F, Goutet JM, Flores Guevara R, Soupre V, Gold F, Vazquez MP. Motor disfunction of the upper digestive tract in Pierre Robin sequence as assessed by sucking-swallowing eletromyography and esophageal manometry. J Pediatr. 2002;140:719–23.

Breugem CC, Evans KN. Best practices for the diagnosis and evaluation of infants with Robin sequence- a clinical consensus report. JAMA Pediatr. 2016;170(9):894–902.

Bromley B, Benacerraf BR. Fetal micrognathia: associated anomalies and outcome. J Ultrasound Med. 1994;13(7):529–33.

Bronshtein M, Blazer S, Zalel Y, Zimmer EZ. Ultrasonographic diagnosis of glossoptosis in fetuses with Pierre Robin sequence in early and mid pregnancy. Am J Obstet Gynecol. 2005;193(4):1561–4.

Brouillette RT, Morielli A, Leimanis A, Waters KA, Luciano R, Ducharme FM. Nocturnal pulse oximetry as an abbreviated testing modality for pediatric obstructive sleep apnea. Pediatrics. 2000;105(2):405–12.

Bush PG, Williams AJ. Incidence of the Robin anomalad (Pierre Robin syndrome). Br J Plast Surg. 1983;36:434–7.

Carpes AF. Avaliação polissonográfica e endoscópica em pacientes com Sequência de Robin isolada submetidas à palatoplastia. [tese]. São Paulo: Hospital das Clínicas da Faculdade de Medicina, Universidade de São Paulo; 2011.

Chung MT, Levi B, Hyun JS, Lo DD, Montoro DT, Lisiecki J. Pierre Robin sequence and Treacher Collins hypoplastic mandible comparison using three-dimensional morphometric analysis. J Craniofac Surg. 2012;23(7 Suppl 1):1959–63.

Cohen MM Jr. The Robin anomalad: its nonspecificity and associated syndromes. J Oral Surg. 1976;34:587–93.

Cohen MM Jr. Syndromology's message for craniofacial biology. J Maxilofac Surg. 1979;7:89–109.

Cohen MM Jr. Robin sequences and complexes: casual heterogeneity and pathogenetic/phenotypic variability. Am J Med Genet. 1999;84(4):311–5.

Edwards JR, Newall DR. The Pierre Robin syndrome reassessed in the light of recent research. Br J Plast Surg. 1985;38(3):339–42.

Elliot MA, Studen-Pevovich DA, Ranalli DN. Prevalence of selected pediatric conditions in children with Pierre Robin sequence. Pediatr Dent. 1995;17(2):106–11.

Evans AK, Rahbar R, Rogers GF, Mulliken JB, Volk MS. Robin sequence: a retrospective review of 115 patients. Int J Pediatr Otorhinolaryngol. 2006;70(6):973–80. Epub 2006 Jan 26

Evans KN, Sie KC, Hopper RA, Glass RP, Hing AV, Cunningham ML. Robin sequence: from diagnosis to development of an effective management plan. Pediatrics. 2011;127(5):936–48.

Fletcher MM, Blum SL, Blanchard CL. Pierre Robin syndrome pathophysiology of obstructive episodes. Laryngoscope. 1969;79:547–59.

Freed G, Pearlman MA, Brown AS, Barot LR. Polysomnographic indications for surgical intervention in Pierre Robin sequence: acute airway management and follow-up studies after repair and take-down of tongue-lip adhesion. Cleft Palate J. 1988;25(2):151–5.

Freeman MK, Manners JM. Cor pulmonale and the Pierre Robin anomaly. Airway management with a nasopharyngeal tube. Anaesthesia. 1980;35(3):282–6.

Glander K 2nd, Cisneros GJ. Comparison of the craniofacial characteristics of two syndromes associated with the Pierre Robin sequence. Cleft Palate Craniofac J. 1992;29(3):210–9.

Hong P, Bezuhly M, Mark Taylor S, Hart RD, Kearns DB, Corsten G. Tracheostomy versus mandibular distraction osteogenesis in Canadian children with Pierre Robin sequence: a comparative cost analysis. J Otolaryngol Head Neck Surg. 2012;41(3):207–14.

Izumi K, Konczal LL, Mitchell AL, Jones MC. Underlying genetic diagnosis of Pierre Robin sequence: retrospective chart review at two children's hospitals and a systematic literature review. J Pediatr. 2012;160(4):645–50 e2.

Jakobsen LP, Knudsen MA, Lespinasse J, García Ayuso C, Ramos C, Fryns JP. The genetic basis of the Pierre Robin sequence. Cleft Palate Craniofac J. 2006;43:155–9.

Jakobsen LP, Ullman R, Christensen SB, Jensen KE, Molsted K, Henriksen KF, Hansen C, Knudsen MA, Larsen LA, Tommerup N, Tümer Z. Pierre Robin sequence may be caused by dysregulation of SOX9 and KCNJ2. J Med Genet. 2007;44:381–6.

Jarrahy R. Controversies in the management of neonatal micrognathia: to distract or not to distract, that is the question. J Craniofac Surg. 2012;23(1):243–9.

Lidsky ME, Lander TA, Sidman JD. Resolving feeding difficulties with early airway intervention in Pierre Robin sequence. Laryngoscope. 2008;118:120–3.

Luedders DW, Bohlmann MK, Germer U, Axt-Fliedner R, Gembruch U, Weichert J. Fetal micrognathia: objective assessment and associated anomalies on prenatal sonogram. Prenat Diagn. 2011;31(2):146–51.

Macedo EF. Avaliação endoscópica da deglutição com nasofaringolaringoscópio (FEESH) na abordagem da disfagia orofaríngea. In: Castro LPS-RP, Melo JCR, Costa MMB, editors. Tópicos em gastroenterologia: deglutição e disfagia. Rio de Janeiro: Medsi; 2000. p. 71–82.

Marques IL, Barbieri MA, Bettiol H. Etiopathogenesis of isolated Robin sequence. Cleft Palate Craniofac J. 1998;35:517–25.

Marques IL, de Sousa TV, Carneiro AF, Barbieri MA, Bettiol H, Gutierrez MR. Clinical experience with infants with Robin sequence: a prospective study. Cleft Palate Craniofac J. 2001;38:171–8.

Marques IL, Peres SP, Bettiol H, Barbieri MA, Andrea M, Souza L. Growth of children with isolated Robin sequence treated by nasopharyngeal intubation: importance of a hypercaloric diet. Cleft Palate Craniofac. 2004;41:53–8.

Marques IL, Souza TV, Carneiro AF, Peres SP, Barbieri MA, Bettiol H. Seqüência de Robin-Protocolo único de tratamento. J Pediatr. 2005;81:14–22.

Marques IL, Prado-Oliveira R, Leirião VH, Jorge JC, Souza L. Clinical and fiberoptic endoscopic evaluation of swallowing in Robin sequence treated with nasopharyngeal intubation. The importance of feeding facilitating techniques. Cleft Palate-Craniofac J. 2010;47(5):523–9.

Monasterio FO, Molina F, Berlanga F, Lopez ME, Ahumada H, Takenaga RH. Swallowing disorders in Pierre Robin sequence: its correction by distraction. J Craniofac Surg. 2004;15(6):934–41.

Nassar E, Marques IL, Trindade AS Jr, Bettiol H. Feeding–facilitating techniques for the nursing infant with Pierre Robin sequence. Cleft Palate Craniofac J. 2006;43:55–60.

Printzlau A, Andersen M. Pierre Robin sequence in Denmark: aretrospective population-based epidemiological study. Cleft Palate Craniofac J. 2004;41(1):47–52.

Rogers GF, Lim AA, Mulliken JB, Padwa BL. Effect of a syndromic diagnosis on mandibular size and sagittal position in Robin sequence. J Oral Maxillofac Surg. 2009;67(11):2323–31.

Rogers GF, Murthy AS, LaBrie RA, Mulliken JB. The GILLS score: part I. Patient selection for tongue-lip adhesion in Robin sequence. Plast Reconstr Surg. 2011;128(1):243–51.

Salmen ICM. Sequencia de Robin: estudo retrospective dos lactentes internados no HRAC-USP [dissertação]. Bauru: Hospital de Reabilitação de Anomalias Craniofaciais, Universidade de São Paulo; 2011.

Scott AR, Tibesar RJ, Sidman JD. Pierre Robin sequence: evaluation, management, indications for surgery, and pitfalls. Otolaryngol Clin N Am. 2012;45(3):695–710.

Sher AE. Mechanisms of airway obstruction in Robin sequence: implications for treatment. Cleft Palate Craniofac J. 1992;29(3):224–31.

Sher AE, Shprintzen RJ, Thorpy MJ. Endoscopic observations of obstructive sleep apnea in children with anomalous upper airways: predictive and therapeutic value. Int J Pediatr Otorhinolaryngol. 1986;11(2):135–46.

Shprintzen RJ. The implications of the diagnosis of Robin sequence. Cleft Palate Craniofac J. 1992;29(3):205–9.

Singer L, Sidoti EG. Pediatric management of Robin sequence. Cleft Palate Craniofac J. 1992;29:220–3.

Society AT. Cardiorespiratory sleep studies in children. Establishment of normative data and polysomnographic predictors of morbidity. American Thoracic Society. Am J Respir Crit Care Med. 1999;160(4):1381–7.

de Sousa TV, Marques IL, Carneiro AF, Bettiol H, Freitas JA. Nasopharyngoscopy in Robin sequence: clinical and predictive value. Cleft Palate Craniofac J. 2003;40(6):618–23.

Souza TV, Marques IL, Carneiro AF, Bettiol H, Freitas JA. Nasopharyngoscopy in Robin sequence: clinical and predictive value. Cleft Palate Craniofac J. 2003;40(6):618–23.

Spina V, Psillakis JM, Lapa FS, Ferreira MC. Classification of cleft lip and cleft palate. Suggested changes. Rev Hosp Clin Fac Med Sao Paulo. 1972;27(1):5–6.

Vandenplas Y, Goyvaerts H, Helven R, Sacre L. Gastroesophageal reflux, as measured by 24-hour pH monitoring, in 509 healthy infants screened for risk of sudden infant death syndrome. Pediatrics. 1991;88(4):834–40.

Bone Graft in Alveolar Cleft Lip and Palate

16

Nivaldo Alonso, Renato da Silva Freitas, Julia Amundson, and Cassio Eduardo Raposo-Amaral

16.1 Introduction

In the beginning of the twentieth century descriptions about alveolar bone graft were reported but only in the middle of this century it became to be more studied (Daw and Patel 2004). Just after basic principles for bone graft integration were very well established bone graft for alveolar cleft became to be used by surgeon worldwide. Alveolar bone grafting in secondary dentition is considered nowadays the golden standard for cleft patient rehabilitation.

There are two very important aspects for cleft patient rehabilitation. Maxillary arch stabilization and tooth preservation are key points that must be emphasized (Daw and Patel 2004).

In 1972, Boyne and Sands found that marrow cancellous cells could survive in fresh autograft when used in alveolar area if they were well covered by local flaps. They proposed the technique that is still used today for most of the cleft team (Boyne and Sands 1972; Boyne 1974). Abyholm subsequently demonstrated that secondary alveolar bone grafting and orthodontic treatment resulted in space closure in 90% of cleft patients and had no impairment to the facial growth.

N. Alonso, M.D., Ph.D. (✉)
Divisao de Cirurgia Plastica e Queimaduras, Hospital das Clínicas da Faculdade de Medicina da Universidade de São Paulo, São Paulo, Brazil
e-mail: nivalonso@gmail.com

R. da Silva Freitas, M.D., Ph.D.
Plastic Surgery Department at Federal University of Paraná, Curitiba, Parana, Brazil

J. Amundson, B.S.
Miller School of Medicine, University of Miami, Miami, FL 33136, USA

C.E. Raposo-Amaral, M.D., Ph.D.
Institute of Plastic and Craniofacial Surgery, SOBRAPAR Hospital, Campinas, São Paulo 13084-880, Brazil

Universidade de São Paulo, São Paulo, Brazil

They concluded that the optimum age for grafting would be between 9 and 11 years, when the facial sutures involved in the surgical procedure could not be disturbed (Abyholm et al. 1981).

The orthodontic treatment and facial growth analysis have shown the importance of the alveolar bone grafting in the mixed dentition before the canine eruption. Today, it is widely considered an essential step in the treatment process of patients with facial clefts (Eppley and Sadove 2000).

The goals and well-established benefits of alveolar bone grafting for the repair of maxillary defects include the stabilization of the maxillary arch (Skoog 1965; Epstein et al. 1970), the elimination of the oronasal fistula (Jolleys and Robertson 1972), the creation of bone support for permanent tooth eruption, and the reconstruction of the pyriform aperture. As these changes lead to better support for the soft tissues of the nasal base, any patient with a facial cleft is a candidate for alveolar bone grafting (Waite DEK 1980).

There are many possible variations in the extent of the alveolar defect, ranging from only one notch on the incisal side of the alveolar process to large defects with widely separated alveolar segments.

In unilateral clefts, the cleft side is usually named as a minor segment of the maxilla. Due to the lack of continuity and stability, cross-sectional collapse of the jaw is quite common. These patients have crossbite due to the collapsed arch, which is particularly noticeable in the projection of the canine and first premolar on the cleft side. Premaxilla position is also variable, with either normal or rotated alignment. The central incisor adjacent to the cleft is usually rotated and set at an angle. The lateral incisor may be absent (between 10 and 30% absent (da Silva Filho et al. 2013)), but it is often hypoplastic, malformed, or substituted by a supernumerary tooth. Sometimes, the tooth may erupt in the alveolar cleft region, or it may be present in the nasal cavity or palate.

Bilateral clefts also have variable presentations. These clefts may be of different lengths and widths, and are not necessarily symmetrical. The pre-maxilla is usually rotated in relation to the lateral segments due to excessive and uncontrolled growth of the vomer-pre-maxillary suture. The pre-maxilla may also be placed inferiorly (overbite) or aberrantly rotated in the coronal and sagittal planes.

The embryological development of facial processes and primary dental germ occurs simultaneously. Thus, it is not uncommon to have tooth malformation or absence adjacent to the cleft. These teeth can be malformed, misplaced, or missing, as in the agenesis of the lateral incisor, with or without the presence of supernumerary teeth. Moreover, the patient's pattern of deciduous dentition will predict the permanent dentition, although the permanent dentition is more significantly altered.

The objectives of alveolar bone grafting include both functional and aesthetic aspects (Wood et al. 1997). Functional objectives include:

1. Allowing the eruption of permanent tooth (canine) in the grafted area
2. Providing bone support to the teeth adjacent to the cleft
3. Creating a continuous and stable maxillary arch, allowing security in orthodontic mobilization
4. Closing the oronasal fistula
5. Facilitating oral hygiene

The maintenance of the oronasal fistula and chronic nasal regurgitation of fluids usually leads to chronic inflammation of the nasal mucosa with continuous secretions. This can cause significant psychosocial issues.

The aesthetic goals include filling the nostril, restructuring the nasal base, and creating a maxillary arch, all of which contribute to a more satisfactory aesthetic appearance and a more beautiful smile.

Some authors prefer conducting gingivoperiosteoplasty only at the time of primary lip treatment. This creates a cavity that can then be filled with bone created due to the effects of local growth factors (Wood et al. 1997; Cohen et al. 1989). Many studies showed no neo-bone formation or even some studies presented important disturbance in facial growth (Friede and Johanson 1974). Preoperative orthopedic alignment of the teeth is necessary to allow for better visualization of the size of the gap in the maxilla and then provide good reestablishment of the alveolar ridge (Cohen et al. 1993).

Alveolar bone grafting can be performed at different times during facial and dental development. This procedure is called *primary bone grafting* when it is performed on children under 2 years old, and *secondary bone grafting* after this age. Secondary bone grafting can be subdivided into three phases: *early secondary*, when the patient still has its deciduous teeth (between 2 and 5 years old); *transitional secondary*, before the eruption of the definitive canines (between 6 and 12 years); and *late secondary or tertiary*, after the eruption of the canines (after age 12) (Eppley and Sadove 2000; Rosenstein et al. 1991).

The ideal age for alveolar bone grafting still remains in discussion, but most of the cleft centers used the age between 8 and 12 years before the canine eruption as the landmark. The few groups that use primary grafting argue that it both reduces the need for orthognathic surgery and leads to lower rates of cross-jaw collapse, thereby decreasing the time needed for orthodontic upper arch correction (Eppley and Sadove 2000; Rosenstein et al. 1991). Those teams in favor of secondary grafting believe that gingivoperiosteoplasty and primary bone grafting lead to a higher incidence of occlusal changes and maxillary growth deficiencies (Jolleys and Robertson 1972; Friede and Johanson 1974). In addition, they believe that the quality of bone formed or grafted from primary grafting is not suitable for orthodontic restoration.

Most treatment centers believe that the best time for grafting should be based on a combination of factors: tooth development, orthodontic state, no disturbance for facial growth, and good surgical conditions. Of these, tooth development, more than chronological age, should be the main factor when determining the appropriate time for bone grafting. It is widely accepted that bone grafting should be conducted during the initial phase of mixed dentition—after the eruption of the permanent medial incisor but before the final canine eruption. This helps to preserve the largest possible number of adult teeth. At this time—usually around age 9—the sagittal and transverse maxillary growth is complete, and the vertical growth remaining requires the eruption of permanent teeth to occur (Bjork and Skieller 1974). In patients with tooth bud of lateral incisor, bone grafting may be performed earlier, between 7 and 8 years of age, to preserve this tooth.

16.2 Orthodontic Management

The orthopedic approach for maxilla is generally started around 5 years of age. The principle is to allow for better alignment of the upper dental arch and to minimize maxillary collapse.

Prior to bone grafting, the alveolar arches should be aligned. In this sense, it is advisable to place a palatal device to increase the transverse diameter of the maxilla, adjusting it to the lower dental arch. This will facilitate the surgical procedure. However, maxillary expansion can be performed after the alveolar grafting, but with more difficulty, since alveolar continuity was created. It is clear that alveolar grafting without prior orthopedic treatment leads to poor results, with bad bone alignment maintenance, maxillary collapse, and posterior crossbite (Vlachos 1996) (Fig. 16.1).

Bone grafting surgery is only postponed in the case of bad dental conditions such as cavities and gingivitis. These must be treated before surgery to minimize the risk

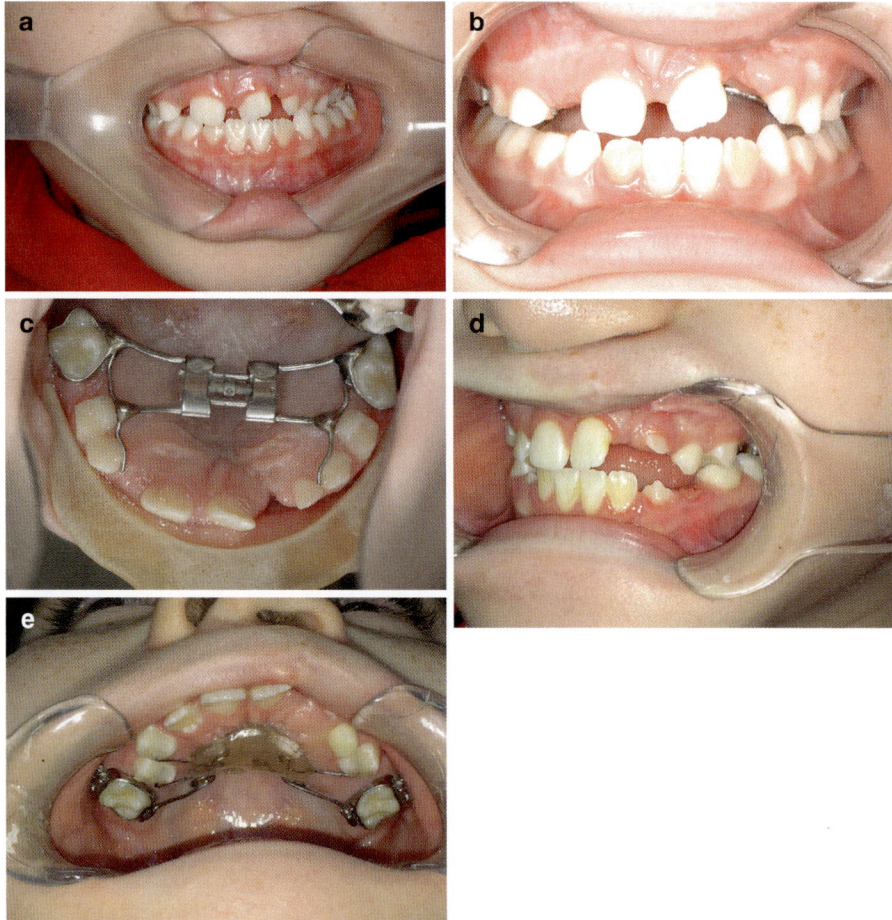

Fig. 16.1 Preorthodontic treatment before and after ABG. (**a**) Unilateral left cleft, (**b**) maxilla expansion, (**c**) intraoral view of the device, (**d**) after expansion with ABG, (**e**) contention after ABG and maxillar expansion

of postoperative infections and subsequent bone grafting failure. If dental extraction is required, it should be done 8 weeks prior to grafting to provide adequate time for the manipulated alveolar region to heal.

The orthodontist has a fundamental role in the treatment of these patients, with different techniques necessary during different stages of facial growth. In childhood, maxillary orthopedics may be necessary to improve arch alignment by shaping the maxillary arch. After alveolar grafting, the orthodontist continues treatment by correcting the remaining crossbites, aligning or rotating the incisors, and improving function and dental aesthetics.

16.3 Selection of Bone Donor Site

Initially, surgeons utilized cortical bone blocks from the iliac and ribs, with the main goal of horizontal stabilization of the jaw to prevent jaw collapse and crossbite. Subsequently, however, it was noticed that using cancellous bone would lead to better results because it would be more readily incorporated into adjacent bone (Boyne and Sands 1972; Boyne 1974). Cancellous bone provides more uniform grafting integration and allows more effective tooth eruption. The most commonly used local donor sites are now the iliac crest (Abyholm et al. 1981) and the cranium (Abyholm et al. 1981; Kalaaji et al. 1994). The iliac crest contains a large amount of bone marrow and can be collected simultaneously with the grafting procedure. Using the cranium enables retrieval of a large amount of bone from the same embryological lineage as the transplant site (membranous bone), and it is virtually painless; however, this bone needs to be crushed. There are also centers using tibial grafts, rib, and chin (Sindet-Pedersen and Enemark 1990; Witsenburg et al. 1990).

The current gold standard for cellular grafting is the bone marrow collected from the iliac crest. This is because the iliac crest provides the greatest amount of bone marrow out of all possible donor sites and has a success rate greater than 80% (Forte et al. 2012). The biggest criticism of the use of the crest is out of concern for morbidity of the donor site, which can be minimized by limiting the detachment of muscle and periosteum adjacent to the bone marrow collection site (Rudman 1997) (Fig. 16.2).

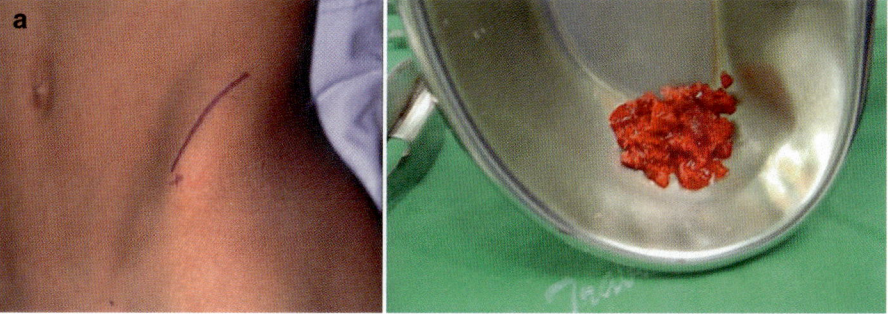

Fig. 16.2 Bone donor-site iliac crest. (**a**) Position of the incision. (**b**) Internal cortical of ilium bone. (**c**) General view of donor site

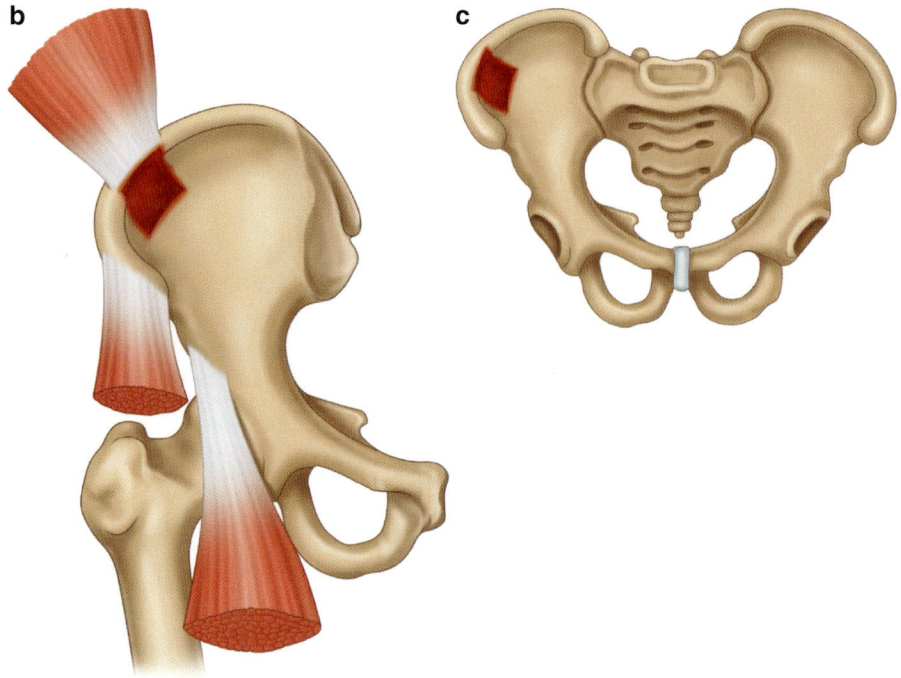

Fig. 16.2 (continued)

Some bone substitutes such as bone morphogenetic protein (BMP) are also in use today. BMP is a member of the transforming growth factor (TGF) group, which stimulates cells—osteocytes—to multiply and produce bone. These bone substitutes are placed in the cleft area, which is then closed through periosteoplasty (Alonso et al. 2010). Although bone substitutes have led to excellent results, their high cost still restricts use.

16.4 Surgical Technique

Patients undergo general anesthesia with local anesthetic using a solution of saline, bupivacaine, and epinephrine in a dilution of 1:120,000 U.

The surgical procedure is conducted using the technique described by Boyne and Sands (1972). The general principle is to manufacture a tissue layer that can fully cover the graft, therefore avoiding its exposure to the oral cavity (Fig. 16.3).

After the incision on the margins of the alveolar cleft, the mucoperiosteous flaps are elevated to the anterior alveolar surface, on the vestibular side of the gingivolabial mucosa. The lateral incision extends into the vestibule on the upper projection of the permanent molars, making that the flap's point of rotation, with an incision parallel to the teeth roots. The next step is to proceed to broad detachment and

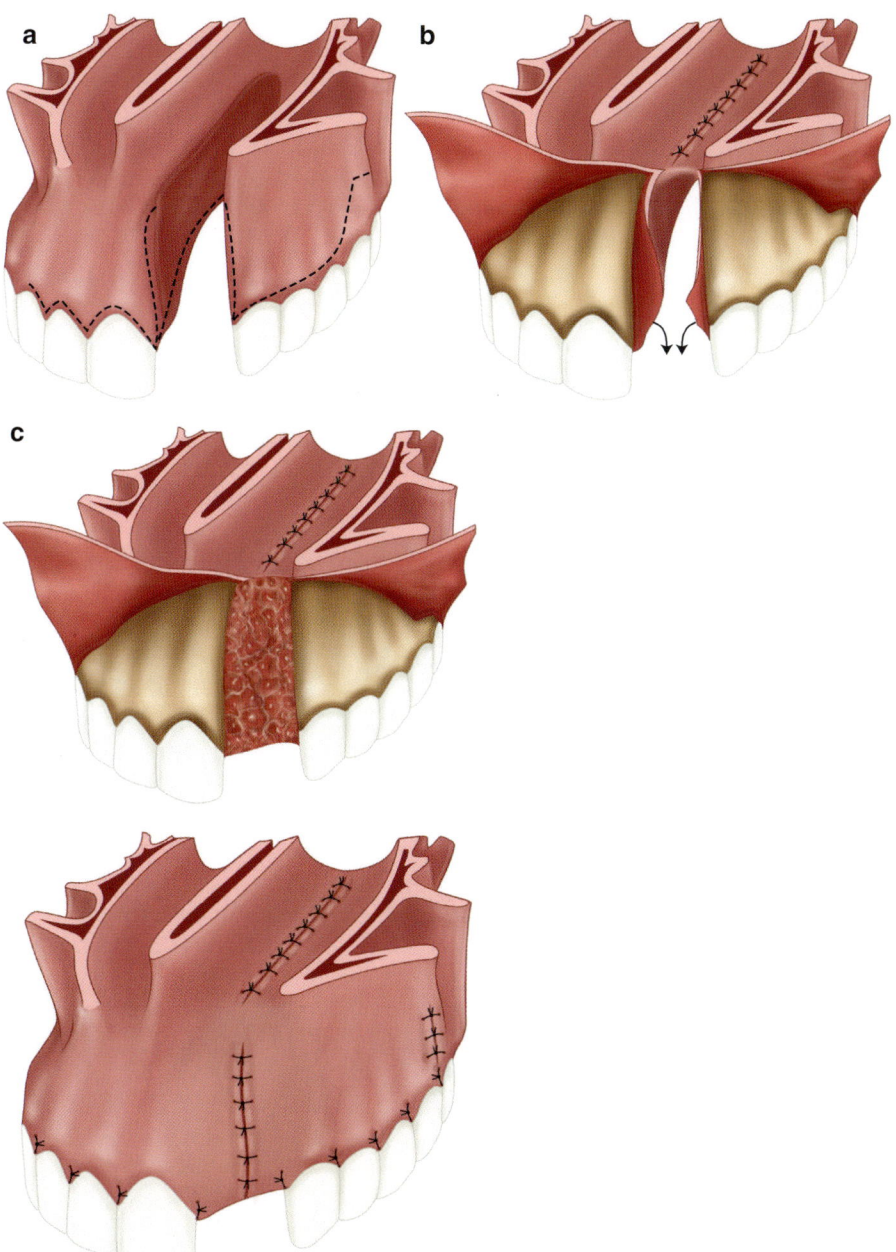

Fig. 16.3 Alveolar bone grafting technique. (**a**) Demarcation of the incision oral and nasal site. (**b**) Three flaps raised. (**c**) Closure of the flap with bone graft chips

maxilla exposure in the anterior region with the nostril opening. The cleft edges are elevated, separating the alveolar flaps laterally and the septum medially.

These flaps should be divided on each side near the hard palate to create two flaps to close the nasal floor superiorly, and two flaps to close the palatal mucosa inferiorly. This creates a space surrounded by alveolar bone on each side, above and below, with flaps separating the nasal and oral cavities. The iliac crest bone graft is then placed through the anterior opening.

The suture of gingival periosteal flap should be performed without tension through periosteal incision inside the flap side, allowing its medial rotation and advancement.

With the patient positioned supine with a pad in the gluteal region to raise the iliac spine and anterior superior iliac crest, a 4-cm incision is made in a lateral line parallel to iliac crest. It is important to avoid the area just below the anterior superior iliac spine, through which the lateral femoral cutaneous nerve traverses. With an electric cautery, dissect the subcutaneous plane, fascia, muscle, and periosteum overlying the iliac crest. Care must be taken in children, in whom there is cartilage in the upper portion of the iliac crest. In these cases, the osteotomy is performed more internally, below the growth plate. Detachment of periosteum on the internal side of the crest is performed to allow access to the cortical surface. An osteotome is used to make a window into the cortical bone, exposing the bone marrow that can then be collected with curettes and stored in a sterile tank with saline.

After removing a sufficient amount of bone graft, hemostasis should be achieved using bone wax and reposition the cortical bone. The fascial planes are closed with continuous suture with 3.0 polygalactin stitches and the subcutaneous and deep dermis with interrupted sutures. The superficial skin is closed with intradermal continuous suture of 4.0 polygalactin.

Little importance was initially given to planning the mucoperiosteal flap that would be used to cover the grafted bone but this is crucial for the final functional result (Backdahl 1961). Histologically, the masticatory mucosa is composed of a keratinized squamous epithelium layer and a dense, firm lamina propria layer with static ligaments towards the alveolar bone and tooth roots. This structure provides support and protects the masticatory apparatus from minor damage and bacterial contamination (Friede and Johanson 1974).

The mucoperiosteal flaps are the best option for covering bone grafts. These flaps allow cleft reconstruction using tissue that is similar to the adjacent structures in terms of color, texture, and strength. Moreover, the tooth can then erupt through keratinized tissue, which does not occur if the tissue is only composed of mucosa (Cohen et al. 1989).

In the first week after surgery, patients are placed on a cold liquefied diet and receive analgesics and symptomatic medication. After 2 weeks, patients can be advanced to a soft diet for 4 weeks. They are advised to avoid biting with their incisors for 4 weeks. Oral hygiene is encouraged after each meal by rinsing their mouths with 0.12% chlorohexidine gluconate solution. Due to the graft withdrawal from the iliac crest, patients are suspended from physical activities for 2 months. Stitches on the donor area are removed about 7 days after surgery (Fig. 16.4).

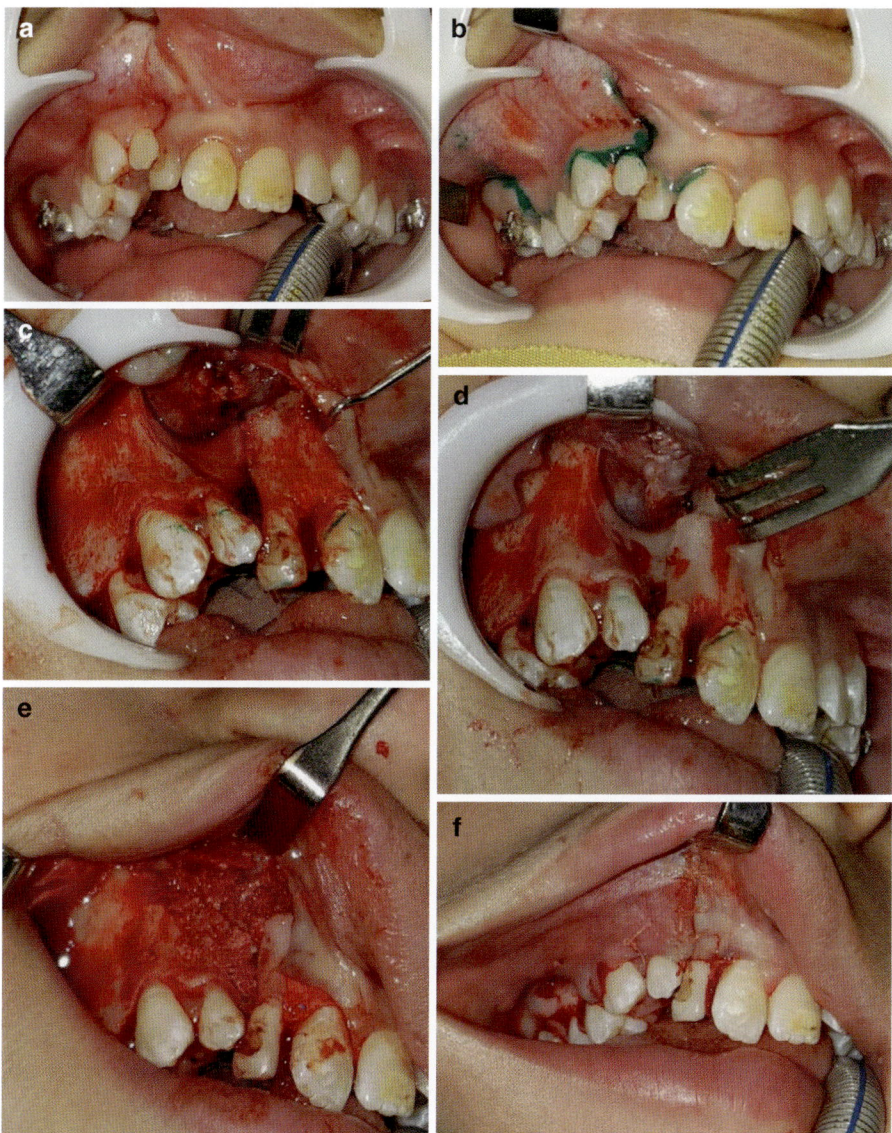

Fig. 16.4 Intraoperative steps of ABG surgery. (**a**) Right alveolar cleft, (**b**) demarcation of gingival flap, (**c**) bone cleft exposed, (**d**) closure of nasal lining, (**e**) medullary bone chips in the defect, (**f**) final aspects of the flap rotation

Outpatient follow-up consists of weekly revaluations in the first month. In each visit, patients are assessed for pain, signs of fever, edema, and erythema beyond the mucosa, and potential graft exposure due to evolution of the scar.

After the first month, reassessments should be made in 3 months to monitor mucogingival healing and tooth eruption. After 3 months, patients can resume periodic evaluations with the orthodontic team (Fig. 16.5).

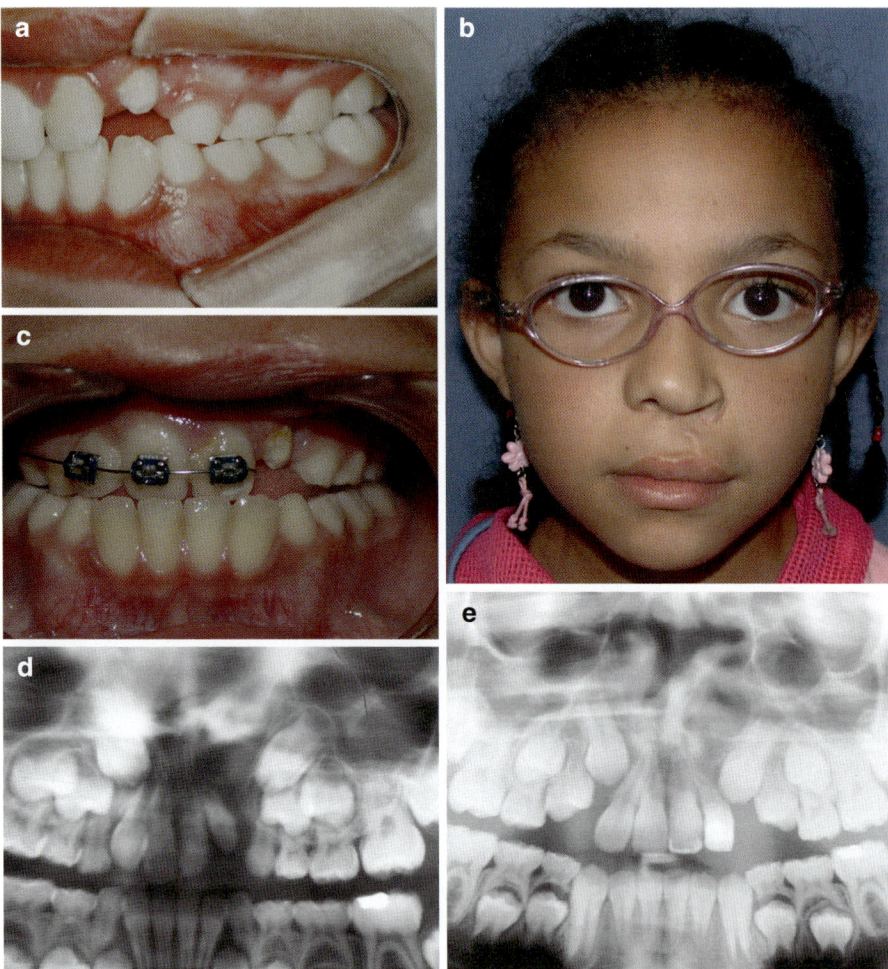

Fig. 16.5 Long-term outcomes of ABG with images. (**a**) Left alveolar cleft at mixed dentition, (**b**) cleft patient, (**c**) orthodontic preparation for ABG, (**d**) panorex at 7 years old, (**e**) panorex after ABG, (**f**) panorex after ABG with canine in position, (**g**) panorex 8 years late, (**h**) final occlusion at 16 years old, (**i**) CT scan at 17 years old, (**j**) final facial appearance

16 Bone Graft in Alveolar Cleft Lip and Palate

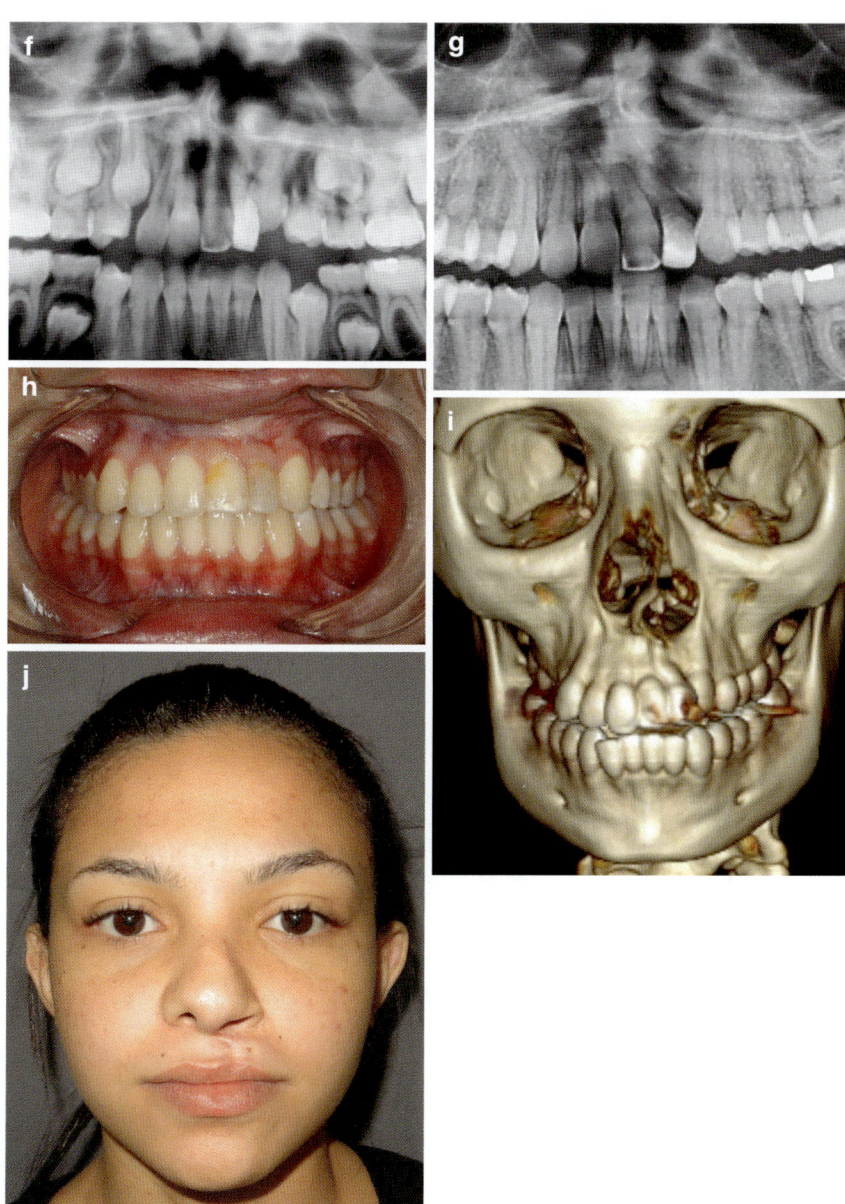

Fig. 16.5 (continued)

However, some authors preferred to use minimally invasive techniques for iliac bone graft harvesting. Consistently lower morbidity (e.g., donor-site pain and gait disorders) in patients who underwent closed techniques has been shown by our group (SOBRAPAR) and others (Sharma et al. 2011; McCanny and Roberts-Harry 1998; Raposo-Amaral et al. 2015).

Surgery using minimally invasive techniques has been performed with patients in the supine position under general anesthesia. Two techniques have been used to harvest medullar bone for alveolar grafting. The techniques varied by the extent of periosteal elevation and diameter of the extractor devices. Incision of 1.5 to 2 cm and subcutaneous undermining allowed the inclusion of bone extractor on the surface of the iliac crest with minimal periosteal flap elevation. Following, a periosteal flap elevation (or not) was preceded until at least 4 cm deep from the most superficial point of the anterior-superior iliac crest where the presence of bone could be detected by subtle pressure of the instrument against the bone structure. Rotational movements of the extractor were performed until the absence of resistance and then a block of cancellous bone was obtained to be used in the alveolar region (Raposo-Amaral et al. 2015) (Fig. 16.6).

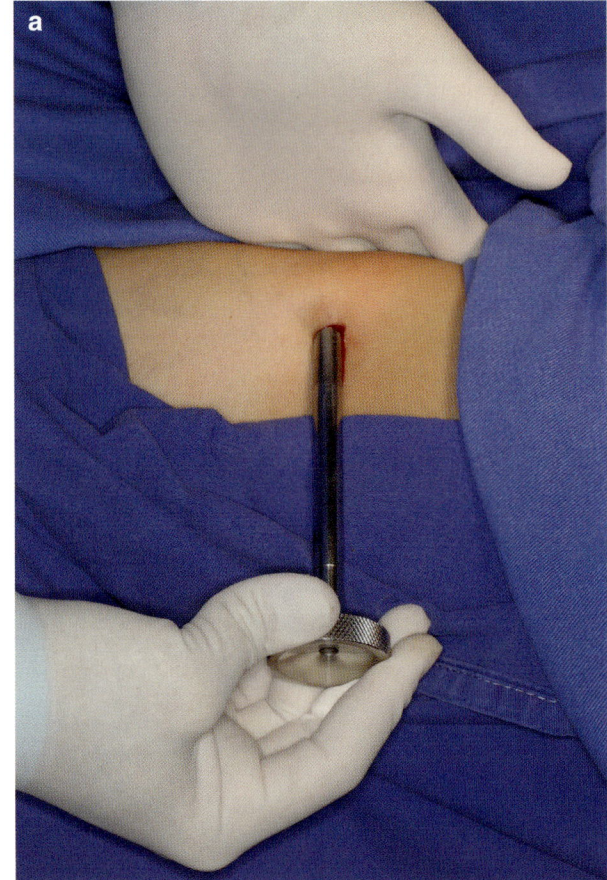

Fig. 16.6 Minimal invasive bone grafting harvesting. (**a**) Cylinder bone extractor devices. (**a**) Both devices present a metallic cylindrical rod with a cutting edge and the other edge with "T" or "circle" cable that allows firm grip during iliac crest bone graft harvesting. (**b**) Note the differences in diameter (5 mm [*left*] and 8 mm [*right*]). (**b**) Minimal incision marked at iliac crest and rotational movements of the extractor were performed until the absence of resistance and then a block of cancellous bone was obtained. (**c**) The harvested bone inside the metallic cylindrical rod. Note that 3–5 blocks of bone can be easily removed

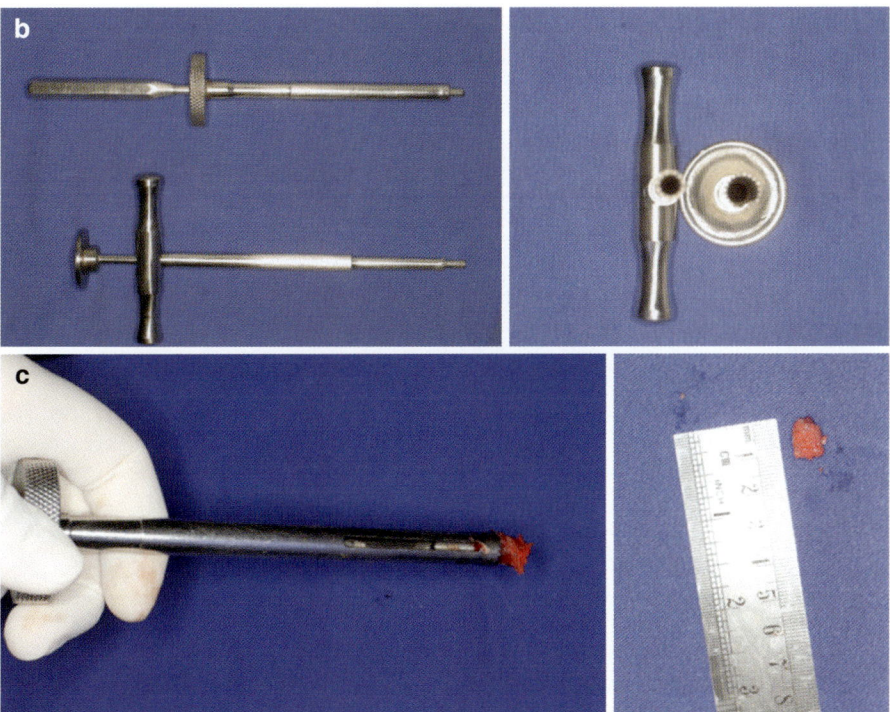

Fig. 16.6 (continued)

In Brazil, as spending of specialized centers in the multidisciplinary management of craniofacial deformities has been financed only partially (50–60% of overall costs) by the Unified Health System (SUS; Ministry of Health, Brazil), any factors that may impact the overall costs of treatment of cleft patients should be considered when choosing between different surgical devices. Thus, we have adopted both surgical devices due to low financial cost to obtain and maintain the materials, if compared, for example, to the industrial electrical devices that have greater financial cost (Raposo-Amaral and Raposo-Amaral 2012).

16.5 Future Perspectives

Tissue engineering has had significant advancements in protein factors with the potential to induce osteogenesis and inhibition in order to maximize the action of BMPs. Studies on stem cells with osteogenic potential from bone marrow or pluripotent cells harvested by liposuction and other sources as muscle of the elevator *palatine* are also promising in the future acquisition of techniques for bone reconstruction in patients with craniofacial deformities (Raposo-Amaral et al. 2014; Freihofer et al. 1993) (Fig. 16.7).

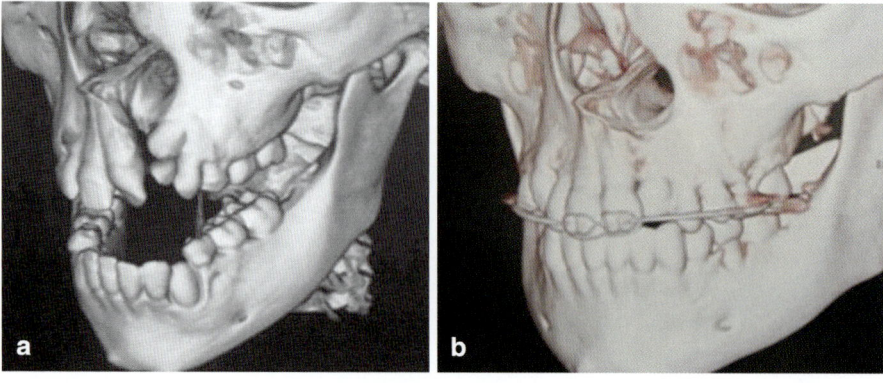

Fig. 16.7 Future bone substitutes. (**a**) Preoperative computerized tomography imaging of the craniofacial skeleton of a patient with complete unilateral cleft lip and palate. (**b**) Postoperative computerized tomography imaging of the craniofacial skeleton after alveolar reconstruction utilizing BMP

References

Abyholm FE, Bergland O, Semb G. Secondary bone grafting of alveolar clefts. A surgical/orthodontic treatment enabling a non-prosthodontic rehabilitation in cleft lip and palate patients. Scand J Plast Reconstr Surg. 1981;15(2):127–40.

Alonso N, Tanikawa DY, Freitas Rda S, Canan L Jr, Ozawa TO, Rocha DL. Evaluation of maxillary alveolar reconstruction using a resorbable collagen sponge with recombinant human bone morphogenetic protein-2 in cleft lip and palate patients. Tissue Eng Part C Methods. 2010;16(5):1183–9.

Backdahl M. Nordinke. Replacement of the maxillary bone defect in cleft palate. A new procedure. Acta Chir Scand. 1961;122:131–7.

Bjork A, Skieller V. Growth in width of the maxilla studied by the implant method. Scand J Plast Reconstr Surg. 1974;8(1–2):26–33.

Boyne PJ. Use of marrow-cancellous bone grafts in maxillary alveolar and palatal clefts. J Dent Res. 1974;53(4):821–4.

Boyne PJ, Sands NR. Secondary bone grafting of residual alveolar and palatal clefts. J Oral Surg. 1972;30(2):87–92.

Cohen M, Figueroa AA, Aduss H. The role of gingival mucoperiosteal flaps in the repair of alveolar clefts. Plast Reconstr Surg. 1989;83(5):812–9.

Cohen M, Polley JW, Figueroa AA. Secondary (intermediate) alveolar bone grafting. Clin Plast Surg. 1993;20(4):691–705.

Daw JL Jr, Patel PK. Management of alveolar clefts. Clin Plast Surg. 2004;31(2):303–13.

Eppley BL, Sadove AM. Management of alveolar cleft bone grafting--state of the art. Cleft Palate Craniofac J. 2000;37(3):229–33.

Epstein LI, Davis WB, Thompson LW. Delayed bone grafting in cleft palate patients. Plast Reconstr Surg. 1970;46(4):363–7.

Forte AJ, da Silva FR, Alonso N. Use of three-dimensional computed tomography to classify filling of alveolar bone grafting. Plast Surg Int. 2012;2012:259419.

Freihofer HP, Borstlap WA, Kuijpers-Jagtman AM, Voorsmit RA, van Damme PA, Heidbuchel KL, et al. Timing and transplant materials for closure of alveolar clefts. A clinical comparison of 296 cases. J Craniomaxillofac Surg. 1993;21(4):143–8.

Friede H, Johanson B. A follow-up study of cleft children treated with primary bone grafting. 1. Orthodontic aspects. Scand J Plast Reconstr Surg. 1974;8(1–2):88–103.

Jolleys A, Robertson NR. A study of the effects of early bone-grafting in complete clefts of the lip and palate--five year study. Br J Plast Surg. 1972;25(3):229–37.

Kalaaji A, Lilja J, Friede H. Bone grafting at the stage of mixed and permanent dentition in patients with clefts of the lip and primary palate. Plast Reconstr Surg. 1994;93(4):690–6.

McCanny CM, Roberts-Harry DP. A comparison of two different bone-harvesting techniques for secondary alveolar bone grafting in patients with cleft lip and palate. Cleft Palate Craniofac J. 1998;35(5):442–6.

Raposo-Amaral CE, Raposo-Amaral CA. Changing face of cleft care: specialized centers in developing countries. J Craniofac Surg. 2012;23(1):206–9.

Raposo-Amaral CE, Bueno DF, Almeida AB, Jorgetti V, Costa CC, Gouveia CH, et al. Is bone transplantation the gold standard for repair of alveolar bone defects? J Tissue Eng. 2014;5:2041731413519352.

Raposo-Amaral CA, Denadai R, Chammas DZ, Marques FF, Pinho AS, Roberto WM, et al. Cleft patient-reported postoperative donor site pain following alveolar autologous iliac crest bone grafting: comparing two minimally invasive harvesting techniques. J Craniofac Surg. 2015;26(7):2099–103.

Rosenstein S, Dado DV, Kernahan D, Griffith BH, Grasseschi M. The case for early bone grafting in cleft lip and palate: a second report. Plast Reconstr Surg. 1991;87(4):644–54. discussion 55-6

Rudman RA. Prospective evaluation of morbidity associated with iliac crest harvest for alveolar cleft grafting. J Oral Maxillofac Surg. 1997;55(3):219–23. discussion 23-4

Sharma S, Schneider LF, Barr J, Aarabi S, Chibbaro P, Grayson B, et al. Comparison of minimally invasive versus conventional open harvesting techniques for iliac bone graft in secondary alveolar cleft patients. Plast Reconstr Surg. 2011;128(2):485–91.

da Silva Filho OG, Ozawa TO, Bachega C, Bachega MA. Reconstruction of alveolar cleft with allogenous bone graft: clinical considerations. Dental Press J Orthod. 2013;18(6):138–47.

Sindet-Pedersen S, Enemark H. Reconstruction of alveolar clefts with mandibular or iliac crest bone grafts: a comparative study. J Oral Maxillofac Surg. 1990;48(6):554–8. discussion 9-60

Skoog T. The Management of the Bilateral Cleft of the primary palate (lip and alveolus). Ii. Bone grafting. Plast Reconstr Surg. 1965;35:140–7.

Vlachos CC. Orthodontic treatment for the cleft palate patient. Semin Orthod. 1996;2(3):197–204.

Waite DEK RB. Residual alveolar and palatal clefts. In: Bell WHP WR, White RP, editors. Correction of Dentofacial deformities. 1. Philadelphia USA: W.B. Saunders; 1980. p. 1329–67.

Witsenburg B, Peter H, Freihofer M. Autogenous rib graft for reconstruction of alveolar bone defects in cleft patients. Long-term follow-up results. J Craniomaxillofac Surg. 1990;18(2):55–62.

Wood RJ, Grayson BH, Cutting CB. Gingivoperiosteoplasty and midfacial growth. Cleft Palate Craniofac J. 1997;34(1):17–20.

Bone Substitute: Alveolar Bone Grafting (ABG) with rhBMP-2 (Recombinant Bone Morphogenic Protein-2)

Nivaldo Alonso and Julia Amundson

Alveolar bone grafting was first introduced to Brazil by the Bauru Cleft Team in 1993, brought from Oslo, Norway (Abyholm et al. 1981a). Since that time, the use of autologous bone grafting harvested from the iliac crest using Boyne's technique has become the gold standard for the rehabilitation of the vast majority of cleft patients worldwide (Boyne and Sands 1972). Secondary alveolar bone grafting is ideally performed at 8–10 years of age, when dental development is finishing and the canine is partially formed, with a root of at least 2/3 of final size, ready to erupt into the maxilla. Preoperatively, the use of transverse maxillary expansion and orthodontics for dental alignment facilitates greatly the alveolar bone grafting procedure (Abyholm et al. 1981a, b).

As this procedure is often performed in children under 10 years of age, alternatives to the use of an iliac crest donor site must be considered. Complications at the donor site are quite common with incidence rates reported to be between 2.5 and 40%, ranging from surgical site infection to pain (Ochs 1996; Hall and Posnick 1983; Daw and Patel 2004; Clarke et al. 2015). Beyond the risk of surgical complications, there is also a risk of encountering a lack of sufficient bone for grafting, and a need for secondary and tertiary intervention in the future (David et al. 2005). Patient's parents are always very concerned when the necessity of a donor site is mentioned for children in this age group. Scars and pain are the main concern for then.

Many studies have evaluated possible alternatives to bone substitution and have suggested the use of stem cells, tricalcium phosphate, and bovine bone among others, especially useful when there isn't a sufficient donor site to be harvested. These

---

N. Alonso, M.D., Ph.D. (✉)
Divisao de Cirurgia Plastica e Queimaduras, Hospital das Clínicas da Faculdade de Medicina da Universidade de São Paulo, São Paulo, Brazil
e-mail: nivalonso@gmail.com

J. Amundson, B.S.
Miller School of Medicine, University of Miami, Miami, FL 33136, USA
e-mail: jamundson2@gmail.com

alternatives show promise for the future but raise many concerns regarding the quality of newly formed bone, mainly in children (Raposo-Amaral et al. 2014; de Mendonca et al. 2008; Bueno et al. 2009).

Since 1965 when M. Urist first described a new protein from the family of growth factors that could induce bone formation many improvements in bone healing have happened. Just because this protein had the ability to direct the formation of bone from neighboring cells many researchers felt that would be the solution for bone substitution in the future (Urist 1965). The very first use in clinical cases was done in tibial nonunion and spinal fusions in 2001and 2002 (Baskin et al. 2003; Boden et al. 2000). In maxillofacial defects the approval of FDA occurred in 2007 with many restrictions (Carstens et al. 2005a, b; Chin et al. 2005).

Studies evaluating the use of recombinant bone morphogenic protein 2 (rhBMP-2) for cleft patients in Brazil began in 2008, based off of previous work done by Chin et al. (2005), Carstens et al. (2005a, b).

Initially described by Chin et al., rhBMP-2 was used (Carstens et al. 2005a, b; Chin et al. 2005) at very early age replacing alveolar bone graft at mixed dentition. Our protocol started as was described by Boyne and Sands (1972) ensuring that any failure of BMP-2 implantation could be followed by an ABG. At the Hospital das Clinicas, University of São Paulo Medical School, a prospective randomized study was performed with eight patients, comparing rhBMP-2 and ABG. The methodology to compare both groups was radiologic and clinical evaluation of the patients (Fig. 17.1).

CT scan was taken pre- and 1 year postoperative, and bone volume and alveolar height were measured. On clinical evaluation, complication in donor site, pain and infection, and hospital stay were used for final comparison. The canine eruption and correction of oronasal fistula were compared. The final results after 1 year showed no significant differences with respect to the three primary outcomes of interest: quality and quantity of newly formed bone, tooth eruption, and complications related to rhBMP-2 (Alonso et al. 2010). Canan et al. presented a comparative study among rhBMP-2, ABG, and gingivoperiosteoplasty and found better performance of rhBMP-2 when the bone volume was evaluated (Canan et al. 2012) (Fig. 17.2).

Beginning in 2010, the cost-effectiveness of rhBMP-2 was studied in 23 consecutive patients operated on with the same technique. These patients included unilateral cleft, bilateral cleft, secondary, and tertiary alveolar bone grafting patients. Differences were found with regard to late postoperative edema, which was dose dependent (Leal et al. 2015) (Fig. 17.3).

Leal et al. found late facial edema higher in rhBMP-2 than ABG in 150 patients (Leal et al. 2015).

At 8-year follow-up, no major complications have been recorded. Recent long-term evaluation is being done to evaluate the cost-effectiveness and the rate of success of BMP-2 maxillary alveolar implants in cleft patients. Interim results show high-quality neo-bone formation, elimination of the need for a donor site, a shorter hospitalization, less operative time, and fewer long-term problems in rhBMP-2 patients compared to ABG patients (Lima Junior 2014).

Repair of maxillary cleft is important for final cosmetic outcomes in cleft lip and palate patients, and patients with defects in their maxillary alveolar bone will often

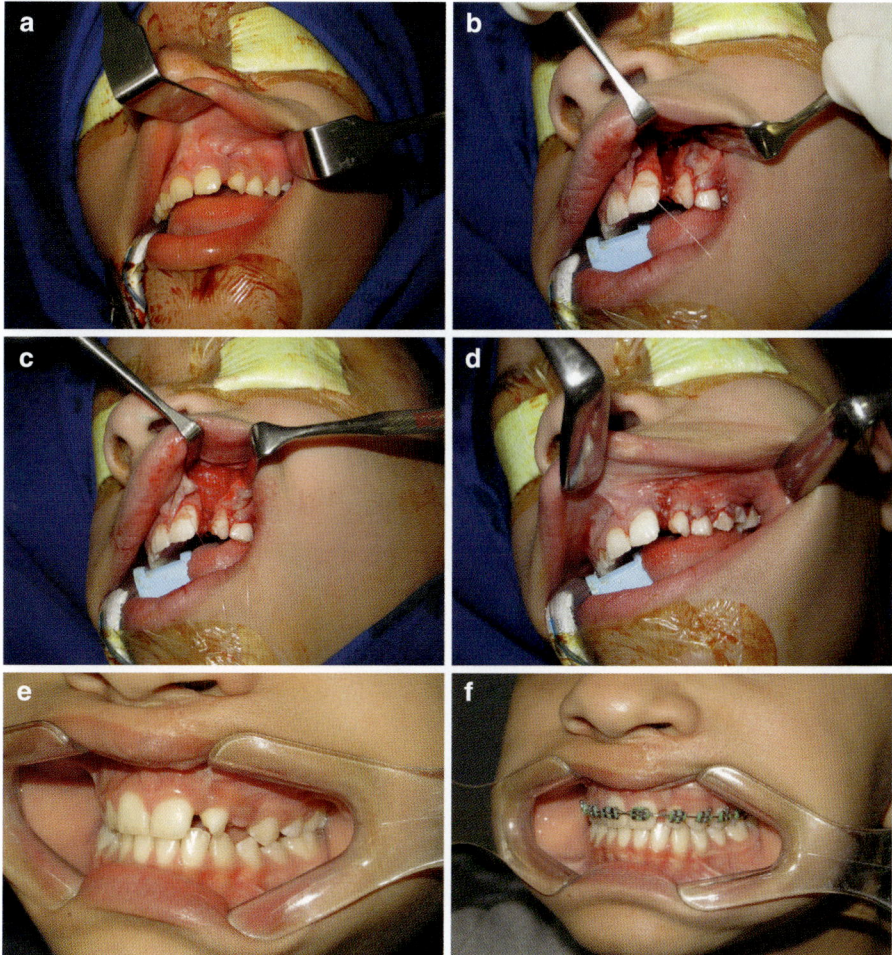

Fig. 17.1 Left unilateral cleft patient age of mixed dentition 10 years old. (**a**) Intraoperative view of the cleft, (**b**) gingivoperiosteal flap raised and nasal mucosa sutured, (**c**) rbBMP-2 with collagen sponge in place without any fixation, (**d**) oral flap in place final suture, (**e**) 6 months after surgery, (**f**) permanent canine irrupted and orthodontic treatment started, (**g**) final dental occlusion 4 years after ABG

Fig. 17.1 (continued)

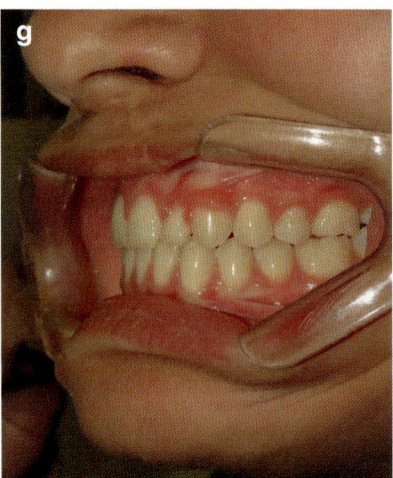

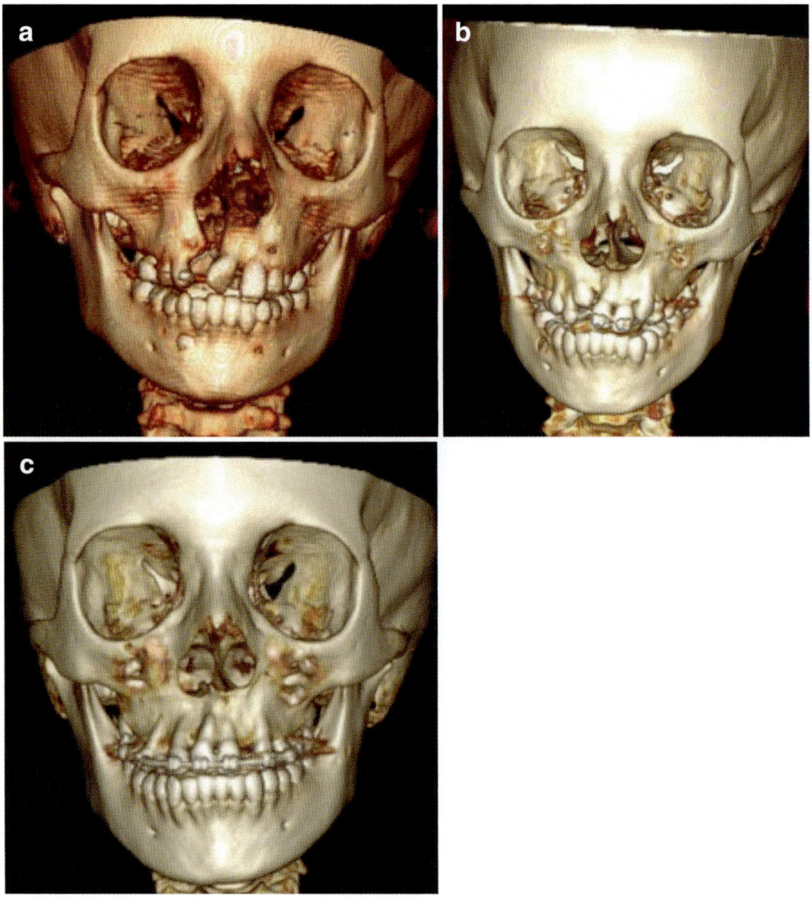

Fig. 17.2 Right unilateral cleft patient before canine eruption. (**a**) CT scan preoperative, (**b**) CT scan during canine eruption, (**c**) CT scan at the end of eruption

Fig. 17.3 At 5 days PO large facial edema

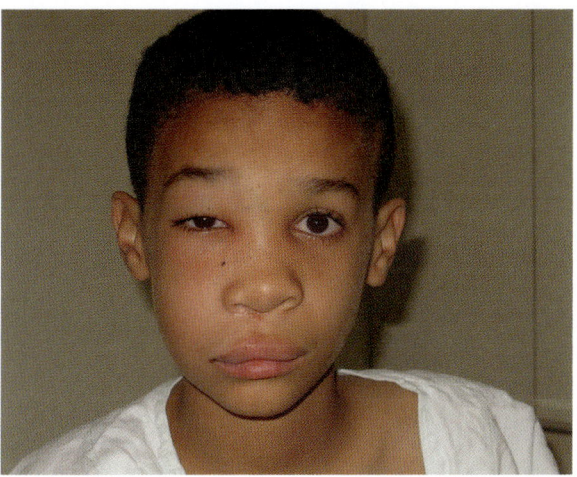

come in requesting rhinoplasty. If rhinoplasty is performed without first correcting the bony defect, the patient will continue to return at intervals ranging from months to years requesting follow-up rhinoplasty. A preferred sequence is to first correct the alveolar maxillary defect using either an ABG or an rhBMP-2, and then perform a staged rhinoplasty. Several studies at our institution have shown no difference in nasal symmetry and overall cosmetic outcomes between ABG and rhBMP-2 for maxillary cleft repair (Alonso et al. 2014; Raposo-Amaral et al. 2015, 2016).

Bone donor site in children will be always a great challenge not just for lack of available bone but also for the complications related to its local harvesting. New bone substitutes have very good perspectives with new tissue engineering technique associated with genetic stem cell studies (Bueno et al. 2009; Tissiani and Alonso 2016; Tanikawa et al. 2013).

References

Abyholm FE, Bergland O, Semb G. Secondary bone grafting of alveolar clefts. A surgical/orthodontic treatment enabling a non-prosthodontic rehabilitation in cleft lip and palate patients. Scand J Plast Reconstr Surg. 1981a;15(2):127–40.

Abyholm FE, Borchgrevink HC, Eskeland G. Cleft lip and palate in Norway. III. Surgical treatment of CLP patients in Oslo 1954-75. Scand J Plast Reconstr Surg. 1981b;15(1):15–28.

Alonso N, Tanikawa DY, Freitas Rda S, Canan L Jr, Ozawa TO, Rocha DL. Evaluation of maxillary alveolar reconstruction using a resorbable collagen sponge with recombinant human bone morphogenetic protein-2 in cleft lip and palate patients. Tissue Eng Part C Methods. 2010;16(5):1183–9.

Alonso N, Risso GH, Denadai R, Raposo-Amaral CE. Effect of maxillary alveolar reconstruction on nasal symmetry of cleft lip and palate patients: a study comparing iliac crest bone graft and recombinant human bone morphogenetic protein-2. J Plast Reconstr Aesthet Surg. 2014;67(9):1201–8.

Baskin DS, Ryan P, Sonntag V, Westmark R, Widmayer MA. A prospective, randomized, controlled cervical fusion study using recombinant human bone morphogenetic protein-2 with the CORNERSTONE-SR allograft ring and the ATLANTIS anterior cervical plate. Spine (Phila Pa 1976). 2003;28(12):1219–24. discussion 25

Boden SD, Zdeblick TA, Sandhu HS, Heim SE. The use of rhBMP-2 in interbody fusion cages. Definitive evidence of osteoinduction in humans: a preliminary report. Spine (Phila Pa 1976). 2000;25(3):376–81.

Boyne PJ, Sands NR. Secondary bone grafting of residual alveolar and palatal clefts. J Oral Surg. 1972;30(2):87–92.

Bueno DF, Kerkis I, Costa AM, Martins MT, Kobayashi GS, Zucconi E, et al. New source of muscle-derived stem cells with potential for alveolar bone reconstruction in cleft lip and/or palate patients. Tissue Eng Part A. 2009;15(2):427–35.

Canan LW Jr, da Silva FR, Alonso N, Tanikawa DY, Rocha DL, Coelho JC. Human bone morphogenetic protein-2 use for maxillary reconstruction in cleft lip and palate patients. J Craniofac Surg. 2012;23(6):1627–33.

Carstens MH, Chin M, Li XJ. In situ osteogenesis: regeneration of 10-cm mandibular defect in porcine model using recombinant human bone morphogenetic protein-2 (rhBMP-2) and Helistat absorbable collagen sponge. J Craniofac Surg. 2005a;16(6):1033–42.

Carstens MH, Chin M, Ng T, Tom WK. Reconstruction of #7 facial cleft with distraction-assisted in situ osteogenesis (DISO): role of recombinant human bone morphogenetic protein-2 with Helistat-activated collagen implant. J Craniofac Surg. 2005b;16(6):1023–32.

Chin M, Ng T, Tom WK, Carstens M. Repair of alveolar clefts with recombinant human bone morphogenetic protein (rhBMP-2) in patients with clefts. J Craniofac Surg. 2005;16(5):778–89.

Clarke A, Flowers MJ, Davies AG, Fernandes J, Jones S. Morbidity associated with anterior iliac crest bone graft harvesting in children undergoing orthopaedic surgery: a prospective review. J Child Orthop. 2015;9(5):411–6.

David L, Argenta L, Fisher D. Hydroxyapatite cement in pediatric craniofacial reconstruction. J Craniofac Surg. 2005;16(1):129–33.

Daw JL Jr, Patel PK. Management of alveolar clefts. Clin Plast Surg. 2004;31(2):303–13.

Hall HD, Posnick JC. Early results of secondary bone grafts in 106 alveolar clefts. J Oral Maxillofac Surg. 1983;41(5):289–94.

Leal CR, Calvo AM, de Souza Faco RA, da Cunha Bastos Junior JC, Yaedu RY, da Silva Dalben G, et al. Evolution of postoperative edema in alveolar graft performed with bone morphogenetic protein (rhBMP-2). Cleft Palate Craniofac J. 2015;52(5):e168–75.

Lima Junior JEAN. O uso de rhBMP-2 para enxerto osseo alveolar em fissurados. Relação custo efetividade. 51 Congresso Brasileiro de Cirurgia Plastic. Bahia, Brasil; 2014.

de Mendonca CA, Bueno DF, Martins MT, Kerkis I, Kerkis A, Fanganiello RD, et al. Reconstruction of large cranial defects in nonimmunosuppressed experimental design with human dental pulp stem cells. J Craniofac Surg. 2008;19(1):204–10.

Ochs MW. Alveolar cleft bone grafting (part II): secondary bone grafting. J Oral Maxillofac Surg. 1996;54(1):83–8.

Raposo-Amaral CE, Bueno DF, Almeida AB, Jorgetti V, Costa CC, Gouveia CH, et al. Is bone transplantation the gold standard for repair of alveolar bone defects? J Tissue Eng. 2014;5:2041731413519352.

Raposo-Amaral CE, Denadai R, Alonso N. Three-dimensional changes of maxilla after secondary alveolar cleft repair: differences between rhBMP-2 and autologous iliac crest bone grafting. Plast Reconstr Surg Glob Open. 2015;3(7):e451.

Raposo-Amaral CE, Denadai R, Alonso N. Three-dimensional upper lip and nostril sill changes after cleft alveolus reconstruction using autologous bone grafting versus recombinant human bone morphogenetic protein-2. J Craniofac Surg. 2016;27(4):913–8.

Tanikawa DY, Aguena M, Bueno DF, Passos-Bueno MR, Alonso N. Fat grafts supplemented with adipose-derived stromal cells in the rehabilitation of patients with craniofacial microsomia. Plast Reconstr Surg. 2013;132(1):141–52.

Tissiani LA, Alonso N. A prospective and controlled clinical trial on stromal vascular fraction enriched fat grafts in secondary breast reconstruction. Stem Cells Int. 2016;2016:2636454.

Urist MR. Bone: formation by autoinduction. Science. 1965;150(3698):893–9.

Orthodontic Treatment of Patients with Orofacial Cleft

18

Paulo Camara, Endrigo Oliveira Bastos, Daniel Curi, and Nivaldo Alonso

18.1 Introduction

Cleft lip and cleft palate are major public health problems that should receive a comprehensive treatment (Freitas et al. 2012). These defects arise on intrauterine development of the face and may have long-standing implications on dental arch morphology and impair facial growth as well. Cleft correction itself may also harm facial growth potential, even if performed properly (Mølsted et al. 2005). Anatomical and physiological cleft-related problems can have implications on speech, eating, and aesthetic, sometimes leading to deep psychological consequences. Proper dental care from birth to adulthood is necessary to overcome these conditions while avoiding further harm. In this setting, the orthodontist plays an important role in the prevention, correction, and reduction of the consequences of cleft lip and cleft palate (Long et al. 2000).

Orthodontic treatment within the interdisciplinary team that takes care of children with cleft lip and cleft palate has a role to counteract the morphological impact on transverse, vertical, and anteroposterior maxillary dimensions imposed by reconstructive surgeries or by underdevelopment intrinsic to the pathology.

P. Camara, D.D.S. (✉) • E.O. Bastos, M.D., D.D.S., M.Sc.
N. Alonso, M.D., Ph.D.
Divisao de Cirurgia Plastica e Queimaduras, Hospital das Clínicas da Faculdade de Medicina da Universidade de São Paulo, São Paulo, Brazil
e-mail: prpcamara@gmail.com

D. Curi, M.D., D.D.S.
Fellow Craniofacial Surgery, Department of Plastic Surgery at University of São Paulo, São Paulo, Brazil

© Springer International Publishing AG 2018
N. Alonso, C.E. Raposo-Amaral (eds.), *Cleft Lip and Palate Treatment*, https://doi.org/10.1007/978-3-319-63290-2_18

Treatment as a whole should do a care protocol in order to harmonize the face and improve dental positioning.

One of the sought-after results for these patients is a good relation between upper and lower dental arches. In some cases, minor orthodontic treatment is sufficient to provide good occlusion. However, specially in patients operated too early or in more severe cases, good occlusion achievement may require quite complex treatment by the orthodontist, extensive orthopedics, or even surgical repositioning of the jaws through orthognathic surgery. Previous cephalometric studies have shown that primary surgery tends to affect the facial growth and dental development (Capelozza Filho et al. 1996). Therefore, a close follow-up by the orthodontist is of paramount importance to achieve a satisfactory outcome.

There are mainly three phases in which interventions in this area may take place. First one should be even before tooth eruption, when maxillary orthopedics can be applied in order to minimize deformities on alveolar bone ridge. This phase will not be covered in this chapter and its classical approach is nasoalveolar molding (Grayson et al. 1999). A second time window is during early mixed dentition, when orthopedics and orthodontics are used mainly to provide space for adequate permanent dentition. Finally on the end of facial growth, orthodontics may be necessary for final compensation or for decompensation in preparation for orthognathic surgery. At any time, the main goal is to maximize final esthetics and function. Nevertheless, successful treatment depends on the degree of skeletal and dental commitment that the patient presents.

18.2 Classification

In order to improve results in cleft management, it is important to apply periodic protocols and evaluations of the treatments employed. Some interventions will take many years to show their consequences. Therefore, classification methods and evaluation parameters were developed to compare intervention protocols and prognosis regarding facial skeletal growth. When comparing results from different approaches, used for instance by different centers, it is important to be sure that one is comparing patients of the same severity (Mølsted et al. 2005). Outcome studies based on classifications can provide information that clinicians may use in order to preview treatment difficulties and limitations of each case (Gray and Mossey 2005).

For unilateral clefts, which comprise the majority of cases, the most commonly used index is the Goslon yardstick, which analyzes the occlusal relationship through plaster models and clinical analysis (Mars et al. 1987). More recently, virtual tools based on dentofacial scanning were added. In bilateral clefts, the analysis proposed by Ozawa and colleagues in 2005 is the method most commonly used (Ozawa et al. 2011). These indexes classify patients according to features such as sagittal, transverse, and vertical relations between dental arches into categories with different prognosis.

Goslon yardstick was originally designed to classify patients during mixed and early permanent dentition (Mars et al. 1987). Later, adaptations for patients around

5 years were published (Atack et al. 1997; Mars et al. 2006). These systems divide patients into five groups:

- Group 1: Positive overjet with average inclined or retroclined incisors with no crossbite or open bite. Long-term outcome: excellent.
- Group 2: Positive overjet with average inclined or proclined incisors with unilateral crossbite or crossbite tendency with or without open-bite tendency around cleft site. Long-term outcome: good (Fig. 18.1).
- Group 3: Edge-to-edge bite with average inclined or proclined incisors or reverse overjet with retroclined incisors. Unilateral crossbite with or without open-bite tendency around cleft site. Long-term outcome: fair.
- Group 4: Reverse overjet with average inclined or proclined incisors. Unilateral crossbite with or without bilateral crossbite tendency with or without open-bite tendency around cleft site. Long-term outcome: poor (Fig. 18.2).
- Group 5: Reverse overjet with proclined incisors, bilateral crossbite, and poor maxillary arch form and palatal vault anatomy. Long-term outcome: very poor.

Ozawa et al. published the Bauru index, with the same purpose of Goslon yardstick, but designed for patients with bilateral complete clefts (Ozawa et al. 2011). It's interesting to note that this index changes little from the mixed to permanent dentition. It also consists of a scale of 1–5 with increasing severity degree, considering interarch relationship, shape of the upper dental arch, and inclination of upper incisors:

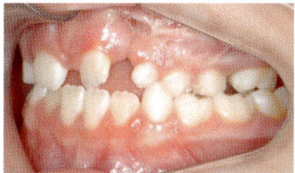 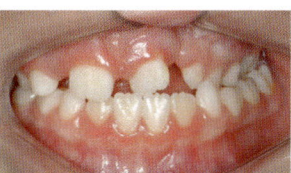 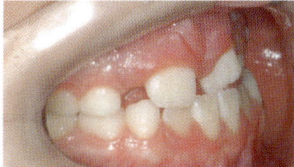

Fig. 18.1 Patient classified as group 2 according to Goslon yardstick. Maxilla is sagittally well positioned in relation to mandible. Despite the need for transverse expansion to correct unilateral posterior crossbite, prognosis is good. Probably, orthognathic surgery will not be needed in the future; therefore dental compensation can be used if necessary in order to correct occlusion

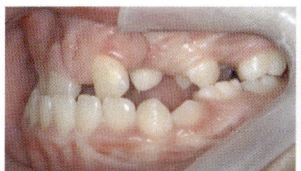 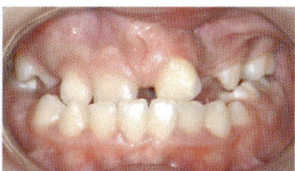 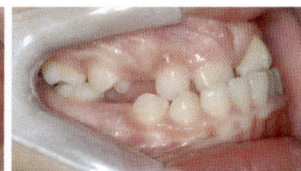

Fig. 18.2 Patient classified as group 4 according to Goslon yardstick. Maxilla retracted in relation to mandible. Prognosis is fair, but probably orthognathic surgery will be advisable in the future. Maxillary expansion, leveling, and alignment must be performed, having in mind that there is a high chance that this maxilla will be brought forward during orthognathic operation and therefore decompensation would be needed as preparation

18.3 Dental Peculiarities

The development of primary dentition around the cleft region may be delayed. Teeth in this area may also show abnormalities in shape, structure, number, and position (Haque and Alam 2015; Galante et al. 2005). Usually, the more extensive the cleft, the more frequent these abnormalities are. Due to some of these irregularities, proper oral hygiene maintenance may be impaired, leading to cavities and early teeth loss. Preservation of teeth next to the cleft is very important, as their presence helps to maintain bony structure in the area.

Supernumerary teeth may be present in unilateral or bilateral cleft regions. Primary tooth eruption is delayed (Kobayashi et al. 2010). On the other hand, in patients with cleft lip and palate, natal and neonatal teeth occur more often and, because of their typical extreme mobility, extraction is indicated (Cabete et al. 2000).

Eruption of permanent teeth is also delayed by 6 months in average (de Carvalho Carrara et al. 2004). Permanent lateral and central incisors may have alterations in enamel structure (Gomes et al. 2009). Permanent lateral incisors are the most frequently absent teeth in patients with complete unilateral cleft (da Silva et al. 2008). Great care with oral hygiene is advised in order to prevent further teeth decay (Freitas et al. 2012).

18.4 Orthodontic Treatment

The goal of orthodontic treatment in cleft patients should be to counter the dental problems and incorrect relationships between alveolar bone bases. Orthodontic treatment in these children has a complexity related to the type and size of the cleft. Teeth may be analyzed according to their intra-arch and interarch relationships. In unilateral clefts, there may be a midline shift towards the cleft, often leading to the need for asymmetric extractions for correction. Extractions may also be necessary in order to correct crowding, which is a common feature on the maxilla due to poor sagittal and transverse growth (Capelozza Filho et al. 1996). When the cleft involves the alveolar ridge, the neighboring teeth show changes in their mesiodistal angulation added to abnormalities previously described. Central incisors are especially prone to present giroversion.

One great improvement on cleft lip and palate treatment was the introduction of secondary alveolar bone grafting. This procedure rebuilds bone anatomy of the alveolar cleft, allowing tooth movement in the region of the lateral incisors and making room for eruption of permanent canines (Bergland et al. 1986).

Over the years several studies have reported that patients with complete unilateral cleft had progressive restriction of anteroposterior maxillary growth, mainly due to consequences of primary surgery. The tension exerted by a rebuilt lip and the scar can be caused by cheiloplasty restricting growth and anterior maxillary development. Early palatoplasty also seems to have a restrictive influence on sagittal growth of the maxilla; thereby, in both unilateral and bilateral clefts, we often observe an anterior crossbite as a consequence of these constraining factors

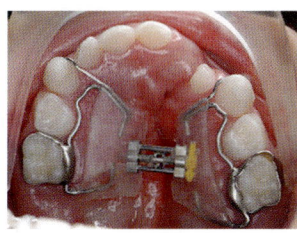 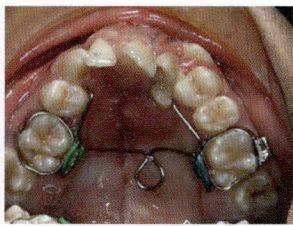 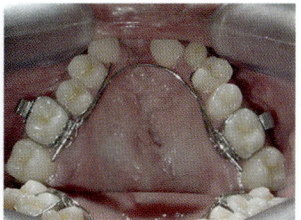

Fig. 18.3 Examples of different palatal expansion devices that may be employed, depending on factors like rate and vector of expansion

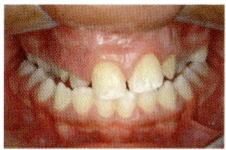 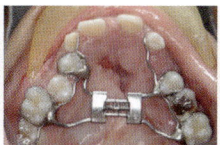 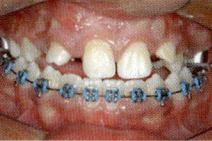 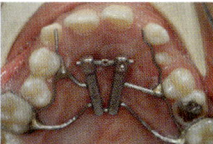

Fig. 18.4 From *left* to *right*: Patient with bilateral cleft, with posterior crossbite. Hyrax expander in place. Postexpansion transversal gain. Device in place to promote transversal gain in anterior region

(Nollet et al. 2005; Liao and Mars 2006). Due to the restraining action of palatoplasty and the absence of midpalatal suture, there is a lack of maxillary development in the transversal direction. This maxillary atresia leads to a posterior crossbite, making maxillary expansion procedures a routine therapy in cleft patients (Capelozza Filho et al. 1996; Liao and Mars 2006) (Figs. 18.3–18.4).

Diagnosis and treatment plan for cleft patients are based on the same diagnostic methods used for noncleft patients, meaning facial analysis, plater models, and radiologic as tomographic analysis. Classification of the case according to Goslon yardstick for unilateral clefts and Bauru method for bilaterals can help on prediction of the outcome.

Treatment may involve the steps described in the following protocol (Freitas et al. 2012):

1. Orthodontics before alveolar bone grafting
2. Secondary alveolar bone grafting
3. Orthodontics after alveolar bone grafting
4. Orthognathic surgery
5. Finalization and containment

Pre-alveolar bone graft orthodontic treatment aims to promote maxillary transverse gain in order to align the teeth and the alveolar bone ridge. As a side result, there is a widening of the cleft, where the bone graft will be placed. The ideal age for secondary alveolar grafting is about 8–12 years old, on a moment just previous to canine eruption, as controlled by radiographic means. Surgery at this age also proves convenient because vertical and anteroposterior growth of the maxilla may be quite stabilized by then. Commencement of pre-grafting orthodontics must be planned having this time frame in mind. Orthodontic appliances are used, such as Hyrax expanders, Haas, or quad-helix. After expansion, a fixed containment device is provided in order to minimize relapse. Expanders allow an improvement in maxillary transverse deficiency but sagittal deficiency should be treated by means of devices that provide stimulus in this direction. Protraction masks can be used with this intention, but should only be applied to cases where there is a palatal inclination of the alveolar process. Fixed orthodontic appliances may be used in this step, but care should be taken on the periodontal limitations mainly in complete bilateral clefts. Repositioning of the premaxilla may also be necessary, in which case it should be performed at this phase.

In orthodontics after alveolar bone grafting, a quantitative and qualitative assessment of the grafted bone through clinical and radiographic examination of the area should be conducted while monitoring of the nonerupted canine; if the canine has already erupted, one must wait for 60–90 days after bone grafting surgery, before preforming orthodontic movement (Freitas et al. 2012).

Orthodontic treatment of patients that will not require orthognathic surgery involves the elimination of problems in the cleft region. If lateral incisors are present and have appropriate root and crown length, they must be correctly positioned. If they are missing, one must decide if the space will be closed by mesial movement of canine or if the space will be maintained for future prosthetic rehabilitation. This decision is based on the position canine eruption, on intermaxillary relationship, and on tooth size discrepancy. In patients with unilateral cleft, asymmetric extractions of premolars or laterals may be necessary for correction of deviated midline (Freitas et al. 2012).

Patients with complete bilateral clefts or unilateral clefts classified as Bauru or Goslon 3–5, by the end of facial growth, will probably present anterior crossbite and require orthognathic surgery. Orthodontic preparation on these patients involves alignment and leveling of both dental arches. Incisor decompensation is not necessary on the maxilla since superior incisors are usually already vertical, due to the restraining force of operated superior lip. Inferior incisors must be decompensated from their lingual inclination, provided that periodontal tissue is healthy and allows for the movement. Early classification, during childhood, is important to keep the orthodontist from compensating cases like Goslon 4–5 that will require orthognathic surgery in the future. After alignment, leveling, and decompensation, model cast analysis is performed to simulate final intercuspation. When this analysis shows that surgery is already viable, orthodontist and surgeon can decide on the magnitude and direction of movements of the jaws at the operation, always involving maxillary advancement. After postsurgical bone consolidation has occurred, orthodontic finalization can take place (Figs. 18.5–18.7).

As on any orthodontic treatment, appliance removal must be done when esthetic and functional goals are achieved. Nevertheless, some adaptations may be necessary. If a canine had to be moved into lateral incisor position, the protection provided by canine contact during lateral excursion is lost. In these cases, contacts of posterior teeth in group function must be able to provide protection on lateral excursion.

Orthodontic relapse is a concern in cleft patients. Therefore, usage of containing devices is of paramount importance. Upper containment device (Hawley plate) must be used 24 h a day for 1 year. After this period, the removable device can be used during the night. Inferior fixed lingual container from canine to canine should be placed when fixed appliance is removed and must be left in place indefinitely. Prosthodontics and periodontal care may be necessary and the patient must be educated about the need for continuation of oral hygiene for maintenance of oral health.

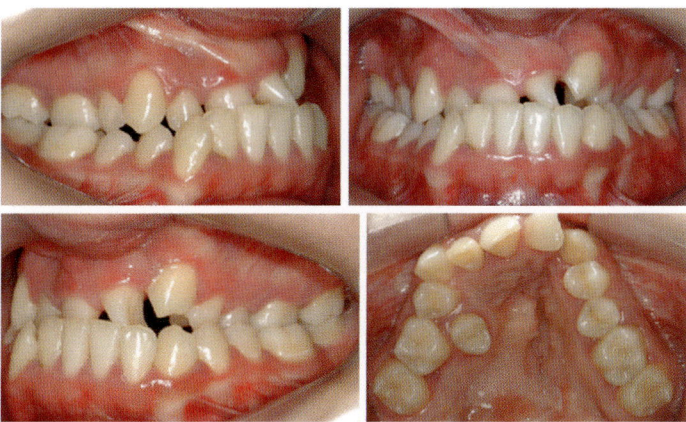

Fig. 18.5 At the end of facial growth, this unilateral cleft patient shows posterior crossbite and dental crowding due to maxillary transverse deficiency along with reduced maxillary dimensions as a whole. This Angle class III occlusion must be corrected surgically. Orthodontics in preparation for orthognathic surgery must involve extraction of superior malpositioned premolar, transverse expansion, alignment, leveling, and decompensation, which is performed mainly for correction of lingual inclination of inferior incisors

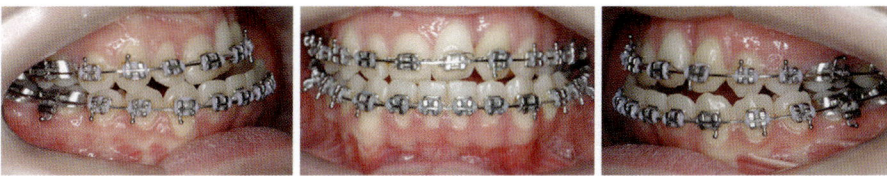

Fig. 18.6 Case shown in Fig. 18.5 just before maxillary advancement. Negative overjet after decompensation reflects sagittal malposition. Arches are leveled and aligned. Residual posterior crossbite will be corrected by the advancement itself

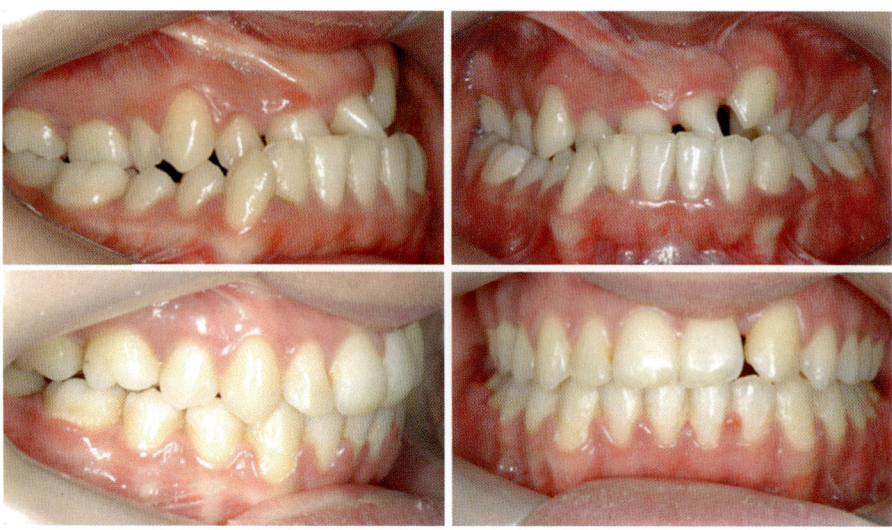

Fig. 18.7 Case shown in Fig. 18.5 before and after orthodontic and surgical treatment. Canine in position of lateral must receive esthetic treatment in order to mimic lateral shape

References

Atack NE, Hathorn IS, Semb G, Dowell T, Sandy JR. A new index for assessing surgical outcome in unilateral cleft lip and palate subjects aged five: reproducibility and validity. Cleft Palate Craniofac J. 1997;34:242–6.

Bergland O, Semb G, Abyholm FE. Elimination of the residual alveolar cleft by secondary bone grafting and subsequent orthodontic treatment. Cleft Palate J. 1986;23:175–205.

Cabete HF, Gomide MR, Costa B. Evaluation of primary dentition in cleft lip and palate children with and without natal/neonatal teeth. Cleft Palate Craniofac J. 2000;37:406–9.

Capelozza Filho L, Normando AD, da Silva Filho OG. Isolated influences of lip and palate surgery on facial growth: comparison of operated and unoperated male adults with UCLP. Cleft Palate Craniofac J. 1996;33:51–6.

de Carvalho Carrara CF, de Oliveira Lima JE, Carrara CE, Gonzalez VB. Chronology and sequence of eruption of the permanent teeth in patients with complete unilateral cleft lip and palate. Cleft Palate Craniofac J. 2004;41:642–5.

Freitas JA, Garib DG, Oliveira M, et al. Rehabilitative treatment of cleft lip and palate: experience of the Hospital for Rehabilitation of craniofacial anomalies-USP (HRAC-USP)--part 2: pediatric dentistry and orthodontics. J Appl Oral Sci. 2012;20:268–81.

Galante JM, Costa B, de Carvalho Carrara CF, Gomide MR. Prevalence of enamel hypoplasia in deciduous canines of patients with complete cleft lip and palate. Cleft Palate Craniofac J. 2005;42:675–8.

Gomes AC, Neves LT, Gomide MR. Enamel defects in maxillary central incisors of infants with unilateral cleft lip. Cleft Palate Craniofac J. 2009;46:420–4.

Gray D, Mossey PA. Evaluation of a modified Huddart/Bodenham scoring system for assessment of maxillary arch constriction in unilateral cleft lip and palate subjects. Eur J Orthod. 2005;27:507–11.

Grayson BH, Santiago PE, Brecht LE, Cutting CB. Presurgical nasoalveolar molding in infants with cleft lip and palate. Cleft Palate Craniofac J. 1999;36:486–98.

Haque S, Alam MK. Common dental anomalies in cleft lip and palate patients. Malays J Med Sci. 2015;22:55–60.

Kobayashi TY, Gomide MR, Carrara CF. Timing and sequence of primary tooth eruption in children with cleft lip and palate. J Appl Oral Sci. 2010;18:220–4.

Liao YF, Mars M. Hard palate repair timing and facial growth in cleft lip and palate: a systematic review. Cleft Palate Craniofac J. 2006;43:563–70.

Long RE, Semb G, Shaw WC. Orthodontic treatment of the patient with complete clefts of lip, alveolus, and palate: lessons of the past 60 years. Cleft Palate Craniofac J. 2000;37:533–42.

Mars M, Plint DA, Houston WJ, Bergland O, Semb G. The Goslon yardstick: a new system of assessing dental arch relationships in children with unilateral clefts of the lip and palate. Cleft Palate Craniofac J. 1987;24:314–22.

Mars M, Batra P, Worrell E. Complete unilateral cleft lip and palate: validity of the five-year index and the Goslon yardstick in predicting long-term dental arch relationships. Cleft Palate Craniofac J. 2006;43:557–62.

Mølsted K, Brattström V, Prahl-Andersen B, Shaw WC, Semb G. The Eurocleft study: intercenter study of treatment outcome in patients with complete cleft lip and palate. Part 3: dental arch relationships. Cleft Palate Craniofac J. 2005;42:78–82.

Nollet PJ, Katsaros C, Van't Hof MA, Kuijpers-Jagtman AM. Treatment outcome in unilateral cleft lip and palate evaluated with the GOSLON yardstick: a meta-analysis of 1236 patients. Plast Reconstr Surg. 2005;116:1255–62.

Ozawa TO, Shaw WC, Katsaros C, et al. A new yardstick for rating dental arch relationship in patients with complete bilateral cleft lip and palate. Cleft Palate Craniofac J. 2011;48:167–72.

da Silva AP, Costa B, de Carvalho Carrara CF. Dental anomalies of number in the permanent dentition of patients with bilateral cleft lip: radiographic study. Cleft Palate Craniofac J. 2008;45:473–6.

Orthognathic Surgery in Cleft Patients

19

Nivaldo Alonso, Endrigo Oliveira Bastos, and Geraldo Capuchinho Jr.

Despite the development of specialized treatment centers and establishment of treatment protocols for patients with cleft lip and/or palate, surgical interventions are initiated at an early age and involve numerous procedures to obtain complete rehabilitation, which can cause restrictions on facial growth (Bardach and Eisbach 1977).

Thus, at the end of facial growth, a significant proportion of patients undergoing surgical treatment in childhood will present with dentofacial deformities not amenable to orthodontic treatment and possibly will require supplementary treatment with orthognathic surgery (Good et al. 2007).

Figure 19.1 Midface retrusion in bilateral cleft patients.

19.1 Anatomical Considerations

The anatomical characteristics of cleft patients are peculiar according to the cleft type (unilateral or bilateral). Thus, the maxilla may be divided into two or three segments, which may lead to tissue changes in three levels: bone structure, muscle tissue, and skin/mucous tegument. Moreover, bilateral cleft has the prolabium and pre-maxilla originating embryologically nasofrontal process structures that direct treatment in some protocols (Victor 1973).

N. Alonso, M.D., Ph.D. (✉) • E.O. Bastos, M.D., D.D.S., M.Sc.
Divisao de Cirurgia Plastica e Queimaduras, Hospital das Clínicas da Faculdade de Medicina da Universidade de São Paulo, São Paulo, Brazil
e-mail: nivalonso@gmail.com

G. Capuchinho Jr., M.D.
Department of Plastic and Reconstructive Surgery, Hospital Universitário Risoleta Tolentino Neves, Universidade Federal de Minas Gerais, Belo Horizonte, Brazil

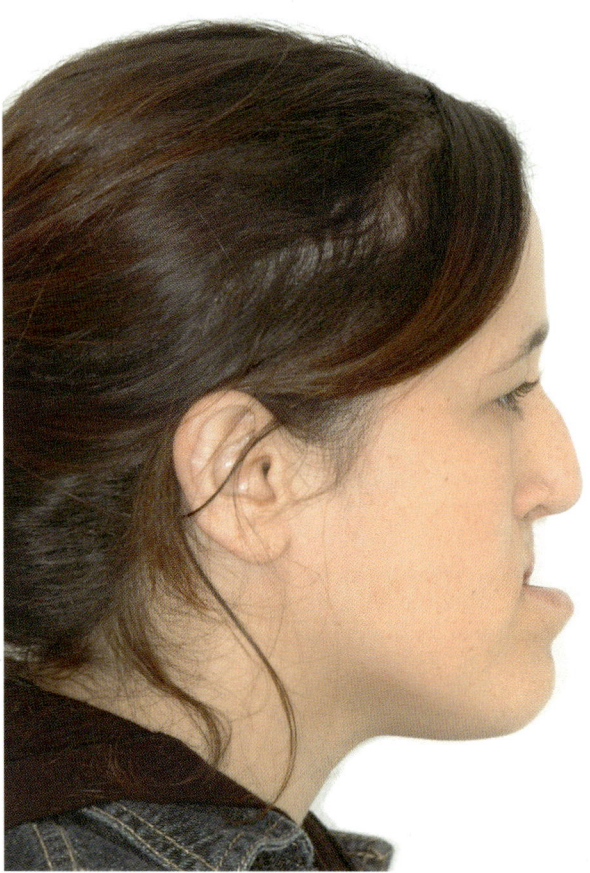

Fig. 19.1 Severe midface retrusion in bilateral cleft patients after lip and palate repair

Some points are responsible for the growth and development of the facial skeleton. When analyzing normal facial growth between 3 and 18, it can be noted that there is a large displacement of the upper jaw forward and down driven by different factors. Among them, we highlight the bone centers of growth, tooth eruption, breathing, and chewing. However, growth abnormalities and development of craniofacial structures are frequent findings in patients with cleft lip and palate previously operated (Shetye 2004; Semb 1991).

Figure 19.2 Normal facial growth (Silva Filho 2007).

The main deformity found in cleft patients occurs in the upper jaw, which is the first bone affected by cleft, with inhibition of their previous growth and its translation (Bardach and Eisbach 1977). Thus, patients present with concave face, middle third of disability, and occlusion class III Angle (Shetye 2004). In addition, there is a palatal inclination of the upper incisors, which contributes to the anterior crossbite; the lateral strands in unilateral cleft are often uneven; the absence of teeth in the alveolar is common slot; and sometimes it can be observed changing the exclusive occlusal plane on the side of the cleft, with deviation from the dental midline (Fig. 19.3).

Specifically in patients with bilateral clefts, the pre-maxilla may be poorly positioned both in the vertical plane and the horizontal plane. The collapse of the side

Fig. 19.2 Superimposition of cephalometrics images between 3 and 18 years old in facial growth showing the direction of jaw growth

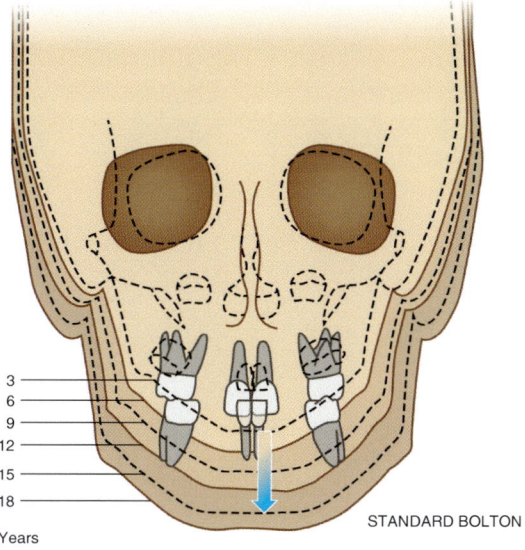

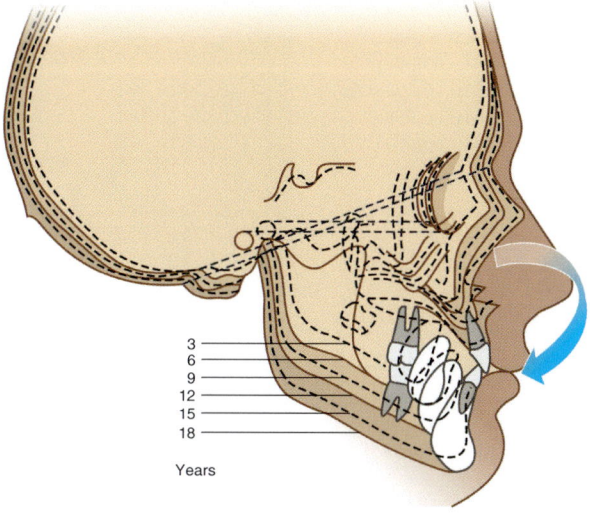

segments often prevents the pre-maxilla repositioning damaging alignment and proper leveling of the arches and the existence of horizontal overlap with decreased transverse diameter of the jaw with the collapse of the maxillary posterior segments leads to posterior crossbite. The profile analysis demonstrates the lack of projection of the upper lip often with thin vermilion, and an excessive emphasis of the lower lip. Finally, the presence of oronasal fistulas and scars, the quality of the gingiva, and the presence or absence of the upper gingiva-labial groove are important points to be evaluated in planning (Fig. 19.4a, b).

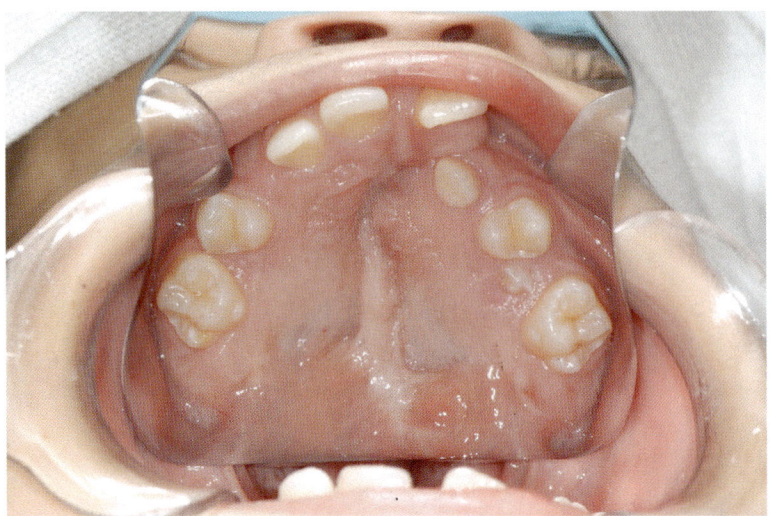

Fig. 19.3 Crossbite in maxillar arch of unilateral cleft with lip repair

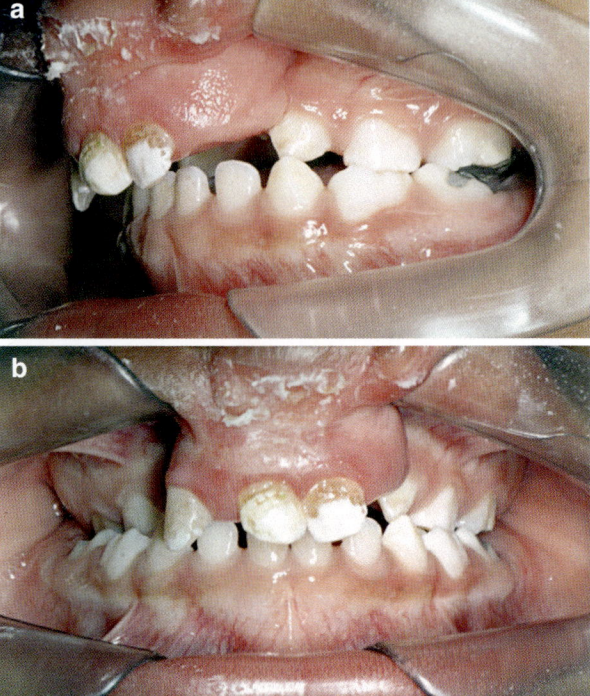

Fig. 19.4 (**a**, **b**) Frontal and lateral views of the dental occlusion—bilateral cleft with nasal-oral fistula, posterior crossbite, and protruding pre-maxilla

Regarding the lateral cephalometric, in nonoperated patients NSA angle is normal or increased, although the determination of the point A in the maxilla is quite difficult (Laspos et al. 1997a, b; Mars and Houston 1990; Capelozza Junior et al. 1993).

The jaw also shows some variations of its morphology and such deformities may become more evident with the lack of upper third of the projection. The NSB angle shows a discrete retrognathia (Shetye 2004; Capelozza Junior et al. 1993; Bishara 1973a, b; Yoshida et al. 1992), although the body size and mandibular branch can be normal. In addition, the goniac angle can be obtuse and the angle of the mandibular plane relative to the cranial base is increased.

19.2 Craniofacial Growth

Factors that may affect the facial growth in cleft can be attributed to (1) intrinsic deficiency secondary to the cleft; (2) inhibition of the growth resulting from the surgical correction of cleft lip and palate at an early age; and (3) genetic inheritance for maxillary hypoplasia of both parents. Clinical examination of untreated patients may elucidate the genetically determined components of craniofacial growth, differentiating them from disorders caused by surgical procedures (Shetye 2004).

Factors that may determine the degree of facial retrusion of these patients are dentofacial configuration, which can be genetically influenced, and the shape of the cleft. This can be observed in patients with rather large clefts and those with cutaneous epithelial bands (Simonart's bands). More recently, genetic factors have also been implicated as a cause of more late sequelae. Patients with genetic alterations, such as van der Woude syndrome (IRF6 deficiency), may have worse final results than nonsyndromic cleft patients (Jugessur et al. 2008).

Classically, there is a facial bone growth very close to normal in nonoperated cleft lip and palate patients. Studies comparing these two groups show that there is minimal difference of maxillary growth (Shetye 2004; Capelozza Junior et al. 1993). There are only tooth position changes and distortions of alveolar arch due to the absence of muscular mouth strap. The non-cleft segment is usually protruded, while the fissured thread is collapsed. This is due to the absence of modeling the oral orbicularis muscle and tissue continuity. The tongue presses the teeth and the alveoli previously. The cleft jaw segment is pulled superiorly, contributing to the occurrence of bite anterior open.

Figure 19.5a, b Nonoperated cleft patients and its maxillar arch compared to normal growth expected.

Patients with cleft lip and palate who had only repaired lips have the same kind of anteroposterior growth of non-treated patients due to remodeling of the alveolar segments caused by muscular belt created. Studies comparing these two groups show that there is minimal difference of maxillary growth. Therefore, the lip

Fig. 19.5 (**a**, **b**) Maxillar arch of nonoperated cleft patient at the age of 10 years old compared to the expected one

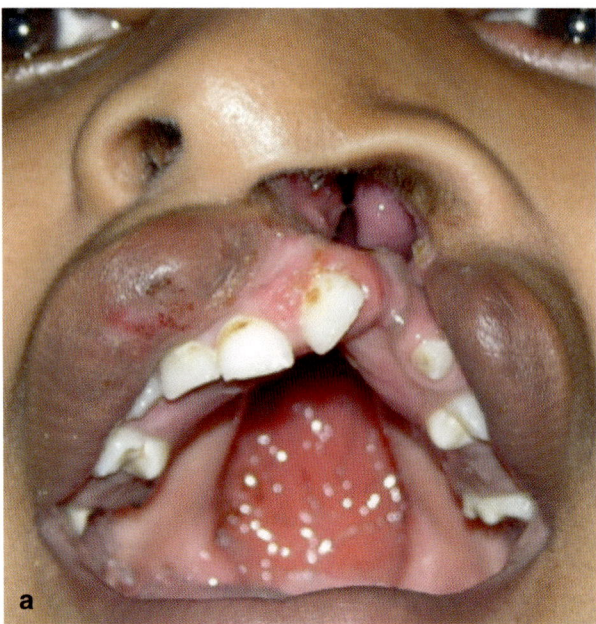
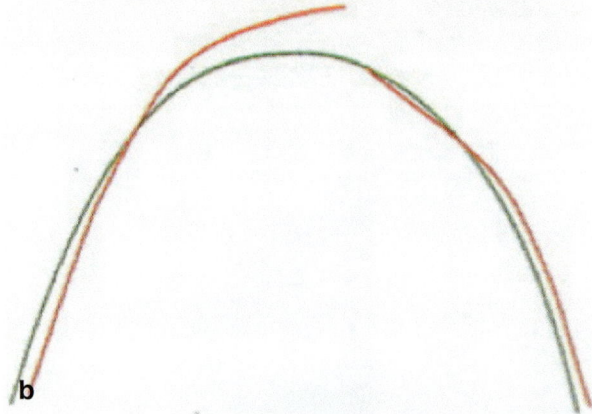

surgery would have little effect on the growth of the maxilla and minimal effect on dentition. Only when the lip repair is very tense, the incisors may be positioned higher. Moreover, palatal surgery is known to be a primary etiologic factor in inhibiting the growth of the facial medium third. However, it is very difficult to isolate the effect of palatal repairs and labial (Daskalogiannakis and Ross 1997).

The primary lip and palate surgery appear to have a restrictive effect to the growth of the maxilla previously targeted by the deformity, so that care during the initial surgery is essential for the ultimate success of the treatment. The maxilla in operated cleft tends to have deficiencies in three directions: transverse, anteroposterior, and sagittal, being higher in the last plan (da Silva Filho et al. 2007). It is said that the effects on the jaw growth are more related to the surgeon's skill than the technique used (Jugessur et al. 2008). But numerous studies have shown the negative effect of surgery on facial growth and development. The curve of evolution facial growth in operated cleft patients is clearly impaired compared to normal growth (Bardach and Eisbach 1977; Semb 1991).

Surgical treatment of cleft should consider the inverse relationship between surgery and facial growth and some principles: minimal tissue resection, nontraumatic technique, and avoiding tension in the operated areas. Although it has been understood that external forces (such as statements with tissue adhesives or traditional cards) may restrict the facial growth in cleft patients, these resources together with sequential surgeries can be used to prevent further restrictions on facial growth forces in very large clefts.

19.3 Indications

The data regarding the percentage indication of orthognathic surgery in cleft patients are diverse, ranging from 6 to 48%; however, it is considered acceptable rates between 1 and 10% of patients who underwent osteotomy face corrections for dentoskeletal deformities (Ross 1987). This variation is mainly in unilateral/bilateral clefts, being more common in bilateral patient. Furthermore, Ross cited that even in patients treated in the ideal age, approximately 20% of patients required orthognathic surgery because the unique orthodontic treatment was not possible. More recent data from HRAC/USP Bauru show that between 20 and 30% of patients with unilateral transforamen cleft underwent orthognathic surgery (da Silva Filho et al. 2007).

Severe hypoplasia of the jaw, causing alteration of dental occlusion and modification of facial profile, is initially the main indication for orthognathic surgery. However, some of these patients have as main changes the presence of oronasal fistulas and septal deviation. The surgeon should observe the presence of permanent dentition and skeletal maturity, so you can start surgical planning and orthodontic preparation. One very important point when we observe the high incidence of orthognathic surgery is to consider that facial appearance must be harmonic and also the occlusion adequate. Many times the orthodontist could achieve very good dental occlusion with disharmonic profile.

19.4 Treatment Planning

Count on the assistance of an integrated team of professionals from different areas from the beginning is essential in the proper planning of these patients. Preoperative medical documentation includes quality photos with view of face and occlusion, lateral and front X-rays for cephalometry, CT scans if necessary, and speech therapy approach, including nasoendoscopy.

The speech pathologist performs, both in the initial stage and during growth, a very important, vital role for the ultimate success. The treatment of velopharyngeal dysfunction (VPD) is initiated in the early stages of facial development, between 5 and 7 years old, but some of these patients may require bone surgery jaws at age 15, when phonation structures can be changed again. Velopharyngeal function tends to suffer from deterioration after jaw osteotomy with great maxillar advancements. Patients with suitable speech before surgery may become adjacent after the breakthrough, and borderline cases with preoperative closure can become incompetent after bone surgery (Posnick and Ricalde 2004).

In general, orthodontic preparation involves maxillary expansion and alignment and levelling of the alveolar slopes, leading to a coordination of the maxillary and mandibular arches. Levelling the lateral bone segments in bilateral should be done isolated. It is very important to have the upper jaws prepared for orthognathic surgery without any discontinuity; for this, alveolar bone grafting in early age is crucial; if it was not done previously we prefer to bone graft 01 year before the orthognathic surgery.

This preparation requires a large degree of expertise and has two distinct phases. In the early stages the concern should be to maintain the transverse diameter of the maxilla and avoid breakdowns caused by surgical scars of the lip and palate previous corrections. Often external traction devices play an important role at this stage. In the next phase, when the hypoplastic facial middle third has already established itself, the ortho-surgical preparation begins (Fig. 19.6a, b, c).

Surgical correction of deformities of the jaws is best performed when the skeleton is mature and the teeth were orthodontically aligned. The craniofacial growth is usually complete between the ages of 14 and 16 years in women and between 16 and 18 years for men. However, skeletal growth is variable, and an evaluation of closing the epiphyseal growth plate must be made through a specific ray. Wolford has shown that very early surgery in cleft determines high recurrence rate, requiring further surgical revision (Wolford 1992). Another risk associated with surgery in very young patients is damage to permanent teeth germs.

If the alveolar process has been adequately treated in the mixed dentition, the canine erupts in the grafted area. So, as the lateral incisor is often absent, the canine can be used to disguise the failure dental or orthodontic be pulled distally, making room for a future implant in the bone fissure.

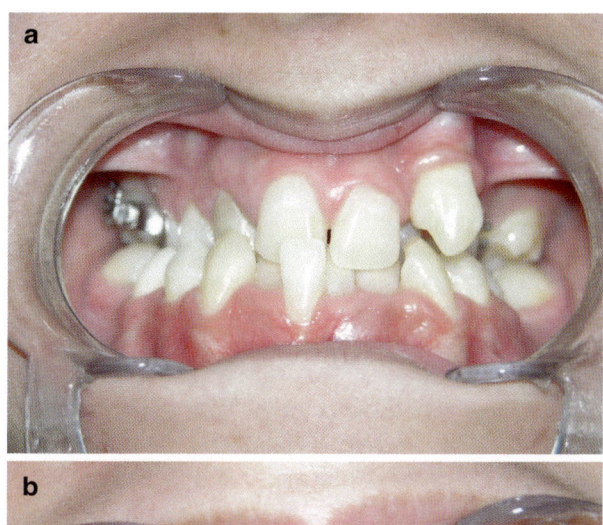
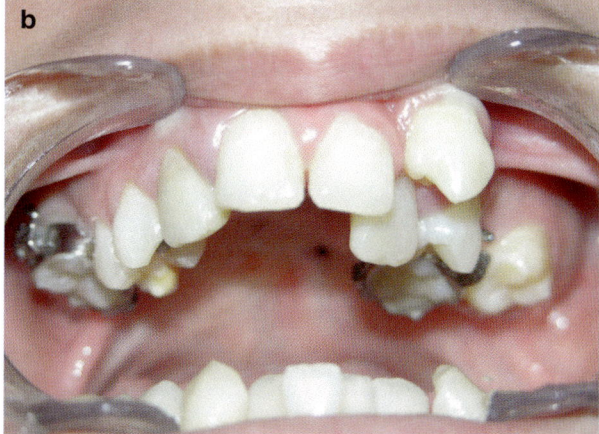
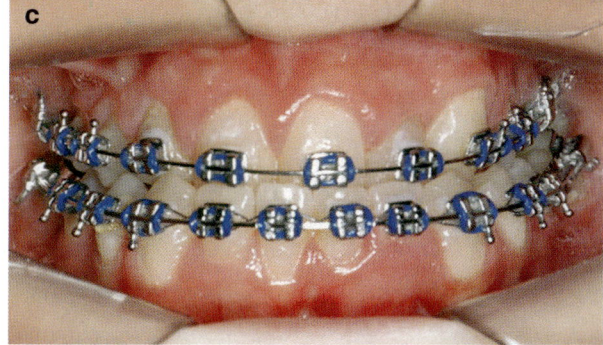

Fig. 19.6 (a–c) Cleft palate patient with small palate fistula dental occlusion pre- and during preparation of orthognathic surgery

19.5 Surgical Technique

The most commonly used maxillary osteotomy in cleft patients is Le Fort I type, described initially by Wasmund. Despite the well-documented blood supply of mucoperiosteal flaps, revascularization, and bone healing in maxillary osteotomy Le Fort I, there is much discussion about the technical difficulties and possible complications of this surgical technique in cleft patients, due to the possibility of total or partial necrosis of the mobilized segments (Posnick and Tompson 1995). Thus, Bell showed that the preservation of large mucoperiosteal lateral pedicle is critical in this type of osteotomy. In addition, he demonstrated that the blood supply of the upper jaw is maintained by the palatal mucosa and mainly by the periosteum of the lateral segments. On the other hand, the pre-jaw is nourished primarily by the labial mucosa and also by the periosteum of the bone central portion of the septum (Phillips et al. 2005) (Figs. 19.7a–g, 19.8a–d).

Posnick and Tompson(1995) introduced important technical changes in the osteotomy of the maxilla, both in unilateral cleft patients and in bilateral. For patients where bone grafting was not performed or where he did not get proper result, the author simultaneously used the previous mobilization of lateral segments of jaw for closing fistulas' mesial and anteroposterior projection of the bone segment (Posnick and Ricalde 2004; Posnick and Tompson 1995). In our service we have used, whenever possible, bone grafting in the same procedure for the closure of oronasal fistula previously. The maxillary osteotomy is performed after at least 1 year after bone graft, as we believe that there is greater stability, ability to work with single-jaw segment, faster operation, and reduced risk of aseptic necrosis jaw.

However, sometimes the jaw is targeted by both the alveolar cleft and the absence of bone grafting, and there are greater difficulties than the classically

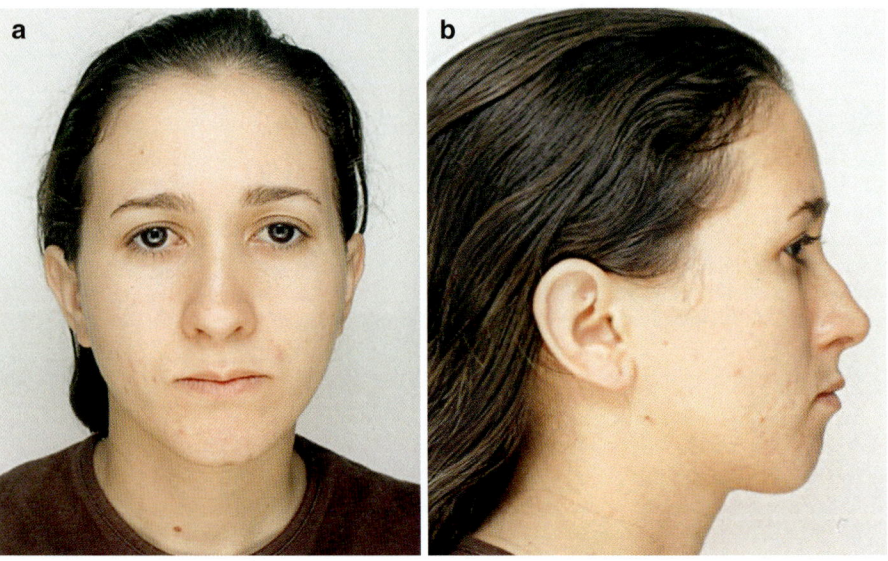

Fig. 19.7 (**a–f**) Le Fort I advancement with chin advancement in a cleft patient

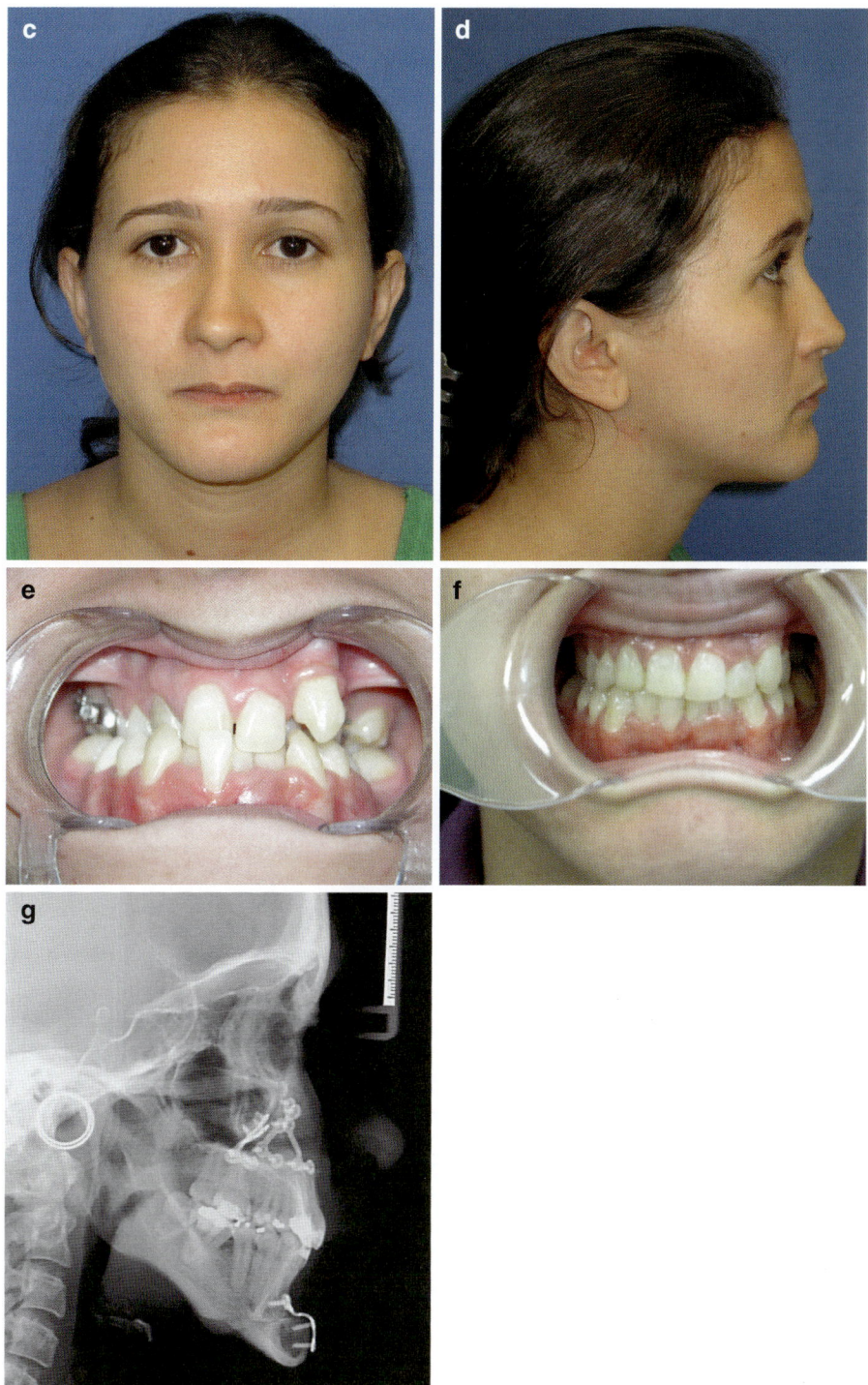

Fig. 19.7 (continued)

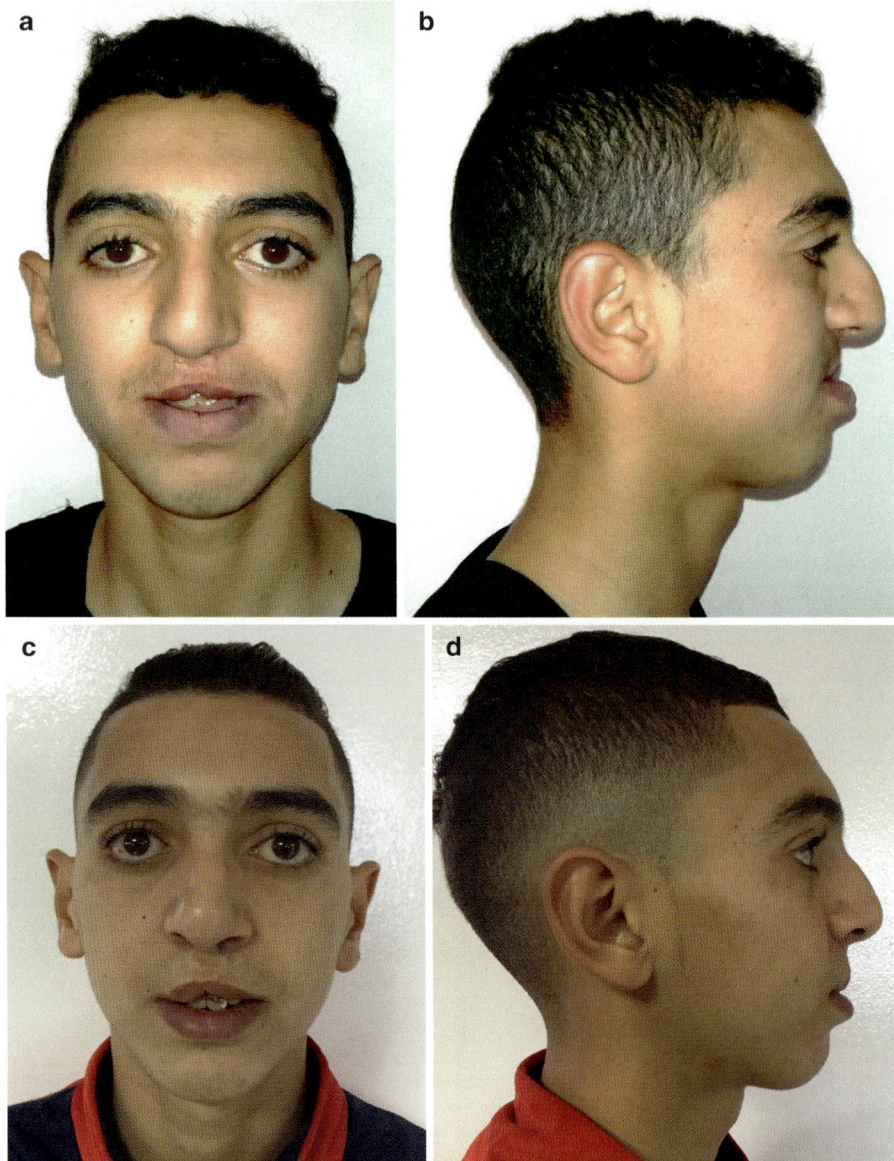

Fig. 19.8 (**a–d**) (**a, b**) Bilateral cleft patients pre-op frontal and profile view (**c, d**) after Le Fort I advancement of 12 mm frontal and profile views

employed maxillary osteotomy. In these cases, the preparation is used for a specific surgical guide to prevent internal rotation of the segments and proceeds to the correction of fistulas in the same surgery. The preservation of lateral mucoperiosteal vascular pedicles is essential to the nutrition of the bone jaw structure. In bilateral cases, the pre-maxilla osteotomy is performed in its posterior region to preserve vascularity. The arc of rotation and advancement of the pre-maxilla are always limited to its vascular pedicle. In special cases, the maxillary advancement associated with oronasal fistula repair with bone grafting preserving the superior pedicle soft tissue, in addition to holding tunnel to complete the osteotomy, can be used (Figs. 19.9a–g, 19.10a–f).

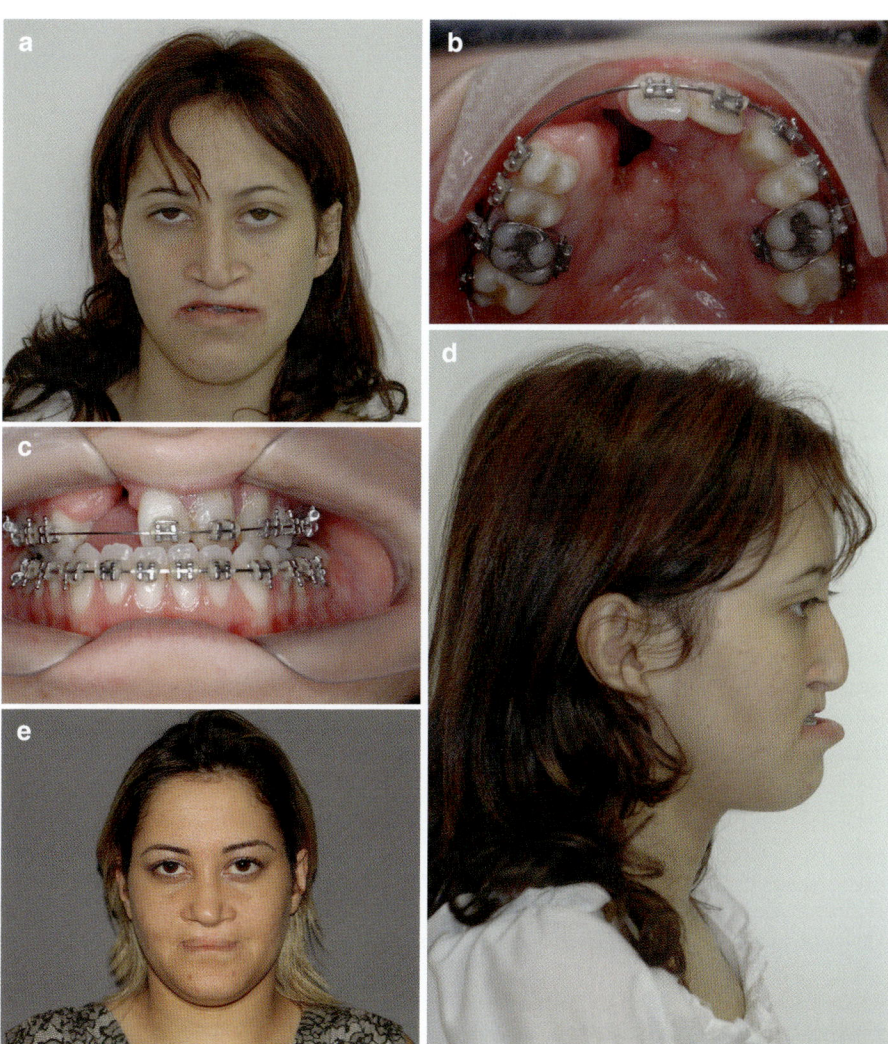

Fig. 19.9 (**a–h**) Bilateral cleft patient with anterior oral fistula. (**a, b, c, d**) Preoperative. (**e, f, g, h**) Postoperative after Le Fort I as described by Posnick with closure of the fistula at the same time

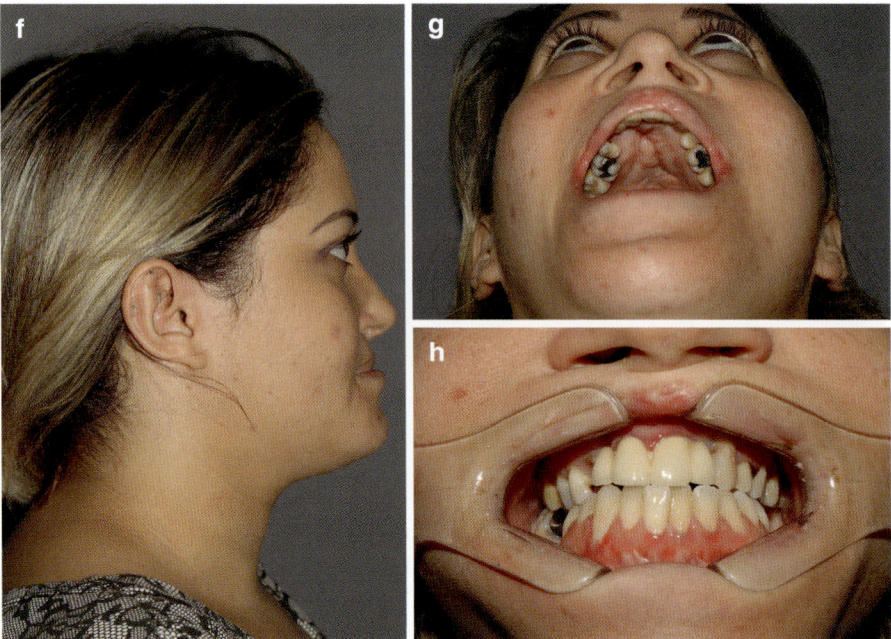

Fig. 19.9 (continued)

19.6 Specific Difficulties

19.6.1 Distraction Osteogenesis

When an upper jaw is set forward 10 mm the use of bone distractors for the gradual anterior traction of the jaw and soft tissue should be considered. Its main advantages are less invasive surgery, lower morbidity, possibility of early treatment, and recurrence rate. However, with respect to the prevention of velopharyngeal incompetence and speech disorders, distraction was not superior than isolated orthognathic surgery in moderate advances. It can be used in internal or external devices, but the latter are the most used worldwide. Distraction osteogenesis allows adjustments to be made during bone elongation. Association jaw breaker can be performed, enabling the improvement in transverse relation at the same time correcting the anteroposterior and sagittal advance by bone distractor (Chua et al. 2010a).

19.6.2 Velopharyngeal Dysfunction

Some peculiarities must be observed in patients with maxillary hypoplasia associated with velopharyngeal dysfunction or even previously submitted to pharyngeal flap patients. There may be changes in speech after maxillary advancement, which

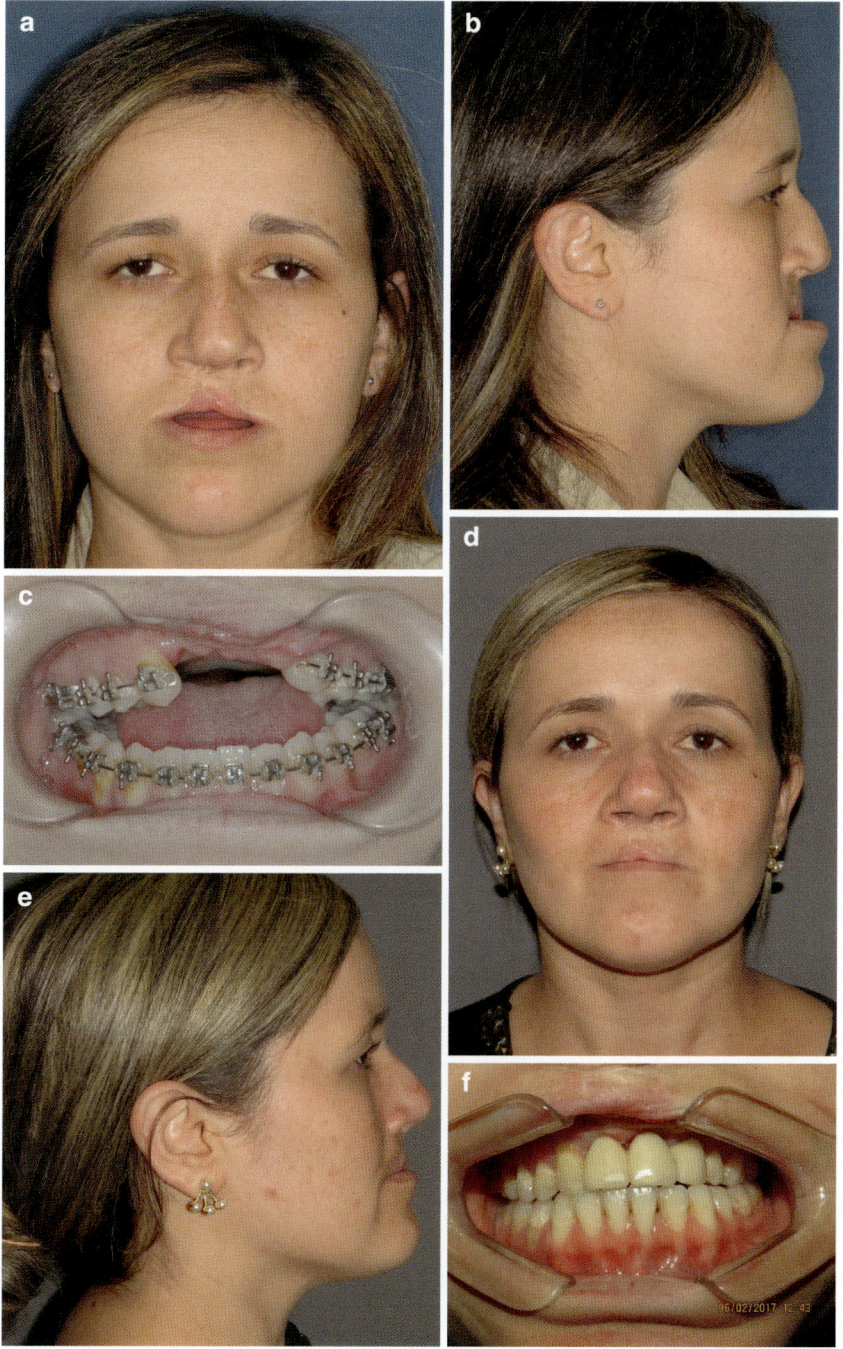

Fig. 19.10 (**a–f**) Bilateral cleft patient with oral fistula and without pre-maxilla. (**a, b, c**) Preoperative view and (**d, e, f**) postoperative view after maxillar advancement and rhinoplasty

even worsen it. However, patients with normal vocal resonance have a very low risk of postoperative hypernasality. Moreover, the presence of a short palate and a deep pharynx, identified by preoperative cephalometric, is the most important measure of the sagittal maxillary advancement as risk predictors of IVF (Chua et al. 2010a, b; Phillips et al. 2005).

19.6.3 Other Peculiarities

Another point to consider is the presence of pharyngeal flaps, which may limit the maxillary advancement. During the surgery, if there is no possibility of tracheal intubation by side holes to the flap, one can perform the pedicle section of the pharyngeal flap or perform intubation via submandibular. These are items to be discussed with the patient and their families preoperatively in conjunction with speech therapists.

In the tense lips, lacking tissues and absence of superior gingivolabial groove always consider the previous preparation with the use of lower lip flap, Abbé flap, and then later perform the maxillary advancement.

19.6.4 Final Considerations

Assessment protocols and conduct of primary surgery by experienced surgeons can avoid late bone surgery. The coordinated multidisciplinary team should always aim for the monitoring of growth and facial development of these individuals, performing the procedures in the ideal age.

During the planning and preparation of cleft patients for orthognathic surgery, there are major differences in relation to orthognathic surgery in other dento-skeletal deformities. Thus, you should always consider the presence of scars from previous surgeries and oronasal fistulas and also evaluate the velopharyngeal function and associated respiratory disorders (deviated nasal septum, hypertrophy of the turbinates, and obstructive sleep apnea) to achieve a degree of excellence in the treatment and improve the quality of life in patients.

References

Bardach J, Eisbach KJ. The influence of primary unilateral cleft lip repair on facial growth. Cleft Palate J. 1977;14(1):88–97.
Bishara SE. The influence of palatoplasty and cleft length on facial development. Cleft Palate J. 1973a;10:390–8.
Bishara SE. Cephalometric evaluation of facial growth in operated and non-operated individuals with isolated clefts of the palate. Cleft Palate J. 1973b;10:239–46.
Capelozza Junior L, Taniguchi SM, da Silva Junior OG. Craniofacial morphology of adult unoperated complete unilateral cleft lip and palate patients. Cleft Palate Craniofac J. 1993;30(4):376–81.
Chua HD, Hagg MB, Cheung LK. Cleft maxillary distraction versus orthognathic surgery--which one is more stable in 5 years? Oral Surg Oral Med Oral Pathol Oral Radiol Endod. 2010a;109(6):803–14.

Chua HD, Whitehill TL, Samman N, Cheung LK. Maxillary distraction versus orthognathic surgery in cleft lip and palate patients: effects on speech and velopharyngeal function. Int J Oral Maxillofac Surg. 2010b;39(7):633–40.

Daskalogiannakis J, Ross RB. Effect of alveolar bone grafting in the mixed dentition on maxillary growth in complete unilateral cleft lip and palate patients. Cleft Palate Craniofac J. 1997;34(5):455–8.

Good PM, Mulliken JB, Padwa BL. Frequency of le fort I osteotomy after repaired cleft lip and palate or cleft palate. Cleft Palate Craniofac J. 2007;44(4):396–401.

Jugessur A, Rahimov F, Lie RT, Wilcox AJ, Gjessing HK, Nilsen RM, et al. Genetic variants in IRF6 and the risk of facial clefts: single-marker and haplotype-based analyses in a population-based case-control study of facial clefts in Norway. Genet Epidemiol. 2008;32(5):413–24.

Laspos CP, Kyrkanides S, Tallents RH, Moss ME, Subtelny JD. Mandibular asymmetry in noncleft and unilateral cleft lip and palate individuals. Cleft Palate Craniofac J. 1997a;34(5):410–6.

Laspos CP, Kyrkanides S, Tallents RH, Moss ME, Subtelny JD. Mandibular and maxillary asymmetry in individuals with unilateral cleft lip and palate. Cleft Palate Craniofac J. 1997b;34(3):232–9.

Mars M, Houston WJ. A preliminary study of facial growth and morphology in unoperated male unilateral cleft lip and palate subjects over 13 years of age. Cleft Palate J. 1990;27(1):7–10.

Phillips JH, Klaiman P, Delorey R, MacDonald DB. Predictors of velopharyngeal insufficiency in cleft palate orthognathic surgery. Plast Reconstr Surg. 2005;115(3):681–6.

Posnick JC, Ricalde P. Cleft-orthognathic surgery. Clin Plast Surg. 2004;31(2):315–30.

Posnick JC, Tompson B. Cleft-orthognathic surgery: complications and long-term results. Plast Reconstr Surg. 1995;96(2):255–66.

Ross RB. Treatment variables affecting facial growth in complete unilateral cleft lip and palate. Cleft Palate J. 1987;24(1):5–77.

Semb G. A study of facial growth in patients with bilateral cleft lip and palate treated by the Oslo CLP team. Cleft Palate Craniofac J. 1991;28(1):22–39. discussion 46-8

Shetye PR. Facial growth of adults with unoperated clefts. Clin Plast Surg. 2004;31(2):361–71.

Silva Filho OG. Crescimento Facial. In: Ltda LS, editor. Fissuras Labiopalatinas: uma abordagem interdisciplinar. 1. Sao Paulo: Trindade, I.E.K. e Silva Filho, O.G; 2007. p. 173–98.

da Silva Filho OG, Rosa LA, Lauris RC. Influence of isolated cleft palate and palatoplasty on the face. J Appl Oral Sci. 2007;15(3):199–208.

Victor S. A proposed modification for the classification of cleft lip and cleft palate. Cleft Palate J. 1973;110:251–2.

Wolford LM. Effects of orthognathic surgery on nasal form and function in the cleft patient. Cleft Palate Craniofac J. 1992;29(6):546–55.

Yoshida H, Nakamura A, Michi K, Wang GM, Liu K, Qiu WL. Cephalometric analysis of maxillofacial morphology in unoperated cleft palate patients. Cleft Palate Craniofac J. 1992;29(5):419–24.

Secondary Unilateral Cleft Rhinoplasty

20

Cesar Augusto Raposo-Amaral, Rafael Denadai,
Cassio Eduardo Raposo-Amaral, and Celso Luiz Buzzo

20.1 Introduction

Unilateral cleft nose repair is challenging because of the complexity of the deformity. This three-dimensional deformity involves several structures such as the lower lateral cartilage (the medial and lateral crus), the nasal dome, the columella, the nasal septum, and the skeletal platform, which includes the alveolus, maxillary segments, and palate (Fisher et al. 2014; Byrd et al. 2007). Thus, to obtain the realistic treatment goal (normal appearance and function, with better symmetry, balance, and less scarring), both skeletal and soft-tissue structures must be adequately managed. Although the primary cleft rhinoplasty has currently been performed at the time of cleft lip repair, the longitudinal follow-up usually revels a residual (from minor to major) nasal deformity (Freeman et al. 2013; Haddock et al. 2012; Chang et al. 2010; Salyer et al. 2004), regardless of surgeon's skills. Therefore, secondary (definitive or final) cleft nose repair with a greater number and complexity of maneuvers is needed after the completion of facial growth to correct aesthetic and functional issues (Hwang et al. 2012; Masuoka et al. 2012; Turkaslan et al. 2008; Bashir et al. 2011; Guyuron 2008; Stal and Hollier 2002).

In this chapter, we include an overview of secondary unilateral cleft rhinoplasty including a brief history, the anatomy of deformity, and the surgical approach.

C.A. Raposo-Amaral, M.D. (✉) • R. Denadai, M.D. • C.L. Buzzo, M.D.
Institute of Plastic and Craniofacial Surgery, SOBRAPAR Hospital,
Campinas, São Paulo, Brazil
e-mail: cesaraugustoraposo@hotmail.com

C.E. Raposo-Amaral, M.D., Ph.D.
Institute of Plastic and Craniofacial Surgery, SOBRAPAR Hospital,
Campinas, São Paulo 13084-880, Brazil

Universidade de São Paulo, São Paulo, Brazil

20.2 Brief History of Cleft Nose Repair

In 1932, Gillies and Kilner (1932) introduced a superior advancement of the composite chondrocutaneous hemicolumella flap using a midcolumellar incision. In 1964, Converse (1964) provided the first major modification of this technique by replacing the midcolumellar incision with a marginal incision; the medial crura composite flap was advanced superiorly and sutured to the contralateral dome, and the defect at the base of the columella was repaired with an auricular composite graft. In 1954, Potter (1946) advocated a similar concept but from the opposite direction, using a lateral-to-medial advancement of the lateral crural composite chondrocutaneous flap; the resultant defect created in the lateral vestibular skin was closed in a V-to-Y fashion. In 1977, Tajima and Maruyama (1977) described the reverse-U incision to address two classic cleft problems, namely obliteration of the soft triangle and nostril apex overhang. This incision starts inferomedially at the junction of the columella and membranous septum, and continues superiorly into the depressed dome skin, creating an arc similar in shape to the nostril on the noncleft side, and returning into the mucosa of the nostril. After wide undermining of the nasal skin envelope, the cartilages are repositioned and the excess skin of the nostril apex is rolled into the nostril. Closure of the skin edges creates a soft triangle on the cleft side. In 1982, Dibbell (1982) proposed incisions within the nostril rim and excision of soft tissue to correct medial rotation of the lower lateral cartilage, lateral displacement of the alar base, twisting of the domes, columellar asymmetry, and overhang of the ala. This technique is accomplished through the creation of a double-pedicled composite flap of lower lateral cartilage, mucosa, columella, and nasal floor, followed by superior and medial rotation of the flap, resulting in an anatomical repositioning of the displaced lower lateral cartilage. In 2009, Flores et al. (2009) reported the Cutting's experience adopting an open rhinoplasty approach using a combination of both the Dibbell and Tajima techniques to correct the nostril apex overhang and reposition the depressed lower lateral cartilage and laterally displaced ala on the cleft side. They reported that avoidance of an upper lip incision with this technique is an advantage, particularly in those patients who have a well-healed lip scar from primary lip repair. Historically, numerous other techniques have been described for cleft nose repair, including suture, flaps, and cartilage grafting techniques (Hwang et al. 2012; Masuoka et al. 2012; Turkaslan et al. 2008; Bashir et al. 2011; Guyuron 2008; Stal and Hollier 2002).

20.3 Unilateral Cleft Nose Deformity

To repair the cleft nose, plastic surgeons should become familiar with the abnormalities and dysmorphology associated with the specific deformity and its effects on nose physiology resulting in nasal dysfunction (Guyuron 2008; Kaufman et al. 2012). It is important to recognize that the nasal deformity at the time of primary cleft repair may vary significantly from the secondary deformity seen in adulthood (Guyuron 2008; Kaufman et al. 2012).

20.3.1 Primary Cleft Nose Deformity

The primary unilateral cleft nose deformity is characterized by the following features: the columella is shorter on the cleft side; the base of the columella is deviated to the noncleft side; the lateral crus of the lower lateral cartilage is longer on the cleft side; the nasal tip is displaced in both the frontal and the horizontal planes; the nasal tip is asymmetric; the ala is flattened, resulting in horizontal orientation of the nostril; the nostrils are asymmetric; the entire nostril is retropositioned because of the deficiency in the underlying frame; the base of the ala is displaced laterally and/or posteriorly and sometimes inferiorly; the nasal floor is caudal on the cleft side; a nasolabial fistula could be present; the septum and anterior nasal spine are shifted toward the noncleft vestibule; the nasal septum is deviated, resulting in a varying degree of nasal obstruction; the inferior turbinate on the cleft side is hypertrophic; the maxilla is hypoplastic on the cleft side; and the premaxilla and the maxillary segments are displaced (Bardach and Cutting 1990).

20.3.2 Secondary Cleft Nose Deformity

Features of the primary deformity complicated by the influence of primary rhinoplasty and facial growth eventually determinate a complex and wide spectrum of secondary cleft nasal deformities (Figs. 20.1, and 20.2). The cleft ala lies caudal and lateral to the noncleft side. It rests on an underdeveloped maxilla, which partly accounts for alar base lowering and horizontal nostril seating. The cleft ala may be underdeveloped and weak and exhibit a convoluted shape. This contributes further to dome lowering on the cleft side. Malfunction of the cleft ala external valve is caused by alar base malposition, imbalanced muscular pull, and abnormal attachment of the cheek muscles to the lateral crus. Tip projection is further compromised by a foreshortened columella that lies obliquely with its base directed away from the cleft side. The caudal septum is associated with the anterior nasal spine, which is deviated off facial midline to the noncleft side. The cartilaginous mid-septum and the osseous posterior septum (perpendicular plate of the ethmoid bone) deviate significantly toward the cleft side, resulting in a complex C-shaped deformity both craniocaudally and anteroposteriorly. The deviation of the cartilaginous septum toward the cleft side narrows the cleft-side airway while enlarging the noncleft cross-sectional area. The noncleft-side turbinate hypertrophies to occupy this space on the noncleft side. The nasal bones are frequently widened both at the dorsum and at the frontal process of the maxilla. Deviation may affect the bony and the cartilaginous segments. Generally, midvault curvature is present with collapse on the concave side and fullness on the convex side. Furthermore, smaller airways as demonstrated in rhinometry and external valve malfunction may add to the airway problem (Fisher et al. 2014; Byrd et al. 2007).

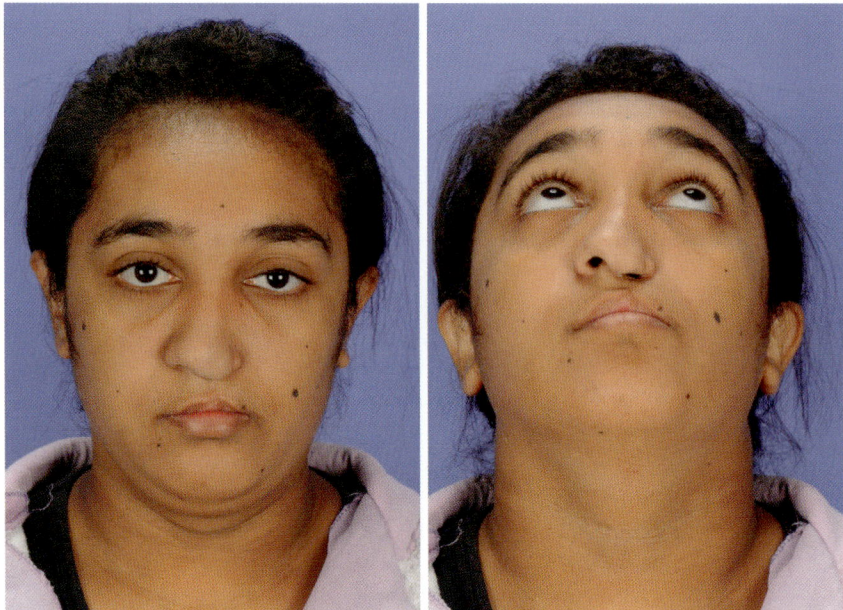

Fig. 20.1 (*Left*) Full-face front and (*right*) basal views of a skeletally mature patient with unilateral complete cleft lip and palate illustrating the secondary unilateral cleft lip nasal deformity: nasal tip deviated; alar cartilage displaced caudally; angle between medial and lateral crura more obtuse buckling in lateral crura; the alar base deviated posteriorly, inferiorly, and laterally when compared with the noncleft side; flattened alar facial angle; widened nostril floor; columella and anterior caudal septal border deviated on noncleft side

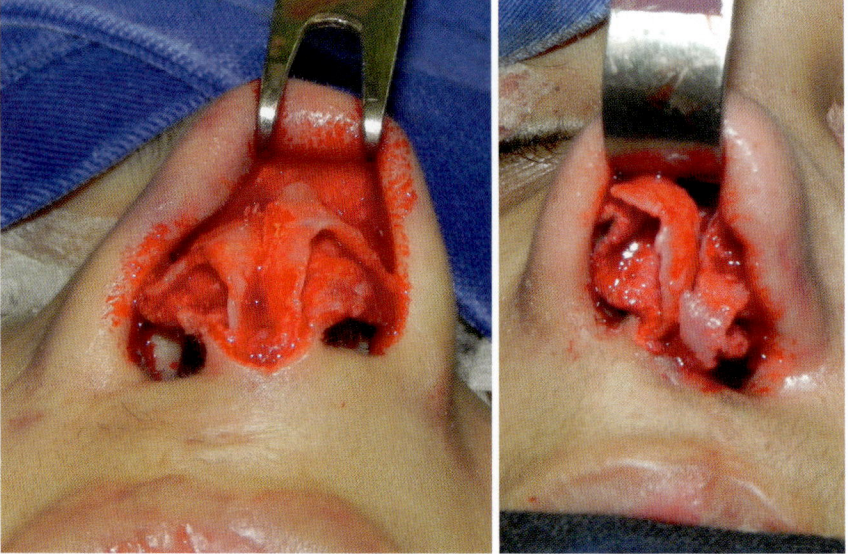

Fig. 20.2 Intraoperative basal photographs of two skeletally mature patients with unilateral complete cleft lip and palate illustrating the different patterns of secondary unilateral cleft lip nasal deformity

20.4 Surgical Management

The goals of cleft nose repair include final creation of lasting symmetry, achieving definition of the nasal base and nasal tip, relief of nasal obstruction, and management of nasal scarring and webbing. In the literature (Fisher et al. 2014; Byrd et al. 2007; Guyuron 2008; Stal and Hollier 2002; Wolfe et al. 2016; Sykes et al. 2016), there are an enormous variation in techniques and treatment protocols for the cleft nose. In fact, as the clinical presentation of cleft nose deformities varies widely, each particular cleft patient presents a unique challenge and an arsenal of well-orchestrated maneuvers can be used with slight variations from patient to patient. As complete correction of all of the cleft nose deformities remains a challenge for plastic surgeons, a standardized surgical approach based on the severity of soft-tissue and skeletal deformities as well as previous procedures performed is important to outline the predilection of the results and their limitations.

20.4.1 Timing

Relevant standardized surgical steps (namely, primary rhinocheiloplasty, alveolar bone grafting, and Le Fort I advancement) from the comprehensive rehabilitate longitudinal cleft care are extremely relevant prior to the secondary cleft rhinoplasty as it may directly influence the surgical approach and outcomes.

Performing primary cleft rhinoplasty at the same setting as the cleft lip repair had been accepted worldwide and the traditional concern for disruption of growth centers in the nose has waned (Millard and Morovic 1998; McComb and Coghlan 1996). The principal goal of primary nasal correction has been to produce a more symmetrical nasal form (closure of the nasal floor and sill, repositioning of the alar base, and repositioning of the lower lateral cartilages) and to reduce the stigma that is often experienced during childhood. It may also provide a less complicated secondary revision, which is required by many patients in late adolescence (Byrd et al. 2007; Haddock et al. 2012). At our craniofacial plastic surgery center, primary cleft lip nose repair is typically performed at 3 months of age; we adhere to the conventional rule of 10s, and surgery is deferred until the child is 10 pounds in weight, at or after 10 weeks of age, with a hemoglobin concentration of 10 g/dL. We (Buzzo 2010; Raposo-Amaral et al. 2014, 2012; Raposo-Amaral 2010; Somensi et al. 2012) have particularly adopted two primary cleft lip repairs (namely, modified Göteborg technique and modified Cutting extended Mohler technique according to author's experience) without presurgical nasoalveolar molding. The treatment of the unilateral cleft nose has been according to McComb primary nasal reconstruction principles (McComb and Coghlan 1996; Buzzo 2010; Raposo-Amaral et al. 2014, 2012; Raposo-Amaral 2010; Somensi et al. 2012): using the existing cleft lip incisions, wide undermining of the nasal cartilages from the nasal skin is undertaken from the nostril rim to the nasion; and the lower lateral cartilages are then supported in proper position with sutures. Further relevant modifications were compiled in the "fifty years of the Millard rotation-advancement" article (Stal et al. 2009).

As the interplay of anatomy variables between maxillary advancement and rhinoplasty is inseparable (Davidson and Kumar 2015), secondary cleft nasal reconstruction should not be performed without first evaluating and correcting any significant problems with the skeletal base under the nose (Cutting 2000). Restoration of the continuity of the maxillary arch with alveolar bone grafting allows closure of oronasal fistulae, proper platform for tooth eruption, and alar base and pyriform aperture augmentation (Alonso et al. 2014; Raposo-Amaral et al. 2015a). In our center, cleft patients have preferably undergone transferring of secondary alveolar bone graft (between 7 and 12 years old) immediately before the cleft-side canine eruption and with previous orthodontic management. Late secondary alveolar bone grafting (>12 years) has been implemented in delayed referral. We adopted well-described principles (Alonso et al. 2014; Raposo-Amaral et al. 2015a; Santiago et al. 2014) including appropriate flap design, wide exposure, nasal floor reconstruction without tension, closure of oronasal fistula, packing bony defect with cancellous bone, and coverage of bone graft with gingival mucoperiosteal flaps. Bone grafts have been harvested from the anterior superior iliac crest by minimal access using two different techniques (Raposo-Amaral et al. 2015b).

Once skeletal growth nears completion, patients with repaired cleft lip and palate often exhibit a characteristic concave facial profile, which requires correction by Le Fort I osteotomy and maxillary advancement (Good et al. 2007). Le Fort I internal distraction presents better dental occlusion, less relapse, and better speech results than conventional orthognathic procedure, particularly in cleft patients with severe maxillary deficiency (Kumar et al. 2006), and the gradual advancement produced by distraction osteogenesis may result in greater facial soft-tissue changes and nasal projection than similar advancements using conventional maxillary advancement (Chua and Cheung 2012). At our center, Le Fort I internal distraction is adopted for surgical correction of the class III malocclusion secondary to maxillary hypoplasia in cleft patients with established severe negative overjet near the time of maxillary growth completion (11–12 years of age) and in cleft patients with maxillary retrusion (10 mm or higher of discrepancy between jaws) who have reached skeletal maturity. On the other side, conventional maxillary advancement (combined or not with mandibular setback) has been adopted in selected skeletal maturity patients with cleft maxillary hypoplasia according to the availability of devices and potential to adhere to the institutional protocol of distraction osteogenesis.

Finally, we perform the secondary cleft rhinoplasty at 14–16 years of age in female patients and at 16–18 years of age in male patients, as it allows the completion of the postpubertal growth spurt in the maxillary and nose (anterior septum and bony dorsum). Rhinoplasty at this time is definitive and more aggressive surgical maneuvers (e.g., septoplasty, cartilage grafting, and osteotomies) may be performed without concerns for affecting maxillary and nasal growth. In selected situations (i.e., severe nasal obstruction due to caudal septal deviation; and severe emotional distress from peer psychological pressure even with all the multidisciplinary support including longitudinal psychological care), an intermediate rhinoplasty (generally more conservative) is performed before the completion of nasal growth. In addition, if a cleft patient with significant dentofacial deformities (typically class III malocclusion) refuses to undergo maxillary reconstruction, their secondary rhinoplasty is delayed until this patient with aid of psychological support accepts the correction of the underlying skeletal base by alveolar bone grafting and/or Le Fort I advancement according to their individual needs.

20.4.2 Preoperative Characterization of Deformity

To make an accurate diagnosis of secondary cleft nose deformity, the skin (thickness), the nasal bones (symmetry, length, and distance from the midline; the depth of the radix; and the presence or absence of a dorsal hump), the midvault (upper lateral cartilage collapse and vertical symmetry), the nasal tip (asymmetry or fullness; projection; bulbous, boxy, narrow, or parenthesis deformity), the alar base (width), the alae (thickness, vertical position), the nasal sill (configuration), the nasolabial angle, the internal and external valves (stenosis), the septum (deviation, perforation), and the turbinates (size and shape) should be examined and documented in detail (Fisher et al. 2014; Guyuron 2008). Nasal endoscopy and computed tomographic scans provide visualization beyond that which is visible on anterior rhinoscopy and are useful in surgical planning (Fisher et al. 2014). Some of the cardinal deformities proposed by Lee et al. (2011) and the key points described by Byrd et al. (2007) are extremely useful and complementary in the characterization of the deformity, contributing to elucidation of a specific anatomic pattern, and allow plastic surgeons to perform the most effective and directed correction procedures based on the formulation of a patient-customized surgical plan (Table 20.1).

Table 20.1 Useful notes for the elucidation of a specific cleft nose pattern, allowing the formulation of a patient-customized surgical plan

Lee's cardinal deformities (Lee et al. 2011)	Byrd's key points (Byrd et al. 2007)
Caudal deflection of the nasal septum to the noncleft side	Was primary cleft nose rhinoplasty performed?
Deviation of the nasal dorsum	Is the nasal lining deficient?
Low setting of the medical crus	Is the external valve patent and functional?
Tethering deformity of the lateral crus	Is tip projection adequate?
Discontinuity of the orbicularis oris muscle	Is the cleft lateral crus deformed by persisting alar crease or buckle?
Long or short lip deformity	Is the alar base recessed and tethered to the pyriform?
Absence of a philtral column	Is projection of the bony dorsum deficient, normal, or overprojecting?

20.5 Secondary Unilateral Cleft Rhinoplasty

The surgical reconstruction of cleft nose deformity borrows from a large number of historical and innovative surgical principles as stated by Wolfe (2004). We compile the previously described surgical maneuvers (Fisher et al. 2014; Byrd et al. 2007; Guyuron 2008; Stal and Hollier 2002; Potter 1946; Tajima and Maruyama 1977; Flores et al. 2009; Kaufman et al. 2012; Wolfe et al. 2016; Sykes et al. 2016; Cutting 2000; Basta et al. 2014; Chang et al. 2011; Wang 2010; Cho 2007) which our group have adopted in secondary unilateral cleft rhinoplasties.

20.5.1 Inferior Turbinate Hypertrophy

We preferably perform selective submucosal resection of bone combined with lateral out-fracture and lateral displacement on one or both sides depending on the degree of obstruction. Performing this first will avoid trouble with bleeding in the remaining surgical intervention.

20.5.2 Open Approach

An open rhinoplasty approach facilitates nasal correction as it allows maximal visualization for accurate diagnosis, and adequate exposure for placement and suturing of structural grafts. We adopted a standard inverted V-shaped incision or a prior transcolumellar incision. In asymmetric nostrils, we connect the inferior/medial pole of the Tajima inverted-U nostril apex incision with the transcolumellar incision to reposition the alar cartilage and recontour the soft-tissue envelope of the nose on the cleft side. Subsequently, the nasal tip and nasal dorsum are degloved in a supraperichondrial and subperiosteal plane. Next, the septum is approached by dividing the interdomal ligament of the lower lateral cartilages. A submucoperichondrial dissection is performed, beginning at the anterior septal angle. Bilateral mucoperichondrial tunnels are dissected deep to the upper lateral cartilages, and a scalpel is used to separate the upper lateral cartilages from the dorsal septum, taking care not to disrupt the k-area and lose the anchoring point of the upper lateral cartilages.

20.5.3 Dorsum

Dorsal humps are usually not a significant issue for cleft patients, but if a dorsal humpectomy is indicated, conservative excision is advisable at the outset of the surgical procedure because additional excision is always possible. If a bone hump is to be reduced, a subperiosteal pocket should be created; if osteotomies are expected, this dissection should not be carried out laterally to preserve soft-tissue support of the nasal bones. The cartilaginous dorsum is sharply excised with a number 11 blade under direct vision, followed by a series of graded fomon rasps for mild-to-moderate osseous hump reduction. For large dorsal humps, an en bloc bone and cartilaginous dorsal hump reduction is performed with a 10-mm nasal osteotome. Care is taken not to disrupt the upper lateral cartilage attachments to the undersurface of the nasal bones. Nasal rasps can be further used to soften any jagged, asymmetrical, or irregular edges; it should be performed at an oblique angle to again avoid loss of upper lateral cartilage attachment and direct trauma to these cartilages themselves.

If the dorsum is deficient or the nose is short, osseocartilaginous dorsal onlay rib graft is our choice for reconstruction of the dorsum. The harvested rib segment is shaped to span the entire length of the nasal dorsum, from the radix to the septal angle, to minimize the risk for palpable irregularities. In addition, the recipient bed must be made as flat and as smooth as possible to give the greatest surface area for the dorsal onlay graft to contact.

20.5.4 Septum

Having achieved a smooth dorsum, comprehensive treatment of the septum is undertaken. The bowing midportion of the cartilaginous septum is resected, leaving behind a 12–15 mm L-strut; it not only treats the septal deformity but also provides graft material. Deviated portions of the perpendicular plate of the ethmoid bone are carefully resected, avoiding transmission of forces cephalad that can injure the cribriform plate. A typically lengthy spur along the maxillary crest is also resected using a combination of a 2 mm osteotome and Kerrison rongeurs. Next, the caudal portion of the L-strut is disarticulated from the osseocartilaginous junction with the anterior nasal spine and maxillary crest in the noncleft side, the degree of vertical excess is then excised as indicated, and it is finally anchored at the midline into the periosteum of the anterior nasal spine.

20.5.5 Middle Nasal Vault

If the internal valve has collapsed, suturing Sheen's spreader grafts (contoured in a rectangular shape with variable length, 1–4 mm in width, and no more than 5 mm in height so as not to impinge on the nasal airway) between the dorsal septum (2 mm below the septal border) and the anterior aspect of the upper lateral cartilages reconstructs the midvault (close the open-roof deformity, if present) while improving the internal valve and straightening the dorsal angle. Depending on the amount of deviation and asymmetry, bilateral or asymmetric spreader grafts are applied; a thicker graft can be placed on the cleft side to address concavity, if present. In selected patients, caudally extended bilateral spreader grafts is a very useful technique for nasal lengthening and controlling of tip projection, rotation, and shape; stability is optimized when these grafts are integrated with a columellar strut. We prefer harvesting the spreader grafts from the cartilage of the septum. If the quadrangular cartilage is insufficient, the costal cartilage grafts are harvested from the sixth or seventh ribs. The segment of the rib harvested can be up to 3.5–4 cm in length (it generally provides sufficient cartilaginous tissue for both the dorsal graft and the columellar strut) (Figs. 20.3 and 20.4) and be delivered through an inframammary

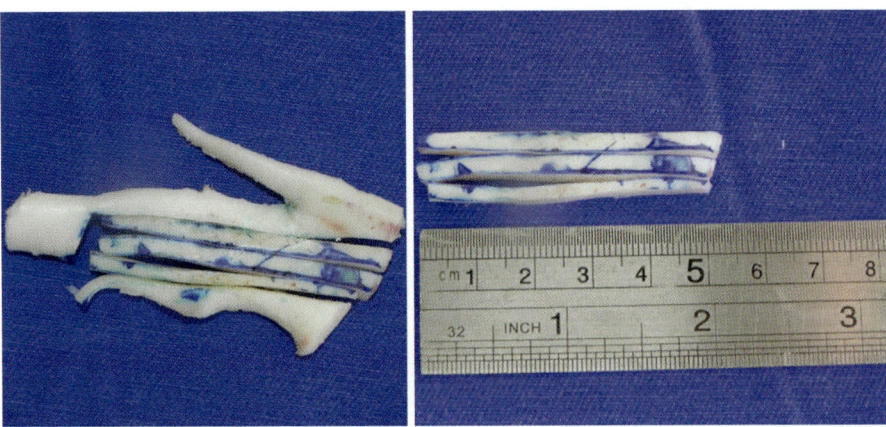

Fig. 20.3 Only the central portion of the harvested rib cartilage was applied for the fabrication of the strut columellar graft and the spreader grafts

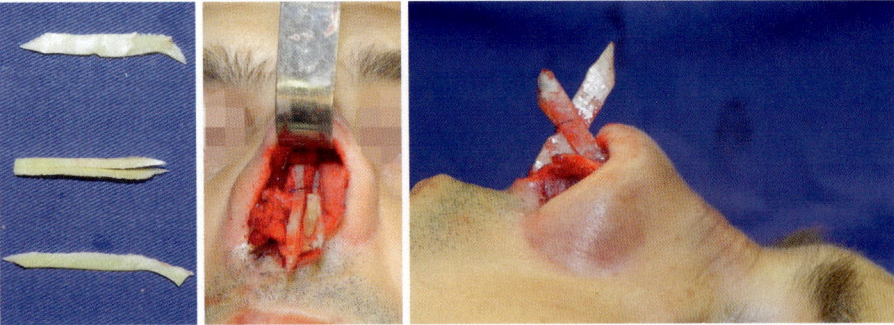

Fig. 20.4 (*Left*) Rib cartilage grafts (strut columellar and spreader grafts). (*Central*) Basal and (*right*) lateral intraoperative views of bilateral spreader grafts and strut columellar graft inset. The columellar strut placed between the paired intermediate and medial crura provides structural support to the nasal tip and improves tip projection. Spreader grafts placed along either side of the septum correct internal nasal valve dysfunction. Clinical photographs of the patient in Figs. 20.27–20.31

incision in female (marked approximately 5 mm above the fold) or subcostal incision in male with variable dimensions according to the surgical technique and patients' characteristics.

Spreader flaps, also known as autospreader flaps or turnover flap, entail mucosal elevation as with normal spreader grafts, then use of the medial aspect of the upper lateral cartilages themselves as a spreader; this is accomplished with either complete separation, a partial-thickness incision and hinged placement, or folding of the medial aspect of the cartilage without any incisions. It adjusts the height of the upper lateral cartilages in a precise and safe manner while preserving the function of the internal valve. These flaps are secured in the same fashion as standard spreaders.

20.5.6 Nasal Tip

A variety of surgical maneuvers can be used to enhance or improve the nasal tip. The tongue-in-groove technique allows the nasal tip to be resuspended on the septum (i.e., fixation of the medial crura of the lower lateral cartilages to the caudal end of the nasal septum) to improve tip support and projection; the cleft alar cartilage has to be advanced more than the noncleft side to improve the flattening of the cleft lower lateral cartilage and enhance overall tip symmetry. As an alternative, we prefer to advance and fix the medial crura on the columellar strut cartilage graft to enhance projection and support according to the Anderson's tripod theory of nasal tip support.

Once the central limb of the tripod is stabilized, attention is directed to its lateral limbs. The cleft lateral crus of the lower lateral cartilage is usually concave and often associated with alar malposition, with the cartilage often being inferiorly displaced in relation to the position of the noncleft lower lateral cartilage. An alar margin (rim) graft (placed inferior to the existing cartilage in a nonanatomic position) or a Gunter's lateral crural strut graft (placed on the deep surface of the lower lateral cartilage, with the graft sutured to the undersurface of the cartilage, and the lateral extent positioned in a pocket at the pyriform aperture) can be adopted for supporting the alar rim, elevating the level of the alar rim, and repositioning the rim laterally. Importantly, the lateral crural strut graft is well suited to the thin-skinned patient who has a moderate degree of alar collapse and in whom an unfavorable aesthetic result would be expected with alar batten grafting (placed cephalad to the alar rim for correction of external nasal valve collapse; the exact position of the graft is determined by the site of maximal collapse). An alar turn-in flap (the cephalic portion of the lower lateral cartilage is transposed on a pedicle and sutured to the undersurface of the remaining lower lateral cartilage) or the flip-flop technique (dissecting the lateral crura off the underlying vestibular skin, excising this portion, turning it over, and resuturing it to the vestibular lining) can also be adopted to strengthen and support the lower lateral cartilage and to flatten the preexisting concavity. A superomedially based V-Y chondromucosal composite flap of the cleft-side lateral crus of the lower lateral and its attendant nasal mucosa in association with an interdomal suture (to advance the cleft-side lower lateral cartilage flap) and a Tajima-type suture (to suspend the lower lateral cartilage to the contralateral upper lateral cartilage) can also be an option to achieve symmetric tip contour and projection.

If the tip cartilages have been damaged in the previous rhinoplasty procedures, we adopt the "Golden Arch" procedure described by Wolfe. A whole new alar structure (septal or costal cartilage) is sutured to the tip of the columellar strut and folded over to make a new ala, ignoring the native cartilage still tethered below. Instead, one-half of the arch can be sutured to the columellar strut and the underlying native ala (Figs. 20.5, 20.6, and 20.7).

In addition, intradomal, interdomal, and/or transdomal sutures can be used for improvement of alar contour as indicated. Imbrication of the cleft-side scroll area can also be executed by placing mattress sutures internally to raise the lateral crus cephalad, if needed. The glabella, dorsum, tip, and/or infratip lobule can be filled with diced cartilage to camouflage irregularities, especially in cleft patients with thin or inelastic skin. Further cartilaginous tip graft can be added to camouflage irregularities and improve tip definition or according to specific diagnosis,

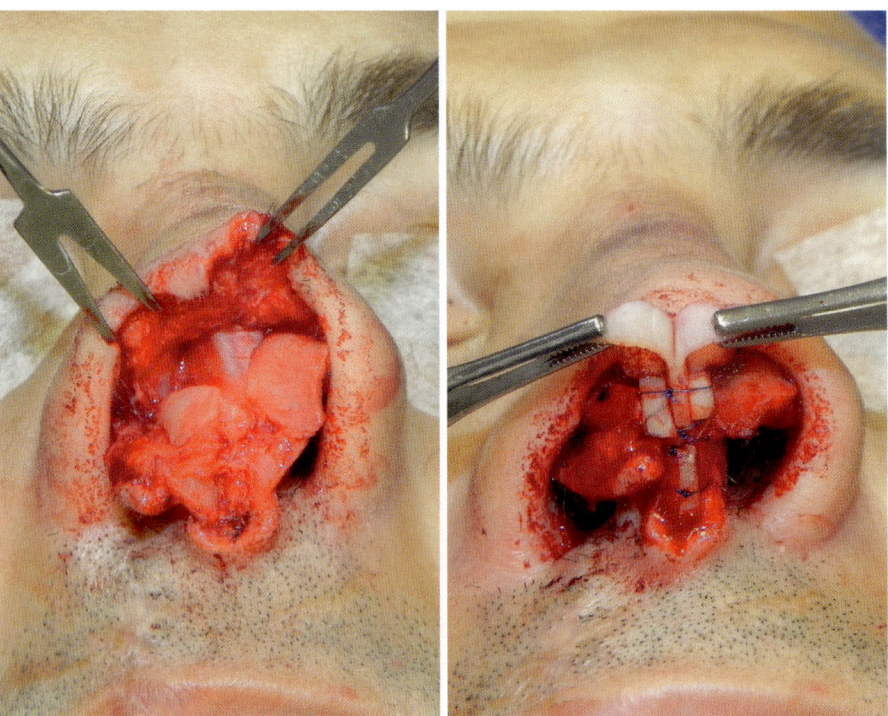

Fig. 20.5 A completely new alar cartilage framework was fabricated overlying the native alar cartilages, with a columellar strut and spreader grafts. Clinical photographs of the patient in Figs. 20.27–20.31

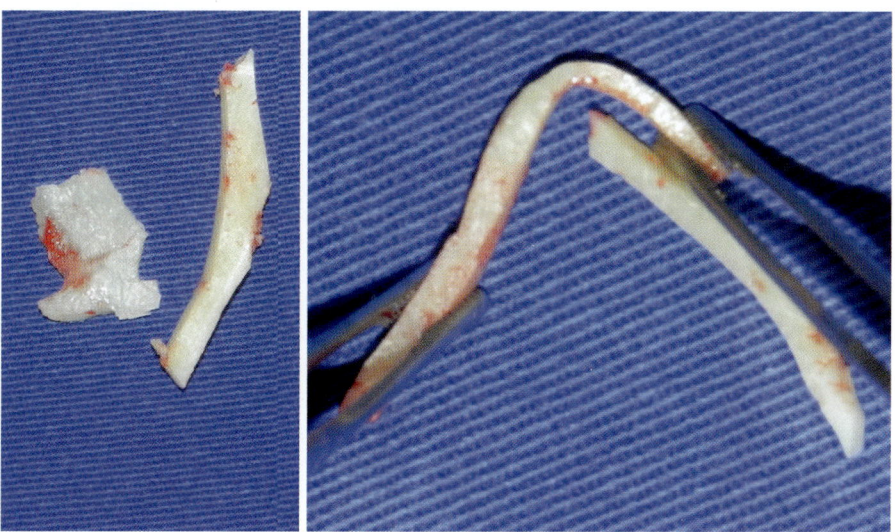

Fig. 20.6 A new alar cartilage framework and a shield graft were fabricated with rib cartilage and septal cartilage, respectively. Clinical photographs of the patient in Figs. 20.24–20.26

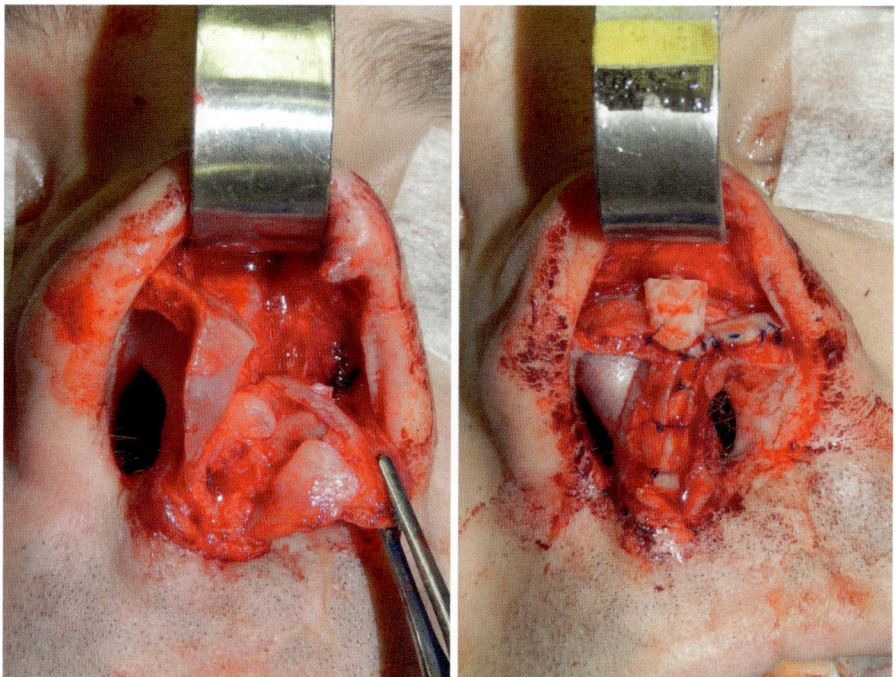

Fig. 20.7 (*Left*) Intraoperative basal photograph of a skeletally mature patient with unilateral complete cleft lip and palate illustrating the commitment of the cleft-side alar cartilage. (*Right*) Intraoperative basal photograph demonstrating a new cleft-side alar cartilage framework fabricated overlying the native alar cartilage, a septal cartilage shield tip graft, and rib cartilage strut columellar graft. Clinical photographs of the patient in Figs. 20.24–20.26

individual needs and/or prevent postoperative abnormalities. Overall, placement of tip grafts over the tip-defining points will increase tip projection and definition, whereas placement of these grafts at and below the tip-defining points will increase projection and add volume to the infratip lobule. The Sheen's shield graft (or infralobular graft) may be inserted at the tip-columellar junction (anterior to the intermediate crura) to define the "double-break" columellar profile; beveling of edges is important to avoid a visible "tombstone" appearance through skin. The anchor graft, a modified infratip shield graft, may be adopted to enhance tip projection, improve alar rim position, and augment the infratip region. Peck's onlay graft may be placed on the domal area to increase of tip projection in occasion of a thick fatty skin and this graft also permits variation of tip rotation, in relation to its more cranial or caudal placement. In a different maneuver, the cephalic trim portion of lower lateral cartilages can be left attached medially and then be used as an onlay tip graft. Another option is the umbrella graft which integrates an onlay tip graft with a columellar strut. The columella is sutured first with deep 5–0 mononylon (or polypropylene) then 6–0 mononylon in the skin; the intranasal incisions are closed with 5–0 catgut.

20.5.7 Nasal Bone Osteotomies

Nasal osteotomies are performed to straighten and narrow the nasal bridge and align the nasal profile; in cleft patients, abnormalities in the bony vault typically include a deviation to the noncleft side and a broad and flattened dorsum. We preferentially perform lateral osteotomies via an intranasal approach as a final surgical maneuver in our surgical rationale. A high-to-low lateral osteotomy (begins 3–4 mm anteriorly on the aperture and is continued in a posterocephalic direction up to the level of the medial canthus) is generally followed by a digital compression to produce a transverse greenstick fracture. If greater movement is required, we adopt a transverse percutaneous osteotomy (to insure that the thick frontal process of the maxilla breaks at the desired level) followed by a low-to-low lateral osteotomy (begins at the junction of the pyriform aperture and frontal process of the maxilla and is continued cephalically as close to the maxilla as possible up to the medial canthus), which results in a continuous osteotomy and a complete movement. If an open roof deformity is present after dorsal humpectomy, it needs to be corrected by low-to-low lateral osteotomies. At the end of the surgical procedure, home-customized internal paraseptal splints are sutured in position using transseptal nonabsorbable sutures and maintained for 1 month to coapt the mucosal flaps, keep the repositioned septal structures in the midline, and prevent synechiae. Packing (gauze with antibiotic ointment in the nasal cavity for 24 to 48 h), external taping, and dorsal nasal splinting (for 1–2 weeks) are also placed. Finally, we provide a wide spectrum of clinical examples (Figs. 20.8, 20.9, 20.10, 20.11, 20.12, 20.13, 20.14, 20.15, 20.16, 20.17, 20.18, 20.19, 20.20, 20.21, 20.22, 20.23, 20.24, 20.25, 20.26, 20.27, 20.28, 20.29, 20.30 and 20.31) surgically treated with a combination of surgical principles and maneuvers detailed in this chapter.

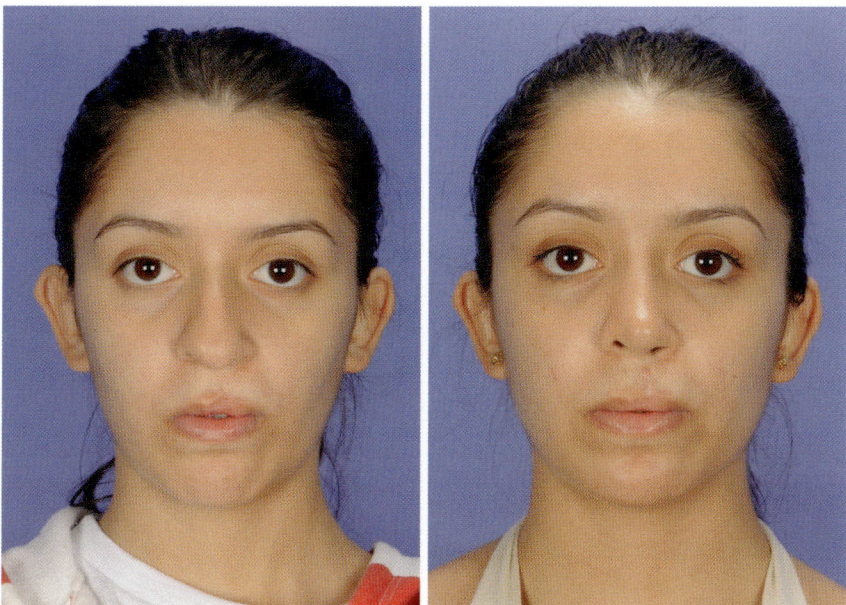

Fig. 20.8 (*Left*) Preoperative full-face front view of a skeletally mature patient with unilateral complete cleft lip and palate requesting secondary rhinoplasty. (*Right*) Late postoperative full-face front photographs after secondary cleft rhinoplasty

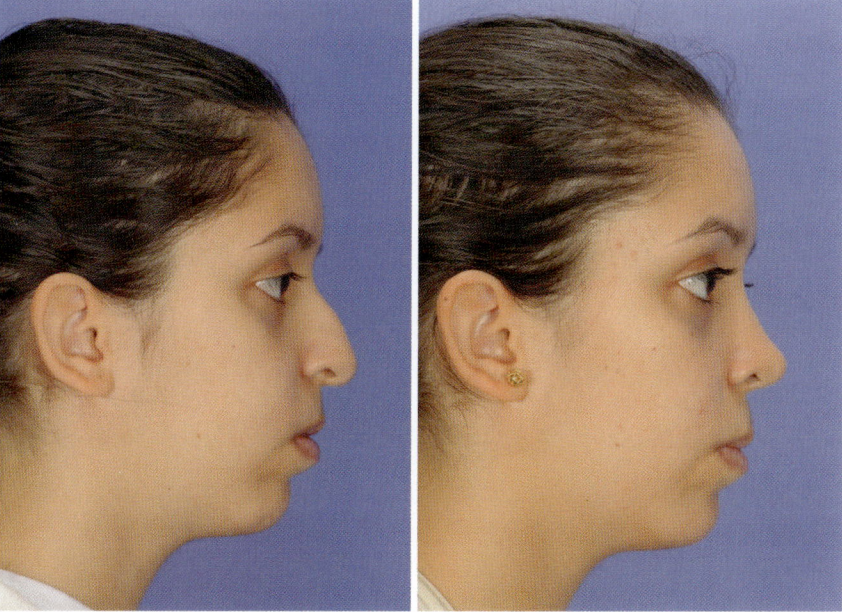

Fig. 20.9 (*Left*) Preoperative and (*right*) postoperative right profile photographs of the patient in Fig. 20.8

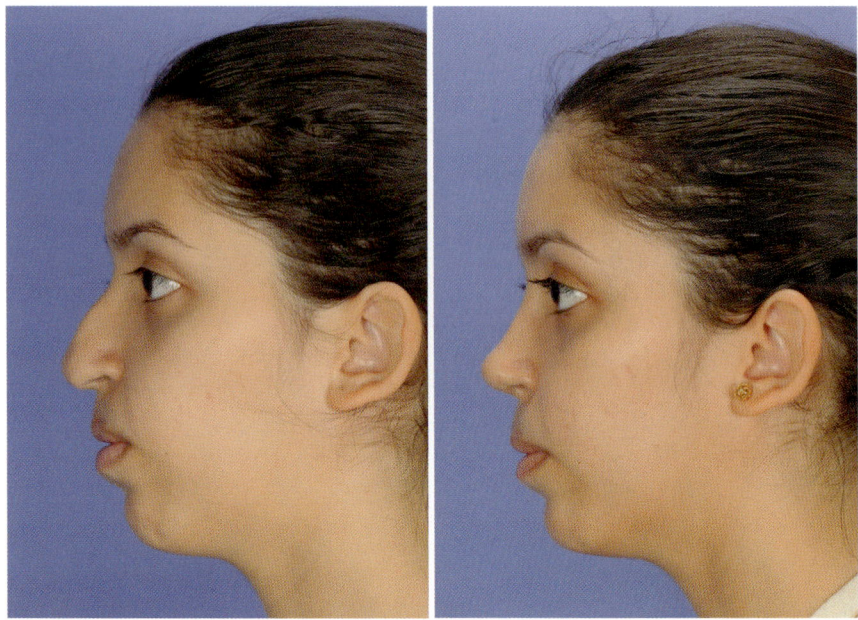

Fig. 20.10 (*Left*) Preoperative and (*right*) postoperative left profile photographs of the patient in Figs. 20.8, 20.9

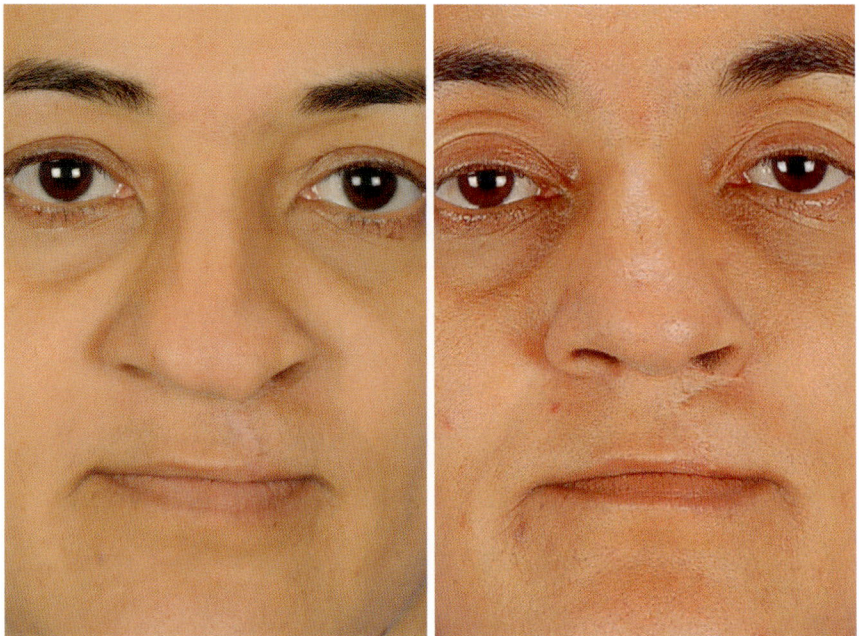

Fig. 20.11 (*Left*) Preoperative close-up front view of a skeletally mature patient with unilateral complete cleft lip and palate. (*Right*) Late postoperative full-face photographs after cleft nasal deformity repair

20 Secondary Unilateral Cleft Rhinoplasty

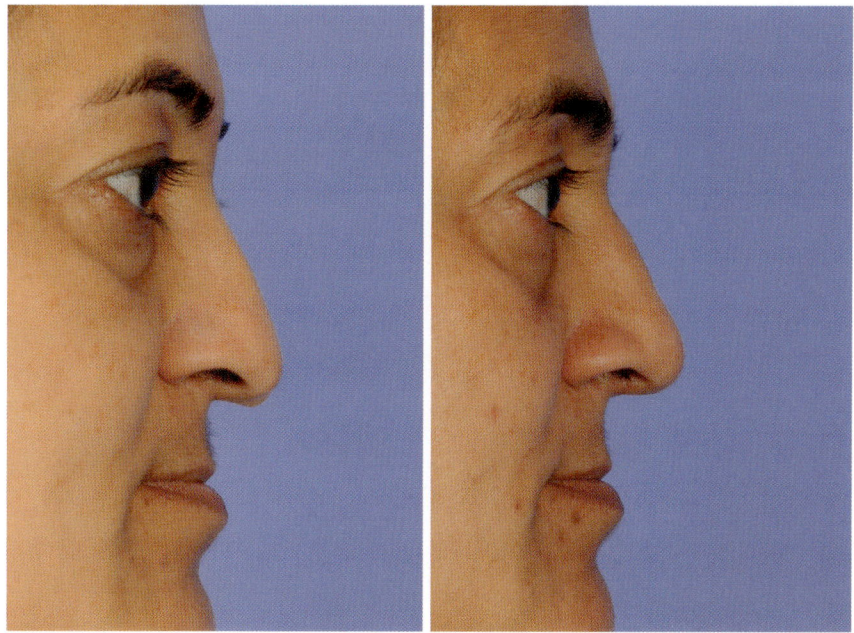

Fig. 20.12 (*Left*) Preoperative and (*right*) postoperative close-up right profile photographs of the patient in Fig. 20.11

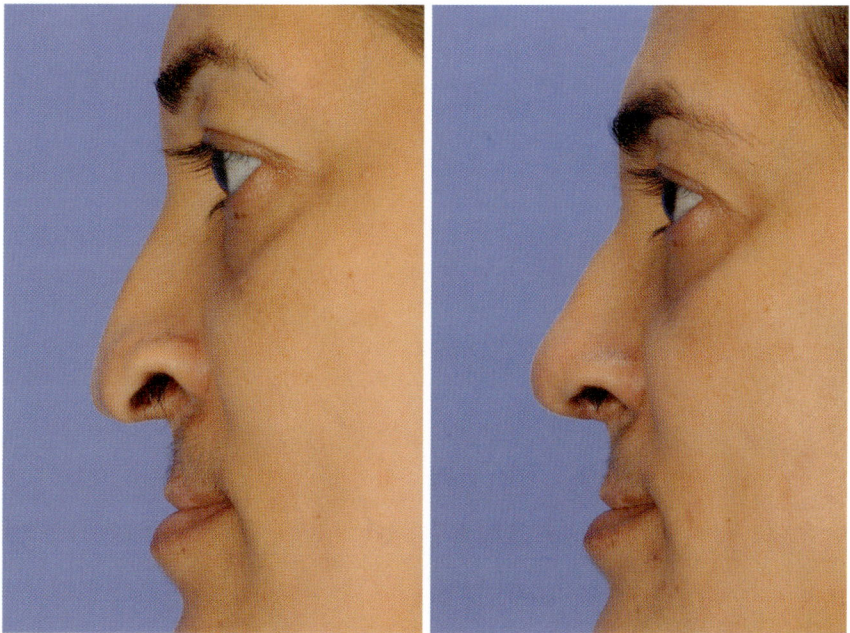

Fig. 20.13 (*Left*) Preoperative and (*right*) postoperative close-up left profile photographs of the patient in Figs. 20.11, 20.12

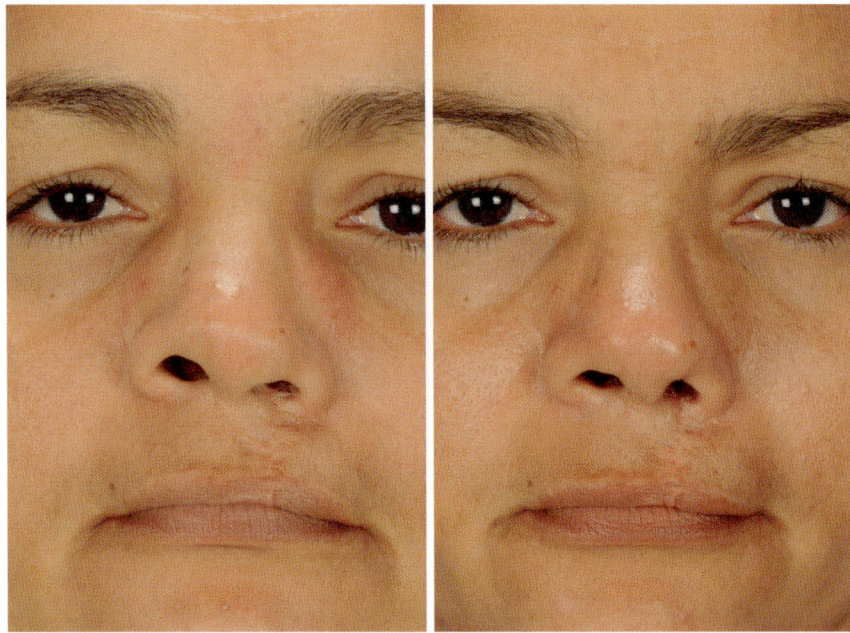

Fig. 20.14 (*Left*) Preoperative close-up front view of a patient with unilateral complete cleft lip and palate requesting secondary rhinoplasty. (*Right*) Late postoperative close-up photographs after secondary rhinoplasty

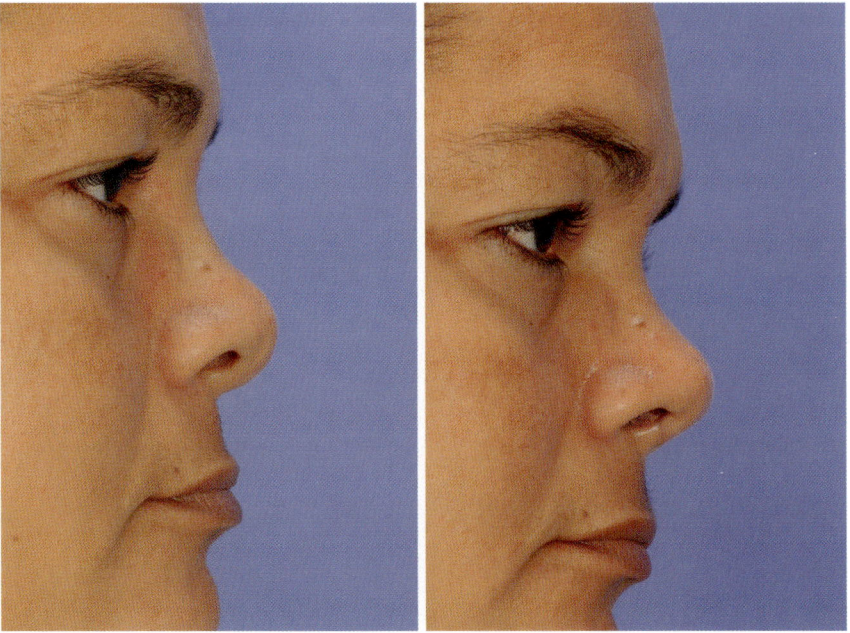

Fig. 20.15 (*Left*) Preoperative and (*right*) postoperative close-up right profile photographs of the patient in Fig. 20.14

20 Secondary Unilateral Cleft Rhinoplasty

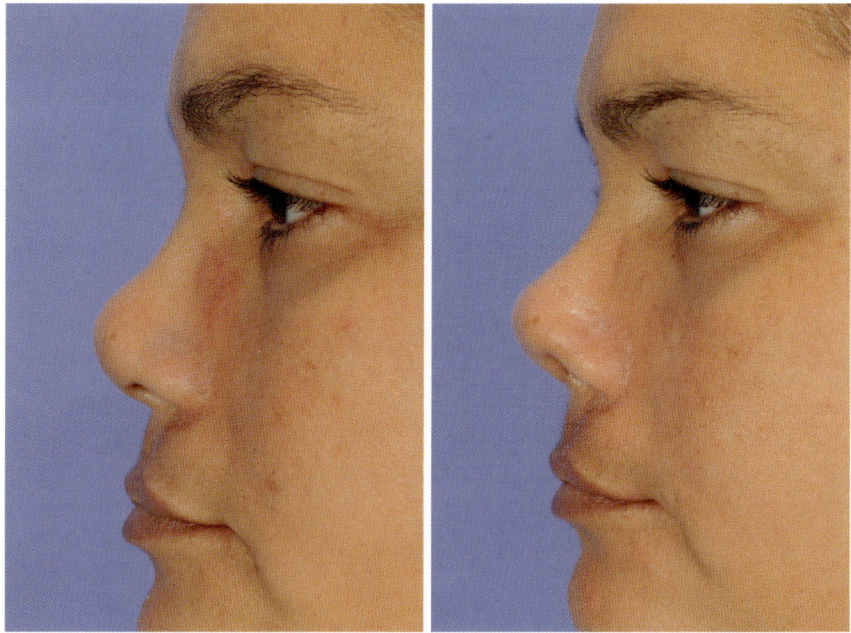

Fig. 20.16 (*Left*) Preoperative and (*right*) postoperative close-up left profile photographs of the patient in Figs. 20.14, 20.15

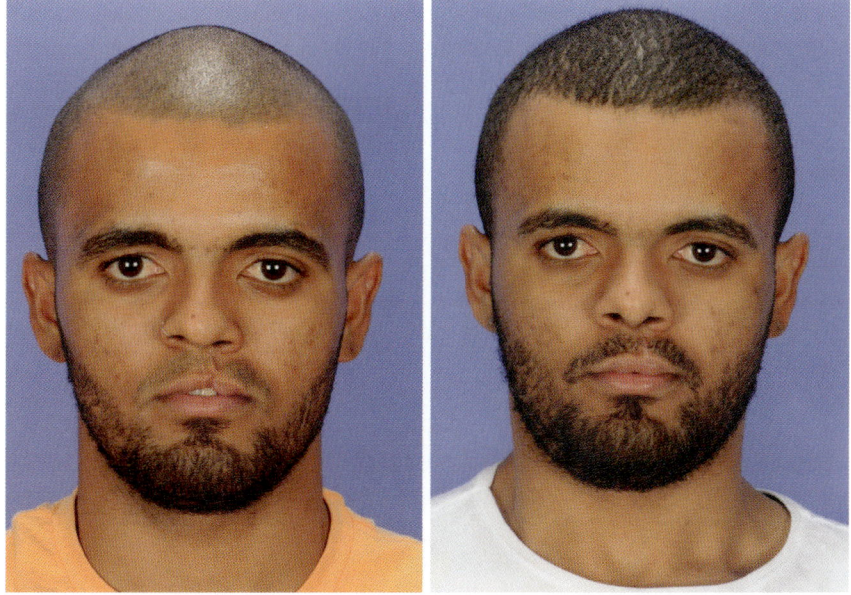

Fig. 20.17 (*Left*) Preoperative full-face front view of a skeletally mature patient with unilateral complete cleft lip and palate. (*Right*) Late postoperative full-face photographs after correction of secondary cleft nasal deformity

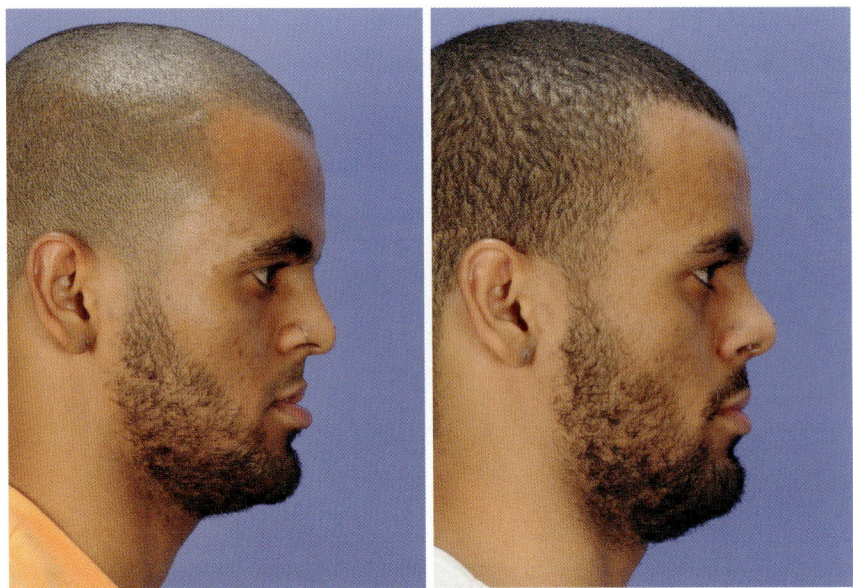

Fig. 20.18 (*Left*) Preoperative and (*right*) postoperative right profile photographs of the patient in Fig. 20.17

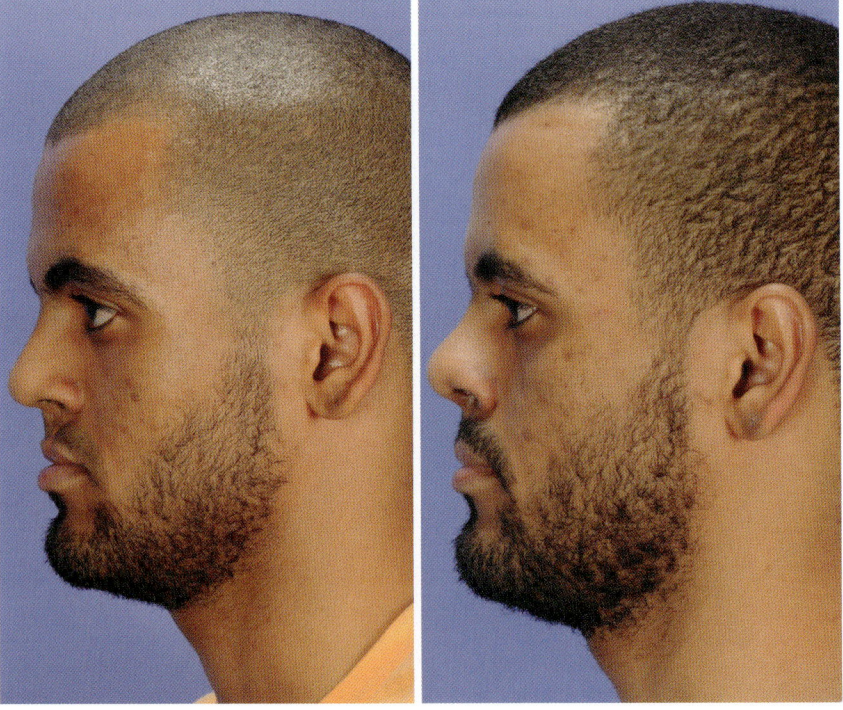

Fig. 20.19 (*Left*) Preoperative and (*right*) postoperative left profile photographs of the patient in Figs. 20.17, 20.18

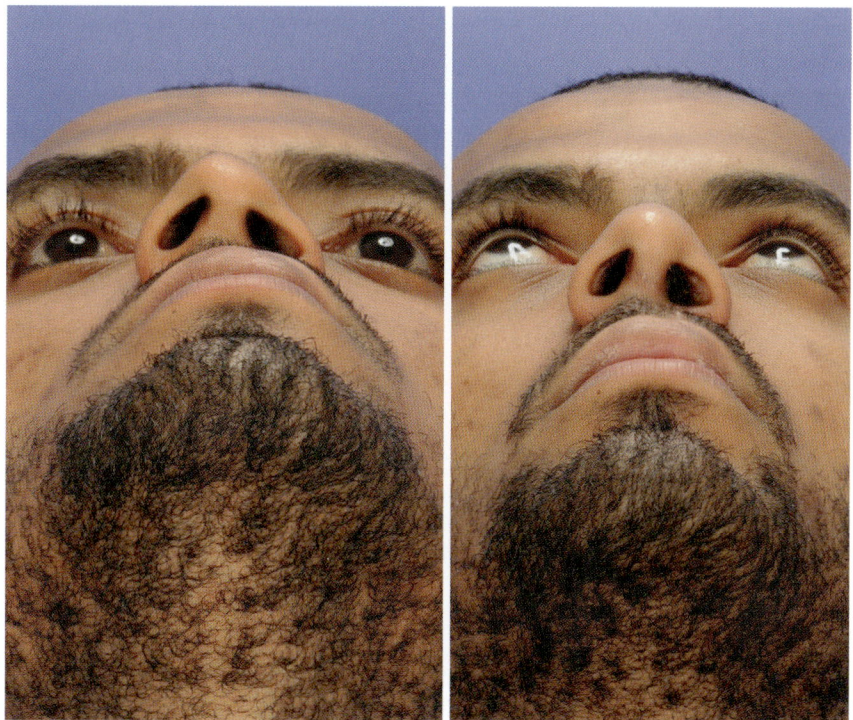

Fig. 20.20 (*Left*) Preoperative and (*right*) postoperative close-up submental oblique photographs of the patient in Figs. 20.17–20.19

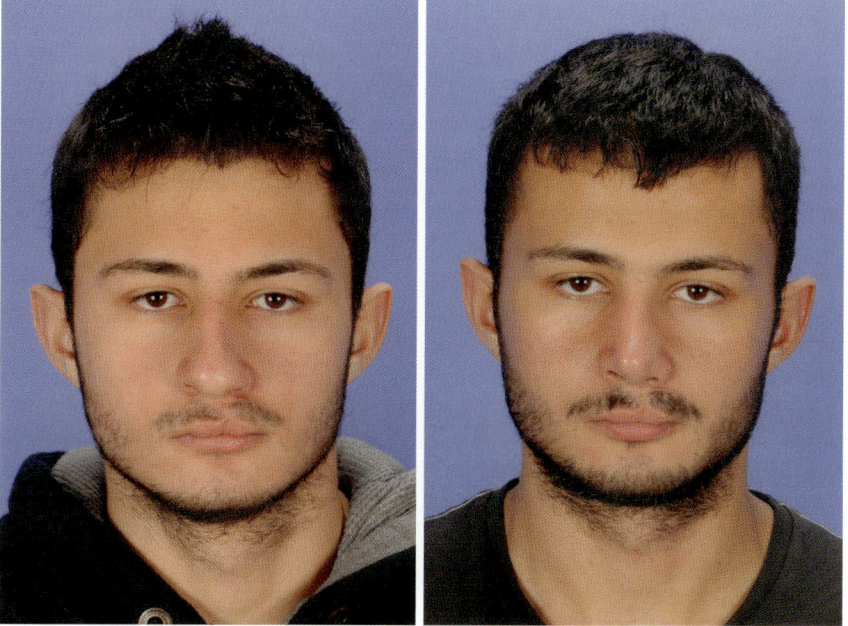

Fig. 20.21 (*Left*) Preoperative full-face front view of a unilateral complete cleft lip and palate patient illustrating the secondary unilateral cleft lip nasal deformity. (*Right*) Late postoperative full-face photographs after secondary cleft nasal reconstruction

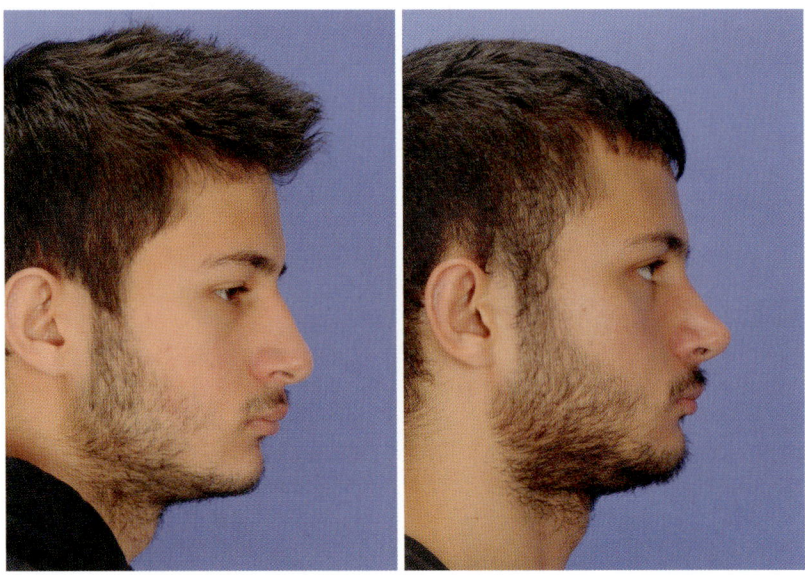

Fig. 20.22 (*Left*) Preoperative and (*right*) postoperative right profile photographs of the patient in Fig. 20.21

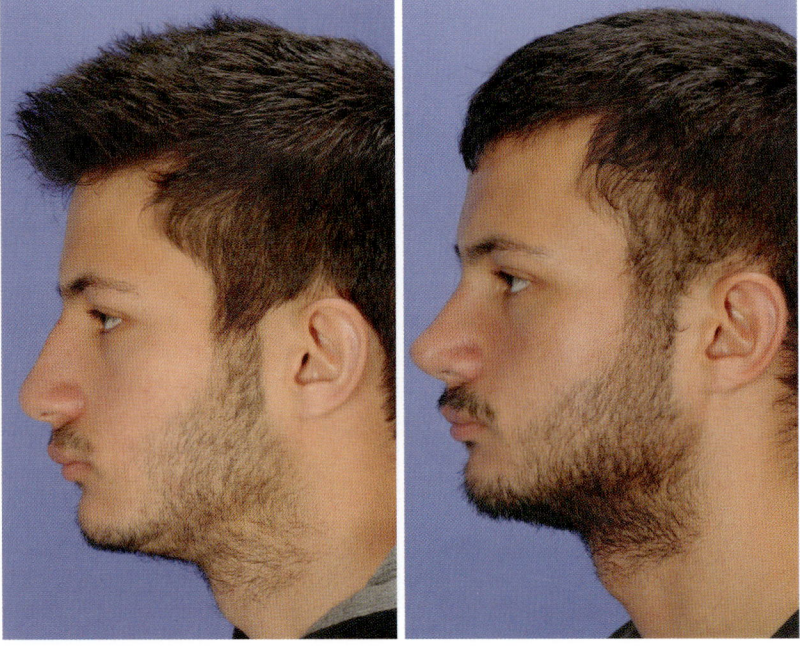

Fig. 20.23 (*Left*) Preoperative and (*right*) postoperative left profile photographs of the patient in Figs. 20.21 and 20.22

20 Secondary Unilateral Cleft Rhinoplasty

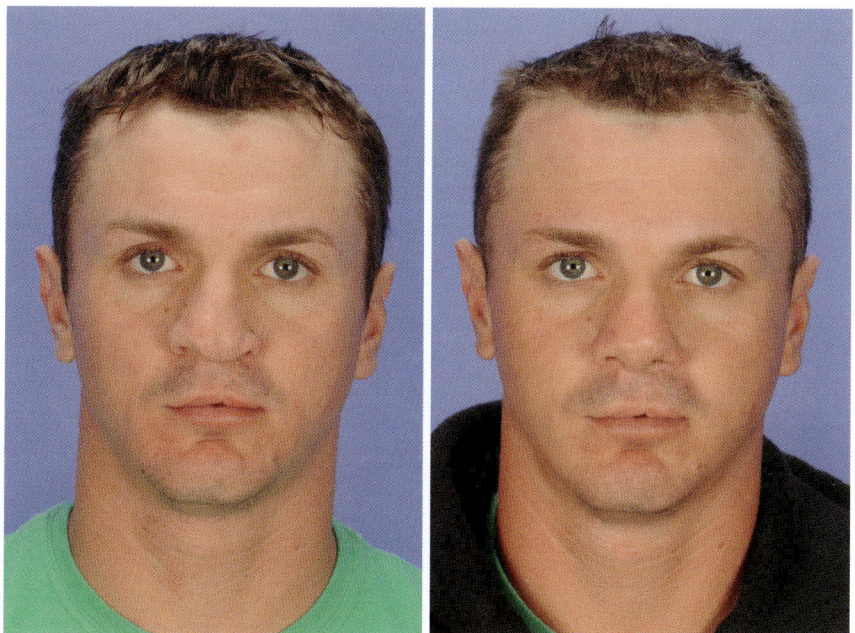

Fig. 20.24 (*Left*) Preoperative full-face view of a patient with secondary unilateral cleft lip nasal deformity. (*Right*) Late postoperative full-face photographs after secondary rhinoplasty

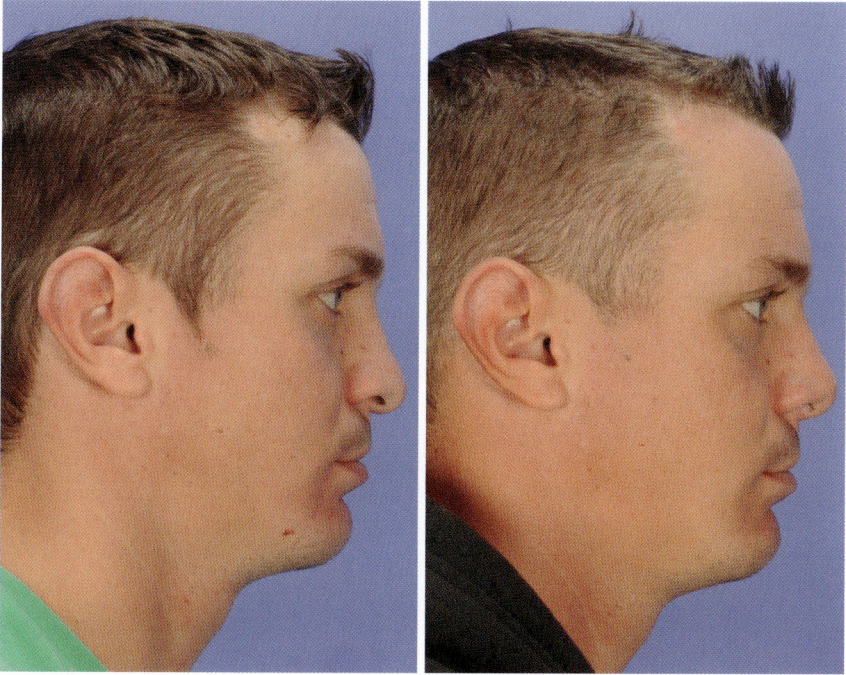

Fig. 20.25 (*Left*) Preoperative and (*right*) postoperative right profile photographs of the patient in Fig. 20.24

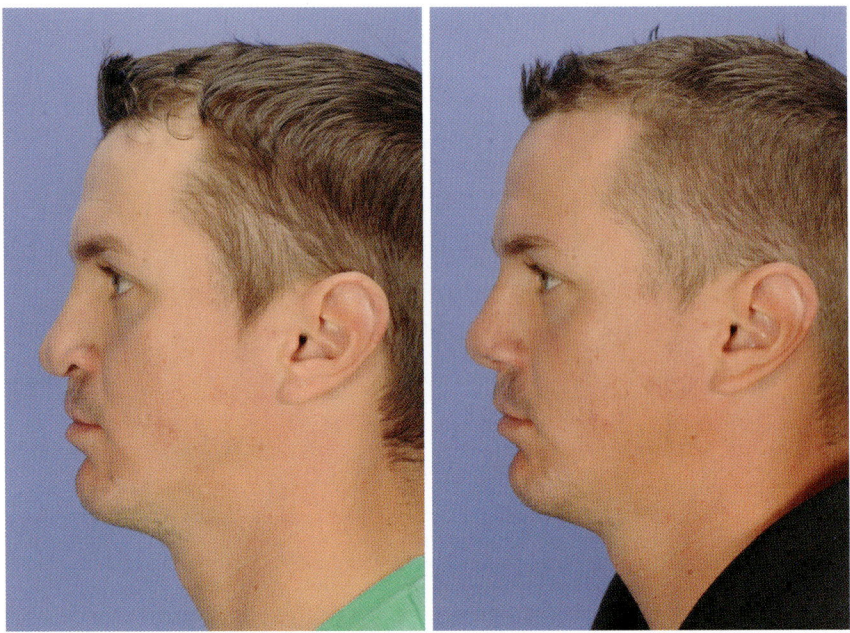

Fig. 20.26 (*Left*) Preoperative and (*right*) postoperative left profile photographs of the patient in Figs. 20.24–20.26

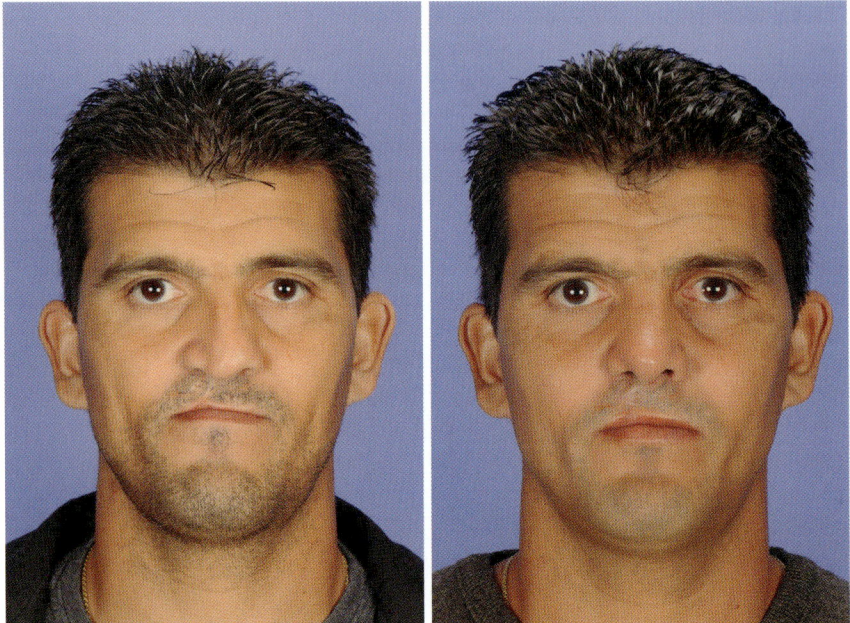

Fig. 20.27 (*Left*) Preoperative full-face view of a unilateral complete cleft lip and palate patient illustrating the secondary unilateral cleft lip nasal deformity. (*Right*) Late postoperative full-face photographs after secondary repair of unilateral cleft nose

20 Secondary Unilateral Cleft Rhinoplasty

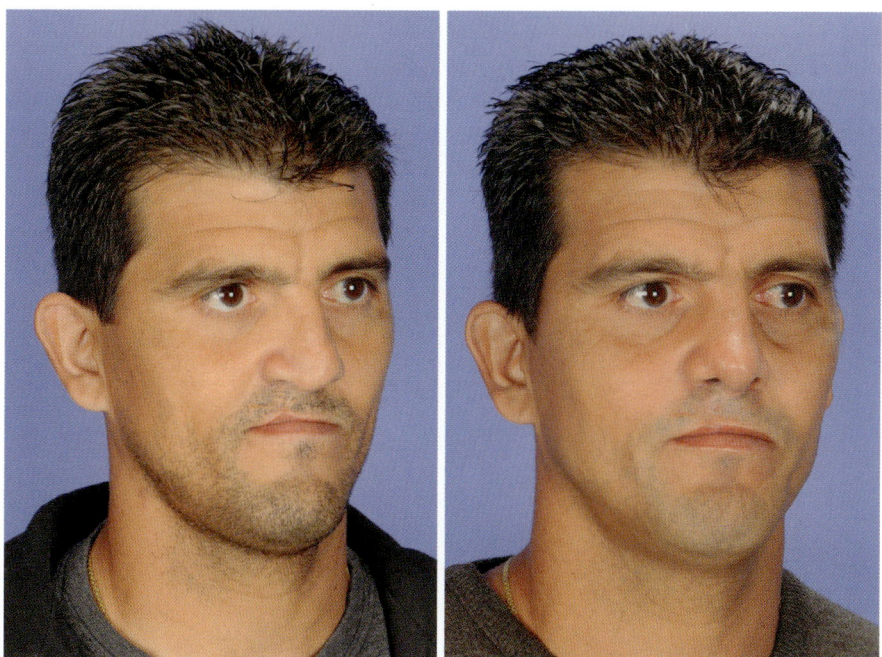

Fig. 20.28 (*Left*) Preoperative and (*right*) postoperative right oblique photographs of the patient in Fig. 20.27

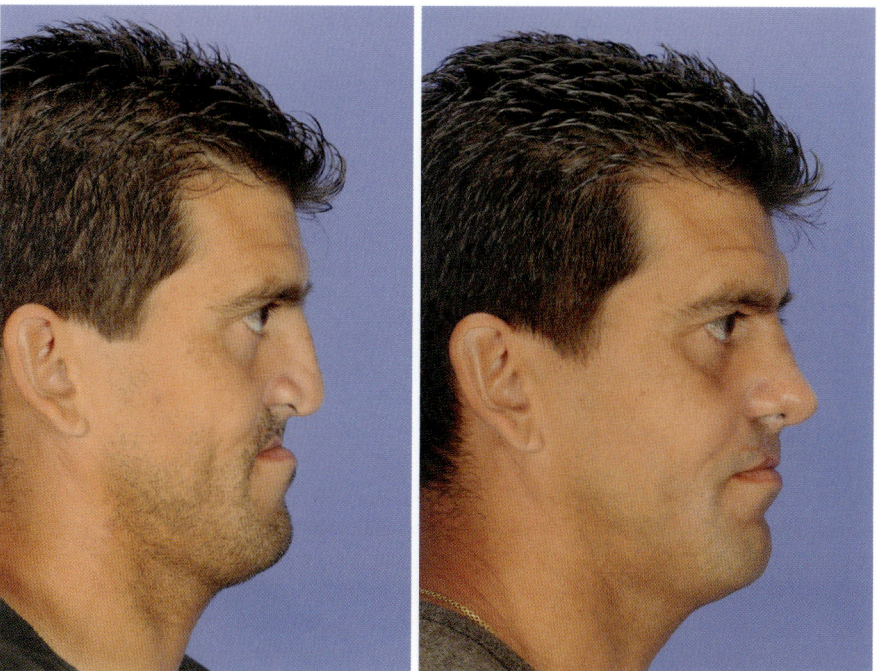

Fig. 20.29 (*Left*) Preoperative and (*right*) postoperative right profile photographs of the patient in Figs. 20.27 and 20.28

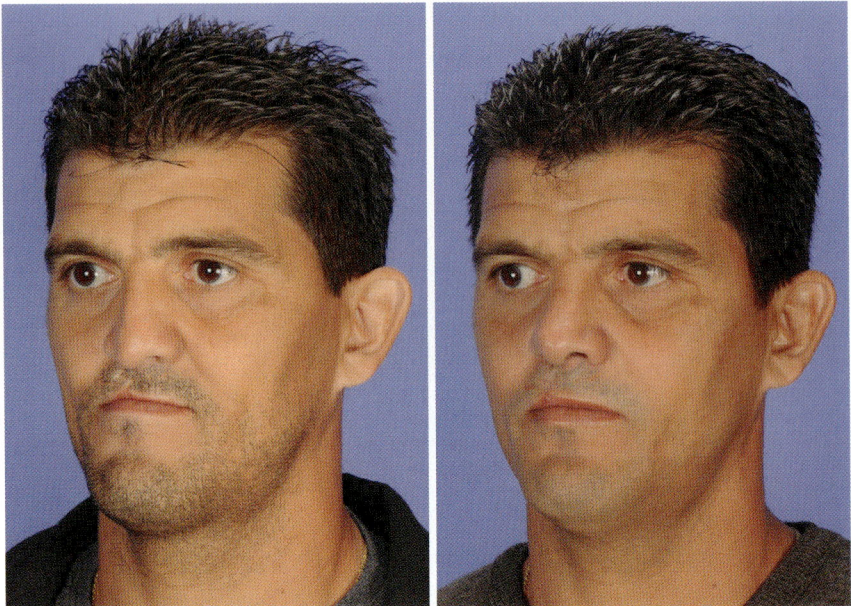

Fig. 20.30 (*Left*) Preoperative and (*right*) postoperative left oblique photographs of the patient in Figs. 20.27–20.29

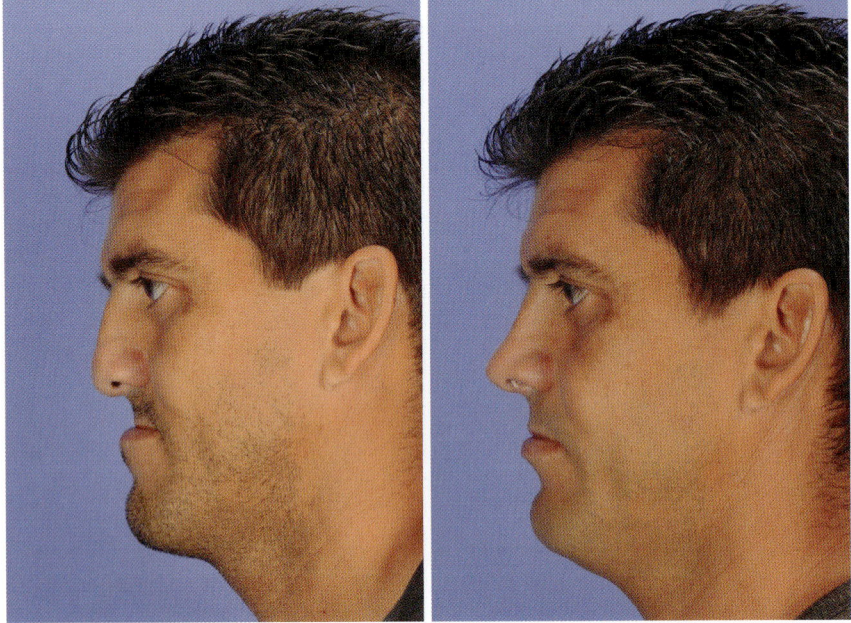

Fig. 20.31 (*Left*) Preoperative and (*right*) postoperative left profile photographs of the patient in Figs. 20.27–20.30

References

Alonso N, Risso GH, Denadai R, Raposo-Amaral CE. Effect of maxillary alveolar reconstruction on nasal symmetry of cleft lip and palate patients: a study comparing iliac crest bone graft and recombinant human bone morphogenetic protein-2. J Plast Reconstr Aesthet Surg. 2014;67:1201–8.

Bardach J, Cutting C. Anatomy of unilateral and bilateral cleft lip and nose. In: Bardach J, Morris HL, editors. Multidisciplinary Management of Cleft lip and Palate. Philadelphia: Saunders; 1990. p. 154–8.

Bashir M, Malik A, Khan FA. Comparison of suture and graft techniques in secondary unilateral cleft rhinoplasty. J Craniofac Surg. 2011;22:2172–5.

Basta MN, Goldstein JA, Wilson AJ, Taylor JA. A modified V-Y chondromucosal composite flap for correction of secondary cleft nasal deformity: photogrammetric analysis of a case-control study. Plast Reconstr Surg. 2014;134:94–101.

Buzzo CL. Surgical treatment of the cleft lip by Göteborg technique: 7 years follow up. Rev Bras Cir Plást. 2010;25:251–9.

Byrd HS, El-Musa KA, Yazdani A. Definitive repair of the unilateral cleft lip nasal deformity. Plast Reconstr Surg. 2007;120:1348–56.

Chang CS, Por YC, Liou EJ, Chang CJ, Chen PK, Noordhoff MS. Long-term comparison of four techniques for obtaining nasalsymmetry in unilateral complete cleft lip patients: a single surgeon's experience. Plast Reconstr Surg. 2010;126:1276–84.

Chang CS, Bergeron L, Chen PK. Diced cartilage rhinoplasty technique for cleft lip patients. Cleft Palate Craniofac J. 2011;48:663–9.

Cho BC. Correction of unilateral cleft lip nasal deformity in preschool and school-aged children with refined reverse-U incision and V-Y plasty: long-term follow-up results. Plast Reconstr Surg. 2007;119:267–27.

Chua HD, Cheung LK. Soft tissue changes from maxillary distraction osteogenesis versus orthognathic surgery in patients with cleft lip and palate-a randomized controlled clinical trial. J Oral Maxillofac Surg. 2012;70:1648–58.

Converse JM. Reconstructive plastic surgery, vol. 1. Philadelphia, PA: WB Saunders; 1964.

Cutting CB. Secondary cleft lip nasal reconstruction: state of the art. Cleft Palate Craniofac J. 2000;37:538–41.

Davidson E, Kumar AR. A preliminary three-dimensional analysis of nasal aesthetics following le fort I advancement in patients with cleft lip and palate. J Craniofac Surg. 2015;26:e629–33.

Dibbell DG. Cleft lip nasal reconstruction: correcting the classic unilateral defect. Plast Reconstr Surg. 1982;69:264–71.

Fisher MD, Fisher DM, Marcus JR. Correction of the cleft nasal deformity: from infancy to maturity. Clin Plast Surg. 2014;41:283–99.

Flores RL, Sailon AM, Cutting CB. A novel cleft rhinoplasty procedure combining an open rhinoplasty with the Dibbell and Tajima techniques: a 10-year review. Plast Reconstr Surg. 2009;124:2041–7.

Freeman AK, Mercer NS, Roberts LM. Nasal asymmetry in unilateral cleft lip and palate. J Plast Reconstr Aesthet Surg. 2013;66:506–12.

Gillies H, Kilner TP. Hare-lip: operations for the correction of secondary deformities. Lancet. 1932;220:1369–75.

Good PM, Mulliken JB, Padwa BL. Frequency of le fort I osteotomy after repaired cleft lip and palate or cleft palate. Cleft Palate Craniofac J. 2007;44:396–401.

Guyuron B. MOC-PS(SM) CME article: late cleft lip nasal deformity. Plast Reconstr Surg. 2008;121:1–11.

Haddock NT, McRae MH, Cutting CB. Long-term effect of primary cleft rhinoplasty on secondary cleftrhinoplasty in patients with unilateral cleft lip-cleft palate. Plast Reconstr Surg. 2012;129:740–8.

Hwang K, Kim HJ, Paik MH. Unilateral cleft nasal deformity correction using conchal cartilage lily flower graft. J Craniofac Surg. 2012;23:1770–2.

Kaufman Y, Buchanan EP, Wolfswinkel EM, Weathers WM, Stal S. Cleft nasal deformity and rhinoplasty. Semin Plast Surg. 2012;26:184–90.

Kumar A, Gabbay JS, Nikjoo R, Heller JB, O'Hara CM, Sisodia M, Garri JI, Wilson LS, Kawamoto HK Jr, Bradley JP. Improved outcomes in cleft patients with severe maxillary deficiency after le fort I internal distraction. Plast Reconstr Surg. 2006;117:1499–509.

Lee DW, Choi BK, Park BY. Seven fundamental procedures for definitive correction of unilateral secondary cleft lip nasal deformity in soft tissue aspects. J Oral Maxillofac Surg. 2011;69:e420–30.

Masuoka H, Kawai K, Morimoto N, Yamawaki S, Suzuki S. Open rhinoplasty using conchal cartilage during childhood to correct unilateral cleft-lip nasal deformities. J Plast Reconstr Aesthet Surg. 2012;65:857–63.

McComb HK, Coghlan BA. Primary repair of the unilateral cleft lip nose: completion of a longitudinal study. Cleft Palate Craniofac J. 1996;33:23–30.

Millard DR Jr, Morovic CG. Primary unilateral cleft nose correction: a 10-year follow-up. Plast Reconstr Surg. 1998;102:1331–8.

Potter J. Some nasal tip deformities due to alar cartilage abnormalities. Plast Reconstr Surg. 1946;13:358–66.

Raposo-Amaral C. Assessment of lip and nasal asymmetry after primary cleft lip repair. Rev Bras Cir Plast. 2010;25:38–48.

Raposo-Amaral CE, Giancolli AP, Denadai R, Marques FF, Somensi RS, Raposo-Amaral CA, Alonso N. Lip height improvement during the first year of unilateral complete cleft lip repair using cutting extended Mohler technique. Plast Surg Int. 2012;2012:206481.

Raposo-Amaral CE, Giancolli AP, Denadai R, Somensi RS, Raposo-Amaral CA. Late cutaneous lip height in unilateral incomplete cleft lip patients does not differ from the normative data. J Craniofac Surg. 2014;25:308–13.

Raposo-Amaral CE, Denadai R, Alonso N. Three-dimensional changes of maxilla after secondary alveolar cleft repair: differences between rhBMP-2 and autologous iliac crest bone grafting. Plast Reconstr Surg Glob Open. 2015a;3:e451.

Raposo-Amaral CA, Denadai R, Chammas DZ, Marques FF, Pinho AS, Roberto WM, Buzzo CL, Raposo-Amaral CE. Cleft patient-reported postoperative donor site pain following alveolar autologous iliac crest bone grafting: comparing two minimally invasive harvesting techniques. J Craniofac Surg. 2015b;26:2099–103.

Salyer KE, Genecov ER, Genecov DG. Unilateral cleft lip-nose repair--long-term outcome. Clin Plast Surg. 2004;31:191–208.

Santiago PE, Schuster LA, Levy-Bercowski D. Management of the alveolar cleft. Clin Plast Surg. 2014;41:219–32.

Somensi R, Giancolli A, Almeida F, Bento DF, Raposo-do-Amaral CA, Buzzo CA, Raposo-do-Amaral CE. Assessment of nasal anthropometric parameters after primary cleft lip repair using the Mohler technique. Rev Bras Cir Plast. 2012;27:14–21.

Stal S, Hollier L. Correction of secondary deformities of the cleft lip nose. Plast Reconstr Surg. 2002;109:1386–92.

Stal S, Brown RH, Higuera S, Hollier LH Jr, Byrd HS, Cutting CB, Mulliken JB. Fifty years of the Millard rotation-advancement: looking back and moving forward. Plast Reconstr Surg. 2009;123:1364–77.

Sykes JM, Tasman AJ, Suárez GA. Cleft lip nose. Clin Plast Surg. 2016;43:223–35.

Tajima S, Maruyama M. Reverse-U incision for secondary repair of cleft lip nose. Plast Reconstr Surg. 1977;60:256–61.

Turkaslan T, Turan A, Yogun N, Ozsoy Z. A novel approach to cleft lip nose deformity: posterior dome graft technique. J Craniofac Surg. 2008;19:1359–63.

Wang TD. Secondary rhinoplasty in unilateral cleft nasal deformity. Clin Plast Surg. 2010;37:383–7.

Wolfe SA. A pastiche for the cleft lip nose. Plast Reconstr Surg. 2004;114:1–9.

Wolfe SA, Nathan NR, MacArthur IR. The cleft lip nose: primary and secondary treatment. Clin Plast Surg. 2016;43:213–21.

The Rare Facial Cleft

21

Cassio Eduardo Raposo-Amaral, Reza Jarrahy, Rizal Lim, and Nivaldo Alonso

Rare facial cleft has a broad spectrum of clinical presentation as soft tissue and bony structures can be malformed, clefting or absent. The face is a complete three-dimensional structure, composed by regions with different topography, skin thickness, texture, and color. In patients with rare facial cleft, hair follicles may accompany the cleft, especially those above the orbit or that are completely absent causing alopecia, absence of eyebrow and eyelash.

Numerous classification systems for the rare craniofacial clefts have been proposed, including those by American Association of Cleft Palate Rehabilitation (AACPR). Boo-Chai 1969, Karfik 1966. Strengths and drawbacks have been observed in these classification systems. Paul Tessier, the father of craniofacial surgery, described his system for classifying rare facial clefts, offering to the surgical community a comprehensive analysis of the wide spectrum of this disease, including a concise way to categorize not only the obvious soft-tissue deformities of the various clefts but also a description of how the soft-tissue defects related to the underlying aberrant bony anatomy associated with the clefts (Tessier 1976). In other

---

C.E. Raposo-Amaral, M.D., Ph.D. (✉)
Institute of Plastic and Craniofacial Surgery, SOBRAPAR Hospital,
Campinas, São Paulo 13084-880, Brazil

Universidade de São Paulo, São Paulo, Brazil
e-mail: cassioraposo@hotmail.com

R. Jarrahy, M.D. • R. Lim, M.D.
Division of Plastic and Reconstructive Surgery, Department of Pediatrics David Geffen School of Medicine at UCLA, Los Angeles, California, USA

N. Alonso, M.D., Ph.D.
Divisao de Cirurgia Plastica e Queimaduras, Hospital das Clínicas da Faculdade de Medicina da Universidade de São Paulo, São Paulo, Brazil

© Springer International Publishing AG 2018
N. Alonso, C.E. Raposo-Amaral (eds.), *Cleft Lip and Palate Treatment*,
https://doi.org/10.1007/978-3-319-63290-2_21

words, he added a practical component to the descriptive narrative that generates clinical significance to the classification system, facilitates diagnosis, and helps guide therapy. Moreover, Tessier's original description was based on the embryological origins of cleft development. For these reasons the rare craniofacial clefts have been come to be commonly known as the Tessier rare craniofacial clefts.

Tessier divided the face into various "time zones" centered on an imaginary equatorial axis running horizontally through the orbits and vertically through the facial midline (Kawamoto 1976). Clefts occurring below the orbits are numbered 0 through 8 and those above 9 through 14, including both soft-tissue and bone defects (Tessier 1976; Kawamoto 1976) (Fig. 21.1a). This numbering system encourages the clinician to evaluate the entire height of the face and more readily identify instances where caudal and cranial facial clefts are coincident. When upper and lower median/paramedian or oblique clefts occur simultaneously, the numbers of the individual upper and lower clefts add up to 14 (e.g., 0–14, 2–12, 4–10 clefts). Deviating from this overall scheme, Tessier defined a cleft of the lower lip, mandible, and associated midline soft-tissue and skeletal structures of the lower face and neck system as a number 30 cleft.

The preoperative surgical planning should be tailored to each individual deformity and it has been impossible to delineate an algorithm or a protocol to approach each specific condition. It has been a consensus among craniofacial plastic surgeons that the craniofacial skeleton should be reconstructed first; however in some major craniofacial cleft treated at 3–4 months of age, the bony reconstruction is postponed at later age and soft tissue has been a priority to offer satisfactory aesthetic and functional outcomes. The treatment of rare facial cleft demands a complete understanding of the concept of the aesthetic units of the face described by Gonzalez-Ulloa (1956, 1958).

Burget and Menick applied this concept to develop a state-of-the-art philosophy for nasal reconstruction (Burget and Menick 1986). We have been using similar principles to avoid multiple scars crossing the face that can be apparent and evident by reflected highlights and cast shadows. Interestingly, a plastic surgeon approaching a rare facial cleft should have in mind that there is a continuous need to construct the congenitally absent structures. Thus, although these terms construct and reconstruct are used interchangeably, in most scenarios one has to create an absent structure using local tissues that may or may not have similar characteristics. In this chapter we aimed to emphasize some of the modern principles and surgical strategies to approach soft-tissue and bony reconstruction in patients with rare facial cleft. Orthodontics and speech pathology are critical fields in the rehabilitation process. However, technical details of both fields are beyond the scope of this chapter. A detailed description of each cleft type will be followed.

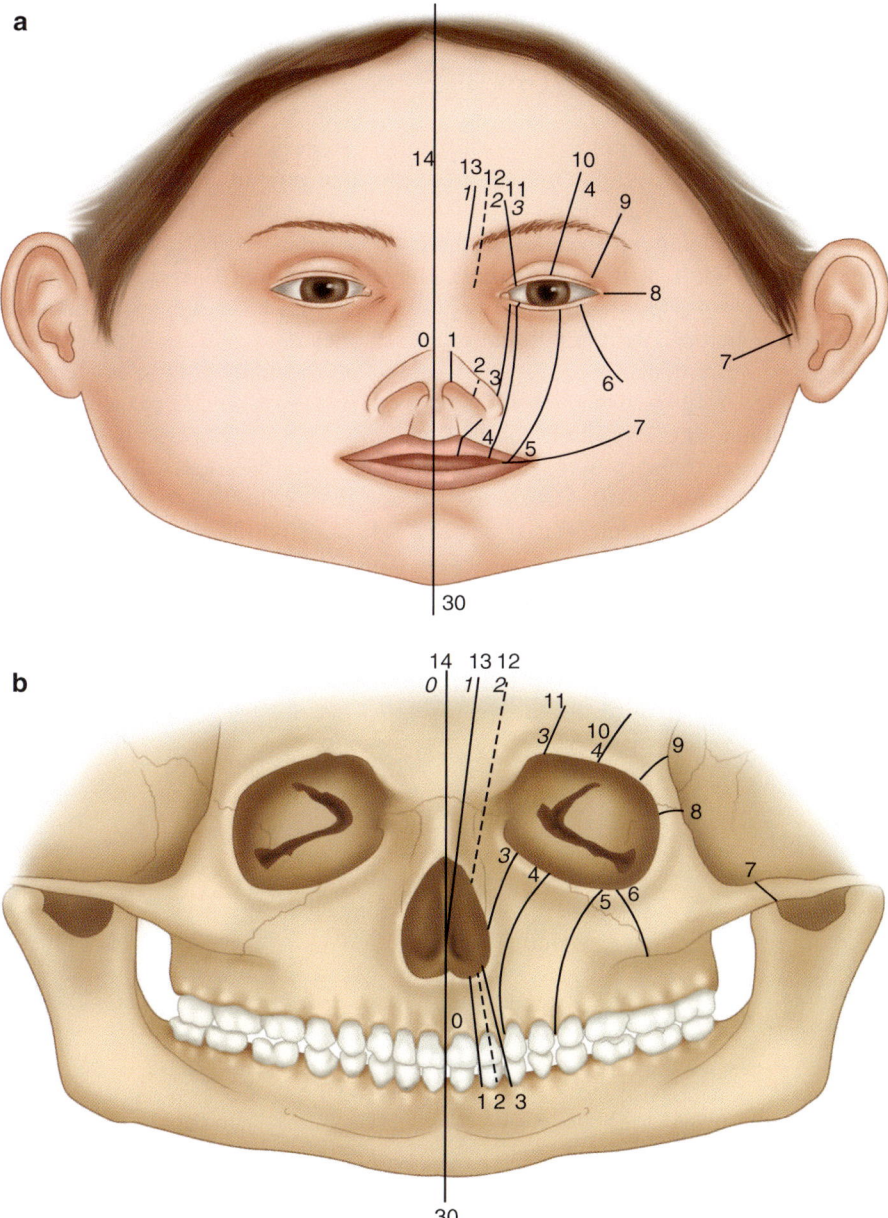

Fig. 21.1 Tessier diagram of rare facial cleft. In the original diagram, Tessier correlates the bony cleft to its associated soft-tissue deformity

21.1 Rare Facial Cleft Number 0

The rare facial cleft number 0 is a midline defect that may involve soft tissue and bone from the central incisors up through the nasal cavity to the perpendicular plate of the ethmoid. These clefts may be characterized by severe tissue deficiency to tissue excess. On one end of the spectrum are deformities that are defined by lack of development of midline facial structures. Mild manifestation may include isolated midline cleft of the lip. The palate may be high and arched or completely cleft, with absent premaxilla and philtrum. A central cleft of the nose, absent columella and nasal septum, hypoplasia of the nasoethmoidal complex, or arrhinia with or without proboscis may contribute to hypotelorism. Associated central nervous system defects can result in holoprosencephaly. Alternatively, midline tissue excess may result in enlarged and broadened nasal bones, widened nasal septum, and enlarged and laterally/superiorly displaced nasal cartilages. Nasofrontal skeletal deficiency may paradoxically present as hypertelorism due to herniation of intracranial contents in the form of frontonasal encephalocele (Pittet et al. 2004; da Silva et al. 2008; Nam and Kim 2014) (Fig. 21.2).

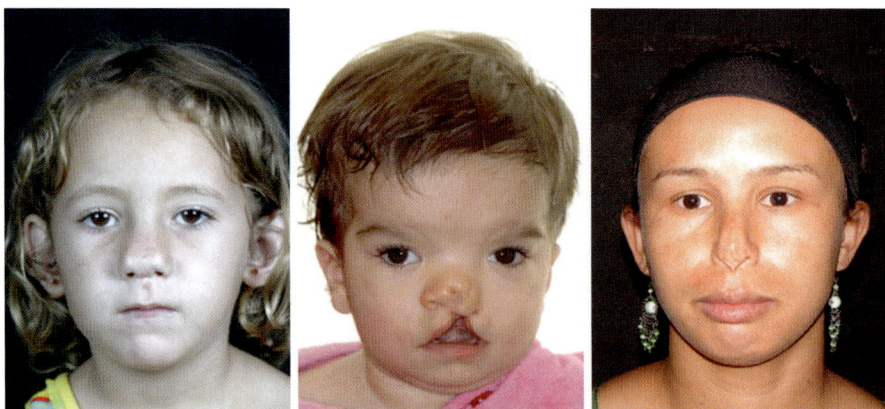

Fig. 21.2 Patient with number 0 Tessier cleft. This cleft crosses the nose and divided it into two equal halves, but not beyond the orbital level. Wide and bifid tip and wide collumela is found in this particular cleft (*left*). Other type of clinical features can be also found (*center*, *right*). Isolated number 0 is very rare as it is usually associated with number 14 Tessier cleft

21.2 Rare Facial Cleft Number 1

The rare facial cleft number 1 is a vertical paramedian cleft characterized by soft-tissue notching through the dome of the nose that extends toward the medial canthus and medial brow. A cleft of the lip may occur in the region of Cupid's bow, where the "traditional" cleft lip manifests. The nasal defect may range from completely missing upper and lower lateral cartilages to paramedian soft-tissue fissures or contour irregularities over the nasal dorsum. A bony cleft between the central and lateral incisors may extend into the pyriform aperture lateral to the anterior nasal spine. The ethmoid sinuses may be involved and the cleft may extend between the nasal bone (which may be notched or absent) and frontal process of the maxilla, resulting in hypertelorism. Heminasal atrophy or a proboscis may be seen in severe forms. The nasolacrimal system is spared in this facial cleft (Kawamoto 1976; Agrawal et al. 1998) (Figs. 21.3–21.6).

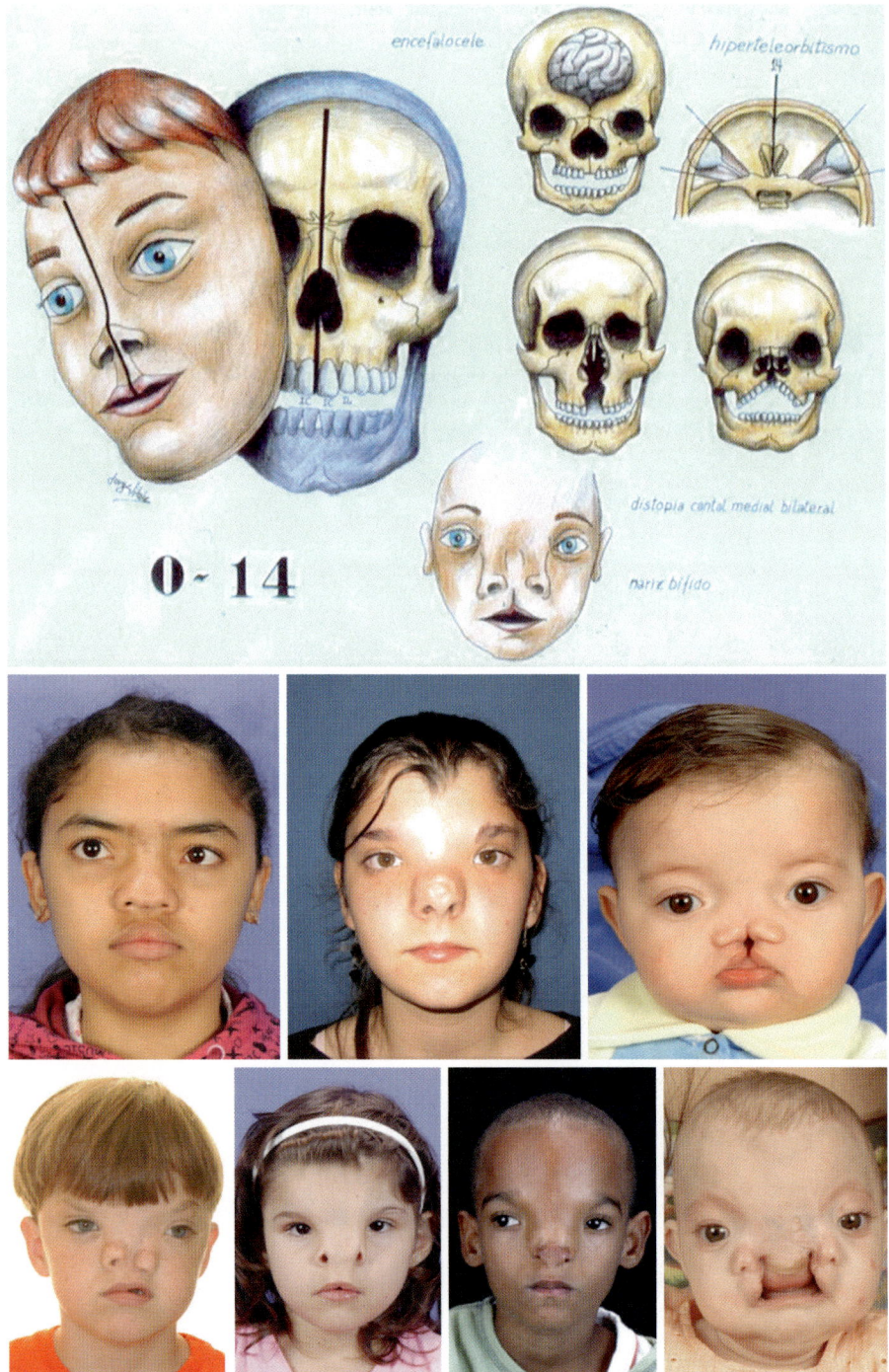

Fig. 21.3 The clinical characteristic of rare facial cleft number 0–14 may broadly vary from a bifid nose from a complete absence of the midline structures with encephalocele

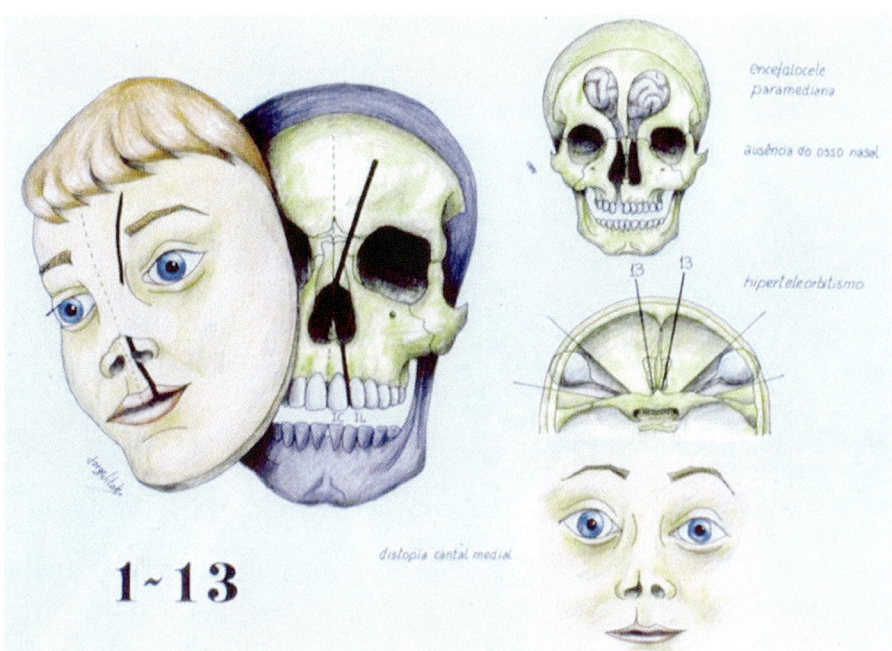

Fig. 21.4 The cleft number 1 crosses the lateral incisor, nasal cavity, and nasal bone. An alternative root is through the region between nasal bone and frontal process of the maxilla. The cranial extension of number 1 is the number 13 Tessier cleft

Fig. 21.5 Patient photograph of cleft number 1

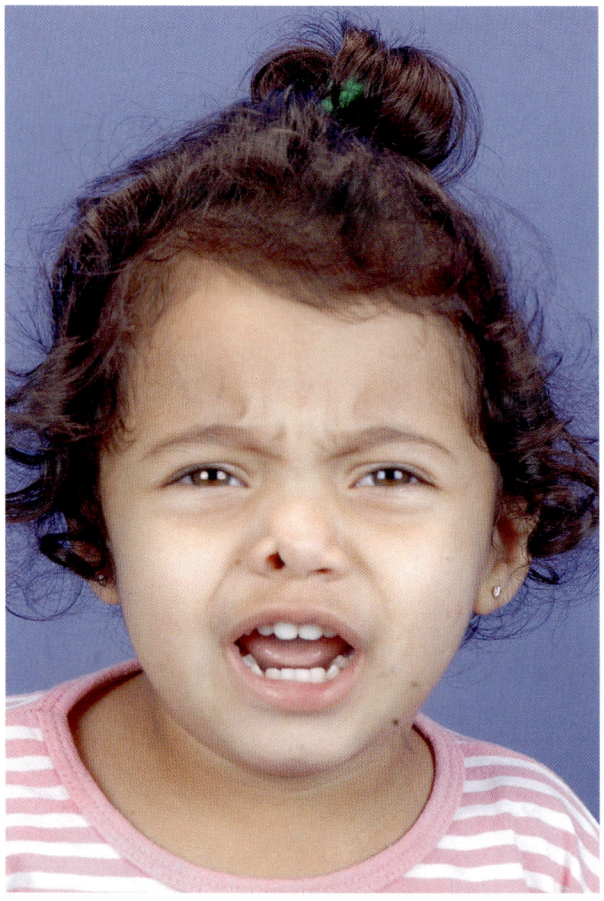

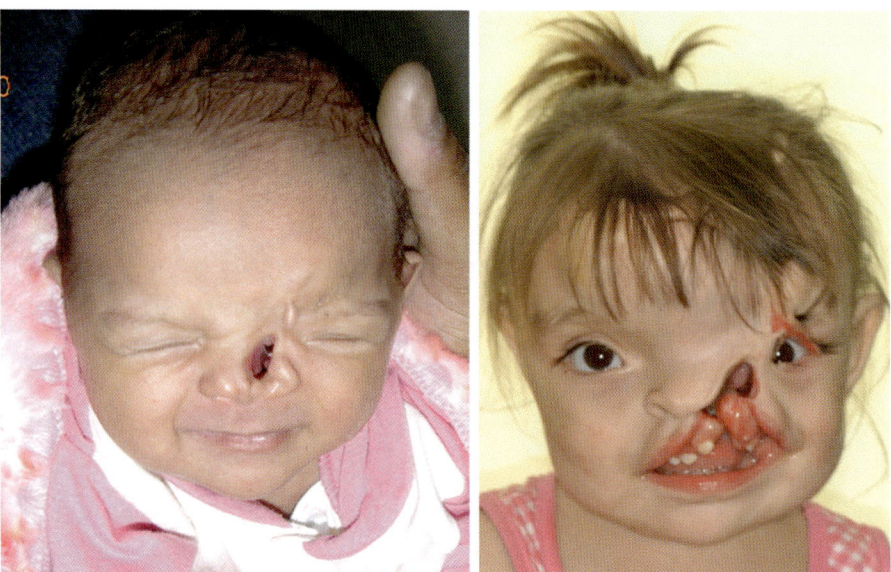

Fig. 21.6 Photograph of patients with number 1 Tessier clefts and its cranial extension number 13

21.3 Rare Facial Cleft Number 2

The rare facial cleft number 2 may be characterized as a transitional or an incomplete form of the number 1 and 3 clefts. It is very rare to identify an isolated number 2 cleft. Similarly to number 1 cleft, the cleft of the lip occurs in the area of Cupid's bow. The medial third of the nasal nostril is flat that can be either apparent without true notching or absent. The nasal dorsum may be widened and the septum may be deviated. The medial canthi and medial brow are intact but may exhibit inferior displacement or epicanthal folding. The bony cleft begins in the region of the lateral incisor and the skeletal fissure extends cephalad into pyriform aperture. The frontal process of maxilla is broad and flat and can be notched. Ethmoid enlargement contributes to hypertelorism, specially in its cranial extension (Kawamoto 1976; Ozek et al. 2001; Tiwari et al. 1991) (Figs. 21.7 and 21.8).

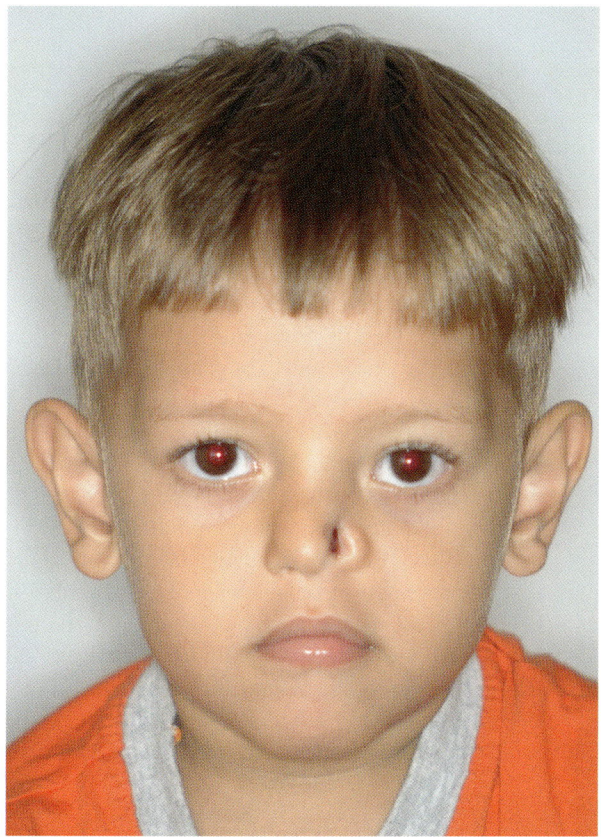

Fig. 21.7 Patient photograph of cleft number 2, more laterally than number 1 with flat nasal nostril and nasal ala clefting

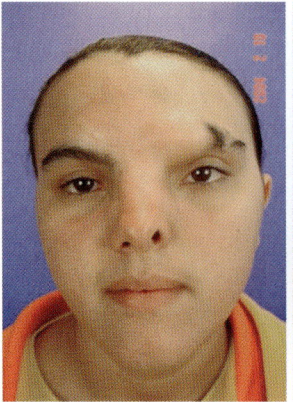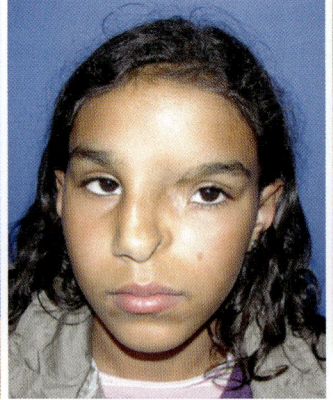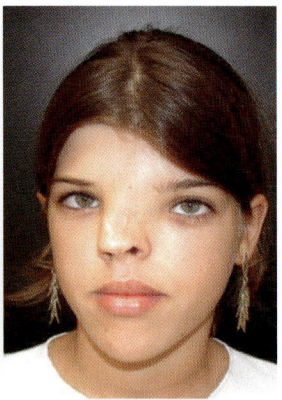

Fig. 21.8 Different clinical presentations of 2–12 Tessier cleft. The hyperlorbitism occurs as a consequence of ethmoidal bone enlargement

21.4 Rare Facial Cleft Number 3

The rare facial cleft number 3 is more frequent than the rare facial cleft number 1 and 2. It has also been referred as oro-naso-ocular cleft or oblique cleft as it involves these anatomical structures leading to oblique facial cavities. The cleft lies in the area of union of the embryologic median nasal, lateral nasal, and maxillary processes and may therefore affect any of the structures that arise from normal fusion of these processes. In addition, failure of the embryonic naso-optic groove to invaginate and form the nasolacrimal drainage system at this confluence of advancing processes may explain the nasolacrimal defects associated with this cleft.

Similarly to rare facial cleft number 1 and 2, the cleft begins at the cleft lip and continues through the alar base toward the medial canthi. The soft-tissue cheek deficiency decreases the distance between the nasal ala to the medial canthi, leading to inferior displacement of the medial canthi, resulting in either vertical orbital dystopia or telecanthus. A lower eyelid coloboma, medial to lacrimal punctum, may also be present, as with agenesis of part or all of nasolacrimal system. Orbital and ocular malformations may include bony defects of the orbital rim and floor, dystopia, microphthalmia, anophthalmia, and epibulbar dermoids. The inferior orbital rim may be incomplete or grooving toward the pyriform aperture, generating a bony communication between the the orbit and nose. The cleft in the alveolus occurs between the lateral incisor and canine and extends through the lateral border of the pyriform into the nasal cavity. The osseous defect can involve the nasal cavity along the nasomaxillary process to the level of the lacrimal bone leading to a compromise of the nasolacrimal system function. The orbital, maxillary, nasal, and oral cavities may be confluent and difficult to distinguish (Allam et al. 2014; Gawrych et al. 2010; Wenbin et al. 2007; Bodin et al. 2006) (Figs. 21.9 and 21.10).

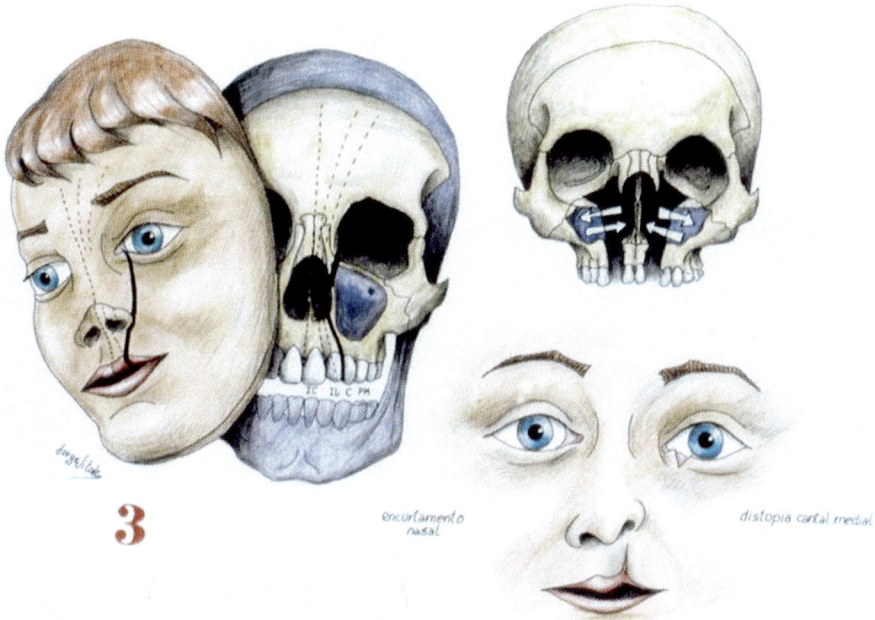

Fig. 21.9 Schematic drawing of number 3 Tessier cleft. The lip cleft is usually located in cupid bow. The base of the nasal ala is involved and the cleft runs toward the medial canthi. In the complete forms the cleft can be seen in the lateral incisors

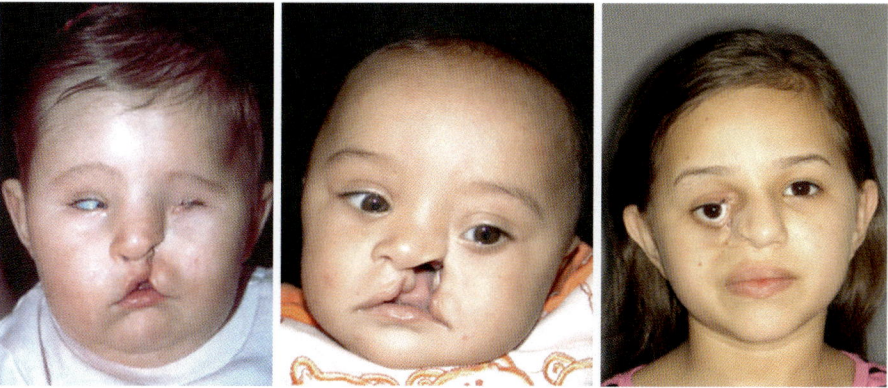

Fig. 21.10 Photographs of patients with Tessier number 3 cleft. All clinical characteristics can be seen in these patients

21.5 Rare Facial Cleft Number 4

The rare facial cleft number 4 is characterized by the soft-tissue involvement laterally to labial philtrum, usually between the philtral ridge and commissure. It differs from the common cleft lip and palate characteristics, as the cleft moves laterally to the common affected structures, affecting the check and lateral nasal aesthetic subunits, sparing the nasal alar base, but shortening the distance between the alar base and medial canthi. The medial canthus are not involved, as the cleft continues from the cheek onto the lower lid lateral to the punctum. The lacrimal drainage structures are therefore intact, but often dysfunctional. The globe can show anophthalmia, microphthalmia, or normal anatomy. Similarly to the rare facial cleft number 3, the cleft alveolus occurs between the lateral incisor and canine, sparing the pyriform aperture. The infraorbital foramen is an anatomical landmark for separation of cleft numbers 4 and 5, as number 4 moves medially to the foramen and then to the orbital rim and floor. Orbital contents may be herniated into the maxillary sinus and the bony orbit may be hypoplastic and dystopic as the eyeball can also be smaller. In the complete form of the number 4 cleft, the oral, maxillary, orbital cavities are confluent, for which this cleft has been referred to as the oro-ocular oblique cleft (Abdollahifakhim et al. 2013; Laure et al. 2010; Portier-Marret et al. 2008; Tokioka et al. 2005; Kale and Pakhmode 2000; Akoz et al. 1996) (Figs. 21.11–21.13).

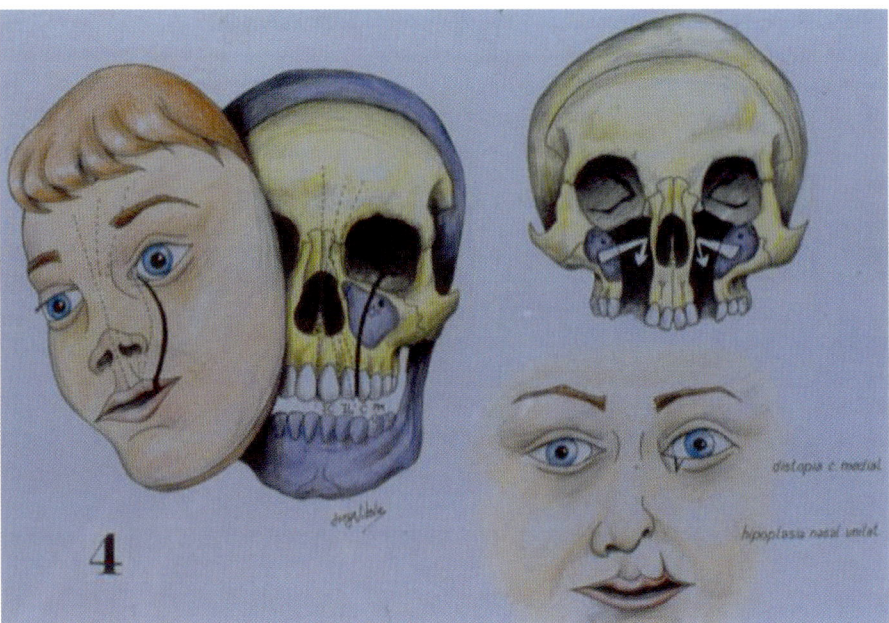

Fig. 21.11 Schematic drawing of Tessier number 4 cleft. (**a**) Patient's photograph of number 4 Tessier cleft. The cleft crosses laterally to the cupid bow. The nose may be distorted and the cleft crosses the medial canthi ligament. (**b**) Patient's photographs of severe forms of number 4 Tessier cleft (*left, center*) and unusual presentation of number 4 Tessier cleft (*right*)

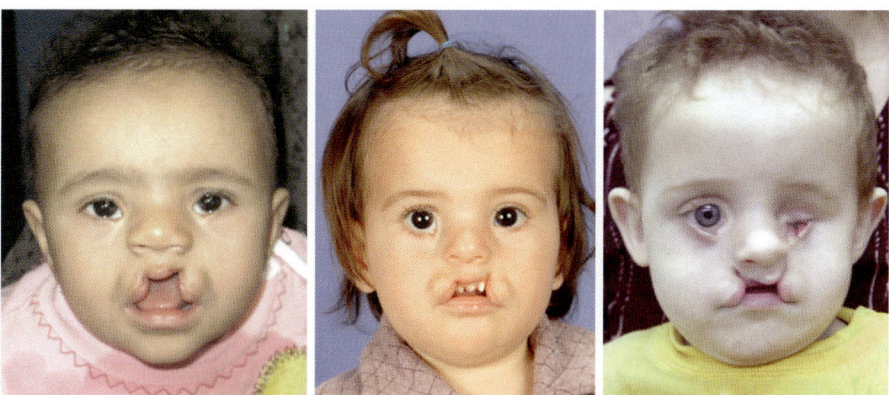

Fig. 21.12 Patients photograph of number 4 Tessier cleft. The cleft crosses laterally to the cupid bow. The nose may be distorted and the cleft crosses the medial canthi ligament

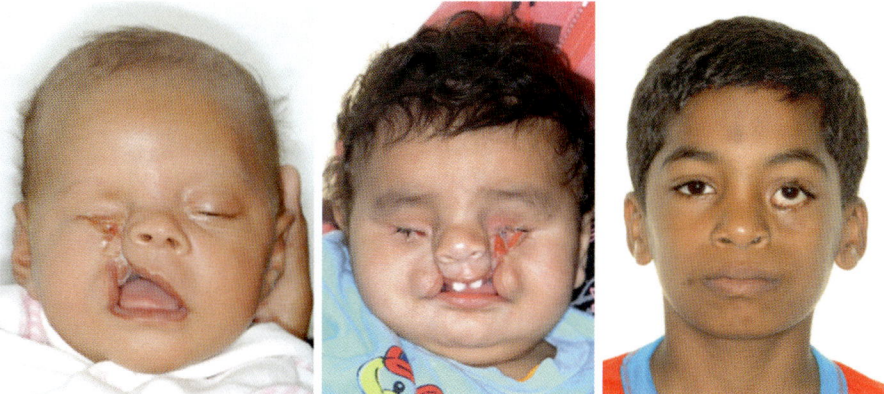

Fig. 21.13 Patient's photograph of number 4 Tessier cleft. The cleft crosses laterally to the cupid bow. The nose may be distorted and the cleft crosses the medial canthi ligament. Patient's photographs of severe forms of number 4 Tessier cleft (*left*, *center*) and unusual presentation of number 4 Tessier cleft (*right*)

21.6 Rare Facial Cleft Number 5

The rare facial cleft number 5 is the rarest of the oblique facial clefts and is rarely seen in isolation. The cleft of the lip occurs medial to the oral commissure and continues cephalad with a curvilinear trajectory on the lateral cheek toward the lower lid at the junction of its median and lateral thirds. Oblique clefts and abnormal muscle attachments of the soft palate may be identified. The lateral oro-ocular height is shortened. The skeletal defect is characterized by an alveolar cleft that occurs distal to canine and extends superiorly along the anterior maxillary wall lateral to the infraorbital foramen and then across the rim and onto the lateral orbital floor. Similar to orbital floor defects seen in the number 3 and 4 facial cleft, herniation of orbital contents into the maxilla can occur, along with orbital hypoplasia and dystopia with associated microphthalmia or anophthalmia (Abdollahifakhim et al. 2013; Garg and Goyal 2009; Galante and Dado 1991) (Figs. 21.14–21.16).

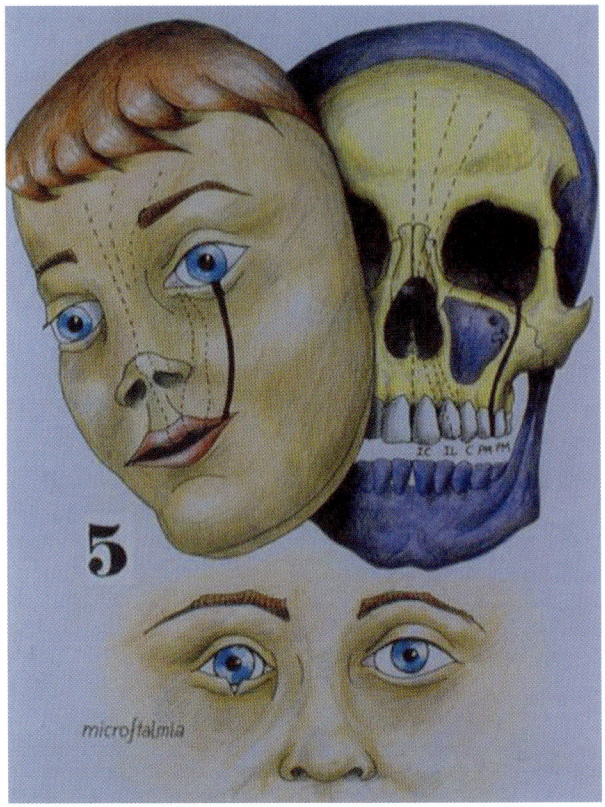

Fig. 21.14 Schematic drawing of severe forms of number 5 Tessier cleft. The cleft of the lip occurs medial to the oral commissure and continues cephalad with a curvilinear trajectory on the lateral cheek toward the lower lid at the junction of its median and lateral thirds. Oblique clefts and abnormal muscle attachments of the soft palate may be identified. The lateral oro-ocular height is shortened

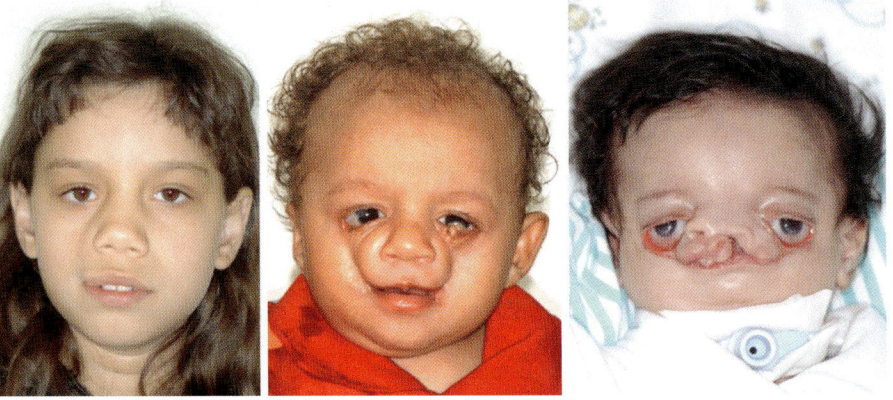

Fig. 21.15 Photographs of patients with number 5 Tessier cleft showing main clinical characteristics of this very rare cleft

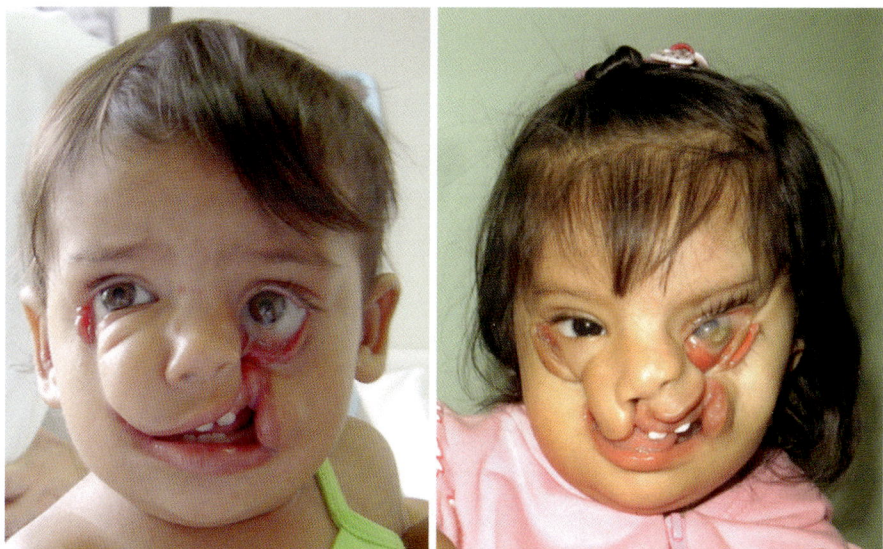

Fig. 21.16 Photographs of a very rare forms of number 5 Tessier cleft on the right side and number 4 on the left side

21.7 Rare Facial Cleft Number 6

The association of the number 6, 7, and 8 rare craniofacial clefts is known as Treacher Collins syndrome (TCS), characterized by the absence of the zygoma. Tessier defines the TCS as a confluence of clefts at the maxillary zygomatic, temporozygomatic, and frontozygomatic regions.

The isolated form of number 6 cleft is described as an incomplete form of TCS but authors have identified very rare forms of complete number 6.

Macrostomia and soft palate are almost always present. An isolate number 6 can be seen as uni- or bilateral when not associated to TCS. There is a fusion between the corner of the mouth and the soft palate. The cleft bone in the retro molar area is responsible for the abnormal insertion of the palate muscles. Palatopharyngeal muscle is not inserted in the central part of the soft palate. Velopharyngeal incompetence is very difficult to solve because the soft palate is too short and the muscles are inserted in a wrong direction. When the cleft continues until the orbit facial, mimic muscles can be damaged. It is unusual to observe facial palsy. Lower eye lid retraction is not related just to lack of fusion of facial soft tissue but also for cleft or absence of zygomatic bone. The frontal process of the zygomatic bone is absent but sometimes is present; for this reason there is no antimongoloid slant in few cases. The number 6 is always parallel to number 5 but more laterally displaced. The infraorbital foramen is in a medial position. Tessier cleft number 6 could be present in Treacher Collins syndrome associated with number 7 and 8 cleft. In this association the phenotype is a little

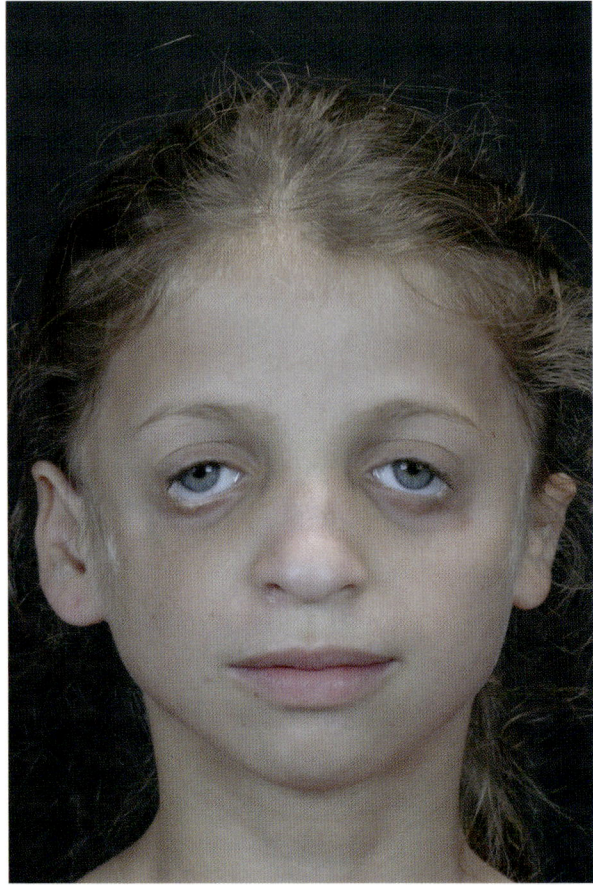

Fig. 21.17 Patient with number 6 Tessier cleft. Those are the incomplete form of Treacher Collins syndrome. Lower eyelid coloboma is seen, but the lateral canthi is less severely dystopic in comparison to Treacher Collins syndrome. These patients are characterized by a tight soft-tissue envelope in the zygomatic region and hypoplastic or clefting zygomatic bone is seen

bit different from the isolated ones. Maxillary duplication is seen in bilateral number 6 (Fig. 21.17).

In contrast to the complete TCS, characterized by absence of the zygoma and its arch, the isolated number 6 cleft is defined by a present but hypoplastic zygomatic body and an intact zygomatic arch. The bony cleft occurs at the junction of the malar bone and maxilla, the zygomaticomaxillary suture. Soft-tissue manifestations are similar to some of those seen in TCS patients, but more mild in nature. These can include external ear deformities, lower lid colobomas at the junction of the median and lateral thirds of the lower eyelids, and hypoplastic or absent lateral canthal tendons. The resultant midface hypoplasia, negative palpebral cant, and inferior displacement of the lateral canthi are reminiscent of the syndromic presentation (Ligh et al. 2015; Nguyen et al. 2016; Plomp et al. 2016).

21.8 Rare Facial Cleft Number 7

The number 7 cleft is the most common isolated rare craniofacial cleft. It has a variable clinical presentation, with a diversity of anatomical structures that may be involved in the clefting. This might explain the numerous ways the number 7 cleft is referred to, including craniofacial microsomia, microtia, otomandibular dysostosis, first and second branchial arch syndrome, and oromandibular-auricular syndrome. Macrostomia is the main feature of the cleft, but soft-tissue involvement can affect all tissue layers of the face. Presentation may range from small preauricular skin tags to mild facial asymmetry to significant soft-tissue hypoplasia that includes the cheek, tongue, soft palate, parotid gland, trigeminal and facial nerves, and muscles they innervate. External ear deformities include the entire spectrum from mild microtia to complete anotia. The cardinal bony defects are centered around the zygomaticotemporal suture, with resultant absence or hypoplasia of the body and arch of the zygoma. As with the soft-tissue deficiency, the mandibular hypoplasia also occurs on a gradient, ranging from a structurally normal but small mandible to complete absence of the mandibular condyle and ramus. Zygomatic arch may be absent and zygoma may terminate in a stump (Bodin et al. 2006; Presti et al. 2004; Woods et al. 2008; Horgan et al. 1995; Poon et al. 2003) (Figs. 21.18–21.20).

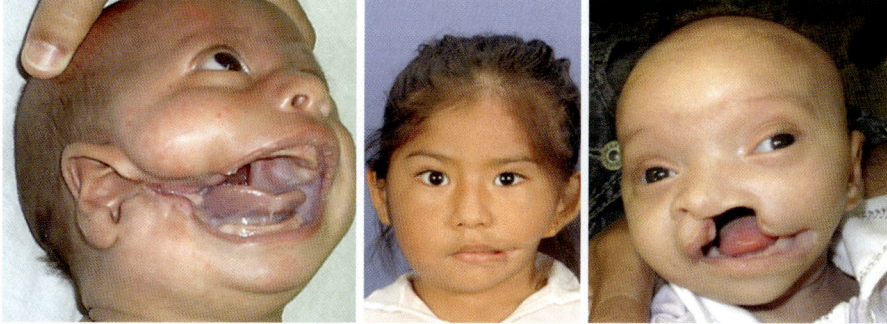

Fig. 21.18 Photographs of patient with number 7 Tessier cleft

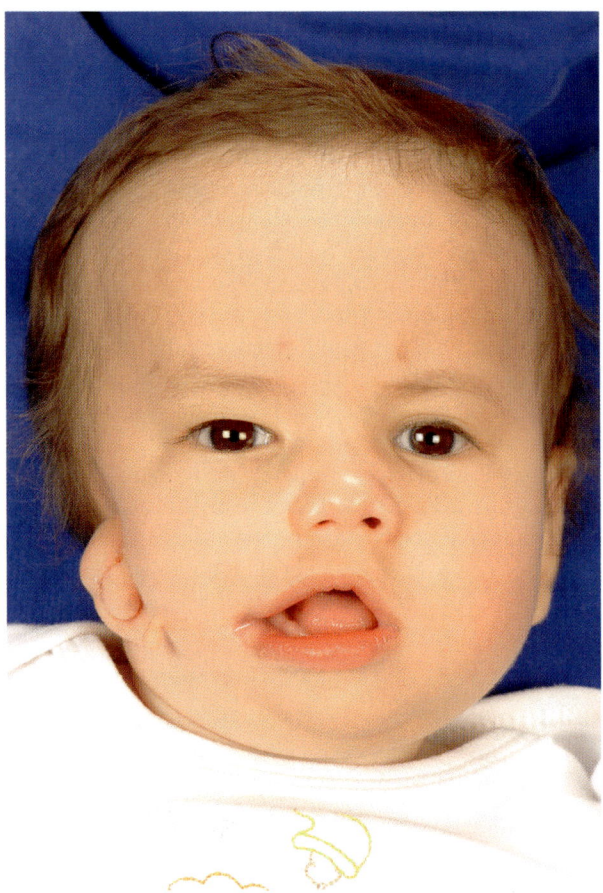

Fig. 21.19 Photograph of a patient with hemifacial microsomia

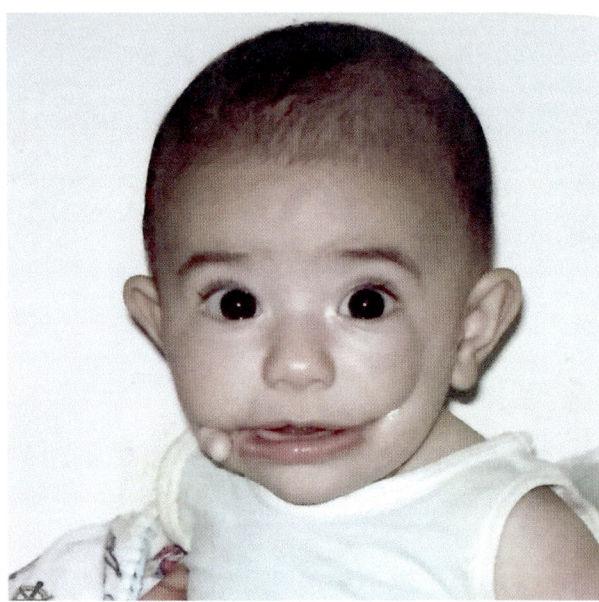

Fig. 21.20 Frontal photograph of a patient with an unusual presentation of number 6 and 7 Tessier cleft

21.9 Rare Facial Cleft Number 8

While commonly associated with the number 6 and 7 rare facial clefts in Treacher Collins syndrome, an isolated number 8 cleft is a rare entity. Centered on the frontozygomatic suture, the cleft begins at the lateral palpebral fissure and extends to temporal region. The bony defect manifests as bone loss of the lateral orbital rim at the level of the suture. More severe forms of bony involvement are likely representative of Treacher Collins syndrome; when these are present defects in the areas of the number 6 and 7 clefts should be sought out. Soft-tissue deficits affect the lateral canthal tendon and its insertion, ranging from a furrow in the lateral palpebral area with discontinuity of the orbicularis oculi ring to a coloboma of the lateral canthus, to a dermatocele (Kawamoto 1976; Fuente-del-Campo 1990) (Figs. 21.21–21.23).

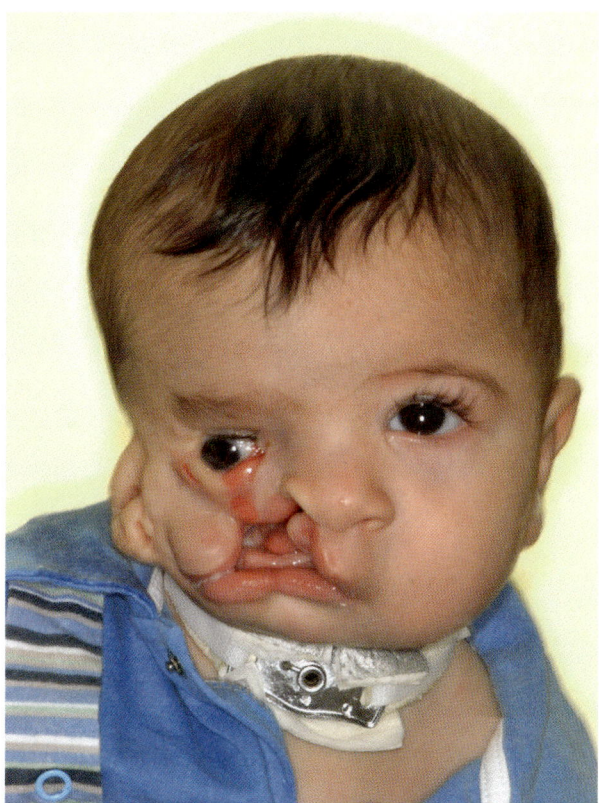

Fig. 21.21 Photograph of a patient with an unusual presentation of number 8 Tessier cleft with hemifacial microsomia and cleft lip. This cleft affects the lateral palpebrum commissure that can be occupied by a dermatocele

Fig. 21.22 Schematic drawing of number 6, 7, 8 Tessier cleft known as Treacher Collins syndrome

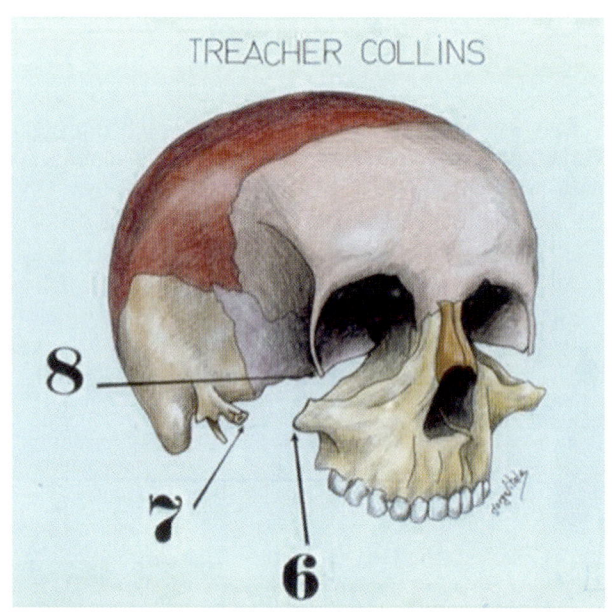

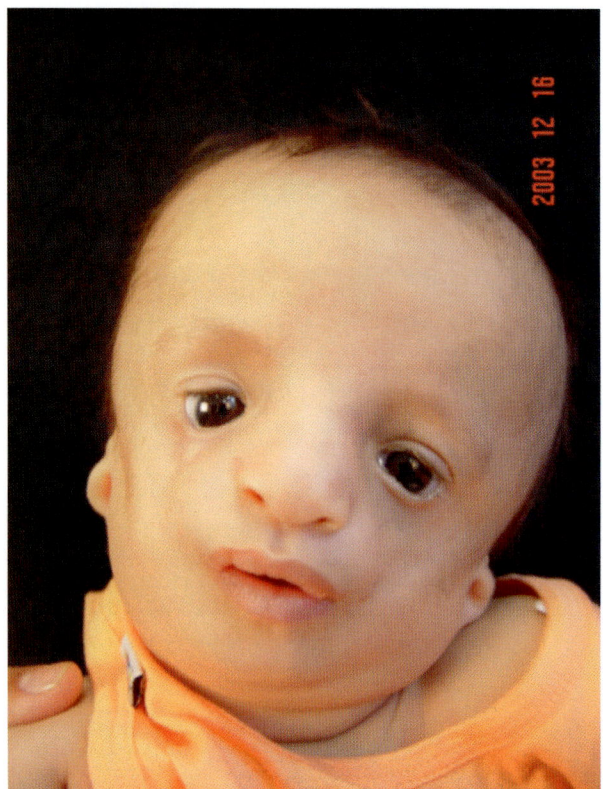

Fig. 21.23 This particular patient shows a complete form of Treacher Collins syndrome

21.10 Rare Facial Cleft Number 9

The isolated number 9 cleft is extremely rare. The cleft is located at the superolateral angle of orbit. As a result, the upper eyelid may exhibit full-thickness tissue loss between its median and lateral thirds. This defect may extend through the brow and obliquely toward the hairline and involve the underlying orbit and forehead (David et al. 1989; Dumortier et al. 1999) (Fig. 21.24).

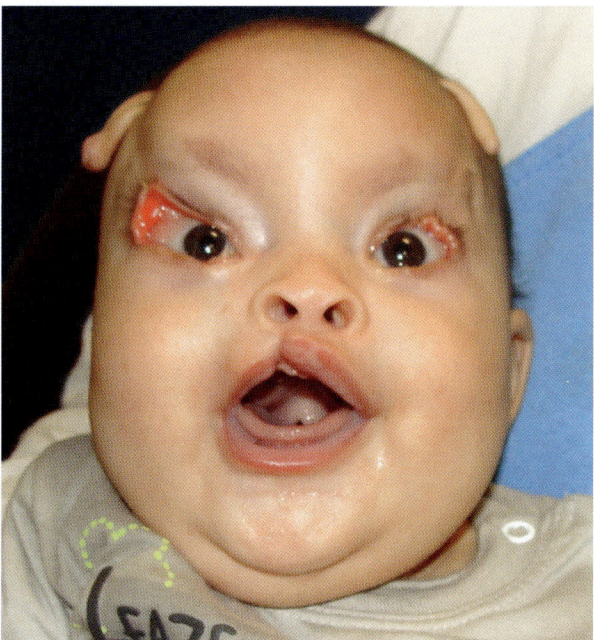

Fig. 21.24 Frontal photograph of a patient with number 9 Tessier cleft, a very rare condition

21.11 Rare Facial Cleft Number 10

This cleft represents the cranial extension of the number 4 cleft. A coloboma of middle third of eyelid with disruption of middle third of brow and continuation to the hairline is possible. A whorl of hair-bearing scalp may be seen in the frontal region. The underlying skeletal defect can include absence of the middle orbital rim and roof as well as adjacent frontal bone, resulting in a fronto-orbital encephalocele of varying size. With herniation of intracranial contents through the bony defect, the orbit is rotated laterally and inferiorly (Kawamoto 1976; Lee et al. 2012) (Figs. 21.25 and 21.26).

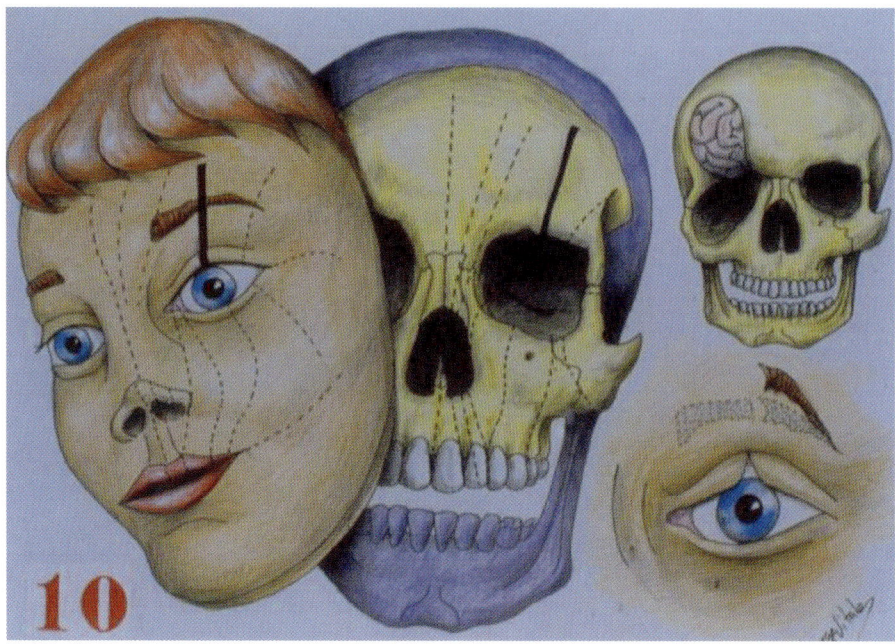

Fig. 21.25 Schematic drawing of number 10 Tessier cleft. Note the presence of the encephalocele

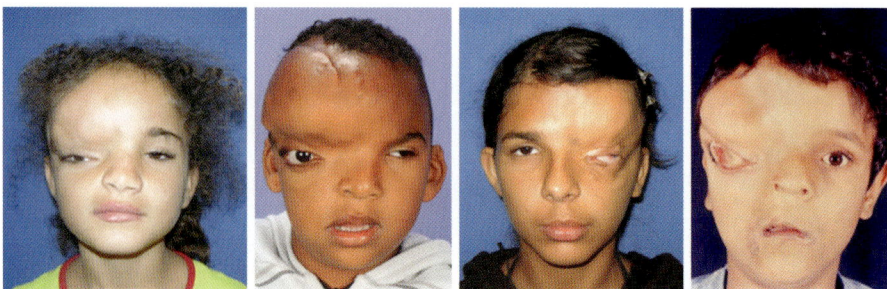

Fig. 21.26 Photographs of patients with number 10 Tessier cleft. Encephalocele and upper-lower eyelid distortion and absent eyebrow are seen

21.12 Rare Facial Cleft Number 11

The number 11 cleft usually occurs along with the number 3 facial cleft, and rarely occurs alone. It passes through the medial third of the upper eyelid and eyebrow, extending to the frontal hairline. At the level of the orbit, it can pass through the orbit itself, causing a defect of the medial orbital rim. Alternatively it can pass through the ethmoid complex, leading to hypertelorism (Kawamoto 1976; Bodin et al. 2006) (Fig. 21.27).

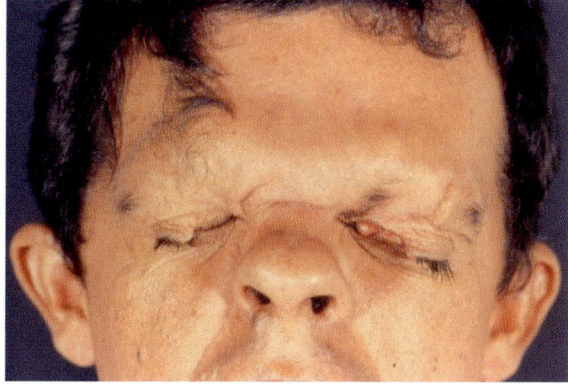

Fig. 21.27 Photograph of patient with number 11 Tessier cleft. This cleft crosses the medial portion of eyelid and eyebrow bilaterally toward the frontal hair line

21.13 Rare Facial Cleft Number 12

The number 12 cleft represents the cranial extension of the number 2 cleft. It passes either through the frontal process of the maxilla or between this process and the nasal bone, with continuation of the bony defect seen in its facial counterpart. Due to increase in the width of the ethmoid sinuses, hypertelorism is a hallmark characteristic. The olfactory organs and cribriform plate are spared. The overlying soft tissue may include brow irregularities immediately lateral to its medial edge (Fig. 21.28).

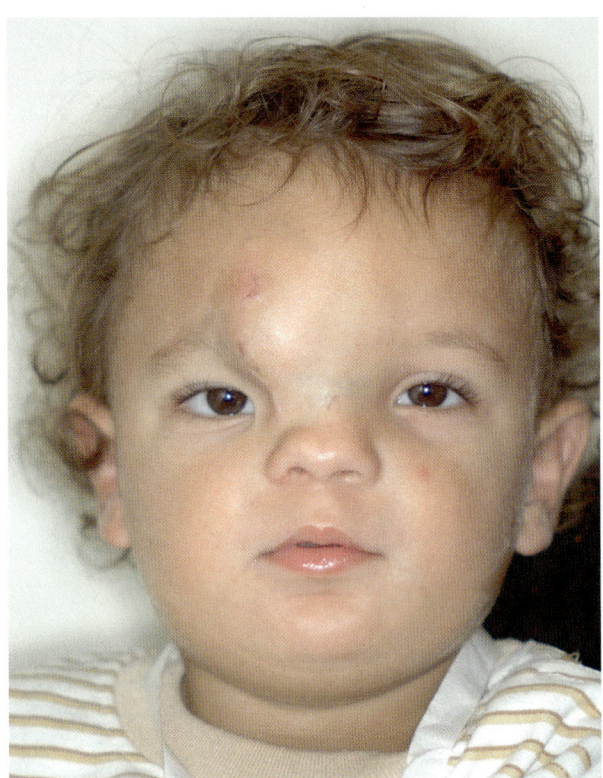

Fig. 21.28 Photograph of a patient with isolated number 12

21.14 Rare Facial Cleft Number 13:

Displacement of an otherwise uninterrupted medial brow is a characteristic of a number 13 cleft. The underlying skeletal anomaly is consistent with the facial number 1 cleft: the cleft may extend between the nasal bone and frontal process of the maxilla. Cranially, the cleft passes through the cribriform plate, widening the olfactory grooves. The concurrent presence of a frontal encephalocele can cause inferior displacement of the cribriform plate as well. The ethmoids may also be increased in their transverse dimension. Collectively, these skeletal components result in hypertelorism, and in the bilateral form the hypertelorism can be remarkable (Kawamoto 1976; Gargano et al. 2015) (Fig. 21.29 and 21.30).

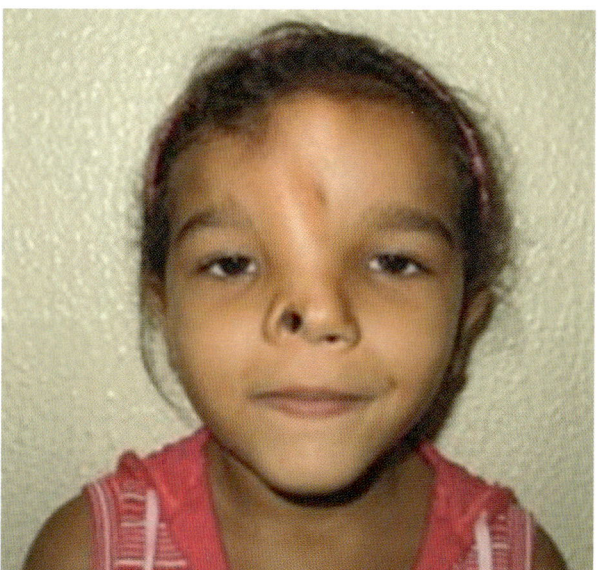

Fig. 21.29 Photograph of a patient with number 1–13 Tessier cleft

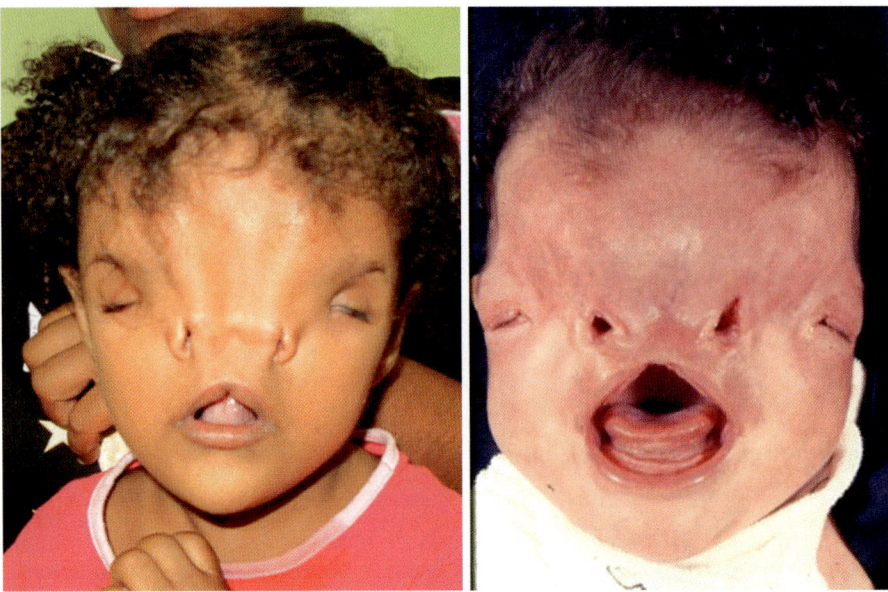

Fig. 21.30 Photographs of patients with 2–12 and 1–13 Tessier clefts. This combination brings the most severe forms of hypertelorism

21.15 Rare Facial Cleft Number 14

The zero cleft continues onto the central forehead as the number 14 cleft, which has a variety of presentations. When tissue agenesis is pathogenetically implicated, clinical manifestations can include hypotelorism that is defined by severe underdevelopment of midline frontal and orbital structures, such as cyclopia, ethmocephaly, cebocephaly, and a single central orbit. In these circumstances, the brain can be significantly hypoplastic in its development, resulting in holoprosencephaly and microcephaly. As Kawamoto describes, the more severe the brain deformity, the more severe the facial appearance, and the more limited life expectancy and meaningful neurologic function (Kawamoto 1976). Paradoxically, the 14 cleft may also be characterized by hypertelorism. Improper migration of the frontonasal process, a bifid cranium, or the presence of a frontal and ethmoid encephalocele may contribute to arrested medial migration of the embryological orbits and an ultimate lateralized position. An enlarged or a duplicated crista galli, widened olfactory grooves, inferiorly displaced cribriform plates, and enlarged ethmoids are also characteristic. The cranial sequelae are wide bossed forehead with midline furrow, depressed nasal root, protrusion of the lateral forehead, or encephalocele (Nam and Kim 2014; Pidgeon et al. 2014; Raposo-Amaral et al. 2011) (Fig. 21.27).

21.16 Rare Facial Cleft Number 30

Cleft of the lower lip and mandible may fall on the same axis as 0 cleft and involve the tongue, hyoid bone, and midline structure of the neck down to the sternum but mandibular involvement classified as distinct **30 cleft** by Tessier (Kececi et al. 1994; Morioka et al. 2003; Bhattacharyya et al. 2012) (Fig. 21.31).

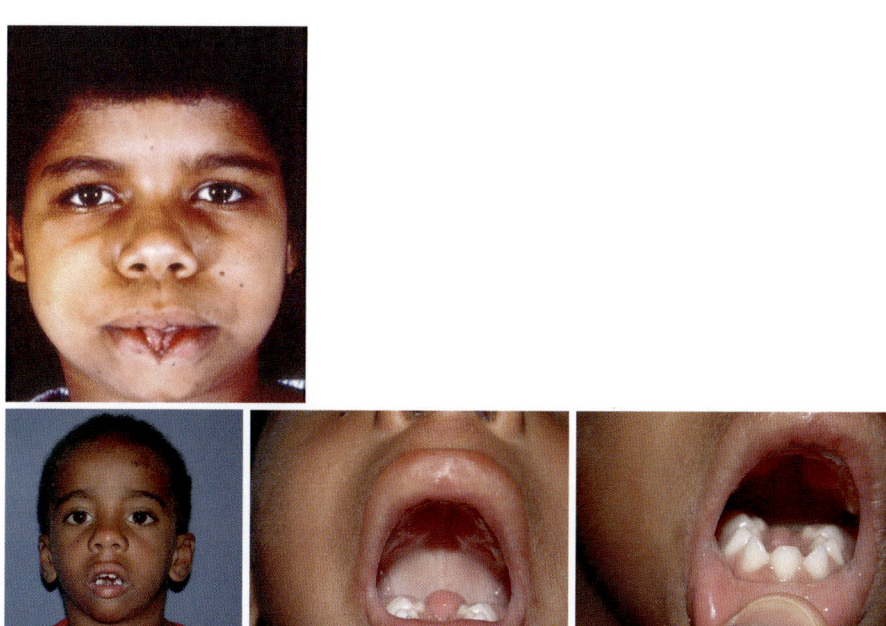

Fig. 21.31 Patients with number 30 Tessier cleft

21.17 Treatment

21.17.1 Nonoperative Management

Definitive management of rare craniofacial clefts is surgical in nature. Nonsurgical care of patients with rare craniofacial clefts is generally supportive in nature and helps facilitate successful surgical outcomes. Under ideal circumstances, patients are treated in a multidisciplinary craniofacial clinic with close coordination among all involved caregivers.

21.17.1.1 Feeding and Nutrition
In the immediate postnatal period, rare facial clefts that involve the upper lip and/or palate may pose challenges to feeding and potentially contribute to dehydration and malnutrition. Parents must be provided with education and guidance on techniques and materials that can facilitate adequate oral feeds. Consultation with an occupational therapist who is experienced in the management of children with facial clefts may be indicated. This support should coincide with a larger more holistic approach to providing longitudinal psychosocial support to patients and their families.

21.17.1.2 Neurological Assessment
Children with rare craniofacial clefts with any suggestion of encephalocele, holoprosencephaly, or other structural cranial deformity should undergo neurological and neurosurgical assessment. These evaluations should include radiographic examination of the craniofacial skeleton via CT scan and of the brain via MRI.

21.17.1.3 Dentistry/Orthodontia
Virtually all patients with rare craniofacial clefts will require attention from a pediatric dentist and an orthodontist during their growth and development. Orthodontic treatment should be tailored to each individual's needs, as hypodontia, alveolar misalignment, malocclusion, and even orthodontic sequelae of surgical interventions can have aesthetic and functional consequences upon occlusal relationships.

21.17.1.4 Speech
Cleft patients may have difficulties with speech stemming from structural abnormalities or from learned misarticulations. The speech pathologist plays a critical and ongoing role in identifying undesirable speech patterns early in language development, providing speech therapy, and monitoring speech patterns throughout childhood and young adulthood.

21.17.2 Operative Management

Due to the wide breadth of clinical diversity that is inherent to the rare craniofacial clefts, it is impossible to define specific algorithms or protocols for any one specific cleft entity. Tessier's ordered classification system, however, allows us to draw upon well-established basic principles of cleft, craniofacial, and general plastic surgery to address the complex defects we encounter in these patients. Below is first a summary of general approaches to surgical management, followed by some cleft-specific considerations. While by no means comprehensive, this overview provides a template for developing surgical treatment plans.

The rare facial cleft number 1 and number 2 require a nasal reconstruction with local flaps. We have been using a nasal reconstruction in two or three stages using a paramedian flap. Nasal lining is usually required with folded paramedian flap or local transpositioning flap. Costal and conchal cartilages are used for adding nasal support to the reconstructed nose (Tessier 1976; Kawamoto 1976; Ozek et al. 2001; Tiwari et al. 1991; da Silva et al. 2010).

The rare facial cleft number 3 is one of the most challenging owing to magnitude of soft-tissue distortion. We aim to construct the lower eyelid and lacrimal system offering ocular protection. The alar base and the lip should be repositioned by enhancing the vertical dimension of the paranasal region. Tessier described a Z-plasty in the medial canthi, positioning one arm of the flap to correct the medial canthi and the other one to fill the vertical dimension of the nose (Tessier 1976). The medial canthi should be elevated by using the contralateral side as a template and a myocutaneous flap can be needed to fill the defect created by the elevation of the medial canthi. The cleft lip can be approached as a common unilateral cleft deformity. The mobilization of the distorted alar base is technically challenging. Glabelar or paramedian forehead flaps can be used to accomplish this task. Kawamoto has used a Z-plasty to gain length of vertical paranasal dimension, and prefer a cheek rotation flap in more severe cases. Elongation of the ala was done by complete degloving of the nose and mucosal lining on that side through an oral vestibular incision. The authors described a detailed approach for each specific spectrum of Tessier number 3 (Allam et al. 2014). We have proposing the unilateral orbital box osteotomy to lift the affected orbit, and completely release the periorbital contents and herniation into the cleft and bone graft in the cleft region and orbital rim. In addition, we also advocate a complete undermining of the medial canthi ligament in the affect side associated with a medial canthopexy with wires. This operation corrects the vertical orbital dystopia commonly found in these patients.

21.18 The Rare Facial Cleft Number 4

Multiple surgical stages are necessary to accomplish a successful clinical rehabilitation in a rare facial cleft number 4. As the oro-ocular distance is deficient, one should aim to construct this dimension by establishing its normal length. Corneal protection is urgent as corneal exposure may jeopardize visual acuity. The patient is usually treated early in life. Tessier, in the late 1970s, described a multiple Z-plasty to approach and reallocate tissue in the clefting region (Tessier 1976). This technique was used by many surgeons as a protocol to approach the number 4. We discard tissue between the philtrum and the cleft edge, offering an aesthetic pleasing lip reconstruction. Instead of sparing tissue one has to discard tissue to obtain better scar positioning into the aesthetic lip unit. This maneuver "discarding tissue where the tissue is already missing" may sound odd. However it is a necessary trade-off to obtain a long-term satisfactory outcome by avoiding the scars crossing the delineations of facial subunits. Alonso has described an approach respecting the aesthetic subunits of the face by using a medially based upper eyelid myocutaneous flap to construct the lower eyelid and lift the medial canthi to the same level (or slightly higher) using the contralateral side as a template. Bone graft has been used primarily or secondarily (Alonso et al. 2008). Millard rotation-advancement principle is used to repair the lip by discarding tissue and placing the scars in the facial subunits (Tessier 1976; Kawamoto 1976; Allam et al. 2014; Kale and Pakhmode 2000; Akoz et al. 1996).

21.19 The Rare Facial Cleft Number 5

Similarly to other oblique facial cleft, corneal exposure should be carefully managed. Radiological imaging is necessary to rule out encephalocele and to define orbital and cranial base anatomy; however soft tissue is approached first, early in life. Z-plasty is usually chosen along the cleft margins and in close proximity to the lower eyelid. Upper eyelid to lower eyelid transpositioning flap can be performed associated to lateral canthopexy as the lateral canthi is usually off. Bone graft can be used in the orbital floor, but in cases of microphthalmia it is extremely difficult to mobilize forward the eyeball as most of the cases there is a certain degree of enophthalmia (Tessier 1976; Kawamoto 1976; Galante and Dado 1991; da Silva et al. 2009).

21.20 The Rare Facial Cleft Number 6

Patients of isolate number 6 present a face that is quite similar to patients with Treacher Collins syndrome. The key point on number 6 is to deal with coloboma, and expand the midface that is tight in all cases. Correction of the coloboma can be accomplished with a combination of Z-plasty and upper to lower eyelid transpositioning flaps. The expansion of craniofacial skeleton is usually performed with parietal bone grating to the zygoma and zygomatic arch. In a second stage, soft-tissue expansion is accomplished using free fat grafting from abdomen, gluteal or thigh regions. Low quantity of free fat, less than 10 cc, is harvested in these regions and injected carefully in the zygomatic region using a 1 cc syringe. The systematization of the technique was previously described in Parry Romberg Syndrome and Hemifacial Microsomia by our group Denadai et al. 2016, 2017, Raposo-Amaral et al. 2013, Plomp et al. 2016.

21.21 The Rare Facial Cleft Number 7

Initial macrostomia repair should not only match the transverse length and wet/dry vermilion orientation of the lip on the uninvolved side, but also reorient the zygomaticus major, risorius, and depressor angulioris muscles to create the absent modiolus. Straight-line and z-plasty skin closure are both acceptable. Microtia repair using either autologous rib cartilage, porous polyethylene implants, or osseointegrated prostheses are all well described.

The technique and timing of skeletal reconstruction of the deficient mandible depend on the degree of hypoplasia, mandibular growth, and secondary effects on the maxilla. Options include rib grafting for the congenitally absent mandible, distraction osteogenesis for the significantly shortened mandibular body or ramus, and conventional orthognathic correction for skeletally mature patients with mandibular asymmetry and malocclusion. Free vascularized bone grafts have also been described for mandibular agenesis (Tessier 1976; Kawamoto 1976; Woods et al. 2008).

21.22 The Rare Facial Cleft Number 8

Soft-tissue reconstruction involves excision of the cleft tissue and repair with tarsopalpebral flaps and laterally based cutaneous flaps. A lateral canthoplasty is performed and covered with adjacent tissue.

21.23 Median and Paramedian Clefts: 0–14, 1–13, 2–12

The rare facial clefts from 8 to 14 are those whose cleft affects all structures above the orbit leading to symmetric and asymmetric hypertelorbitism. Surgical treatment depends on the extent of the deformity. Treatment of the facial and cranial components should be staged, starting with reconstruction of the cleft lip deformity at approximately 3 months of age according to standard cleft lip repair principles. Subsequent repair of the nose can be accomplished with a combination of local and regional tissue advancement, rotation, and transposition flaps in combination with composite or cartilaginous auricular grafts for support. More complex reconstructions are necessary in clefts with cranial extension that affect the orbits and forehead, following the guidelines for management of hypertelorbitism with or without encephalocele as described above. When there is significant deformity of the nose requiring an extensive amount of soft tissue for coverage, initial correction of the hypertelorbitism may provide additional mobile tissue to recruit for nasal reconstruction.

Once the patient presents a mild-to-severe interorbital distance according to Tessier classification, the key point is to medialize the orbit to allow nasal and further soft-tissue reconstruction and refinements.

The current techniques of hypertelorbitism are well described in the literature as well as the best age to perform the surgery to avoid long-term relapse of the orbit positioning (Raposo-Amaral et al. 2011).

In general, adult patients with adequate occlusion underwent an orbital box osteotomy procedure. Skeletally immature patients and patients with rare craniofacial clefts characterized by an inverted-V maxillary morphology underwent a facial bipartition procedure.

21.24 Box Osteotomy

Intracranial and extracranial approaches were used to make orbital box osteotomies. Coronal and gingivobuccal sulcus incisions were used to gain subperiosteal exposure of the frontal bones, orbits, and midface. A bifrontal craniotomy was performed. The interdacyron distance was measured with calipers. Circumferential orbital osteotomies were made with great care to preserve the integrity of the medial canthal tendons. The zygomaticomaxillary and nasomaxillary buttresses were also cut. The planned central frontoethmoidal segment osteotomy was marked and cut with a reciprocating saw, following adequate intracranial midline dissection and retraction. After removal of the median segment, the orbits were translocated medially. The nasofrontal processes of the maxilla were fixed with wires, and the vertical buttresses were rigidly fixed with titanium plates and screws. A pericranial flap was raised and sutured down to the cranial base in the midline before closure (Raposo-Amaral et al. 2011) (Fig. 21.32).

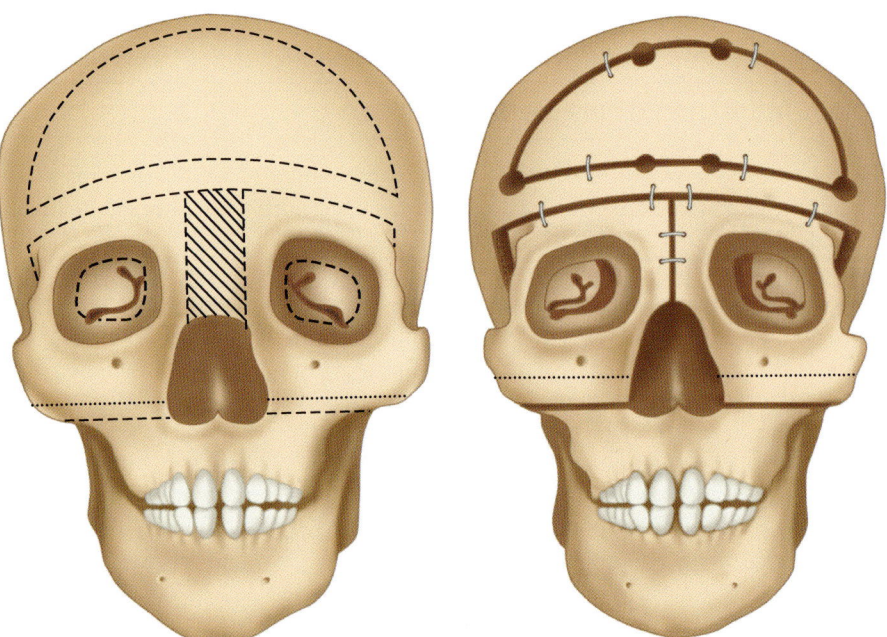

Fig. 21.32 Schematic drawing of a box osteotomy to medialize the orbits and corrects hypertelorism

21.25 Facial Bipartition

For the facial bipartition, pterygomaxillary, septal, and median palatal osteotomies were added to the bone cuts described above to allow complete midface mobilization. Rowe disimpaction forceps were used to downfracture the midface. A wedge of central nasal, frontal, and ethmoid bone was removed, and the hemifacial segments were rotated toward the midline. Preoperative vertical orbital discrepancies were corrected with asymmetric wedge removal. The nasofrontal processes and the lateral aspects of the bipartition halves were fixed to the zygomatic processes with wire. The inferomedial aspects of the bipartition halves were rigidly fixed to one another with plates and screws. Autologous bone grafts were placed at the advanced portions of the lateral orbital rims and zygomatic arches. Where indicated, a cantilever autologous nasal bone graft was placed and rigidly secured (Raposo-Amaral et al. 2011) (Fig. 21.33).

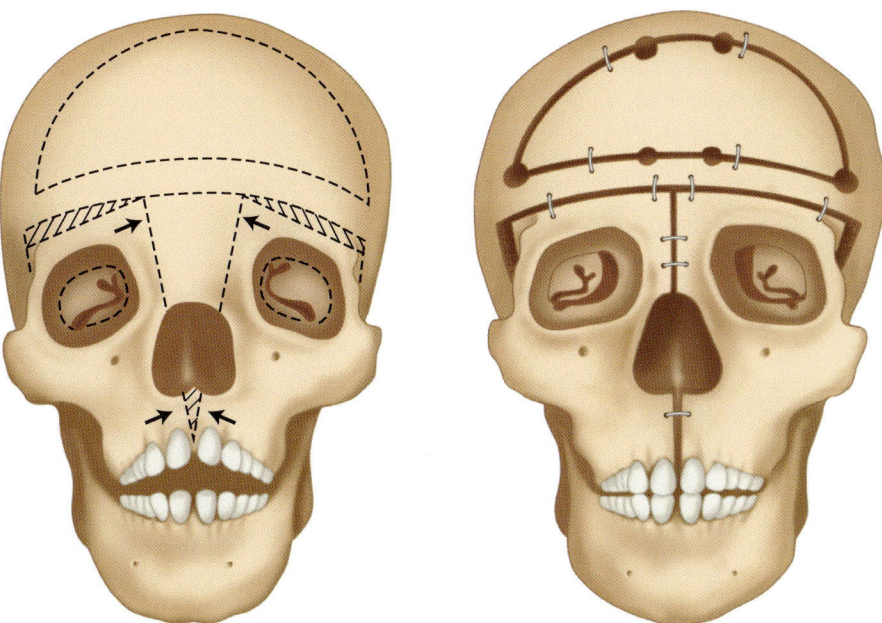

Fig. 21.33 Schematic drawing of facial bipartition osteotomy

21.26 The Rare Facial Cleft Number 10

Patients with gigantic encephalocele, feature commonly found in the number 10 cleft, can be corrected by exenteration of abnormal nonfunctioning brain and autologous bone graft from the parietal region. These procedures can be previously or simultaneously performed to the orbital medialization. After correcting the hypertelorbitism with an asymmetric medial wedge resection, soft-tissue reconstruction using local flaps to lengthen the medial paranasal dimension and to allow medial canthi upward mobilization is fundamental. This can be accomplished with transpositioning flaps. The challenge in this treatment relies on those number 10 patients with complete absence of the eyebrow and inverted eyelash (the upper eyelash with a downward rotation and lower eyelash with an upward rotation). This characteristic can cause corneal irritation in some patients. These distorted eyelash orientations are very difficult to correct.

Similar line of thinking should be used when treating the Tessier 1–13 cleft as similar soft-tissue malformations may be found.

The Tessier number 0–14 is the most common and encephalocele may be accompanied. Patients with complete nasal medial separation and encephalocele as a consequence of a wide hypertelorbitism should be carefully planned. The nose is usually constructed with converse scalping flaps; thus if the encephalocele is needed to be correct at very early age, the incisions should be carefully planned to not jeopardize the vascular pedicle of the scalping flaps based on the superficial and deep temporal arteries. All technical details of bony orbital medialization were extensively described in the literature. Local transpositioning flaps and Z-plastys can be used to adjust the nasal morphology and in most cases to descend the alar base unilaterally or bilaterally to a more gracious positioning (Raposo-Amaral et al. 2017).

21.27 Complications

There are a wide range of complications that may arise from the treatment of these patient populations. Complications may be related to either bone operation or soft-tissue operation. The magnitude of bony movements especially those to treat patients with rare facial cleft above the orbit requires an intracranial route to offer access for the orbital roof cuts and craniofacial disjunction when needed. As a consequence, several complications can be shown that generally occur as a result of severe blood loss or related to the communication between the oral nasal cavity and the anterior cranial fossa. As a result, cerebrospinal fluid leak may occur leading to ascending infection and postoperative meningitis that usually correlated with high morbidity/mortality rates. However, these complications that can be frequently seen in the treatment of syndromic craniosynostosis (Dunaway et al. 2012) are less frequent in the treatment of rare facial cleft mainly because of the normal intracranial pressure seen in these patients and no requirement to bring the face forward. Partial bone flap devascularization may also occur and require second operation for removal of the necrotic bone. Accidental fractures can be seen in patients whose bone cuts are not completely performed especially at the level of the pterygomaxillary junction. During the craniofacial disjunction the fracture can run toward the cranial base causing a CFS or an encephalocele. Orbital translocation carries the additional risk of optic nerve injury, as well as inadvertent medial canthal avulsion. Frontoethmoidal dissection and resection carry the risk of olfactory sensory loss. Soft-tissue complications are more frequently seen than bony complication. Local flaps can be necrotic compromising the postoperative result. Suboptimal result in management of nasal reconstruction and lower eyelid reconstruction and innumerous scars crossing the face can also be seen and this may be a challenge to correct in a later postoperative period.

21.28 Arhinia and Hemi-Arhinia

Congenital absence of nose termed total arhinia have possible genetic component. Gene candidates have been tested; however extended genetic analysis has not been performed in a large series of patients to determine common sporadic mutations. Thus, total arhinia has not been associated to any syndrome and most of the patients described in the literature are sporadic reports of isolated cases in different regions of the world. These patients present with different clinical characteristics and all scientific efforts to classify and grade this striking craniofacial deformity are of paramount importance.

Allam et al. (2011) classified the craniofacial dysplasia into three main division and total arhinia is identified as median craniofacial hypoplasia, described as tissue deficiency or agenesis. A subclassification also proposed by the authors divided the median craniofacial hypoplasia into four subcategories: (1) holoprosencephalic spectrum; (2) median cerebrofacial hypoplasia (lobar brain); (3) median facial hypoplasia; and (4) microforms of median facial hypoplasia. Interestingly, Binder syndrome known as maxillo-nasal dysplasia was included in the last division. Thus, a wide spectrum of bony and soft-tissue deformity makes a surgical algorithm difficult to be developed and proposed (Fig. 21.34).

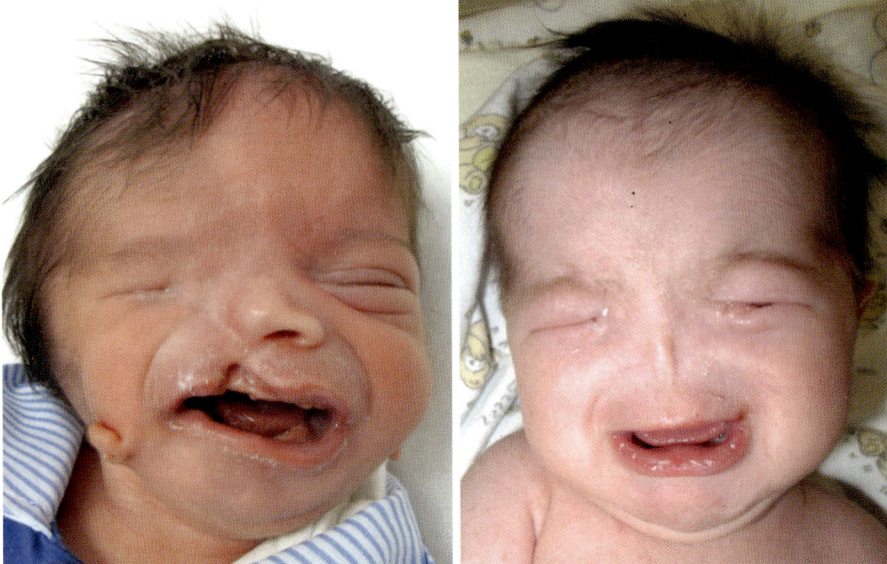

Fig. 21.34 Photographs of patients with facial agenesis, hemi-ahrinia and total ahrinia

21.29 Summary

This chapter highlighted some of very rare clinical examples of Tessier rare facial clefts. Some cases are so unique that similar clinical features may not be seen again in a lifetime.

Acknowledgments The authors thank the plastic surgeon and artist Jorge Vitale for the drawings given to Prof. Dr. Cassio Raposo do Amaral.

References

Abdollahifakhim S, Shahidi N, Bayazian G. A bilateral tessier number 4 and 5 facial cleft and surgical strategy: a case report. Iran J Otorhinolaryngol. 2013;25(73):259–62.

Agrawal K, Panda KN, Prasad S. Isolated Tessier no. 1 cleft of the nose. Ann Plast Surg. 1998;41(3):311–3.

Akoz T, Erdogan B, Gorgu M, Kutlay R, Dag F. Bilaterally involved Tessier no. 4 cleft: case report. Cleft Palate Craniofac J. 1996;33(3):252–4.

Allam KA, Wan DC, Kawamoto HK, Bradley JP, Sedano HO, Saied S. The spectrum of median craniofacial dysplasia. Plast Reconstr Surg. 2011 Feb;127(2):812–21.

Allam KA, Lim AA, Elsherbiny A, Kawamoto HK. The Tessier number 3 cleft: a report of 10 cases and review of literature. J Plast Reconstr Aesthet Surg. 2014;67(8):1055–62.

Alonso N, Freitas RS, de Oliveira e Cruz GA, Goldenberg D, DallOglio Tolazzi AR. Plast Reconstr Surg. 2008;122(5):1505–13.

Bhattacharyya NC, Kalita K, Gogoi M, Deuri PK. Tessier 30 facial cleft. J Indian Assoc Pediatr Surg. 2012;17(2):75–7.

Bodin F, Salazard B, Bardot J, Magalon G. Craniofacial cleft: a case of Tessier no. 3, 7 and 11 cleft. J Plast Reconstr Aesthet Surg. 2006;59(12):1388–90.

Boo-Chai K. The transverse facial cleft: its repair. Br J Plast Surg. 1969;22:119–24.

Burget GC, Menick FJ. Nasal reconstruction: seeking a fourth dimension. Plast Reconstr Surg. 1986;78(2):145–57.

David DJ, Moore MH, Cooter RD, Chow SK. The Tessier number 9 cleft. Plast Reconstr Surg. 1989;83(3):520–7.

Denadai R, Raposo-Amaral CA, Pinho AS, et al. Predictors of autologous free fat graft retention in the management of craniofacial contour deformities. Plast Reconstr Surg. 2017;140:50e–61e.

Denadai R, Raposo-Amaral CA, Buzzo CL, et al. Isolated autologous free fat grafting for management of facial contour asymmetry in a subset of growing patients with craniofacial microsomia. Ann Plast Surg. 2016;76:288–94.

Dumortier R, Delhemmes P, Pellerin P. Bilateral Tessier no. 9 cleft. J Craniofac Surg. 1999;10(6):523–5.

Dunaway DJ, Britto JA, Abela C, Evans RD, Jeelani NU. Complications of frontofacial advancement. Childs Nerv Syst. 2012;28(9):1571–6.

Fuente-del-Campo A. Surgical correction of Tessier number 8 cleft. Plast Reconstr Surg. 1990;86(4):658–61. discussion 62-3

Galante G, Dado DV. The Tessier number 5 cleft: a report of two cases and a review of the literature. Plast Reconstr Surg. 1991;88(1):131–5.

Garg A, Goyal S. Tessier number 5 cleft. Indian Pediatr. 2009;46(10):907.

Gargano F, Szymanski K, Bosman M, Podda S. Tessier 1-13 atypical craniofacial cleft. Eplasty. 2015;15:ic32.

Gawrych E, Janiszewska-Olszowska J, Chojnacka H. Tessier type 3 oblique facial cleft with a contralateral complete cleft lip and palate. Int J Oral Maxillofac Surg. 2010;39(11):1133–6.

Gonzalez-Ulloa M. Restoration of the face covering by means of selected skin in regional aesthetic units. Br J Plast Surg. 1956;9(3):212–21.

Gonzalez-Ulloa M. Selective regional restoration by means of esthetic units. Prensa Med Mex. 1958;23(2):68–73.

Horgan JE, Padwa BL, LaBrie RA, Mulliken JB. OMENS-plus: analysis of craniofacial and extracraniofacial anomalies in hemifacial microsomia. Cleft Palate Craniofac J. 1995;32(5):405–12.

Karfik V. [Proposed classification of rare congenital cleft defects of the face]. Rozhl Chir. 1966;45:518–22.

Kale SM, Pakhmode VK. Bilateral Tessier no. 4 facial cleft with left eye anophthalmos: a case report. J Indian Soc Pedod Prev Dent. 2000;18(3):87–9.

Kawamoto HK Jr. The kaleidoscopic world of rare craniofacial clefts: order out of chaos (Tessier classification). Clin Plast Surg. 1976;3(4):529–72.

Kececi Y, Gencosmanoglu R, Gorken C, Cagdas A. Facial cleft no. 30. J Craniofac Surg. 1994;5(4):263–4.

Laure B, Picard A, Bonin-Goga B, Letouze A, Petraud A, Goga D. Tessier number 4 bilateral orbito-facial cleft: a 26-year follow-up. J Craniomaxillofac Surg. 2010;38(4):245–7.

Lee HM, Noh TK, Yoo HW, Kim SB, Won CH, Chang SE, et al. A wedge-shaped anterior hairline extension associated with a tessier number 10 cleft. Ann Dermatol. 2012;24(4):464–7.

Ligh CA, Swanson J, Yu J, Samra F, Bartlett SP, Taylor JA. A morphological classification scheme for the mandibular hypoplasia in Treacher Collins syndrome. Plast Reconstr Surg. 2015;136(4 Suppl):46.

Morioka D, Simic R, Vlahovic A, Kravljanac D. Tessier 30 median mandibular cleft associated with lower lip hemangioma. Plast Reconstr Surg. 2003;112(3):935.

Nam SM, Kim YB. The Tessier number 14 facial cleft: a 20 years follow-up. J Craniomaxillofac Surg. 2014;42(7):1397–401.

Nguyen PD, Caro MC, Smith DM, Tompson B, Forrest CR, Phillips JH. Long-term orthognathic surgical outcomes in Treacher Collins patients. J Plast Reconstr Aesthet Surg. 2016;69(3):402–8.

Ozek C, Gundogan H, Bilkay U, Cankayali R, Guner U, Gurler T, et al. Rare craniofacial anomaly: Tessier no. 2 cleft. J Craniofac Surg. 2001;12(4):355–61.

Pidgeon TE, Flapper WJ, David DJ, Anderson PJ. From birth to maturity: midline tessier 0-14 craniofacial cleft patients who have completed protocol management at a single craniofacial unit. Cleft Palate Craniofac J. 2014;51(4):e70–9.

Pittet B, Jaquinet A, Rilliet B, Montandon D. Simultaneous correction of major hypertelorism, frontal bone defect, nasal aplasia, and cleft of the upper lip (Tessier 0-14). Plast Reconstr Surg. 2004;113(1):299–303.

Plomp RG, van Lieshout MJ, Joosten KF, Wolvius EB, van der Schroeff MP, Versnel SL, et al. Treacher Collins syndrome: a systematic review of evidence-based treatment and recommendations. Plast Reconstr Surg. 2016;137(1):191–204.

Poon CC, Meara JG, Heggie AA. Hemifacial microsomia: use of the OMENS-plus classification at the Royal Children's Hospital of Melbourne. Plast Reconstr Surg. 2003;111(3):1011–8.

Portier-Marret N, Hohlfeld J, Hamedani M, de Buys Roessingh AS. Complete bilateral facial cleft (Tessier 4) with corneal staphyloma: a rare association. J Pediatr Surg. 2008;43(10):e15–8.

Presti F, Celentano C, Marcazzo L, Dolcetta G, Prefumo F. Ultrasound prenatal diagnosis of a lateral facial cleft (Tessier number 7). Ultrasound Obstet Gynecol. 2004;23(6):606–8.

Raposo-Amaral CE, Raposo-Amaral CM, Raposo-Amaral CA, Chahal H, Bradley JP, Jarrahy R. Age at surgery significantly impacts the amount of orbital relapse following hypertelorbitism correction: a 30-year longitudinal study. Plast Reconstr Surg. 2011;127(4):1620–30.

Raposo-Amaral CE, Denadai R, Camargo DN, et al. Parry-Romberg syndrome: severity of the deformity does not correlate with quality of life. Aesthetic Plast Surg. 2013;37:792–801.

Raposo-Amaral CE, Denadai R, Ghizoni E, et al. Surgical strategies for soft tissue management in hypertelorbitism. Ann Plast Surg. 2017;78:421–27.

da Silva FR, Alonso N, Shin JH, Busato L, Ono MC, Cruz GA. Surgical correction of Tessier number 0 cleft. J Craniofac Surg. 2008;19(5):1348–52.

da Silva FR, Alonso N, Shin JH, Busato L, DallOglio Tolazzi AR, de Oliveira e Cruz GA. The Tessier number 5 facial cleft: surgical strategies and outcomes in six patients. Cleft Palate Craniofac J. 2009;46(2):179–86.

da Silva FR, Alonso N, Busato L, Ueda WK, Hota T, Medeiros GH, Kunz RT. Oral-nasal-ocular cleft: the greatest challeng among the rare clefts. J Craniofac Surg. 2010;21(2):390–5.

Tessier P. Anatomical classification facial, cranio-facial and latero-facial clefts. J Maxillofac Surg. 1976;4(2):69–92.

Tiwari P, Bhatnagar SK, Kalra GS. Tessier number 2 cleft, a variation. Case report. J Craniomaxillofac Surg. 1991;19(8):346–7.

Tokioka K, Nakatsuka T, Park S, Okouchi M, Aiba E. Two cases of Tessier no. 4 cleft with anophthalmia. Cleft Palate Craniofac J. 2005;42(4):448–52.

Wenbin Z, Hanjiang W, Xiaoli C, Zhonglin L. Tessier 3 cleft with clinical anophthalmia: two case reports and a review of the literature. Cleft Palate Craniofac J. 2007;44(1):102–5.

Woods RH, Varma S, David DJ. Tessier no. 7 cleft: a new subclassification and management protocol. Plast Reconstr Surg. 2008;122(3):898–905.

Three-Dimensional Digital Stereophotogrammetry in Cleft Care

22

Rafael Denadai and Cassio Eduardo Raposo-Amaral

22.1 Introduction

Modern cleft reconstruction requires accurate technical skills, in-depth knowledge of the three-dimensional (3D), and functional anatomy of the cleft and noncleft lips, nose, and alveolus, and appreciation of 3D facial aesthetics (Vyas and Warren 2014; Sharma et al. 2012; Sitzman et al. 2014). As the main targets of cleft surgery have been to optimize function, facial aesthetic, and health-related quality of life, there is an intrinsic challenge in the cleft outcome measurements (Vyas and Warren 2014; Sharma et al. 2012; Sitzman et al. 2014).

In this context, the American Cleft Palate–Craniofacial Association (www.acpa-cpf.org) established that "the team has mechanisms to monitor its short-term and long-term treatment outcomes" by documenting "its treatment outcomes, including base-line performance and changes over time" and conducting "periodic retrospective or prospective studies to evaluate treatment outcomes." In addition, the Eurocleft (Shaw et al. 2001) and the Americleft (Long et al. 2011) reports also recommended that documentation and records should be taken at standardized timing points to facilitate research and clinical audit.

Among different outcome tools (Vyas and Warren 2014; Sharma et al. 2012; Sitzman et al. 2014; Shaw et al. 2001; Long et al. 2011), standardized two-dimensional (2D) photography has been historically part of the armamentarium of cleft teams for the longitudinal follow-up of cleft patients according to specific purposes such as indirect anthropometric measurements and aesthetic evaluations (Al-Omari et al. 2005). However, this image modality lacks shape and depth, and flaws are inevitable when

---

R. Denadai, M.D. (✉)
Institute of Plastic and Craniofacial Surgery, SOBRAPAR Hospital, Campinas, São Paulo, Brazil
e-mail: denadai.rafael@hotmail.com

C.E. Raposo-Amaral, M.D., Ph.D.
Institute of Plastic and Craniofacial Surgery, SOBRAPAR Hospital,
Campinas, São Paulo 13084-880, Brazil

Universidade de São Paulo, São Paulo, Brazil

representing a 3D structure in 2D form (Al-Omari et al. 2005; Kuijpers et al. 2014; Chang et al. 2015; Brons et al. 2014; Tzou et al. 2014; Ladeira et al. 2013; Tzou and Frey 2011). To overcome the deficiencies of conventional 2D photography, various 3D surface imaging modalities have been developed (Al-Omari et al. 2005; Kuijpers et al. 2014; Chang et al. 2015; Brons et al. 2014; Tzou et al. 2014; Ladeira et al. 2013; Tzou and Frey 2011). A major advantage of 3D surface imaging over 2D photographs is the ease of capturing a patient in a 3D image, compared with traditional multiview photographs; a single 3D system can generate any 2D view without repositioning the patient. Additionally, these surface imaging modalities have shown accuracy in the submillimeter range when compared with their real-life representations, becoming especially relevant in the field of cleft surgical care as precision is crucial for identification and quantification of particular clinical features, preoperative evaluation, treatment planning (to plan the surgical maneuvers, flap design, and movement), and monitoring of operative outcomes including assessment of longitudinal postoperative changes (Al-Omari et al. 2005; Kuijpers et al. 2014; Chang et al. 2015; Brons et al. 2014; Tzou et al. 2014; Ladeira et al. 2013; Tzou and Frey 2011). However, there is no criterion standard measurement tool to date (Vyas and Warren 2014; Sharma et al. 2012; Sitzman et al. 2014; Shaw et al. 2001; Long et al. 2011; Al-Omari et al. 2005; Kuijpers et al. 2014; Chang et al. 2015; Brons et al. 2014; Tzou et al. 2014; Ladeira et al. 2013; Tzou and Frey 2011).

Various 3D surface imaging technologies have measured the complexities of an object with image subtraction techniques, Moiré topography, liquid-crystal scanning, laser scanning, structured light, stereophotogrammetry, among others (Al-Omari et al. 2005; Kuijpers et al. 2014; Chang et al. 2015; Brons et al. 2014; Tzou et al. 2014; Ladeira et al. 2013; Tzou and Frey 2011). However, most of these systems have not been applied in clinical routine due to time-consuming processes, inconsistent image quality, and unpredictable costs (Al-Omari et al. 2005; Kuijpers et al. 2014; Chang et al. 2015; Brons et al. 2014; Tzou et al. 2014; Ladeira et al. 2013; Tzou and Frey 2011). In addition, all systems are challenged in rendering accurate surfaces for hair and shiny areas (Al-Omari et al. 2005; Kuijpers et al. 2014; Chang et al. 2015; Brons et al. 2014; Tzou et al. 2014; Ladeira et al. 2013; Tzou and Frey 2011). Recently, advances in optical systems including structured light and stereophotogrammetry have made 3D surface imaging less time consuming and generating precise 3D surface images, handling vast data formats efficiently and being more accessible to patient protocols (Al-Omari et al. 2005; Kuijpers et al. 2014; Chang et al. 2015; Brons et al. 2014; Tzou et al. 2014; Ladeira et al. 2013; Tzou and Frey 2011). Both techniques are currently used depending on the application, and have been refined over time (Al-Omari et al. 2005; Kuijpers et al. 2014; Chang et al. 2015; Brons et al. 2014; Tzou et al. 2014; Ladeira et al. 2013; Tzou and Frey 2011).

This chapter provides an overview of a particular 3D surface facial imaging technology, namely 3D digital surface stereophotogrammetry, highlighting the history, the most common devices, the scientific validation and reliability, and the relevant clinical applications in cleft care.

22.2 History

In 1944, Thalmaan (1944) was the first to clinically apply the 3D stereophotogrammetry technology to capture the facial 3D surface of an adult with facial asymmetry and a baby with Pierre Robin sequence. In 1967, Burke and Beard (1967) improved and shortened the time-consuming Thalmaan's method through using simpler and less expensive cameras and applying a multiplex plotting system to analyze facial surface contours and track facial asymmetry over time, including the assessment of facial deformities of patients with cleft palate or cleft lip and palate. In 1972, Dixon and Newton (1972) performed a subjective assessment of 3D stereophotogrammetric models of face of two cleft patients and concluded that stereophotogrammetry can be a valuable method of describing and recording a minimal form of cleft. In 1991, Deacon et al. (1991) drastically shortened the manual analysis of stereophotogrammetry by replacing the precalibrated metric cameras and film emulsion with low-cost charge-coupled device cameras, which offered the advantage of digitized image capture for 3D automatic analysis. In 1995, Ras et al. (1995) concluded that stereophotogrammetry was an appropriate 3D registration method for quantifying and detecting development and changes in facial morphology of 106 subjects, including 16 surgically treated patients with complete unilateral cleft lip and palate. At the beginning of the twenty-first century, Ayoub et al. (2003) presented the reliability of a 3D stereophotogrammetry imaging system in recording cleft deformities and measuring the changes following cleft surgical repair.

22.3 3D Digital Stereophotogrammetry

Stereophotogrammetry uses two or more cameras arranged as a stereo pair to provide points of intersection between disparate images and to allow for depth perception (Fig. 22.1). Corresponding raw images are matched in space to create a 3D image that can be converted into a 3D anatomical model using 3D software. This 3D surface imaging method is millisecond fast and has archival capabilities for subsequent morphometric studies, a good-resolution color representation, and no

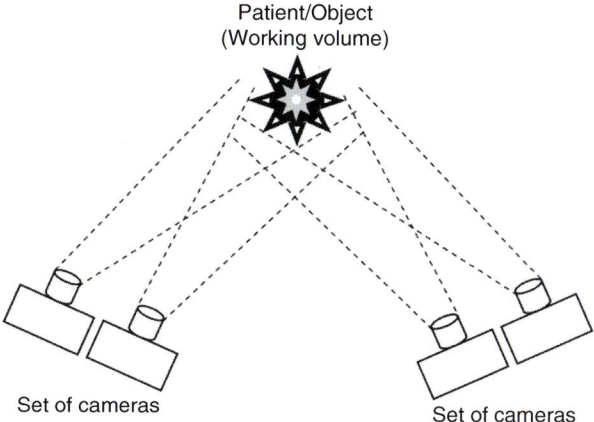

Fig. 22.1 Schematic drawing of a three-dimensional digital stereophotogrammetric device for the analysis of craniofacial soft tissues (*gray zone*). Subject's face should be located within the working volume (*black zone*). Two sets of cameras record the craniofacial characteristics from the right and the left sides. The working volume represents the part of space seen by two or more cameras with nonparallel optical axes. After a calibration procedure, the computer can obtain the metric three-dimensional coordinates of each point of the working volume

exposure to ionizing radiation (Al-Omari et al. 2005; Kuijpers et al. 2014; Chang et al. 2015; Brons et al. 2014; Tzou et al. 2014; Ladeira et al. 2013; Tzou and Frey 2011). In particular, the craniofacial image is visualized as a collection of points in 3D space (termed a "point cloud") resulting from the reconstructed craniofacial surface. The surface data are a collection of points interrelated by their position along an x, y, and z coordinate system, and the distances among these points can be readily computed. At a computer workstation, anthropometric landmarks are identified by the user by marking them on the surface using a "soft" cursor that deforms itself to the facial contour. Landmarks appear as color points with reference coordinates that can be saved for subsequent morphometry sessions. In fact, an advantage of this 3D method is the reduced time of exposure and embarrassment patients (principally children) may feel during measurements; some measurements, such as those around the eyes, are difficult to obtain directly without risk for discomfort (snap shut of the caliper or contact of its tips on the skin can make the subject uncomfortable) or injury to the patient. It also allows the cleft team to take the measurements under proper conditions at a time other than during a patient visit.

Additionally, stereophotogrammetry relies on triangulation, which overlays multiple images of the same object from different angles to form a 3D image. There are two basic triangulation strategies for stereophotogrammetry, namely active and passive. Active stereophotogrammetry deploys the projection of a focused random unstructured light pattern on the actual surface of the target object. It combines this pattern with the visible natural pattern of the object's surface (if any) to give the stereo algorithms as much information as possible to generate a quality 3D geometry. No special external lighting conditions are needed for this technique, and it is resilient to the effects of ambient lighting. In contrast, passive stereophotogrammetry generates 3D geometry solely based on the natural patterns of the target object's surface. High-resolution cameras are needed to ensure that enough surface detail is available to generate the 3D geometry. Care must be taken to avoid the effects of strong directional ambient light to avoid glare on the surface (Al-Omari et al. 2005; Kuijpers et al. 2014; Chang et al. 2015; Brons et al. 2014; Tzou et al. 2014; Ladeira et al. 2013; Tzou and Frey 2011).

In a recent review, Heike et al. (2010) detailed the main technical issues related to the practical use of stereophotogrammetry, including its physical location, suggestions to reduce image artifacts and maximize facial surface coverage, and hints for the analysis of children and persons with special needs. The discussion of all these aspects is beyond the scope of this chapter.

22.3.1 Companies and Products

Currently, three companies provide the most notable commercialized 3D stereophotogrammetry imaging software and hardware that is sold and supported worldwide, and each offers different approaches: 3dMD (3dMD LLC; London, UK, and Atlanta, Georgia, USA; www.3dmd.com); Canfield Imaging Systems (Canfield Research Group LLC; Fairfield, New Jersey, USA; www.canfield.com); and DI3D (Dimensional Imaging Ltd.; Glasgow, Scotland, UK; www.di3d.com). All systems vary in their camera setup, colors, capture time, and computed tomographic image fusion capabilities (Table 22.1). As these systems differ widely in technique and technology, selection is based on intended clinical application (Al-Omari et al. 2005; Kuijpers et al. 2014; Chang et al. 2015; Brons et al. 2014; Tzou et al. 2014; Ladeira et al. 2013; Tzou and Frey 2011).

Table 22.1 Three-dimensional stereophotogrammetry imaging products commercialized worldwide (Al-Omari et al. 2005; Kuijpers et al. 2014; Chang et al. 2015; Brons et al. 2014; Tzou et al. 2014; Ladeira et al. 2013; Tzou and Frey 2011)

Characteristics	Companies (products)		
	3dMD (3dMDface and 3dMDhead)	Canfield (VECTRA H1, M3, XT, and CR3D)	DI3D
Hardware	From 2 to 5 modular units of 6 to 15 machine vision cameras, industrial-grade system synchronized in a single capture with a PC-controller desktop or laptop for portability	From 1 to 3 pods, onboard, intelligent flash units, floor stand with motorized lift to adjust for patient height, and PC + 23″ monitor or laptop	Standard 3D system used 4 Canon EOS 550D 18 MP, 2 head studio flash kit for illumination, laptop with software
Stereophotogrammetry	Hybrid (active and passive)	Passive	Passive
Coverage	190-degree face capture (ear-to-ear) or full 360-degree face capture	Capturing volume (mm): 220x130x70 to 600x550x350 (H---W---D)	~180-degree face capture
Capture speed	~1.5 ms at highest resolution	2–8 ms	Length of a flash ~1 ms
Processing speed	<8–15 s	~20–120 s	60 s
Geometry representation	A continuous point cloud available as a textured mesh and dense textured point model	Mesh	A continuous point cloud converted to mesh later
Error in geometry	<0.2 mm	>0.1 mm	≥0.2 mm
Calibration time	20–90 s	No calibration to <3 min	5 min
Sample density	62 vertices/cm^2	1.2 mm geometry resolution (polygon edge length)	20 to 30 samples/mm^2
CT/CBCT fusion	3dMDvultus and third-party software (e.g., dolphin, maxilim and materialize OMS)	Third-party software (e.g., dolphin)	Third-party software (e.g., dolphin, maxilim, and materialize OMS)
Simulate surgery	Yes	Yes	Third-party software
Real-time 3D volumetric visualization	Yes	Yes	Third-party software
Tissue behavior simulation	Yes	Yes	Third-party software

CT/CBCT, computed tomography/cone beam computed tomography; *3D*, three-dimensional. Note: some characteristics vary according to products within the same company

22.3.2 Scientific Validation and Reliability

In a recent systematic review, Kuijpers et al. (2014) evaluated 3D imaging methods for quantitative analysis of facial soft tissues and skeletal morphology in patients with orofacial clefts and demonstrated that 13 (61.9%) of the 21 studies using stereophotogrammetry have good-quality methodological scores (mean 64%) and 92% presented the highest score. In the following studies (Aldridge et al. 2005; Weinberg et al. 2006; Wong et al. 2008; Plooij et al. 2009; Maal et al. 2010; Lübbers et al. 2010; Metzler et al. 2012, 2014; Nord et al. 2015; de Menezes et al. 2010; Rosati et al. 2010; Othman et al. 2013; Winder et al. 2008; Khambay et al. 2008; Kook et al. 2014; Fourie et al. 2011; Ayoub et al. 2007; Naudi et al. 2013), 3D stereophotogrammetry was found to be an objective, accurate, and reliable system for quantifying the dimension and changes of the soft tissues, particularly of the face region.

3dMD: Aldridge et al. (2005) investigated the precision, error, and repeatability associated with anthropometric landmark coordinate data collected from 3D digital photogrammetric images of children and adults and showed that the data were highly repeatable and precise, and it can be useful for evaluation of clinical dysmorphology and surgery, analyses of genotype-phenotype correlations, and inheritance of complex phenotypes. Weinberg et al. (2006) compared anthropometric measurements obtained by 3dMD, Genex 3D system, and direct anthropometry. Although statistically significant mean differences were observed across methods for nine anthropometric variables, the magnitude of these differences was consistently at the submillimeter level; no significant differences were noted for precision; the magnitude of imprecision was determined to be very small, with technical error of measurement scores well under 1 mm; and intraclass correlation coefficients ranging from 0.98 to 1 (Weinberg et al. 2006). Wong et al. (2008) evaluated the validity and reliability of facial anthropometric linear distances imaged by 3dMDface system with respect to direct anthropometry and 3D assessment of most of the linear distances studied (17 of 18 measurements) was accurate when compared with direct anthropometry; the test-retest reliability of digital measurements was excellent and comparable to direct anthropometry; and 3D digital anthropometry was shown to be as precise as direct measurements. In the study by Plooij et al. (2009), two observers used a 3dMDface system in 20 patients to obtain facial measurements, and the intraobserver coefficient of reliability was as high as 0.97, the interobserver coefficient of reliability was 0.94, and the reproducibility was also high. Maal et al. (2010) analyzed treatment outcomes in oral and maxillofacial surgery by comparing the data captured with 3dMD and Maxilim (Medicim NV, Mechelen, Belgium). The intra- and interobserver error of the reference-based registration method was found to be 1.2 and 1.0 mm, respectively. They (Maal et al. 2010) concluded that surface-based registration is an accurate method to compare 3D photographs of the same individual at different times, and 3D stereophotogrammetry is an accurate tool to evaluate facial changes (surgical or nonsurgical) over time. Lubbers et al. (2010) evaluated data of the 3dMD system and found the system to be reliable for evaluation and documentation of the facial surface, with a mean global error of 0.2 mm for phantom head measurements; and neither the position of the head nor that of the camera influenced these parameters. Metzler et al. (2012) investigated the intraobserver repeatability of 27 craniofacial landmarks in children and showed that the mean 3D repeatability error was 0.82 mm, with no statistical differences from one patient to another. Nord et al. (2015) assessed the repeatability and accuracy of the 3dMDface system when used by different operators and at different times and revealed that virtual 3D models derived from the system provide a high level of not only technical precision but also intra- and interobserver reliability regarding landmark identification.

Canfield Imaging Systems: de Menezes (2010) tested the accuracy and reproducibility of the VECTRA-CR. No systematic errors were found for all tests performed and repeated sets of acquisition showed random errors up to 0.91 mm, without systematic biases. Rosati et al. (2010) evaluated the integration of the dental cast virtual model into soft-tissue facial morphologies created with VECTRA-CR and found that the greatest mean relative error of measurements was <1.2%, with no significant differences in repeatable reproductions. Othman et al. (2013) assessed the reproducibility of facial soft-tissue landmarks using VECTRA-3D and revealed that intraclass correlation coefficients for all 24 landmarks ranged from 0.68 to 0.97, indicating moderate-to-high reliability and reproducibility of all facial soft-tissue landmarks, with no significant differences in all facial soft-tissue landmark measurements. Metzler et al. (2014) analyzed the validity (precision and accuracy) of the VECTRA-3D system for craniofacial anthropometric measurements and suggested its suitability for clinical applications, particularly anthropometric studies.

DI3D: In a study with DI3D system, Wider et al. (2008) assessed geometric accuracy and maximum field of view on phantom head with black ink dots serving as facial landmarks and found a mean error in the 3D surfaces of 0.057 mm, a repeatability error (variance) of 0.0016 mm, and a mean error of 0.6 mm in linear measurements, compared with manual measurements. Khambay et al. (2008) evaluated the accuracy and reproducibility using adult facial plaster casts with landmarks marked and reported that reproducibility of the DI3D capture was 0.13 mm, and the system error averaged 0.21 mm. Kook et al. (2014) analyzed facial soft-tissue measurements performed by the direct anthropometry, digitizer, 3D computerized tomography, 3D scanner, and DI3D system and all methods demonstrated good accuracy and had a high coefficient of reliability (>0.92) and a low technical error (<0.9 mm), and the mean measurement error in every measurement method was low (<0.7 mm). Fourier et al. (2011) demonstrated that the results of accuracy and reliability comparing laser surface scanning (Minolta Vivid 900), cone beam computed tomography, and DI3D system were sufficiently accurate and reliable for research and clinical use. Ayoub et al. (2007) verified the feasibility of merging skeletal and soft-tissue images (captured using 3D computed tomography scanner and DI3D system) to develop a 3D virtual human face model for craniofacial diagnosis and treatment planning with a minimal surface registration error of 1.5 mm. Naudi et al. (2013) revealed that simultaneous capture of the 3D surface of the face using the DI3D and cone beam computed tomography scan of the skull significantly improved the accuracy of superimposition of these image modalities.

22.4 Clinical Applications in Cleft Patients

Digital stereophotogrammetry has an expanding application in cleft arena including different issues (e.g., facial morphology prior to primary surgery; anthropometric measures; asymmetry assessment of the face, nose, and lips; soft-tissue changes after therapeutic interventions; facial aesthetics; facial soft-tissue growth; and stone cast measurements (Hood et al. 2004, 2003; Tse et al. 2014; Ayoub et al. 2011a, b, c; Bugaighis et al. 2010; Krimmel et al. 2011; Kau et al. 2011; Sade Hoefert et al. 2010; van Loon et al. 2010; Stebel et al. 2016; Desmedt et al. 2015; Davidson and Kumar 2015; Brons et al. 2013; Sforza et al. 2012; De Menezes et al. 2016)), which should be considered as integrated and interrelated areas of cleft outcome assessment. Some clinical examples of the applicability of stereophotogrammetry in cleft care are described in this chapter (Hood et al. 2004; Tse et al. 2014; Hood et al. 2003; Ayoub et al. 2011a, b, c; Bugaighis et al. 2010; Krimmel et al. 2011; Kau et al. 2011; Sade Hoefert et al. 2010; van Loon et al. 2010; Stebel et al. 2016; Desmedt et al. 2015; Davidson and Kumar 2015; Brons et al. 2013; Sforza et al. 2012; De Menezes et al. 2016), but without the intent of fully addressing the growing body of pertinent literature.

22.4.1 Nasolabial Anthropometry/Morphology Before Primary Surgical Repair

Hood et al. (2004) characterized the 3D facial soft-tissue features of 3-month cleft children prior to primary surgery and compared with noncleft controls. Significant differences were found between the unilateral cleft lip and palate group and unilateral cleft lip and control groups in anatomical and soft nose width, cleft-side alar wing length, and nasal tip horizontal displacement. Both cleft groups were significantly different from controls and from each other in cleft-side nostril dimensions, alar wing angulation, columella angle, and alar base to corner of mouth dimension; alar base width; and soft-tissue defect in nose and the lip and philtrum length bordering the cleft. Significant differences between clefts and controls were identified in the nostril and philtrum on the noncleft side. They (Hood et al. 2004) concluded that the use of children with unilateral cleft lip as controls for unilateral cleft lip and palate studies is inappropriate. In addition, capturing facial morphology of infants using a noninvasive 3D stereophotogrammetry method overcame the limitations of direct measurement of infant faces to aid the cleft surgeon in the planning and subsequent reevaluation of surgical rationale (Hood et al. 2004).

Tse et al. (2014) assessed the reliability of 3D stereophotogrammetry for anthropometric assessment of the unilateral cleft lip ± palate deformity in infants before cleft lip repair. Regarding intrarater and interrater reliability, most measurements had Pearson coefficients greater than 0.75, mean differences less than 0.8 mm, and mean proportional differences less than 0.1. For measurements involving vermilion height, nostril remnants, or Cupid's bow width, Pearson coefficients ranged from 0.3 to 0.75, mean differences ranged from 0.4 to 0.9 mm, and mean proportional differences ranged from 0.1 to 0.3. Regarding intermethod reliability, correlation coefficients ranged from 0.4 to 0.75 for most measurements. The mean differences for nose and lip measurements were less than 1 mm and between 0.8 and 1.3 mm, respectively. Therefore, the 3D stereophotogrammetry provides a reliable method for many anthropometric measurements of nasolabial form in infants with unrepaired unilateral cleft lip ± palate (Tse et al. 2014).

22.4.2 Nasolabial Anthropometric/Morphologic Changes After Therapeutic Interventions

Hood et al. (2003) evaluated the 3D faces of cleft children, and 20 age-matched, noncleft controls, prior to primary Millard lip and McComb nose repair (at 3 months), at 6 months and at age 1 year. It revealed that the unilateral cleft lip and palate group was more asymmetric than the unilateral cleft lip group, displaying greatest improvement in nasal symmetry following primary repair. Immediate improvement in asymmetry scores in children with unilateral cleft lip and palate is related to the production of a more symmetrical nasal form after primary surgery; in contrast, the nasal asymmetry seen in children with unilateral cleft lip is unchanged despite surgery; and nasal and lip asymmetry should be considered individually (Hood et al. 2003).

Ayoub et al. (2011a) assessed 3D lip scarring and residual dysmorphology following primary repair in 10-year-old cleft children relative to noncleft data. Residual lip dysmorphologies were more pronounced in unilateral cleft lip and palate cases. The width of the Cupid's bow was increased due to lateral displacement of the christa philteri left in both unilateral cleft lip and unilateral cleft lip and palate patients. In the upper part of the lip, the nostril base was significantly wider in unilateral cleft lip and palate cases when compared with unilateral cleft lip cases and controls. Scar redness was more pronounced in unilateral cleft lip than in unilateral cleft lip and palate cases. This group (Ayoub et al. 2011b, c) also evaluated 3D nasal and lip morphology following primary repair in 3-year-old cleft children relative to noncleft data and found significant nasal deformities following the surgical repair of unilateral cleft lip and palate and significant increase of the philtrum width, and the lip appeared flatter and more posterior displaced in unilateral cleft lip and palate patients compared with controls.

Bugaighis et al. (2010) explored 3D facial asymmetry differences in operated 8- to 12-year-old cleft children and compared the results with a sex- and age-matched control group. The unilateral cleft lip and palate and unilateral cleft lip and alveolus patients displayed the greatest asymmetry, followed by the bilateral cleft lip and palate group. The cleft palate group was the least asymmetric among the cleft groups. Shape analysis indicates the possible differences in the etiology and growth pattern of the cleft palate group compared to unilateral cleft lip and alveolus or unilateral cleft lip and palate and bilateral cleft lip and palate groups.

Krimmel et al. (2011) analyzed the 3D facial surface changes (namely, craniofacial landmarks on the nose and the upper lip) after alveolar bone grafting in patients with cleft lip and palate. A significant increase in anterior projection on the operative side was found for the labial insertion points of the alar base (subalare), but no significant changes were detected for the position of the labial landmarks.

Kau et al. (2011) compared landmark versus surface shape measurements in patients with unilateral cleft lip and palate following secondary alveolar bone grafting. Color map surface-to-surface comparison revealed a significant anteroposterior elevation in the nasal region (the ala, alar base, and paranasal areas) of the cleft side after bone grafting. In conclusion, they (Kau et al. 2011) argue that while landmark studies showed not too many clinically significant changes, the 3D surface-to-surface analysis allows for better quantification of treatment changes.

Sade Hoefert et al. (2010) assessed 3D soft-tissue changes in facial morphology of cleft children and Class III malocclusion under therapy with rapid maxillary expansion and Delaire facemask. Significant forward rotation and forward displacement of the soft tissue in the lower midface with the dentoalveolar areas were detected in all patients. No significant asymmetric forward displacement of the soft tissue in the maxilla could be verified in the lower or upper midface. The Class III malocclusion patients showed greater maxillary soft-tissue changes. In their conclusion, the authors (Sade Hoefert et al. 2010) assert that the 3D data allowed to discriminatively interpret the effects of the orthopedic mask on the entire maxillary complex and maxillary alveolar process.

Van Loon et al. (2010) analyzed the results of patients with unilateral cleft who received 3D imaging before and 3 months after rhinoplasty. The images were superimposed to generate a topographic distance map of preoperative and postoperative tissue changes. No statistically significant differences were found within and between observers for the measured volumes and symmetry. Postoperatively, the total volume of the nose increased significantly, especially the volume at the cleft side. No significant volume difference pre- and postoperatively was found for the noncleft side. The symmetry of the nose improved significantly. Therefore, the authors (van Loon et al. 2010) concluded that 3D stereophotogrammetry is a sensitive, quick, noninvasive method for evaluating volumetric changes of the nose in cleft patients (van Loon et al. 2010).

22.4.3 Nasolabial Aesthetics

Stebel et al. (2016) compared reliability of rating nasolabial appearance on 3D images and standard 2D photographs in cleft children. Intrarater agreement demonstrated a better reliability of ratings performed on 3D images than 2D images. 3D images were regarded more informative than 2D images but probably more difficult to evaluate (Stebel et al. 2016). Desmedt et al. (2015) determined the relationship between nasolabial symmetry and aesthetics in 3D facial images of cleft patients and showed that nasolabial appearance was affected by nasolabial asymmetry; subjects with more nasolabial asymmetry were judged as having a less aesthetically pleasing nasolabial area. Davidson and Kumar (2015) evaluated changes in nasal aesthetics using 3D photography after Le Fort I advancement in patients with nonsyndromic cleft-related maxillary hypoplasia. Cleft-related scarring and malposition affect changes in nasal aesthetics following maxillary advancement that are different to the noncleft population, and two-piece Le Fort I increases variability of changes in nasal aesthetics compared with single-piece advancement (Davidson and Kumar 2015).

22.4.4 Facial Soft-Tissue Growth

A recent systematic review (Brons et al. 2014) concluded that stereophotogrammetry seems to be the best 3D method to longitudinally assess facial growth in children younger than 6 years of age. Brons et al. (2013) developed a reference frame for 3D facial soft-tissue growth analysis in cleft children and control children. Results of intraobserver comparisons showed a mean distance of <0.40 mm, distance variability of <0.51 mm, and P95 of <0.80 mm. For interobserver reliability, the mean distance was <0.52 mm, distance variability was <0.53 mm, and P95 was <1.10 mm. Presence of a cleft, age, and absence of one ear on the 3D photograph did not have a significant influence on the reproducibility of placing the reference frame. They (Brons et al. 2013) concluded that children's reference frame is a reproducible method to superimpose on 3D soft-tissue stereophotogrammetry photographs of growing individuals with and without orofacial clefts.

22.4.5 Palatal Casts

Sforza et al. (2012) assessed a 3D stereophotogrammetric method for palatal cast digitization of neonatal patients with unilateral cleft lip and palate. 3D measurements (cleft width, depth, length) were made separately for the longer and shorter cleft segments on the digital dental cast surface between landmarks, previously marked. The 3D method presented good accuracy error (<0.9%) on measuring geometric objects. No systematic errors between operators' measurements were found. Statistically significant differences were noted for different methods (caliper versus stereophotogrammetry) for almost all distances analyzed, with mean absolute difference values ranging between 0.22 and 3.41 mm; caliper values were larger than three-dimensional stereophotogrammetric values. As 3D stereophotogrammetric systems have some advantages over direct anthropometry, the 3D method could be sufficiently precise and accurate on palatal cast digitization of cleft patients (Sforza et al. 2012). In De Menezes et al. (2016) study, the cleft segment delimitation on digital dental casts and area measurements by the 3D stereophotogrammetric system revealed an accurate (true and precise) method for evaluating the stone casts of newborn patients with unilateral cleft lip and palate.

22.5 3D Facial Norms Database

The development of accurate and reproducible 3D facial imaging and analysis has led to the creation of high-quality craniofacial norms based on 3D imaging technology. With these craniofacial databases, patients with craniofacial anomalies can be compared, determining morphologic differences with the ultimate utility of advanced surgical planning. In 2009, the 3D Facial Norms project was created with the goal of generating an interactive, Web-based repository of 3D stereophotogrammetric facial images and measurements to aid the clinical and research community in the assessment of craniofacial dysmorphology (Weinberg et al. 2016). In 2015, the 3D Facial Norms database presented data from 2454 US male and female participants ranging in age from 3 to 40 years (Weinberg et al. 2016). Users can gain access to both summary-level statistics and individual-level data, including 3D facial landmark coordinates, 3D-derived anthropometric measurements (including growth curves for every anthropometric measurement), 3D facial surface images, and genotypes from every individual in the dataset (Weinberg et al. 2016).

22.6 Limitations and Future

Although the clinical applications of 3D digital stereophotogrammetry surface imaging have progressed rapidly over the past years, limitations include cost, ease of use, dimensions, patient applicability, capture and processing speed, interface portability, image quality, and others. Furthermore, early postoperative analysis may not be accurate as postoperative inflammatory edema or fibrosis distorts 3D images and associated analysis. Therefore, advancements must be made in the imaging software to be more user friendly, efficient, and accurate to engage the utility of cleft teams. In addition, over time, the pricing of the device will become more agreeable.

In this context, it is important to emphasize that the imaging and analysis must transition from the cleft team's perspective to the patient's perspective to be truly applicable to the patient's surgical/orthodontics experience. By integrating the technology in the surgical/orthodontics consultation, both the patient and the professional can appreciate the preoperative anatomical aspects and proposed surgical/orthodontics corrections. However, simulations of potential surgical/orthodontics results are only estimates of results based on the collaboration of engineers and cleft teams, and the available software lack evidence-based data (i.e., the impact of age, gender, ethnicity, scars, and professional skills on surgical outcomes). Ultimately, with these factors integrated, outcome simulations will improve patient consultation and enhance preoperative planning in a near future. Moreover, to generate a 3D image database validated worldwide, more data are required from various centers representing all patient demographics (Al-Omari et al. 2005; Kuijpers et al. 2014; Chang et al. 2015; Brons et al. 2014; Tzou et al. 2014; Ladeira et al. 2013; Tzou and Frey 2011; Weinberg et al. 2016).

References

Aldridge K, Boyadjiev SA, Capone GT, DeLeon VB, Richtsmeier JT. Precision and error of three-dimensional phenotypic measures acquired from 3dMD photogrammetric images. Am J Med Genet A. 2005;138A:247–53.

Al-Omari I, Millett DT, Ayoub AF. Methods of assessment of cleft-related facial deformity: a review. Cleft Palate Craniofac J. 2005;42:145–56.

Ayoub A, Garrahy A, Hood C, White J, Bock M, Siebert JP, Spencer R, Ray A. Validation of a vision-based, three-dimensional facial imaging system. Cleft Palate Craniofac J. 2003;40:523–9.

Ayoub AF, Xiao Y, Khambay B, Siebert JP, Hadley D. Towards building a photo-realistic virtual human face for craniomaxillofacial diagnosis and treatment planning. Int J Oral Maxillofac Surg. 2007;36:423–8.

Ayoub A, Bell A, Simmons D, Bowman A, Brown D, Lo TW, Xiao Y. 3D assessment of lip scarring and residual dysmorphology following surgical repair of cleft lip and palate: a preliminary study. Cleft Palate Craniofac J. 2011a;48:379–87.

Ayoub A, Garrahy A, Millett D, Bowman A, Siebert JP, Miller J, Ray A. Three-dimensional assessment of early surgical outcome in repaired unilateral cleft lip and palate: part 1. Nasal changes. Cleft Palate Craniofac J. 2011b;48:571–7.

Ayoub A, Garrahy A, Millett D, Bowman A, Siebert JP, Miller J, Ray A. Three-dimensional assessment of early surgical outcome in repaired unilateral cleft lip and palate: part 2. Lip changes. Cleft Palate Craniofac J. 2011c;48:578–83.

Brons S, van Beusichem ME, Maal TJ, Plooij JM, Bronkhorst EM, Bergé SJ, Kuijpers-Jagtman AM. Development and reproducibility of a 3D stereophotogrammetric reference frame for facial soft tissue growth of babies and young children with and without orofacial clefts. Int J Oral Maxillofac Surg. 2013;42:2–8.

Brons S, van Beusichem ME, Bronkhorst EM, Draaisma JM, Bergé SJ, Schols JG, Kuijpers-Jagtman AM. Methods to quantify soft tissue-based cranial growth and treatment outcomes in children: a systematic review. PLoS One. 2014;9:e89602.

Bugaighis I, O'Higgins P, Tiddeman B, Mattick C, Ben Ali O, Hobson R. Three-dimensional geometric morphometrics applied to the study of children with cleft lip and/or palate from the North East of England. Eur J Orthod. 2010;32:514–21.

Burke PH, Beard FH. Stereophotogrammetry of the face. A preliminary investigation into the accuracy of a simplified system evolved for contourmapping by photography. Am J Orthod. 1967;53:769–82.

Chang JB, Small KH, Choi M, Karp NS. Three-dimensional surface imaging in plastic surgery:foundation, practical applications, and beyond. Plast Reconstr Surg. 2015;135:1295–304.

Davidson E, Kumar AR. A preliminary three-dimensional analysis of nasal aesthetics following Le Fort I advancement in patients with cleft lip and palate. J Craniofac Surg. 2015;26:e629–33.

De Menezes M, Ceron-Zapata AM, Lopez-Palacio AM, Mapelli A, Pisoni L, Sforza C. Evaluation of a 3D stereophotogrammetric method to identify and measure the palatal surface area in children with unilateral cleft lip and palate. Cleft Palate Craniofac J. 2016;53:16–21.

Deacon AT, Anthony AG, Bhatia SN, Muller JP. Evaluation of a CCD-based facial measurement system. Med Inf. 1991;16:213–28.

Desmedt DJ, Maal TJ, Kuijpers MA, Bronkhorst EM, Kuijpers-Jagtman AM, Fudalej PS. Nasolabial symmetry and esthetics in cleft lip and palate: analysis of 3D facial images. Clin Oral Investig. 2015;19:1833–42.

Dixon DA, Newton I. Minimal forms of the cleft syndrome demonstrated by stereophotogrammetric surveys of the face. Br Dent J. 1972;132:183–9.

Fourie Z, Damstra J, Gerrits PO, Ren Y. Evaluation of anthropometric accuracy and reliability using different three-dimensional scanning systems. Forensic Sci Int. 2011;207:127–34.

Heike CL, Upson K, Stuhaug E, Weinberg SM. 3D digital stereophotogrammetry: a practical guide to facial image acquisition. Head Face Med. 2010;6:18.

Hood CA, Bock M, Hosey MT, Bowman A, Ayoub AF. Facial asymmetry--3D assessment of infants with cleft lip & palate. Int J Paediatr Dent. 2003;13:404–10.

Hood CA, Hosey MT, Bock M, White J, Ray A, Ayoub AF. Facial characterization of infants with cleft lip and palate using a three-dimensional capture technique. Cleft Palate Craniofac J. 2004;41:27–35.

Kau CH, Medina L, English JD, Xia J, Gateno J, Teichgraber J. A comparison between landmark and surface shape measurements in a sample of cleft lip and palate patients after secondary alveolar bone grafting. Orthodontics. 2011;12:188–95.

Khambay B, Nairn N, Bell A, Miller J, Bowman A, Ayoub AF. Validation and reproducibility of a high-resolutionthree-dimensional facial imaging system. Br J Oral Maxillofac Surg. 2008;46:27–32.

Kook MS, Jung S, Park HJ, Oh HK, Ryu SY, Cho JH, Lee JS, Yoon SJ, Kim MS, Shin HK. A comparison study of different facial soft tissue analysis methods. J Craniomaxillofac Surg. 2014;42:648–56.

Krimmel M, Schuck N, Bacher M, Reinert S. Facial surface changes after cleft alveolar bone grafting. J Oral Maxillofac Surg. 2011;69:80–3.

Kuijpers MA, Chiu YT, Nada RM, Carels CE, Fudalej PS. Three-dimensional imaging methods for quantitative analysisof facial soft tissues and skeletal morphology in patients withorofacial clefts: a systematic review. PLoS One. 2014;9:e93442.

Ladeira PR, Bastos EO, Vanini JV, Alonso N. Use of stereophotogrammetry for evaluating craniofacial deformities: a systematic review. Rev Bras Cir Plást. 2013;28:147–55.

Long RE Jr, Hathaway R, Daskalogiannakis J, Mercado A, Russell K, Cohen M, Semb G, Shaw W. The Americleft study: an inter-center study of treatment outcomes for patients with unilateral cleft lip and palate part 1.Principles and study design. Cleft Palate Craniofac J. 2011;48:239–43.

van Loon B, Maal TJ, Plooij JM, Ingels KJ, Borstlap WA, Kuijpers-Jagtman AM, Spauwen PH, Bergé SJ. 3D Stereophotogrammetric assessment of pre- and postoperative volumetric changes in the cleft lip and palate nose. Int J Oral Maxillofac Surg. 2010;39:534–40.

Lübbers HT, Medinger L, Kruse A, Grätz KW, Matthews F. Precision and accuracy of the 3dMD photogrammetric systemin craniomaxillofacial application. J Craniofac Surg. 2010;21:763–7.

Maal TJ, van Loon B, Plooij JM, Rangel F, Ettema AM, Borstlap WA, Bergé SJ. Registration of 3-dimensional facial photographs for clinical use. J Oral Maxillofac Surg. 2010;68:2391–401.

de Menezes M, Rosati R, Ferrario VF, Sforza C. Accuracy and reproducibility of a 3-dimensional stereophotogrammetric imaging system. J Oral Maxillofac Surg. 2010;68:2129–35.

Metzler P, Bruegger LS, Kruse Gujer AL, Matthews F, Zemann W, Graetz KW, Luebbers HT. Craniofacial landmarks in young children: how reliable are measurements based on 3-dimensional imaging? J Craniofac Surg. 2012;23:1790–5.

Metzler P, Sun Y, Zemann W, Bartella A, Lehner M, Obwegeser JA, Kruse-Gujer AL, Lübbers HT. Validity of the 3D VECTRA photogrammetric surface imaging system for craniomaxillofacial anthropometric measurements. Oral Maxillofac Surg. 2014;18:297–304.

Naudi KB, Benramadan R, Brocklebank L, Ju X, Khambay B, Ayoub A. The virtual human face: superimposing the simultaneously captured 3D photorealistic skin surface of the face on the untextured skin image of the CBCT scan. Int J Oral Maxillofac Surg. 2013;42:393–400.

Nord F, Ferjencik R, Seifert B, Lanzer M, Gander T, Matthews F, Rücker M, Lübbers HT. The 3dMD photogrammetric photo system in cranio-maxillofacial surgery: validation of interexaminer variations and perceptions. J Craniomaxillofac Surg. 2015;43:1798–803.

Othman SA, Ahmad R, Mericant AF, Jamaludin M. Reproducibility of facial soft tissue landmarks on facial images captured on a 3D camera. Aust Orthod J. 2013;29:58–65.

Plooij JM, Swennen GR, Rangel FA, Maal TJ, Schutyser FA, Bronkhorst EM, Kuijpers-Jagtman AM, Bergé SJ. Evaluation of reproducibility and reliability of 3D soft tissue analysis using 3D stereophotogrammetry. Int J Oral Maxillofac Surg. 2009;38:267–73.

Ras F, Habets LL, van Ginkel FC, Prahl-Andersen B. Method for quantifying facial asymmetry in three dimensions using stereophotogrammetry. Angle Orthod. 1995;65:233–9.

Rosati R, De Menezes M, Rossetti A, Sforza C, Ferrario VF. Digital dental cast placement in 3-dimensional, full-facereconstruction: a technical evaluation. Am J Orthod Dentofac Orthop. 2010;138:84–8.

Sade Hoefert C, Bacher M, Herberts T, Krimmel M, Reinert S, Göz G. 3D soft tissue changes in facial morphology in patients with cleft lip and palate and class III mal occlusion under therapy with rapid maxillary expansion and delaire facemask. J Orofac Orthop. 2010;71:136–51.

Sforza C, De Menezes M, Bresciani E, Cerón-Zapata AM, López-Palacio AM, Rodriguez-Ardila MJ, Berrio-Gutiérrez LM. Evaluation of a 3D stereophotogrammetric technique to measure the stone casts of patients with unilateral cleft lip and palate. Cleft Palate Craniofac J. 2012;49:477–83.

Sharma VP, Bella H, Cadier MM, Pigott RW, Goodacre TE, Richard BM. Outcomes in facial aesthetics in cleft lip and palate surgery: a systematic review. J Plast Reconstr Aesthet Surg. 2012;65:1233–45.

Shaw WC, Semb G, Nelson P, Brattström V, Mølsted K, Prahl-Andersen B, Gundlach KK. The Eurocleft project 1996-2000: overview. J Craniomaxillofac Surg. 2001;29:131–40.

Sitzman TJ, Allori AC, Thorburn G. Measuring outcomes in cleft lip and palate treatment. Clin Plast Surg. 2014;41:311–9.

Stebel A, Desmedt D, Bronkhorst E, Kuijpers MA, Fudalej PS. Rating nasolabial appearance on three-dimensional images in cleft lip and palate: a comparison with standard photographs. Eur J Orthod. 2016;38(2):197–201. doi:10.1093/ejo/cjv024.

Thalmaan D. Die Stereogrammetrie: ein diagnostisches Hilfsmittel in der Kieferorthopaedie (Stereophotogrammetry: a diagnostic device in orthodontology). Zurich: University of Zurich; 1944.

Tse R, Booth L, Keys K, Saltzman B, Stuhaug E, Kapadia H, Heike C. Reliability of nasolabial anthropometric measures using three-dimensional stereophotogrammetry in infants with unrepaired unilateral cleft lip. Plast Reconstr Surg. 2014;133:530e–42e.

Tzou CH, Frey M. Evolution of 3D surface imaging systems in facial plasticsurgery. Facial Plast Surg Clin North Am. 2011;19:591–602. vii

Tzou CH, Artner NM, Pona I, Hold A, Placheta E, Kropatsch WG, Frey M. Comparison of three-dimensional surface-imaging systems. J Plast Reconstr Aesthet Surg. 2014;67:489–97.

Vyas RM, Warren SM. Unilateral cleft lip repair. Clin Plast Surg. 2014;41:165–77.

Weinberg SM, Naidoo S, Govier DP, Martin RA, Kane AA, Marazita ML. Anthropometric precision and accuracy of digital three-dimensional photogrammetry: comparing the Genex and 3dMD imaging systems with one another and with direct anthropometry. J Craniofac Surg. 2006;17:477–83.

Weinberg SM, Raffensperger ZD, Kesterke MJ, Heike CL, Cunningham ML, Hecht JT, Kau CH, Murray JC, Wehby GL, Moreno LM, Marazita ML. The 3D facial norms database: part 1. A web-based craniofacial anthropometric and image repository for the clinical and research community. Cleft Palate Craniofac J. 2016;53(6):e185–97. doi:10.1597/15-199.

Winder RJ, Darvann TA, McKnight W, Magee JD, Ramsay-Baggs P. Technical validation of the Di3D stereophotogrammetry surface imaging system. Br J Oral Maxillofac Surg. 2008;46:33–7.

Wong JY, Oh AK, Ohta E, Hunt AT, Rogers GF, Mulliken JB, Deutsch CK. Validity and reliability of craniofacial anthropometric measurement of 3D digital photogrammetric images. Cleft Palate Craniofac J. 2008;45:232–9.

Standardized Two-Dimensional Photographic Documentation of Cleft Patients

23

Rafael Denadai and Cassio Eduardo Raposo-Amaral

23.1 Introduction

The American Cleft Palate–Craniofacial Association and the Americleft (Daskalogiannakis et al. 2011; Mercado et al. 2011) and the Eurocleft (Brattström et al. 2005; Asher-McDade et al. 1992) have highlighted the importance of longitudinal documentation and records at standardized timing points to monitor short- and long-term treatment outcomes. As two-dimensional (2D) photography has been historically adopted for this longitudinal follow-up of cleft patients (Daskalogiannakis et al. 2011; Mercado et al. 2011; Brattström et al. 2005; Asher-McDade et al. 1992; Jones and Cadier 2004; Vegter and Hage 2000), this chapter delineates our standardized 2D photographic protocol particularly delineated to capture cleft patients' images. We included a set of instructions regarding the photographic equipment, photographic concepts, preparation and positioning of the patients, explanations of the different views, and patient's consent forms to help cleft teams acquire consistent, informative, and accurate photographs.

23.2 Protocol for Photographic Documentation

In SOBRAPAR Hospital, the protocol for standardized 2D photographic documentation has been systematized in order to maintain a longitudinal medical image database of all cleft patients for different purposes including diagnostic and evolutionary

R. Denadai, M.D. (✉)
Institute of Plastic and Craniofacial Surgery, SOBRAPAR Hospital,
Campinas, São Paulo 13084-880, Brazil
e-mail: denadai.rafael@hotmail.com

C.E. Raposo-Amaral, M.D., Ph.D.
Institute of Plastic and Craniofacial Surgery, SOBRAPAR Hospital,
Campinas, São Paulo 13084-880, Brazil

Universidade de São Paulo, São Paulo, Brazil

process, preoperative planning, visual baseline intraoperatively, therapeutic results, ethical and medicolegal issues, medical education, and scientific research (Raposo-Amaral et al. 2014, 2012). Therefore, in addition to the standard photographic documentation (preoperative, intraoperative, and postoperative imaging), all further clinical aspects, surgical steps, surgical details, intraoperative findings, and complications have also been systematically photographed.

23.3 Photographic Studio

In SOBRAPAR Hospital, a dedicated professional photographer and senior plastic surgeons have been responsible for photographic documentation within our multidisciplinary cleft care. For this, a private white-walled room was equipped with blackout curtains (ensuring patient privacy), a swivel chair with an adjustable seat height (and without back rest) for the patient placed at a distance of 30–60 cm from the blue background, a Nikon® D300 interchangeable-lens digital camera, some lenses (AF zoom Sigma® 28/70 mm and AF Nikkor® 105 mm), and a flash photography kit (Nikon® SB-21/AS-14, Nikon® SB-26 and Atek® 160 Plus).

23.4 Basic Concepts

The lenses are the photography key components as the definition and sharpness of the image projected by the lens are the determinants of quality. Fixed focal lens has been the most recommended for capturing craniofacial anatomy, providing a greater depth of field, ensuring that the entire surface is in focus; we prefer focal length between 90 and 105 mm. The macro lens with ring light flash is more suitable for intraoperative documentation (principally, oral cavity) and photographs of scars to eliminate shadows and improve the photographic result (Archibald et al. 2010; Persichetti et al. 2007; Ettorre et al. 2006; Schaaf et al. 2006; Yavuzer et al. 2001; Peck et al. 2010; Neff et al. 2010).

Standardized photographs require appropriate light sources to provide optimal contrast and detail of the patients (Fig. 23.1). The relationship between aperture ("the size of the hole controlling the amount of the light that reaches the sensor"; symbolized by "f" ["focal length of the lens"], ranging from f1.4 [widest open and most light] to f32 [smallest opening and least light]), shutter speed ("how long the shutter opens to expose the sensor to light"), and ISO (International Standards Organization; "the sensitivity of the sensor to light," ranging from 50 to 6400) has been considered the "tripod for photographic exposition." Aperture is important for depth of field ("the part of the image that is in sharp focus"); the larger number "f" (which counter-intuitively allows the least light onto the sensor) will produce the greatest depth of field. For clinical photography (under studio light conditions), high aperture settings ($f > 16$) and short exposure time ($<1/125$ s) can easily be achieved. Additionally, the ideal ISO position is 100–200, which maintains maximum resolution with adequate light and speed. This guarantees appropriate depth of

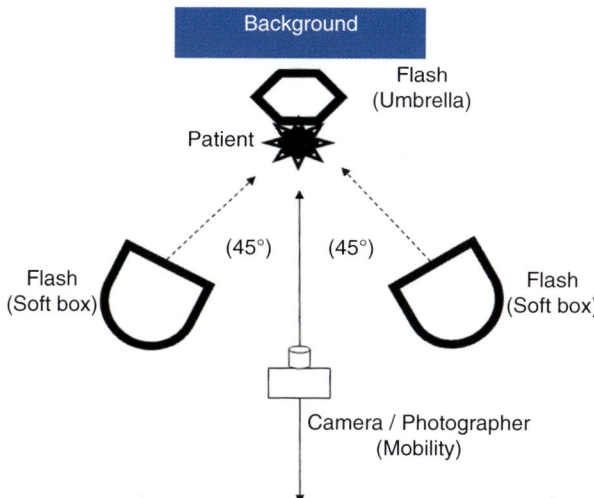

Fig. 23.1 Simplified schematic representation of artificial illumination adopted in our studio for standard photographic documentation. Three flashes were carefully distributed to reflect and diffuse the light. Two flashes with soft boxes on tripods were positioned 1–1.5 m from the patient and at 45° from the camera-subject axis, and one flash with a reflective umbrella was positioned at the top of the patient's head. A distance of 30–60 cm was maintained between the cleft patient and the *blue* background to minimize shadow effects. Flashes were synchronized with the camera shutter. Note: The proportions of the distances and sizes of the scheme are not equivalent to reality

field and prevents loss of sharpness attributable to shaking of the camera. As a result of constant quality and amount of lighting, the white balance of digital cameras can be set on the provided flashlight setting. Adopting the manual mode, one can ideally and consistently regulate the shutter speed, aperture, and ISO to maximize depth of field and resolution according to particular clinical setting. Therefore, as digital pictures can immediately be assessed, several pictures be taken (trial and error) with different aperture settings rather than using a handheld light meter (Archibald et al. 2010; Persichetti et al. 2007; Ettorre et al. 2006; Schaaf et al. 2006; Yavuzer et al. 2001; Peck et al. 2010; Neff et al. 2010).

23.5 Patient Preparation and Positioning

Proper patient preparation and positioning are critical to maintain consistency and standardization between the different views. The patient's hair should be pulled away from the face; eyeglasses, jewelry, collars, and distracting clothing should also be removed. The level of the camera lens should be at the same height as the center of the area being photographed. The distance between the patient and the camera should also be standardized and it may vary according to the photographed anatomical region (Fig. 23.2) (Archibald et al. 2010; Persichetti et al. 2007; Ettorre et al. 2006; Schaaf et al. 2006; Yavuzer et al. 2001; Peck et al. 2010; Neff et al. 2010).

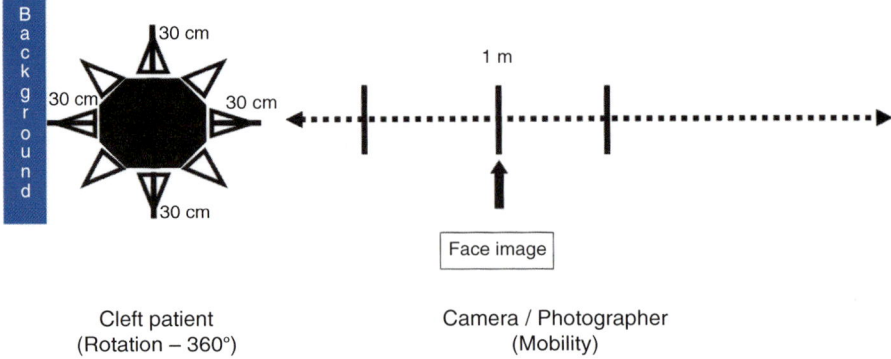

Fig. 23.2 Simplified schematic representation of the patient and the camera (photographer) positioning. The patient should be positioned in the center of an octagon with a radius of 30–60 cm, allowing rotation of 360°. To determine the ideal focal length for specific anatomical regions, experimental shots must be performed at different distances. Once the desired photographic results have been achieved, the position should be recorded on the floor and then documentation of the same anatomical region should always be performed using this mark. In the scheme, the distance of 1 meter (m) between the patient and the camera was standardized to document the full face in our studio (constant lighting; 105 mm lens; ISO 100; 1/125 s; and variable aperture). Note: The proportions of the distances and sizes of the scheme are not equivalent to reality

23.6 Photographic Settings

23.6.1 Preoperative and Postoperative

The surgical results are comparable only when standardization is consistently reproduced. The identical equipment with the same adjustment should be adopted in the preoperative and postoperative photographic documentation. Therefore, there are several differences in interindividual comparisons (mainly children versus adults), but the intraindividual comparisons are completely feasible as the preoperative and postoperative photographs of cleft patients should differ only in the aspect changed by the cleft surgery performed.

23.6.2 Operative Setting

Aperture priority mode with the "macro" setting on can be helpful for intraoperative photography when the camera is positioned close to the patient. A lightweight external flash or ring flash should be considered to help produce acceptable pre-, intra-, and postoperative images. The background should be a clean blue towel with the creases removed by pulling on all four corners. We have systematically removed redundant instruments and excess water, blood, and/or debris whenever possible. It is also important to keep the surgeon's hands out of the surgical field by using hooks and retractors to move nonrelevant tissues from the focus of the image.

23.6.3 Pediatric Patients

Photographing the pediatric cleft patients is challenging as time, photographic skills, and patience are key aspects to obtain uniformity in documentation. Patients who not yet sit or stand up (small children and babies) should be photographed preferably in the parent's lap (sitting squarely on the parent's knees), taking care to wrap the body of parents with a blue fabric (the parent should be out of the image view), maintaining a single blue background. Noises or movements to hold the child's attention and keeping your head in the designated position may be required. Photographic documentation before surgical procedures with children already anesthetized should also be routine.

23.7 Photographic Views

We adopted a standard set of photographic views (Jones and Cadier 2004; Vegter and Hage 2000; Ettorre et al. 2006; Schaaf et al. 2006; Swamy and Most 2010) (Figs. 23.3–23.5, Fig. 23.6). Both neutral expression (instruct cleft patients to relax their faces, with their mouths closed and the lips gently pressed together) and facial animation (patient at rest, whistling or puckering, smiling, and opening their mouth) have been used in this documentation. Anatomical landmarks and limits should be carefully applied to maintain the standardization of photographic views. We use the grid lines on the viewer to ensure optimal head positioning in the midsagittal plane (the point in the middle between the eyes, the middle of the tip of the nose, and the middle of the lips) and Frankfort horizontal plane (the lower margins of the orbits should be on the same level of the upper margins of the ear canals) for full frontal view (face perpendicular to the camera), right and left oblique views (face 45° away from the camera), and right and left profile views (face 90° away from the camera). Submental (aligning the nasal tip evenly with the glabella) view, close-up nose/lips (frontal, oblique, and profile) views, and intra-oral (occlusion, hard palate, and soft palate) views should also be performed. Lip retractors and a mirror can be used for intra-oral views.

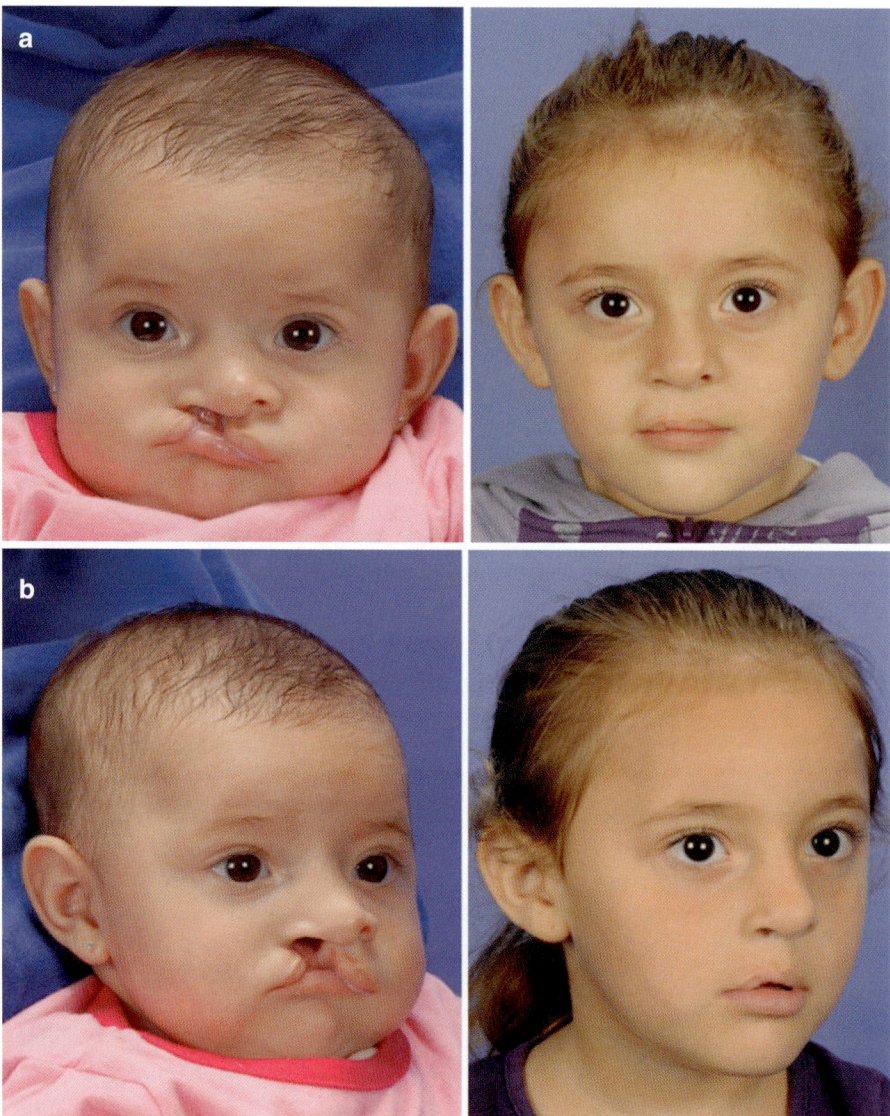

Fig. 23.3 Standard views for preoperative and postoperative photographic documentation. (**a**) Full-face frontal (anteroposterior) view; (**b**) right oblique view; (**c**) right lateral view; (**d**) left oblique view; (**e**) left lateral view; (**f**) submental view

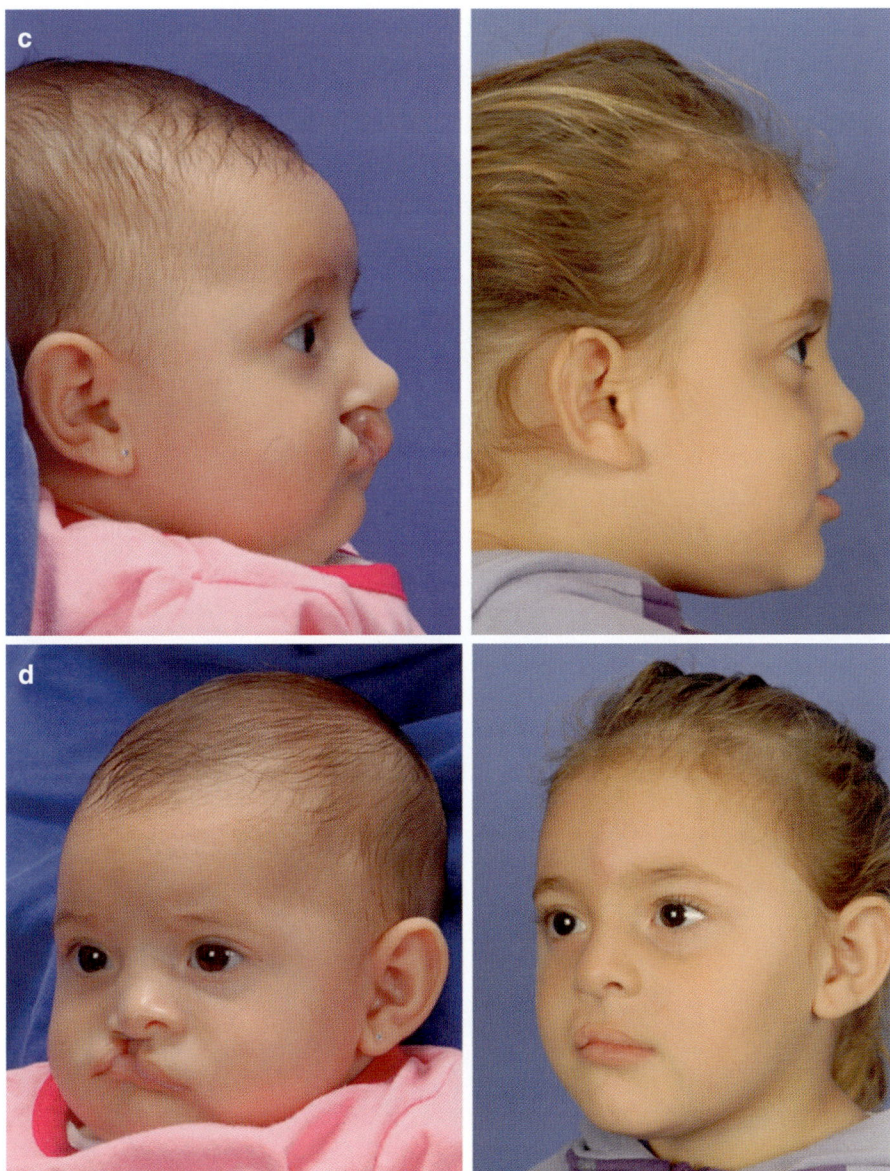

Fig. 23.3 (continued)

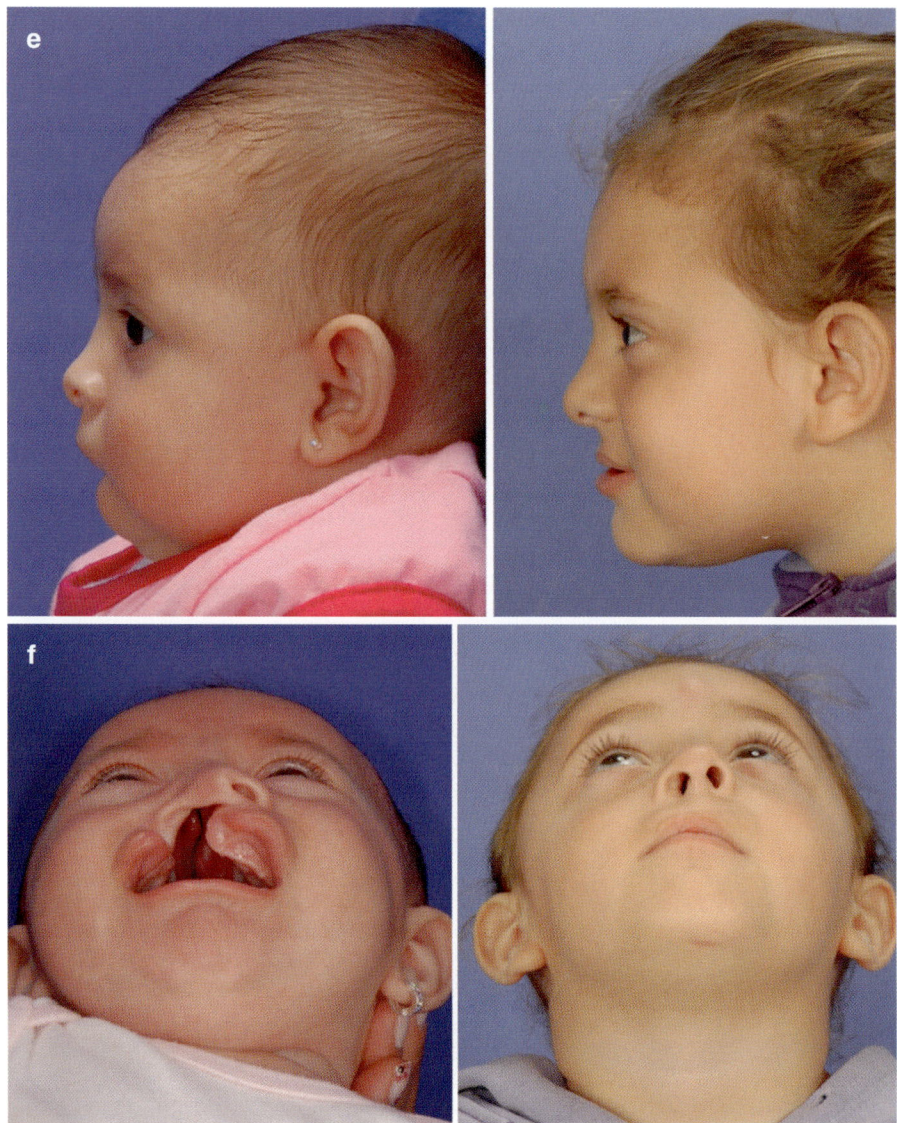

Fig. 23.3 (continued)

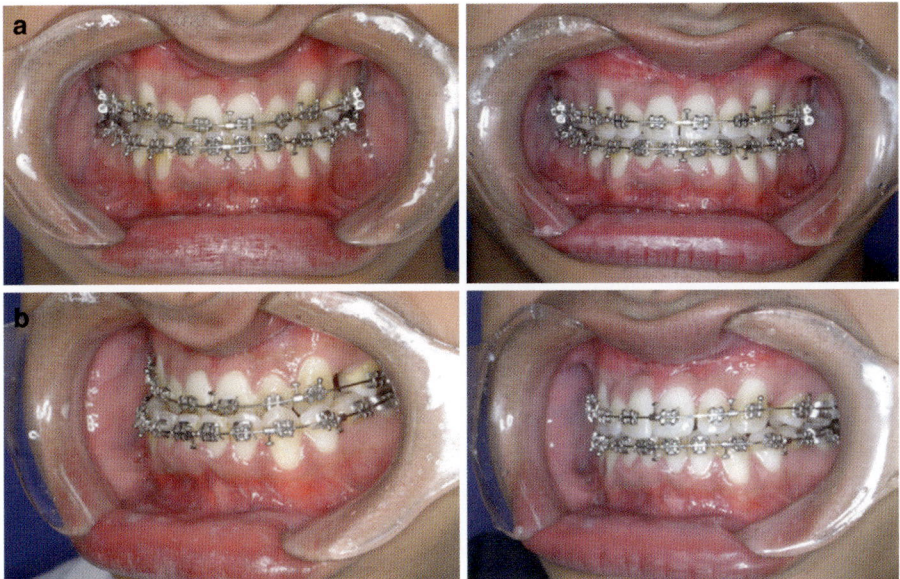

Fig. 23.4 Occlusal views with lip retractors before (class III malocclusion) and after (class I) the LeFort I osteotomy with horizontal advancement. (**a**) Frontal view; (**b**) left oblique view

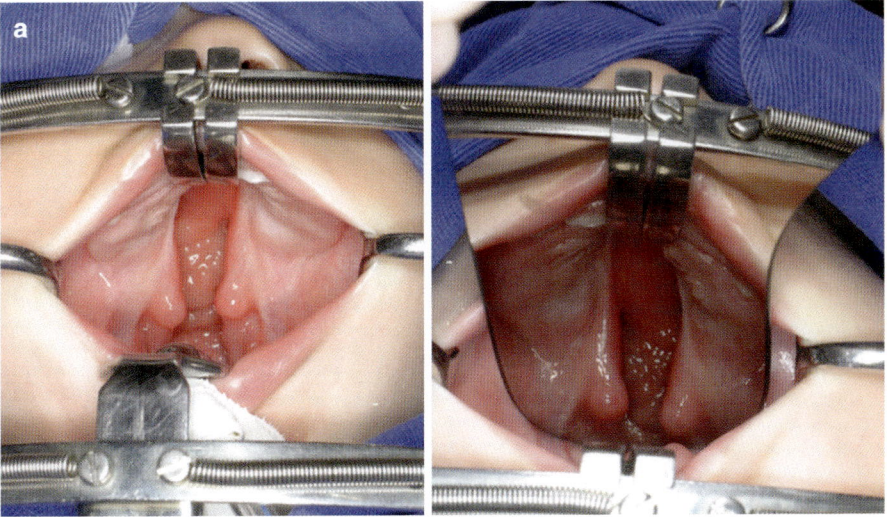

Fig. 23.5 Palatal views with Dingman retractor. (**a**, *left*) Soft and hard palate and (**a**, *right*) palatal images of the soft and hard palate using the mirror that should be positioned to reflect the vomer. (**b**) The camera is positioned in landscape to offer a wider angle of the cleft palate. (**c**) Intraoperative (preoperative and postoperative) palatal images

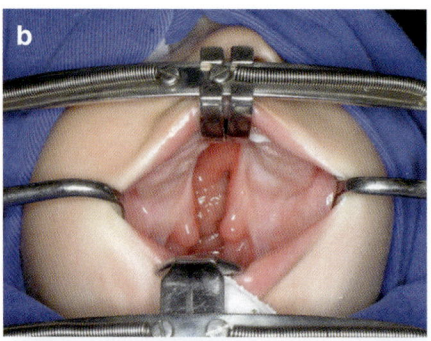

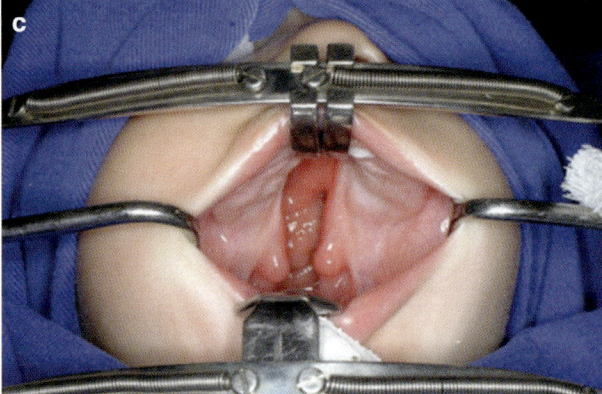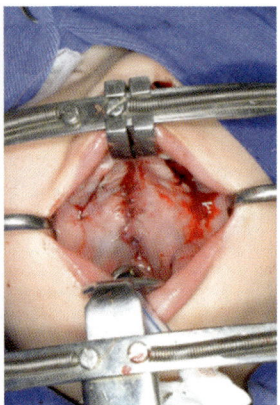

Fig. 23.5 (continued)

23.8 Patient's Consent Forms

In our hospital, consent forms have been signed by all patients or their relatives prior to any photography. The consent form also includes permission to publish all photographs of the patient or use them for academic purposes. As photographic documentation is an integral component of the medical records, maximum security must be guaranteed (Segal and Sacopulos 2010); our database has passwords and restricted access. In addition, our patients have been photographed only according to the present protocol, and we have avoided shooting photographs with personal camera or mobile phones.

References

Archibald DJ, Carlson ML, Friedman O. Pitfalls of nonstandardized photography. Facial Plast Surg Clin North Am. 2010;18:253–66.

Asher-McDade C, Brattström V, Dahl E, McWilliam J, Mølsted K, Plint DA, Prahl-Andersen B, Semb G, Shaw WC, The RP. A six-center international study of treatment outcome in patients with clefts of the lip and palate: part 4. Assessment of nasolabial appearance. Cleft Palate Craniofac J. 1992;29:409–12.

Brattström V, Mølsted K, Prahl-Andersen B, Semb G, Shaw WC. The Eurocleft study: intercenter study of treatment outcome in patients with complete cleft lip and palate. Part 2: craniofacial form and nasolabial appearance. Cleft Palate Craniofac J. 2005;42:69–77.

Daskalogiannakis J, Mercado A, Russell K, Hathaway R, Dugas G, Long RE Jr, Cohen M, Semb G, Shaw W. The Americleft study: an inter-center study of treatment outcomes for patients with unilateral cleft lip and palate part 3. Analysis of craniofacial form. Cleft Palate Craniofac J. 2011;48:252–8.

Ettorre G, Weber M, Schaaf H, Lowry JC, Mommaerts MY, Howaldt HP. Standards for digital photography in cranio-maxillo-facial surgery - part I: basic views and guidelines. J Craniomaxillofac Surg. 2006;34:65–73.

Jones M, Cadier M. Implementation of standardized medical photography for cleft lip and palate audit. J Audiov Media Med. 2004;27:154–60.

Mercado A, Russell K, Hathaway R, Daskalogiannakis J, Sadek H, Long RE Jr, Cohen M, Semb G, Shaw W. The Americleft study: an inter-center study of treatment outcomes for patients with unilateral cleft lip and palate part 4. Nasolabial aesthetics. Cleft Palate Craniofac J. 2011;48:259–64.

Neff LL, Humphrey CD, Kriet JD. Setting up a medical portrait studio. Facial Plast Surg Clin North Am. 2010;18:231–6.

Peck JJ, Roofe SB, Kawasaki DK. Camera and lens selection for the facial plastic surgeon. Facial Plast Surg Clin North Am. 2010;18:223–30.

Persichetti P, Simone P, Langella M, Marangi GF, Carusi C. Digital photography in plastic surgery: how to achieve reasonable standardization outside a photographic studio. Aesthet Plast Surg. 2007;31:194–200.

Raposo-Amaral CE, Giancolli AP, Denadai R, Marques FF, Somensi RS, Raposo-Amaral CA, Alonso N. Lip height improvement during the first year of unilateral complete cleft lip repair using cutting extended Mohler technique. Plast Surg Int. 2012;2012:206481.

Raposo-Amaral CE, Giancolli AP, Denadai R, Somensi RS, Raposo-Amaral CA. Late cutaneous lip height in unilateral incomplete cleft lip patients does not differ from the normative data. J Craniofac Surg. 2014;25:308–13.

Schaaf H, Streckbein P, Ettorre G, Lowry JC, Mommaerts MY, Howaldt HP. Standards for digital photography in cranio-maxillo-facial surgery--part II: additional picture sets and avoiding common mistakes. J Craniomaxillofac Surg. 2006;34:444–55.

Segal J, Sacopulos MJ. Photography consent and related legal issues. Facial Plast Surg Clin North Am. 2010;18:237–44.

Swamy RS, Most SP. Pre- and postoperative portrait photography: standardized photos for various procedures. Facial Plast Surg Clin North Am. 2010;18:245–52.

Vegter F, Hage JJ. Standardized facial photography of cleft patients: just fit the grid? Cleft Palate Craniofac J. 2000;37:435–40.

Yavuzer R, Smirnes S, Jackson IT. Guidelines for standard photography in plastic surgery. Ann Plast Surg. 2001;46:293–300.

Printed by Printforce, the Netherlands